MATERIA MEDICA

OF

HOMOEOPATHIC MEDICINES

MATERIA MEDICA
OF
HOMOEOPATHIC MEDICINES

By

DR. S.R. PHATAK

M.B.B.S.

Author of Concise Homoeopathic Repertory (English),
Repertory of Biochemic Remedies (English),
Homoeopathic Materia Medica and
Repertory of Homoeopathic Medicines (Marathi).

Second edition
Revised & enlarged

B. Jain Publishers (P) Ltd.

USA — Europe — India

MATERIA MEDICA OF HOMOEOPATHIC MEDICINES

Second Revised & Enlarged Edition: 1999
23rd Impression: 2019

Note from the Publishers
Any information given in this book is not intended to be taken as a replacement for medical advice. Any person with a condition requiring medical attention should consult a qualified practitioner or therapist.

Published by Kuldeep Jain for
B. JAIN PUBLISHERS (P) LTD.
B. Jain House, D-157, Sector-63, NOIDA-201307, U.P. (INDIA)
Tel.: +91-120-4933333 • *Email:* info@bjain.com
Website: **www.bjain.com**

ISBN: 978-81-319-0002-4

PREFACE

WHY THIS BOOK

Students of homeopathy who read different materia medicas written by various authors must have observed that some symptoms given under a particular remedy in one materia medica are not given by another. Boger has selected the most important symptoms from various materia medicas and has included them in his Synoptic Key. But while presenting these symptoms he has at times used such words that unless the student has the ability to read between the lines he will miss their hidden meaning. Moreover, Boger has omitted many important symptoms given by other authors. I will give some examples to illustrate my point. Boericke has given "Retention of urine after operation" under Causticum. Boger has not given this symptom. Boger has given "Distension of abdomen after operation" under Carbo animalis which is not given by other authors. Kent has not mentioned the above two symptoms in his repertory. But these two symptoms gave me opportunity to remove these distressing conditions successfully. Dr. Boger has given a very curious symptom "Breathes through a metallic tube, as if" under Merc. cor. which is not given by any other author. Moreover, he has made it a general symptom under the heading — "Tube metallic - Merc. cor." The meaning is obvious. If a person comes and says that while passing stools or urine or even talking, he is doing these functions as if through a tube, Merc. cor. is apt to be useful. I had an occasion to give this remedy to a person who was speaking through a tube.

If well understood, Boger's Materia Medica and Repertory are quite sufficient for most of the cases. But we possess neither his intellect, nor his acumen.

In compiling this materia medica, I have included all the symptoms given by Boger. I have tried to simplify many of his ambiguous words by explaining their meaning. Moreover, I have garnered many useful clinical and other symptoms from other materia medicas (which were not given by Dr. Boger) and have included them here.

The presentation of materia medica is in the usual schematic basis. Under generalities the profile picture of the remedy is given along with the regions on which it acts and how it acts, diseases which it is liable to cure, and causations. Then general modalities of the remedy are given, after that regional symptoms with their particular modalities follow.

It is my belief that Boger wished to compile a concise repertory arranged in alphabetical order rather than a regional one. In the same way a concise materia medica, in which all relevant symptoms pertaining to each remedy are given, was desirable. He has given clues in his Synoptic Key for compiling such books. With my poor intellect and limited knowledge of homeopathy I have tried to fulfil his wish. How far I am successful in my attempt, only time will show.

THANKS - GIVING

My thanks are due to my friend Dr. (Miss) Homai Merchant for typing the manuscript twice without a single murmur. Thanks are also due to my son Dr. D.S. Phatak for correcting first to final proofs several times and for making arrangement to print the book with Mouj Printing Bureau. Mr. Datay who got the composing done and Mr. M.R. Sane who composed the book single-handed deserve my thanks.

Readers are requested to have a look especially "Hints for the Beginners" and "Index of Surgical Remedies."

Finally I am very grateful to God for sparing me in spite of my heart disease and old age to see the book getting completed. I have done whatever I could. Capable young homoeopaths should carry on the work further.

July 1977

S.R. Phatak

HINTS FOR THE BEGINNERS

Materia medica and repertory are the twin pillars on which a successful practice of homeopathy stands. Both are complementary to each other. None is complete in itself.

Study of materia medica is a long drawn out effort. There is no short or easy road to success.

Drugs should become your friends. You can identify your friend from the way he rings the bell, taps or opens the door, climbs the foot-steps, etc. Similarly, you should be able to know the drug even when it is partially studied.

The marks of identification of the drug are found in its Generalities, Modalities (i.e., worse and better) and Mind. A thorough grasp of these headings helps you to identify the drug in relation to the patient.

To achieve this, when you read a drug, each rubric should be seen in the repertory. The relative importance of this drug is to be fixed in your mind by comparing it with other drugs under the same rubric. This appears to be tedious. But the drug picture slowly gets firmly and clearly set in your mind.

SYMPTOMS

The most difficult thing in homeopathy is interpretation of symptoms. When the patient is telling his story in his own words, you should be able to fix these, in terms of rubrics given in the repertory. If you have grasped the materia medica well, certain drugs will automatically come to your mind. Verify them in repertory. Causation, modalities are more important. The peculiar symptom which the underlying pathology fails to explain does many a time point towards the suitable drug.

When a cup is half-full, it is half empty also. While interpreting symptoms, try to look at the same thing from various angles.

While reading materia medica try to remember the peculiar things in the drug. Bland discharges of Pulsatilla, "Can't throw things off" in Zincum met. "Great variety of symptoms" in Mercurius etc. As said before, these are the identification marks of the drug.

Three types are used in this book to show the gradation. Relative importance of different symptoms is given by this. But in a particular patient a low grade symptom may prove to be the most important. So you need not be carried away by the gradations.

Lastly, give respect to the authorities on homeopathy for what they say. But if your experience is contrary to what the authorities say, do not get swayed by their opinions. Ultimately your experience is the best authority as far as you are concerned.

S. R. Phatak

Preface to the Second Edition

`Materia Medica of homoeopathic Medicines' by Dr. S.R. Phatak occupies a very important place in homoeopathic literature.

Internationally it has been ranked alongside Boericke and Clarke's Materia Medica's.

In this edition we have undertaken to correct it, for even the best books have their share of errors. All ambiguous statements have been clarified where possible so has to bring across to the readers what the author was actually trying to express.

For eg: The statement "Metastasis from suppressed milk to the brain, abdominal trouble etc." on page - has been modified to -

Ailments from suppression of milk; resulting in brain, abdominal troubles.

Some symptoms were incomplete and vague. For eg:- Nat-sulph. extremities. "Inflammation around root of nails. Run-arounds. Hang nail pain in hip-joint < rising or sitting down.

"Run-arounds" is incomplete and erroneously situated. In fact in Clarke's Materia Medica it has been used to describe the severity of the pain. Hence the above symptom has been altered to "Pain in hip joint < rising or sitting down compelling the patient to move constantly due to its severity.

Apart from this there are many errors in the original text. For eg: in Veratrum album, page 611 of the original text it says - "Convulsions caused by religious excitement of all Mucous membranes. Burning, children feel better; meant also of children. Post-operative shock. Excessive dry, when carried about quickly.

This has been altered to "Convulsions caused by religious excitement. Excessive dryness of all mucous membranes. Burning - Post-operative shock. Children feel better by being, carried about quickly."

Here I would like to stress that all corrections have been undertaken with great care, and only after verification with other well known texts.

Further, nineteenth century English spelling has been replaced with modern American English spelling.

Words or clinical terminology that are rarely used and are not likely to be understood easily have been replaced by contemporary language.

For eg: "Noma" becomes ulcerative stomatitis and "horripilation" becomes "goose-flesh". etc.

All abbreviations have been standardized in accordance with the "SYNTHESIS" so as to avoid all ambiguity is distinguishing remedy names.

We hope as always that are endeavours to further the cause of homoeopathy shall bear fruit.

Editor

B. Jain Publishers

INDEX

(Drugs Useful to surgeons)

When this book was in press, some surgeons suggested that there should be a short book dealing with drugs useful for pre-and post-operative conditions. There is no such thing in homeopathy as surgical remedies. None the less, certain drugs are useful in such cases. One should never lose sight of the fact that homoeopathy is treating an individual and not a disease entity.

The following list is not exhaustive, but these remedies are more useful in different branches of medicine mentioned.

Name of the drug	Heading	Where useful
ABROTANUM	Generalities	Pediatrics
	Male	Surgery
ACETIC ACID	Generalities	Surgery
ACONITE	Generalities	Surgery
	Urinary	Obstetrics
AETHUSA	Generalities	Pediatrics
	Stomach, Neck & Back	
AGARICUS	Generalities	Pediatrics
ALOE	Generalities	Surgery
	Abdomen	
ALUMEN	Eyes	Eye Surgery
ALUMINA	Female	Gynaecology

AMBRA GRISEA		Lock-jaw of newborn
ARNICA MONTANA	Generalities	Surgery
	Female	Obstetrics
	Eyes	Eye surgery
ARSENIC ALB	Urinary	Obstetrics
BELLIS PERENNIS	Generalities	Surgery
BERBERIS VULGARIS	Generalities	Surgery
	Neck & Back	
BORAX	Female	Gynaecology
CALCAREA CARB.	Female	Gynaecology
CALCAREA FLUOR.	Generalities	Surgery
CALENDULA	Generalities	Surgery
	Female	Obstetrics
CANTHARIS	Generalities	Surgery
CAUSTICUM	Urinary	Surgery
	Female	Gynaecology
CHAMOMILLA	Generalities, Eyes	Obstetrics &
	Female	Pediatrics
CHIMAPHILA	Urinary	Surgery
CICUTA	Injuries (See under-Worse)	Surgery
	Urinary	
COLLINSONIA	Abdomen	Surgery
	Female	Obstetrics
CONIUM	Female	Obstetrics
CROCUS SATIVUS	Stomach	Surgery
	Female	Obstetrics
CYCLAMEN	Female	Obstetrics

DULCAMARA	Urinary	Surgery
ECHINACEA	Generalities	Cancer
		Surgery
ERIGERON	Female	Gynaecology
EUPHRASIA	Eyes	Eye Surgery
FRAXINUS		Gynaecology
GELSEMIUM	Eyes	Eye Surgery
	Female	Gynaecology
HAMAMELIS	Generalities	Surgery
	Eyes	Eye Surgery
HEPAR SULPH	Generalities	Surgery
	Urinary	
	Eyes	Eye Surgery
HYOSCYAMUS	Urinary	Obstetrics
	Female	
HYPERICUM		Surgery
IRIS VERSICOLOR	Stomach	Pediatrics
JABORANDI	Eyes	Eye Surgery
	Stomach	Obstetrics
KALI BROM	Female	Gynaecology
LACHESIS	Generalities	Surgery
LEDUM PAL	Generalities	Surgery
LEPTANDRA	Abdomen	Surgery
LILIUM TIGRINUM	Generalities	Obstetrics
	Urinary	Gynaecology
	Female	
LYCOPODIUM	Urinary	Surgery
	Male	

MAGNESIA MUR	Generalities	Obstetrics
	Female	
MAGNESIA PHOS	Generalities	Surgery
	Urinary	
MERCURIUS	Generalities	Surgery
	Abdomen	
	Urinary, Male	
MEZERIUM	Eyes	Eye Surgery
MILLEFOLIUM	Generalities	Surgery
	Female	Obstetrics
MURIATIC ACID	Abdomen	Surgery
	Urinary	
NAPHTHALINE		Eye Surgery
NATRUM MUR	Female	Gynaecology
NATRUM SULPH	Mind	Surgery
NITRIC ACID	Abdomen	Surgery
	Female	Gynaecology
NUX MOSCHATA	Female	Gynaecology
NUX VOMICA	Abdomen	Pediatrics
OPIUM	Head, Abdomen	Surgery
	Urinary	
PARIS QUADRIFOLIA	Generalities	Surgery
PETROLEUM	Abdomen	Surgery
	Urinary	
	Female	Gynaecology
PETROSELINUM	Pediatrics	
PHOSPHORICUM ACIDUM	Generalities	Surgery
	Stomach	
	Abdomen	
	Female	Gynaecology

PHYSOSTIGMA SURGERY	Eyes	Eyes
PHYTOLACCA	Female	Gynaecology
PLATINUM	Generalities	Gynaecology
	Mind	
	Female	
PLUMBUM	Abdomen	Surgery
	Urinary	
	Female	Gynaecology
PSORINUM	Female	Obstetrics
PULSATILLA	Female	Gynaecology
		Obstetrics
RATANHIA	Generalities	Obstetrics
	Abdomen	Surgery
	Female	Gynaecology
RHEUM	Generalities	Pediatrics
RHODODENDRON	Male	Surgery
RHUS TOX	Abdomen	Surgery
SABAL SERRULATA	Generalities	Surgery
SAMBUCUS	Male	Surgery
SECALE	Urinary	Surgery
	Female	Obstetrics
SENEGA	Generalities	Eye Surgery
	Eyes	
SEPIA	Generalities	Gynaecology
		Surgery
	Female	Gynaecology
		Obstetrics

SILICA	Generalities	Surgery
	Eyes	Eye Surgery
	Urinary	Surgery
	Male	Surgery
	Female	Gynaecology
SPIGELIA	Eyes	Eye Surgery
STANNUM	Female	Gynaecology
STAPHISAGRIA	Generalities	Surgery
	Female	Gynaecology
SULPHURICUM ACIDUM	Generalities	Surgery
	Urinary	
	Eyes	Eye Surgery
	Abdomen	Surgery
SYMPHYTUM	Generalities	Surgery
SYPHILINUM	Eyes	Eye Surgery
	Female	Obstetrics
	Extremities	Surgery
TABACUM	Generalities	Surgery
	Abdomen	
TARENTULA CUBENSIS	Generalities	Cancer
TARENTULA HISPANICA	Generalities	Surgery
	Female	Gynaecology
	Neck and Back	Surgery
TELLURIUM	Generalities	Surgery
	Eyes	Eye Surgery
	Neck and Back	Surgery
	Extremities	
TEREBINTHINA	Female	Gynaecology

THUJA	Eyes	Eye Surgery
	Abdomen	Surgery
	Female	Obstetrics
THYROIDINUM	Generalities	Surgery
TRILLIUM	Female	Obstetrics
		Gynaecology
USTILAGO	Female	Gynaecology
VERBASCUM	Trigeminal neuralgia	
VIBURNUM	Female	Obstetrics
XANTHOXYLLUM	Female	Gynaecology
ZINCUM MET	Concussion of brain	
	Abdomen	Surgery
	Urinary	

Contents

ABIES CANADENSIS

GENERALITIES: It affects the mucous membranes and nerves. In stomach it causes a catarrhal condition, which increases the patient's hunger and craving for coarse food, such as pickles, radishes, turnips, etc. Patient wants to lie down all the time on account of nervous weakness and feels faint. In women it causes uterine displacement due to defective nutrition and debility. Peculiar sensations are — right lung and liver feel hard and small; uterus feels soft. Lies with the legs drawn up.

MIND: Easily fretful or quiet and careless.

HEAD: Feels as if it is light or there is a swimming sensation in the head.

STOMACH: Ravenous appetite. Tendency to eat far beyond the capacity of digestion. Distention of abdomen and stomach, with palpitation.

FEMALE: Sore feeling at the uterus, > pressure. Uterus feels soft and feeble.

FEVER: Cold shivering, sensation as if blood were ice-water.

SKIN: Clammy and sticky.

ABIES NIGRA

GENERALITIES: It is a useful remedy in many diseased conditions when they are associated with gastric symptoms. It causes dyspepsia with functional heart symptoms, especially in the aged persons. It is also useful in indigestion of those who abuse the drinking of tea and smoking, or chewing of tobacco. The chief symptom in dyspepsia is a sensation as if a hard-boiled egg has lodged in the cardiac end of the stomach. Patient describes this sensation: as if a hard lump is felt in the pit of stomach or in the lung which he wants to cough out.

WORSE: After eating.

MIND: Very low-spirited, unable to think or study.

STOMACH: Total loss of appetite in the morning, but craves food at noon and at night. Pain in the stomach always comes on after eating.

CHEST: Difficult breathing < lying down. Heart's action heavy and slow, there may be tachycardia or bradycardia.

ABROTANUM

GENERALITIES: It affects nerves, causing numbness, weakness, trembling and paretic conditions. It is the remedy for marasmus in children when nutrition is affected. Inspite of good appetite children emaciate, especially in lower extremities. It causes *true metastatic condition.* Rheumatism occurs after checked diarrhea. Gout recedes and other troubles follow. It has *exudative tendency.* Exudation may occur, as a metastatic condition or otherwise, into pleura, joints, etc. It also causes alternating conditions, one disease condition disappears and another appears, e.g., piles alternating with rheumatism. It is suitable to newborn or children, especially boys, who suffer from hydrocele, epistaxis; it removes weakness remaining after influenza. Oozing of blood and moisture in newborn from navel. Vomiting of large quantities of offensive fluid. Effects remaining after operation on chest.

WORSE: Cold air; wet. Checked secretions, esp. diarrhea. Night. Fog.

BETTER: Loose stools. Motion.

MIND: Great anxiety and depression. Cross and irritable (children in marasmus). Thinking difficult; loss of comprehension. Inhuman; would like to do something evil, cruel.

HEAD: Cannot hold the head up on account of weakness of neck. Brain feels tired, after conversation or mental effort. Veins distended on forehead.

EYES: Blue ring around the eyes. Hollow.

NOSE: Epistaxis in boys.

FACE: Dry, cold, wrinkled, as if old, in marasmus. Acne, with emaciation. Angioma of the face. Pale.

STOMACH: Emaciation progresses, with good appetite. Food passes undigested. Craving for bread, boiled in milk. Cutting, gnawing, burning pain in stomach at night in gastralgia. Feels as if stomach is swimming in water, with coldness.

ABDOMEN: Hard lumps are felt in different parts of abdomen. It is bloated. Tuberculous peritonitis. Weak, sinking feeling in bowels. Piles, protruding, with burning from touch. Frequent desire to stool but only a little blood passes.

MALE: Hydrocele of children.

FEMALE: Darting pain in left ovary. Menses suppressed.

RESPIRATORY: Dry cough, following diarrhea. Pressing sensation remains after pleurisy in the affected side impeding free breathing.

BACK: Sudden aching pain in the back < night > motion. Pain in sacrum due to piles. Back weak, with ovarian pain.

EXTREMITIES: Pain in shoulders, arms, wrists and ankles. Legs greatly emaciated. Cold, prickling, numb fingers and toes. Inability to move the limbs due to rheumatism. Contraction of limbs, from cramps or following colic.

SKIN: Loose and flabby. Skin becomes purplish, after suppression of eruption. Itching chilblain.

FOLLOWS WELL: Acon. and Bry. in pleurisy.

RELATED: Agar.; Chin.; Led.; Nux-v.

ABSINTHIUM

GENERALITIES: It causes convulsion, preceded by trembling. The patient bites tongue, foams at mouth and makes grimaces. Tremor is a marked feature, tremor of tongue, heart. Sudden and severe giddiness; epileptiform seizures, delirium with hallucinations and loss of consciousness. Attacks occur in rapid succession. It is a useful remedy for nervousness, excitement and sleeplessness, in children. Chorea. Opisthotonos.

MIND: Vertigo, with tendency to fall backward. Forgets what has recently happened, after and before convulsion. Wants nothing to do with anybody. Brutal insanity. Kleptomania.

EAR: Discharge; after headache.

FACE: Spasmodic twitching. Foolish look.

URINE: Very strong urine, of deep yellow colour.

HEART: Tumultuous action, beats can be heard in back.

FEMALE: Menopause, premature.

RELATED: Art-v.; Cic.; Cina.; Hydr-ac.

ACETIC ACID

GENERALITIES: The leading symptoms of this drug are profound anemia, with waxy pallor of the face; excessive emaciation; great debility; frequent fainting; difficult breathing; weak heart; profuse urination, vomiting; and sweat. It antidotes the effects of all anesthetic vapors. In convulsions, patient jumps out of bed like a madman and crawls on the floor. It is a remedy for general anasarca and dropsical affections. Hemorrhage from nose, stomach, rectum, lung, ulcer, etc. Child wants to be carried. Nevi, warts, corns.

MIND: Grieves about his sickness and his children. Worried about business affairs. Borrows trouble. Does not know her own children. Forgets what has recently happened.

HEAD: Aches from abuse of narcotics, tobacco. Child does not let its head be touched.

FACE: Left cheek red during fever. Pale, waxen, emaciated.

NOSE: Epistaxis, esp. from fall or blow.

THROAT: Children thirsty, but swallow with difficulty, even a teaspoonful (diphtheria).

STOMACH: No thirst with fever. Great thirst with dropsy. Violent burning pain in stomach and chest, followed by coldness of skin, and cold sweat on forehead. Vomiting after every type of food. Ulcer, cancer of the stomach. Cold drinks disagree; vegetables, except potatoes disagree. Bread and butter disagree.

ABDOMEN: Tympanitis. Ascites. Hemorrhage from bowels. Chronic diarrhea of emaciated children. Scirrhus of pylorus.

URINARY: Large quantitiy of pale urine. Diabetes, with great thirst and debility.

FEMALE: Metrorrhagia, with great thirst; after parturition. Threatening abscess of the breast. Milk impoverished, bluish, sour; suckling droops, (Sagging breasts due to laxity of muscle fibres) lose flesh, get marasmic.

RESPIRATORY: Cough when inhaling. Hurried and laborious breathing. Rattling in chest.

BACK: Pain (myelitis) relieved only by lying on abdomen; with profuse urination.

EXTREMITIES: Edematous swelling of feet and legs, with diarrhea.

SKIN: Diminished sensibility of the whole body. Burning, dry skin.

FEVER: Hectic, with drenching night sweats; sweat profuse and cold.

RELATED: Follows China after hemorrhage.

ACONITE

GENERALITIES: The rapidity of action of Acon determines its symptomatology. Its symptoms are *acute, violent* and *painful.* They appear *suddenly,* remain for a short while, as a big storm, which soon blows over. Mind is affected by such emotional factors, as FRIGHT, SHOCK,

VEXATION. Nerves are excited and the patient remains under emotional and nervous tension. *Neuralgic pains are very intense. Fear is intense,* so much so that the patient becomes *frantic, screams,* groans, gnaws the fist, bites the nails, wants to die. Fear or fright remains. Fear accompanying most trifle ailments. *Heart* and *arterial circulation* is affected strongly producing congestion to the head (often apoplectic), and chest. It is a remedy for acute *inflammation* and congestion. *Hemorrhages are bright red. Pains are sticking, tearing. Sensations of burning, numbness, tingling, prickling, or crawling is marked.* Parts feel big or deformed. External soreness, with internal heaviness. Sudden loss of strength — *collapse. Special senses acute.* Part remains sore or *numb after the pain.* Convulsion. Faintness. Children put their hands on the affected part. Complaints caused by exposure to cold, dry weather, especially respiratory affections. Gastro-intestinal disturbances are caused by exposure to very hot weather. It is adapted to persons of robust habits. Complaints after surgical shocks and injury, or checked perspiration. Remote effects of fright. Cries out and grasps the genitals. Crepitation.

WORSE: *Violent emotions,* FRIGHT, SHOCK, vexation. *Chilled* by COLD, *dry weather,* while sweating. Pressure, touch. *Night,* in bed, p.m. Lying on side. *Noise. Light.* Dentition. During menses. Sleeping in the sun. Music. Tobacco smoke. Inspiration.

BETTER: Open air. Repose. Warm sweat.

MIND: Great ANXIETY. Agonizing FEAR and RESTLESSNESS accompany every ailment, however trivial. *Fear* of death, of crowds, or crossing the streets, of future, of touching others passing by. *Impatient;* besides himself; *frantic; from intensity of pain.* WITH FEAR *screams, moans, gnaws* the fists, bites the nails; wants to die. Afraid to go out of the house. Forebodings, predicts the time of death.

Terror Stricken. Music makes him sad. Clairvoyance. Feels as if what had just been done were a dream. Delirium. Fitful moods; laughing, singing, then sad and fearful. *Anxious, excited, nervous, feverish.* Imagines some part of the body is deformed. Imagines he does all his thinking from stomach.

HEAD: Heavy, *hot,* bursting. *Burning;* undulating sensation in the head as of a hot band about head, or boiling heat in brain. Violent squeezing or bursting in forehead or eyes. Headache with increased secretion of urine. Vertigo, < on rising or any other motion of the head or of the body as if hair were pulled or stood on end. Crackling in head. Pulsation in forehead. Knocks the head.

EYES: Feel dry and hot as if sand in them. Lids swollen, hard and red. Shooting pain in eyeballs. Cannot bear the reflection of sun from the snow. Conjunctivitis from cinders or other foreign bodies. Eyes glitter, stare, bleary. Aversion or desire for light.

EARS: Very sensitive to noise. Music is unbearable. Sensation as of a drop of water in the ear.

NOSE: Numb with epistaxis. Smell acutely sensitive. Pain at the root of the nose. Nose dry, stopped up or runs, hot scanty watery discharge.

FACE: Anxious expression; becomes pale and red alternately. *Hot, red cheeks.* Red face becomes deathly pale on rising or he becomes dizzy. One cheek red hot, other pale and cold. Neuralgia with restlessness, tingling and numbness. Lips black, dry, peeling off. Heavy feeling of the whole face.

MOUTH: Toothache in sound teeth. Throbbing in teeth and head. Grinding of the teeth. Gums hot and inflamed. Tongue feels as if swollen. Everything tastes bitter except water, which has bad taste. Trembling and temporary stammering. Mouth and tongue numb; dry, burning heat in mouth. Tingling on coughing and swallowing. Chewing motion of lower jaw.

THROAT: Red, dry, hot, constricted, chokes on swallowing. Tonsils swollen and dry.

STOMACH: Vomiting with fear, heat, profuse sweat and increased urination. INTENSE BURNING THIRST. Craving for beer, acids, bitter drinks. Thirst < after iced drinks. Hungry. Milk disagrees. Projectile vomiting. Violent bilious or bloody vomiting. Pressure in stomach with dyspnea. Wine generally >. Nausea and sweating before and after loose stool.

ABDOMEN: Sensitive to touch. Colic, no position relieves. Hot, distended. Jaundice; of newborn; from fright. Incarcerated hernia. *Stools; of pure blood;* slimy, grass green or white, < hot days and cold nights. Dysentery. Watery diarrhea in children in hot days; they cry, feel restless and sleepless. Itching and sticking in anus; sensation as if a warm fluid is oozing especially from the anus.

URINARY: Urine scanty, red, hot, painful. Retention or suppression of urine, in newborns, due to cold exposure, with handling of genitals. Agonizing dysuria. Cystitis. Urethral chill.

MALE: Orchitis, testicles feel swollen and hard.

FEMALE: Suppression of menses from fright or cold, in plethoric patients. Afterpains with fear and restlessness. Maniacal fury on the appearance of menses. Active uterine hemorrhage. Ovaritis from sudden checked menstrual flow. Vagina hot, dry and sensitive. Milk fever with delirium. Increase of milk in breast.

RESPIRATORY: *Hoarse, dry, croupy, painful cough* or short, barking, ringing, or whistling cough, < from every inspiration, at night, drinking; grasps the throat. Cough, > lying on back. Shortness of breath during sleep; sits erect. Laryngitis. *Croup with fever.* Violent congestion of blood in the chest. Pneumonia. Oppression of the chest when moving fast or ascending; in heart disease. Blood comes up on hawking. *Lungs feel hot.* Stitches in chest. Pleurisy. Tingling in chest after coughing.

HEART: Feels swollen — Carditis. Palpitation, with anxiety, fainting and tingling in fingers, pain down left arm. Heart pains into left shoulder, < sitting erect. Tachycardia. Pulse fast, bounding, shaking, forcible and tumultuous or wiry, very irritable. Arterial tension.

NECK & BACK: Pain in the back, prevents taking deep inspiration. Bruised pain between shoulders and in sacrum.

EXTREMITIES: Arms hang down powerless. Numbness of the left arm, tingling in fingers. Finger tips red. Hot hands and cold feet. Red, shining swelling of the joints. Hypothenar eminences bright red. Legs powerless; feel tired during repose. Sensation of drops of water trickling down the thighs. JERKING of left arm. *Palms hot.*

SKIN : DRY, HOT or as if ice water on it . Miliary eruptions. Itching, > by stimulants.

SLEEP: Nightmares. Anxious dreams. Sleeplessness with restlessness and tossing about; caused by fear, fright or anxiety. Insomnia of the aged.

FEVER: CHILL passes through him in waves. Chill or coldness alternating with heat. HIGH FEVER; *dry burning* heat, in eyelids, nose, mouth, throat, lungs and palms, must uncover. *Sweat* drenching, wants to uncover. Sweat on uncovered parts or affected part.

COMPLEMENTARY: Coff.; Sulph.

RELATED: Bell.; Cham.; Coff.

ACTEA SPICATA

GENERALITIES: It acts upon joints, especially small joints. Though it affects wrist joints prominently; other joints like ankles and fingers are also affected. It causes tearing and tingling pains. Joints are swollen and pains are < by touch and movement. Slight fatigue causes swelling of the joints. It causes paralytic weakness of affected part. Symptoms are liable to appear from fright and fatigue. Shortness of breath on exposure to cold. Old age. Hypersensitive to cold. Weakness.

WORSE: Change of weather, slight exertion, cold, night, touch.

EYES: Objects look blue.

EARS: Twitching pain on sneezing or blowing the nose.

COMPLEMENTARY: Caul.; Coloc.; Sabin.; Stict.; Vio-o.

ADONIS VERNALIS

GENERALITIES: It acts predominantly on the heart when it is affected after rheumatism, influenza or nephritis, where the muscles of the heart are in the stage of fatty degeneration. It regulates the pulse, increases the contracting power of the heart, causes increased urinary secretion. It is valuable in cardiac dropsy, hydrothorax; ascites and anasarca. Pains wander from place to place. Arrhythmia. It is not cumulative in action. Compensatory hypertrophy of heart in cardiac stenosis and mitral regurgitation.

WORSE: Cold, lying.

BETTER: Exertion.

HEAD: Vertigo, < on rising, turning the head quickly or lying down; with palpitation. Aching from occiput around temples to eyes. Scalp feels tight.

MOUTH: Tongue sore, feels scalded. No thirst.

STOMACH: Faint feeling in epigastric region with vertigo, > out of doors.

ABDOMEN: Heavy weight; bowels seem as if breaking, < bending.

URINARY: Urging to urinate. Albuminuria; urine scanty, oily pellicle on urine.

RESPIRATORY: Frequent desire to take deep breath. Dyspnea, < touching back. Dry tickling, cardiac cough.

HEART: Weak, fatty, arrhythmic. Precordial pain, palpitation and dyspnea. Pulse rapid, irregular.

BACK: Spine and neck stiff; aching pain with tired feeling.

SKIN: Vesicles on the skin.

SLEEP: Sleeplessness with rambling thoughts, or horrible dreams.

RELATED: Bufo.

COMPARE: Conv., Crat., Dig., Stroph-h.

DOSE: 5 to 10 drops of tincture.

AESCULUS HIPPOCASTANUM

GENERALITIES: It has a marked action on the veins of the lower bowels and pelvic organs causing engorged hemorrhoids. Veins of portal system are also engorged producing soreness and fullness of the liver and abdomen. Many of the symptoms which *Aesc.* produces are due to deranged liver or *reflex from piles.* It causes general venous stasis, making parts purple and puffy, varicose veins become purple. Everything is slowed down—digestion, heart, bowels. In addition to the feeling of fulness in internal parts, it produces sensation of HEAT, DRYNESS, STIFFNESS AND ROUGHNESS in throat, nose, anus, etc. There is a characteristic backache which makes the patient unfit for business. Pains are stitching or flying all over hot like lightning.

WORSE: Morning on awakening. From any motion. Lying; stooping; after stools; urinating. Cold air, and after washing in water. Winter. Standing.

BETTER: Cool open air, bathing. Bleeding (piles); kneeling. Continued exertion. Summer.

MIND: Gloomy and *irritable;* unable to fix his attention. Wake up with confusion of mind; bewildered, especially children.

HEAD: Bruised pain from occiput to the frontal region, with flushes of heat over occiput, neck and shoulders.

EYES: Eyeballs feel heavy, dull, hot and sore, with lachrymation. Blood vessels dilated.

NOSE: Sensitive to cool inspired air, which causes burning, rawness and fluent coryza and sneezing. Obstruction of nose due to hepatic disorders. Congestive catarrh.

MOUTH: Scalded feeling in tongue and mouth. Tongue thickly coated. Salivation. Cannot control the tongue so as to form words rightly. Taste sweet, bitter, metallic. Teeth as if coated with oil.

THROAT: Follicular pharyngitis connected with hepatic congestion. Feeling of roughness, dryness, stitching or burning like fire on swallowing. Neuralgic pains in the fauces. Hawking of ropy mucus of sweetish taste.

STOMACH: Pressure as from a stone with gnawing, aching pain about three hours after meals. Heartburn and gulping up of food after eating. Desire to vomit with constant distress and burning.

ABDOMEN: Throbbing deep in abdomen (hypogastrium and pelvis). Tenderness and fulness in the region of liver. Jaundice.

RECTUM: *Stools dry, hard;* of different colors. Feels full of small sticks. *Piles with sharp shooting pain up the back;* blind and bleeding; *purple, painful, external;* < standing and walking. Constipation: hard, dry, knotty, white stools. Pain long after stool. Sensation as if there is a bug crawling from anus. Stools first part hard and black, then white and soft. Burning in anus, with chill up and down the back. Painful constriction; as of a knife sawing up and down. Piles < during climaxis.

URINARY: Frequent scanty urination; urine muddy, dark, hot.

MALE: Discharge of prostatic fluid at every stool and urination.

FEMALE: Constant throbbing behind symphysis pubis. Leucorrhea with lameness of back across sacro-iliac joint and aching in knees; dark, yellow, sticky, corroding, < after menses.

CHEST: Feels constricted, with a hot feeling. Cough depending upon hepatic disorders. Pain around heart in hemorrhoidal subjects. Audible palpitation, when pulsation extends to extremities.

BACK: *Laming, dull lumbar pain. Small of the back gives out.* Pain as if back would break, has to make repeated efforts at rising, < walking and stooping. Bruised pain affecting sacrum and hips.

EXTREMITIES: Aching and soreness in limbs. Paralytic heaviness of arms, spine, feet. Hands and feet swell and become red after washing. *Spine feels weak.*

SLEEP: Disposition to stretch and yawn.

COMPLEMENTARY: Carb-v., Lach., Mur-ac.

RELATED: Aloe, Coll., Puls.

AETHUSA CYNAPIUM

GENERALITIES: It affects BRAIN and *nervous system,* connected with *gastro-intestinal disturbances. Violence* is one of the key-notes of its action. Violent vomiting, convulsions, pain, delirium. On the other hand, there is *profound prostration* and stupor, and lack of reaction, even speechlessness. Mind and body become weak. It is especially useful in children during dentition and summer complaints when anguish, crying and expression of uneasiness and discontent are present. As the disease progresses the patient becomes more and more retired in his disposition, and *more inclined to weep.* In epileptiform spasms, the thumbs are clenched, face becomes red, eyes turned downwards, pupils dilate and are staring, foam at mouth. Patient cannot stand, sit up or hold the head up. Weak, nervous and prostrated from overwork. Dotage. Lancinating pains. Parts feel screwed together. Improperly fed babies. Children who lack the power to hold their heads up, with no particular ailment; sometimes they can't even stand or bear any weight on their limbs.

WORSE: 3 to 4 a.m. and evening. Warmth; *hot weather.* MILK. Dentition. Frequent eating. Over-exertion.

BETTER: Open air, by walking in open air. Conversation.

MIND: *Inability to think or fix attention,* from overstudy. Delirium, sees cats, dogs, rats, etc. Idiocy alternates with furor. Wants to jump out of bed or out of window. Examination funk from simple sense of incapacity. Idiotic children. Awkward. Loves animals.

HEAD: Distressing pain in the occiput down nape of neck and spine, > lying down and pressure. Head symptoms are > by passing flatus and stool. Hair feels pulled. Vertigo, with sleepiness, with palpitation, with weakness. Cannot raise head. Head hot after vertigo. Squeezing headache, with vertigo < walking and looking upward. Dizzy and drowsy.

EYES: Photophobia (chronic). Eyes brilliant and protruding. Eyes drawn downwards. Cornea sunken. Objects seem larger or double. Swelling of Meibomian glands. Rolling of eyes on falling asleep.

EARS: As if something hot streaming out. Feels obstructed, > by inserting the fingers and drawing the parts apart.

NOSE: Herpetic eruptions on tip of nose. Frequent ineffectual desire to sneeze. *Alae nasi* drawn in.

FACE: Sunken; pale, puffed, spotted, red. *Linea nasalis marked.* Blue white pallor about the lips. Deathly aspect. Chin and corners of mouth feel cold.

MOUTH: Tongue seems too long. Aphthae in the mouth. Speech slow, embarrassed. Speechless. Taste bitter, of onions, of cheese; sweetish in morning.

STOMACH: Nibbling appetite. *Intolerance of milk.* Violent sudden vomiting of milk as soon as swallowed or IN LARGE *curds.* Hungry after vomiting. LIMPNESS AND DEEP SLEEP AFTER VOMITING. DEATHLY NAUSEA. Regurgitation of food long after eating. Vomiting of frothy matter white as milk; or yellow fluid. Stomach feels turned upside down. Digestion affected from brain exhaustion. Retching.

ABDOMEN: Black bluish swelling of abdomen; coldness of abdomen, subjective and objective, with coldness of legs, with aching in bowels, > warm application. Colic, followed by vomiting, vertigo and weakness. Bubbling sensation around navel.

STOOL: Yellow green slimy diarrhea. Stool undigested. Obstinate constipation, with feeling as if all the action of the bowels has been lost. Cholereic affection of old age.

URINARY: Cutting pain in bladder with frequent urging.

MALE: Right testicle drawn up with pain in kidney.

FEMALE: Menses watery. Swelling of mammary glands with lancinating pain. Pimples on external parts; itching on getting warm.

RESPIRATORY: Short breath interrupted by hiccough. Suffering renders the patient speechless. Crampy constriction in chest. Cough causes pain in head. Stitches in left side of chest.

HEART: Violent palpitation, with vertigo, headache and restlessness. Pulse rapid, hard, small, unrhythmical.

NECK & BACK: Want of power to stand, to hold up head. Small of back as if in a vise. Swelling of glands around neck like string of beads. A feeling as if pain in back could be > by straightening out and bending stiffly backwards.

EXTREMITIES: Fingers and thumbs bent inwards or clenched. Sensation as if arms had become much shorter. Numbness of hands and feet. Heaviness, weakness, contraction of fingers. Excoriation of thighs on walking.

SKIN: Lymphatic glands swollen like strings of beads. Skin cold and covered with *clammy sweat.* Eruptions itching; around the joints, > from heat. Ecchymosis. Anasarca. Whole body may be blue, black.

FEVER: Great heat without thirst. Must be covered during sweat. Sweating on slightest physical effort.

SLEEP: Disturbed by violent startings and/or by cold perspiration. Dozing after vomiting or stool. Rolling of the eyes or slight convulsion on falling asleep.

COMPLEMENTARY: Calc.

RELATED: Ant-c., Cic.

AGARICUS MUSCARIUS

GENERALITIES: This poisonous mushroom, acts on CEREBRO-SPINAL AXIS. Its action on brain produces more vertigo and delirium. Affection of spinal cord, nerves and medulla produces IRREGULAR, ANGULAR, UNCERTAIN AND EXAGGERATED MOTIONS; patient reaches too far, staggers or steps too high, *drops things,* etc. Symptoms appear slowly. Patient suffers from MANY AND DIVERSE symptoms. TREMBLING; TWITCHING; JERKINGS or *fibrillar spasms* here and there are very marked, EYELIDS and tongue are specially affected. Symptoms appear diagonally such as in right arm and left leg. Shuddering. Nervousness and restlessness. Chorea, > during sleep. Sensation as if pierced by cold needles or hot needles, a cold drop or cold weight on the parts. Painful twitching, then the parts become stiff and cold. In epilepsy and convulsions physical strength is increased, can lift heavy loads. Twitching ceases during sleep. Convulsion after coition; from suppressed milk; after being scolded or punished. Young nervous, hysterical married women who faint after coition. Children walk and talk late on account of brain complaints. Yawning before complaints.

WORSE: COLD air. FREEZING air. Before thunderstorm. *Mental exhaustion. Coition.* Debauchery. *Alcohol. Pressure on spine. Touch. Morning.* During menses. Sun. Fright.

BETTER: Gentle motion.

MIND: Sings, talks incoherently, changes rapidly from subject to subject but does not answer. *Loquacity.* Indisposed to perform any kind of work, especially mental. Fearlessness. Makes verses. Hilarious. Embraces and kisses hands. Selfish. Indifferent. Dull and dizzy as if drunk. Morose, self willed, stubborn; slow in learning to walk and talk. Awkward, clumsy. Knows no one; throws things. Pressure on spine causes involuntary laughter. Cannot do anything new, cannot do his routine work or does the opposite.

HEAD: Vertigo, from sunlight. Dull headache, must *move the head to and fro.* Headache > after stool or urine; headache with nose-bleed or thick mucus discharge. Pain as from nail in right side of head. Head is in constant motion. Head drawn towards shoulders.

EYES: Reading difficult, as type seem to move, to swim. Double vision, oscillating eyeballs. Gum in canthi. Muscae volitantes; brown. *Twitching of eyelids.* Narrowing of space between eyelids. Nystagmus, squint. Eyelids thick, dry, burning.

EARS: Itching in the ears with redness and burning pain, as if they had been frozen. Twitching of the muscles about the ears. *Noises.*

NOSE: Frequent sneezing, without coryza. Flow of clear water, without coryza. Sneezing after coughing. Itches internally and externally. Fetid dark bloody discharge. Epistaxis in old people. Redness. Obstruction on stooping.

FACE: Facial muscles feel stiff; twitch. Face itches and burns. Pain in the cheeks, as if from splinters. Neuralgia as if cold needles run through nerves. Grimaces. Idiotic expression. Face blue and puffed.

MOUTH: Angles of mouth droop; from paralysis; saliva runs out. Herpes on lips. Taste sweet, bitter. Aphthae on the roof of the mouth. Tongue dry, tremulous; one side numb, with vertigo. Indistinct, jerky speech. Offensive breath. Froth at mouth. Swollen and bleeding gums, with pain.

THROAT: Feels contracted. Small solid balls of phlegm thrown up without coughing. Dryness with difficulty in swallowing. Scratching in Throat; cannot sing a note.

STOMACH: Always thirsty. Eructation; empty, tasting of apple, or of rotten egg; alternating with hiccough. *As of a lump in epigastrium.* Gastric disturbances, with sharp pain in liver region. Vomiting bitter, with prostration, with stitches in rectum and groins.

ABDOMEN: Rumbling and fermenting in bowels. Profuse inodorous flatus. Diarrhea, with much fetid garlicky odor flatus. Diarrhea of children, with grass green bilious stools. Flatus hot. Sensation of writhing. Stitch in the splenic region, in runners.

URINARY: Urine profuse, colorless, clear, lemon colored. Viscid, glutinous mucus from urethra. Frequent urination. Urine cold, flows slowly or in drops; has to press for passing urine.

MALE: Sexual desire increased. After coition, great debility, profuse sweat, burning and itching of the skin; tension and pressure under ribs. Seminal discharge hot. Palpitation during coition; depressed afterwards (in both the sexes). Premature ejaculation. Testes painfully retracted. Old gleet. Complaints after sexual debauches.

FEMALE: Bearing down pain, especially after menopause. Sexual excitement. Menses too profuse. Nipples itch and burn, look red; during pregnancy. Complaints following parturition and coitus. Ailments from suppression of milk; resulting in brain, abdominal troubles. Leukorrhea dark, bloody, excoriating, patient is unable to walk. Itching with sexual desire.

RESPIRATORY: Isolated coughing attacks, then sneezing. Cough comes as if from spine. Easy expectoration of floculi or balls of mucus. Labored, oppressed breathing. Chest seems too narrow.

HEART: Palpitation, during coition. Palpitation irregular, tumultuous; with redness of face, > tobacco. Pressure or burning, sticking from heart to left scapula. Angina pectoris, with excessive pain only. Shock in heart region, from sudden noise, from eructation or coughing.

BACK: Single vertebra sensitive to heat. Pain as from fatigue. Painful weakness and soreness. *Spine sensitive* to pressure and touch. Shooting, burning along spine. Spine seems short. Pain in lumbar region and sacrum, a sort of crick in back, extending to nape of neck, < stooping. Lumbago, < in open air, < sitting. Twitching of cervical muscles. Formication along spine. Muscles of the back feel tight, as if they would break on bending. As if cold air were spreading along the back, like an aura.

EXTREMITIES: Arms restless. Burning, itching of both hands as if frozen. Trembling of the hands. Right hand unsteady while writing; arm feels paralyzed from much writing. Uncertain gait. Itching of toes and feet as if frozen. Cramp in soles and feet. Pain in shin-bone. Violent pain in thigh on crossing them. Paralysis of lower limbs, with slight spasm of arms. Numbness of legs on crossing them. Buttocks cold. Pain in the hips, < lying. Fingers fly spasmodically while holding things. Legs feel heavy. Feels as if her limbs do not belong to her.

SKIN: BURNING, ITCHING, *redness and swelling.* As *if* FROZEN. Chilblain. Itching changing place on scratching. Skin pains when cold. Angio-neurotic edema. Miliary eruptions with intolerable itching and burning. Itching over affected part. Slight blow causes ecchymosis.

SLEEP: *Yawning* frequent; before pain or spasm; as a concomitant. Yawning followed by involuntary laughter. On falling asleep, starts, twitches and awakens often.

FEVER: Chilled easily, sweats easily, sweat on alternate sides. Night-sweat.

COMPLEMENTARY: Calc.

RELATED: Phys., Tub.

AGNUS CASTUS

GENERALITIES: *Agn.*, produces its chief effect on SEXUAL ORGANS of both sexes, also there are characteristic symptoms in the Mental Sphere. It lowers sexual vitality, with corresponding mental depression, and loss of nervous energy. There is a great sadness, with a fixed notion of approaching death. It influences both the sexes, but is more pronounced in men. IMPOTENCY AND PREMATURE OLD AGE from abuse of sexual power. History of repeated gonorrhea. Self-contempt from sexual abuse. Nervous debility in unmarried persons. A prominent remedy for sprains and strains. Gnawing, itching in all parts, especially eyes. Tachycardia caused by tobacco in neurotic young men. *Jaded rakes. Agn.* was used in early days by men and women to suppress sexual desire.

WORSE: SEXUAL EXCESS. Sprains of over-lifting.

MIND: Absent-minded. Despairing sadness with impression of speedy death. Distraction. Unable to recollect things. Lack of courage. Says that she will die soon and there is no use doing anything. Bad Memory.

HEAD: Pain as from staying in room filled with thick and smoky atmosphere, looking at one point >.

EYES: Pupils dilated. Gnawing, itching in eyes.

NOSE: Illusion of smell — of herring, musk. Hard ache on dorsum of nose, > pressure.

FACE: Corrosive itching on the cheeks. Formication in the cheeks. Rending, tearing pains under alveoli of right lower jaw.

MOUTH: Ulcer in the mouth and gums. Teeth are painful when in contact with warm food or drink.

STOMACH: Nausea with a sensation as if intestines were pressed downwards, wants to support bowels with hands.

Only the most simple food agrees. Eructations smell like urine.

ABDOMEN: Rumbling in abdomen during sleep. Spleen swollen and sore. Flatus smells like urine, remaining long on the clothes. Deep fissures in anus. Sensation as of subcutaneous ulceration near the anus only while walking. Bowels as if sinking down, has to support with hands.

URINARY: Passes more urine, frequently.

MALE: Sexual desire almost lost. Testes cold, swollen, hard; penis small, flaccid. Spermatorrhea, with impotency. Loss of prostatic fluid on straining. Yellow discharge from urethra.

FEMALE: A transparent leukorrheal discharge passes imperceptibly from very relaxed genitals. Aversion to coition. Leukorrhea staining yellow. Agalactia, with sadness. Menses suppressed, with abdominal pain. Hysterical palpitation with nose-bleed. Sterility, with suppression of menses and no sexual desire. Sexual thrill absent, from excessive masturbation.

RELATED: Olnd., Ph-ac.

AGRAPHIS NUTANS

GENERALITIES: It relaxes the whole system. Patient is prone to take cold on exposure to cold winds. Adenoids with enlarged tonsils. Throat deafness. Mucus diarrhea following a suppressed cold. Mutism of childhood unconnected with deafness.

AILANTHUS GLANDULOSA

GENERALITIES: It acts upon BLOOD, disorganizing it and producing condition like low fever; low types of eruptive diseases and hemorrhagic diathesis. It affects the THROAT causing diphtheria and follicular tonsillitis. Streptococcus infection. The skin appears LIVID or purplish. *Prostration* is rapid. LIVIDITY. STUPOR. FETOR and MALIGNANCY are marked conditions. Discharges are thin and acrid. Sepsis. Rash often returns annually. It is suited to nervous, sensitive persons. Stout and robust. Bilious temperament.

WORSE: Suppression. Raising up or sitting up. Sight of food. Motion, walking.

BETTER: Hot drinks, lying on right side.

MIND: Stupor, or stoic indifference, with sighing. Dullness, must read a subject several times or figures over and over again. All the antecedents are forgotten. Constant muttering delirium with sleeplessness and restlessness. Raging delirium with brilliant eyes.

HEAD: Ache in frontal region, with dizziness and red hot face; cannot sit up. Faint on rising up or vertigo, < lying.

EYES: Suffused and congested; startled look when roused. Pupils dilated. Photophobia.

EARS: Pain, while swallowing. Parotid glands tender and enlarged.

NOSE: Copious, thin, bloody, ichorous nasal discharge. Nose dry. Itching and uneasy feeling around the nose.

FACE: Mahogany-colored; *dark* and swollen. Chronic speckled spotted face; a kind of acne. Lips swollen and cracked.

MOUTH: Teeth covered with sordes. Tongue dry and brown, parched and cracked.

THROAT: Dry, foul fauces. Throat dark and swollen. Tonsils *studded with many deep ulcers.* (< left), with loose pultaceous discharge. Much swelling internal and external. Lacunar tonsillitis. Irritation and itching of posterior pharynx. Diphtheria.

STOMACH: Sudden violent vomiting when sitting up. Peculiar feeling of emptiness.

ABDOMEN: Diarrhea, dysentery with great weakness. Stools thin, watery, offensive, passing involuntarily with urine. Tapeworm. Sense of insecurity—stool, urine, etc.

URINARY: Urine scanty, suppressed; passed unconsciously.

FEMALE: Malignant puerperal fever.

RESPIRATORY: Breathing hurried, irregular. Dry hacking cough. Lungs sore and tired.

HEART: Pulse rapid, small, weak.

BACK & NECK: Neck tender and very much swollen.

SKIN: *Eruption in dark, sparse patches;* appear slowly; disappear on pressure, but return slowly. Skin mottled. Large blisters filled with dark serum. *Scarlatina maligna.* Petechiae. Crawling all over the body.

SLEEP: Drowsy, restless.

FEVER: Adynamic fever with weak heart. Cold sweat.

RELATED: Arum-t., Bapt., Lac-c.

ALETERIS FARINOSA

GENERALITIES: It affects the female organs. It is a remedy for anemic, debilitated, relaxed females who always feel tired and suffer from prolapsus, leucorrhea, rectal distress. Many symptoms appear due to uterine disorder. *Parts feel heavy.* Suitable for anemic girls and pregnant women. Weak emaciated persons. Hemorrhage.

WORSE: Loss of fluids.

BETTER: Passing flatus. Bending backwards.

MIND: Confused feeling. Cannot concentrate.

HEAD: Weight in occiput; as if it would draw the head backwards. Vertigo with fainting, sleepiness, vomiting or purging.

EARS: Feel as if open through from one to the other.

MOUTH: Much frothy saliva.

STOMACH: Want of appetite; disgust for food. Least food causes distress. Obstinate vomiting of pregnancy. Nervous dyspepsia. Nausea, > by coffee, by dinner; with pressure in forehead.

ABDOMEN: Colic settling in lower part, > passing flatus; scanty diarrheic stools, pain > bending backwards. Terrible pain during passing stools, as if forcing a passage. Stools large, hard, difficult. Constipation as from rectal atony.

URINARY: Involuntary urination on walking fast or sneezing.

FEMALE: Early and profuse menses, with labor-like pain. Menorrhagia, profuse, black with clots. Uterus seems heavy. Leukorrhea white, stringy, due to weakness and anemia. Habitual tendency to abortion. Muscular pains during pregnancy. Menses copious followed by copious watery oozing between periods.

RESPIRATORY: Cough before menses.

NECK & BACK: Sensation as if back would break just above waist. Backache with dragging in sacral region, with stringy colorless leukorrhea.

EXTREMITIES: Leg (R) feels paralyzed below knee; numb, could not bear weight on it.

RELATED: Chin., Helon., Tril-p.

ALFALFA

This medicine favorably influences nutrition, and is considered as a tonic. Appetite and digestion improve, mental and physical vigor returns, with gain in weight. It is a useful remedy for neurasthenia, melancholy, nervousness and insomnia. It increases fat, corrects wasting of tissues. It increases the quality and quantity of milk in nursing mothers. Clinically, it favorably influences diabetes insipidus and phosphaturia. Allays vesical irritability of prostatic hypertrophy. Should be given 5 to 10 drops several times a day.

ALLIUM CEPA (Red onion)

GENERALITIES: It affects the mucous membranes of LEUKORRHEA, NOSE, EYES, LARYNX and bowels, causing increased secretion. Burning and stitches in the eyes, nose, mouth, throat, bladder, skin are marked. Nasal secretion is acrid; secretion from eyes is bland. Neuralgic pains are shooting, *as fine as a thread,* following injuries to the nerves or amputation or other surgical operations. Traumatic chronic neuritis. Symptoms go from left to right. Singer's coryza. Neuroma. Senile gangrene. Sensation of glowing heat in different parts of the body.

WORSE: WARM ROOM. *Wet feet.* Singing. Damp weather. Spring. Evening. Eating spoiled fish, cucumber, salad.

BETTER: Cool open air. Bathing. Motion.

MIND: Fear that pain will become unbearable. Melancholy.

HEAD: Aching in forehead, extending to eyes and face, > free coryza or menses, returns when flow ceases. Electric shock passes through head. Skull bones numb.

EYES: Much burning, smarting; profuse *bland lacrimation,* < coughing, wants to rub them. Near objects seem distant, while yawning.

EARS: Aching extending to throat.

NOSE: FREQUENT, VIOLENT SNEEZING; CORYZA; with FLUENT ACRID DISCHARGE, with burning and smarting in the nose. Nose drips. Sensitive to odors, of flowers and the skin of peach. Acrid discharge when singing.

FACE: Paralysis, left side, also of limbs of the same side.

THROAT: Rawness of the throat. Pain extending to the ear. Dripping from uvula. Sensation as of a lump in throat or as if one has swallowed a large lump.

STOMACH: Craving for raw onion, which agree. Pain in the region of pylorus. Prickling perspiration on bald vertex, < after each meal. Voracious appetite with thirst. Nausea. Eructation.

ABDOMEN: Rumbling, offensive flatus. Flatulent colic, < sitting, motion. Glowing heat in rectum.

MALE: Pain in bladder and prostate gland after coition.

FEMALE: Phlegmasia alba dolens; after instrumental delivery.

URINARY: *Copious urine;* with coryza. Strangury after wet feet. Dribbling of urine in old people.

RESPIRATORY: *Hoarseness; incessant, hacking, tickling cough,* < inspiring cold air; with a sensation *as if larynx is split and torn;* must grasp it. Cough is so troublesome that he wants to hold it back. Larynx is painful when talking. Bronchitis in old people.

EXTREMITIES: Joints feel lame; Ulcers or the skin is rubbed off by the shoes especially on the heels. Limbs, especially arms feel sore and tired. Sore feet from long walking.

SKIN: Red streaks running up; felon; of lying in women.

SLEEP: Yawning, in deep sleep, or with headache and drowsiness, and cramp in stomach.

COMPLEMENTARY: Phos., Puls., Ther.

RELATED: Euphr., Gels., Kali-i.

ALLIUM SATIVUM (Garlic)

GENERALITIES: It acts on intestinal mucous membranes, increasing peristalsis. It is adapted to fleshy persons, used to high living who suffer from dyspepsia and catarrhal affections. People who eat a great deal more, especially meat, than they drink. Digestion is disordered by slightest error in diet. Has vasodilatory properties. Acts better on meat eaters than strictly vegetarians. Child is drowsy, lifeless, extremely pale, bowels torpid, will not walk, and the legs do not grow as rapidly as rest of the body.

WORSE: Change of temperature. Evening and night. Walking. Pressure. Drinking bad water. Gluttony.

BETTER: Sitting bent.

MIND: Fear; he will never get well, nor bear any medicine; of being poisoned. Wants many things, pleased with nothing.

HEAD: Vertigo while reading. Headache before menses, ceases during, < afterwards. Dandruff.

FACE: Spots. Lips dry.

MOUTH: Much sweetish saliva, after meals and at night. Hair sensation on tongue or throat. Tongue pale, papillae red.

STOMACH: Voracious appetite. Desire for butter. Complaints from bad water. Slightest error in diet disturbs the stomach. Feeling of something cold and/or hot ascending esophagus.

FEMALE: Menses profuse. Soreness of vulva and thighs. Mammae swollen and tender, during menses. Swelling of breast after weaning.

RESPIRATORY: Cough in the morning, with much difficult expectoration. Cough when smoking. Bronchiectasis, with fetid sputum. Hemoptysis.

EXTREMITIES: Pain in hips; pain in psoas and iliacus muscles, < crossing legs.

COMPLEMENTARY: Ars.

ALOE

GENERALITIES: It affects ABDOMINAL VEINS, causing congestion, *relaxation* of RECTUM, *liver,* colon and pelvis. It establishes physiological equilibrium when disease and drug symptoms are much mixed. Periodic headaches which alternate with *lumbago*. It is a remedy for bad effects of sedentary life or habits. Adapted to weary people, aged, old beer-drinkers. There is a sensation of *fullness in the parts.* HEAVY, DRAGGING, *as of a load.* Drawing, downward sensation. Discharges; gelatinous—post-nasal, stools, etc. *Sense of insecurity.* General weakness and weariness. Heat external and internal. Children, very emotional, chat and laugh.

WORSE: HEAT, Hot damp weather, Summer. Early morning. After dysentery. Yawning or mastication. Stepping hard. Evening. After eating and drinking.

BETTER: Cool open air. Cold applications. Passing flatus. Closing eyes. Taking tea or stimulants.

MIND: Dissatisfied and angry about himself. Disinclination to mental labor. Hates people, repels everyone. Ill humor, < in cloudy weather or with constipation. Thinks that she would die within a week. Life is a burden. Trembling from musical sounds and other noises. Imagines that persons are stepping hard or quickly.

HEAD: Aches above forehead, with heaviness in eyes, must partially close them. Vertigo with a sense of insecurity. Head symptoms alternating with abdominal or lumbar symptoms, > closing eyes. Heavy pressure on vertex. Clinking, as of some thin glass breaking, extending to ears.

EYES: Pain deep in orbit. Flickering before the eyes. Closes eyes partially from pain in forehead.

EARS: Cracking when chewing.

NOSE: Tip cold. Bleeding from the nose after awakening, in bed.

FACE: Lips markedly red, dry, cracked; bleeding. Pain while yawning or chewing.

MOUTH: Taste bitter and sour. Tongue, mouth dry.

THROAT: Hawking of thick lumps of jelly-like mucus. Raw and swollen feeling.

STOMACH: Desire for juicy things, fruits, especially apple, salty food. Pain in pit, when making false step. Aversion to meat. Eructations, with oppression in stomach. Hungry after stool.

ABDOMEN: Feels full, heavy, hot, bloated. Pain from navel to rectum. Sensation of a plug between symphysis pubis and coccyx, with urging for stool. Heaviness in hypogastrium, in rectum; dragging down in the abdomen. Prolapsus recti. *Rumbling, gurgling in bowels; sudden urging.* SENSE OF INSECURITY, *then hurriedly passes a gushing watery stool.* Uncertain whether gas or stool will come. Diarrhea, with pain in the rectum after stool; lienteric. ANUS WEAK, oozes mucus. Stools escape with flatus or when urinating. Stools mushy, lumpy, watery, gelatinous, bloody; solid stools passed involuntarily, urging to stool but passing flatus only. Piles, like a bunch of grapes, prolapsing, > cold bathing. Burning and stitching in anus and rectum, from piles, preventing sleep. Stool and flatus hot. Burning in rectum. Pulsation in rectum after eating. The child goes around the house, dropping little hard, round, marble-like stools. Diarrhea after eating oysters; in hot season, or of beer-drinkers. A lot of mucus is passed, with pain in rectum, after stool. Lumpy, watery stools.

URINARY: Incontinence in aged. Prostate enlarged. Every time on passing urine, feeling as if thin stool would escape with it. Urine hot.

MALE: Sexual irritability, after eating; after awakening (in children). Involuntary emission during siesta.

FEMALE: Heavy, congested uterus, with labour-like pain, felt in groins and hips, < standing and during menses. Climacteric hemorrhage. Menses too early and last too long. Leukorrhea of bloody mucus, preceded by colic. Dysentery after parturition.

RESPIRATORY: Winter cough, with itching. Difficult respiration, with stitches from liver to chest. Cough when she would sit down, or stand up, after sitting, with tears.

NECK & BACK: Lumbago alternating with headache and piles. Pain in sacrum, < while sitting, > moving about.

EXTREMITIES: Drawing pain in the joints. Lameness in all the limbs. Soles are painful when walking on the pavement.

SLEEP: Dreams of soiling himself.

FEVER: *Internal heat.*

COMPLEMENTARY: Sulph.

RELATED: Lil-t., *Podo.*, Sep., Sulph.

ALUMEN (Alum)

GENERALITIES: It causes paralytic weakness of the muscles in all parts of the body. Tendency to induration of glands and other tissues is very marked. Tongue, rectum, uterus, etc. are hardened; ulcers with indurated base. Adapted to old people suffering from bronchial catarrh. Sensation of dryness and of constriction. Constipation of the most aggravated kind, as in cancer of uterus and rectum. Hemorrhage: from leech bite; with large clots. Sensitive to cold; exposure to air causes roughness and chaps in the skin. Useful after operation on the eyes and teeth. Yellow bland discharge. Sensation of constriction, as of a cord or band around limbs, in paralytic states. Relaxation of muscles.

WORSE: During sleep; lying on right side; cold. Bad news.

MIND: Nervous tremors, from bad news. Doubting people. Lectophobia.

HEAD: Burning pain, as of weight on top of head, > pressure by cold hand. Vertigo with weakness in the pit of stomach, > opening eyes, > turning on right side. Headache, > drinking cold water.

EYES: Prolapse of iris, after cataract operation. Right eye squints towards the nose.

EAR: Hears every noise in sleep. Purulent otorrhea.

THROAT: Enlarged and indurated tonsils, from frequent colds. Uvula elongated, relaxed. Scraping in throat with cough. Spasm of esophagus, liquids can scarcely be swallowed. Complete aphonia.

ABDOMEN: Very obstinate constipation; no desire for days. Hard, marble-like masses passed, but rectum still feels full. Long-lasting pain and smarting in rectum after stools. Hematemesis of hard drinkers. Passes large clots from rectum.

FEMALE: Induration of cervix uteri and mammary glands. Chronic yellow vaginal discharge. Menses watery. Hands weak, drops things during menses.

RESPIRATORY: Copious, ropy expectoration, in a.m. in aged persons. Catarrh of chest; chest weak, hemoptysis; mucus expelled with difficulty.

HEART: Palpitation ; < lying on right side, from thinking of her disease.

SKIN: *Eczema on the back of penis and scrotum.* Alopecia.

ALUMINA

GENERALITIES: It affects the CEREBRO-SPINAL AXIS causing *Disturbances in co-ordination, and paretic effects.* Paresthesia. In mental sphere the consciousness of reality and judgment gets disturbed. It is suitable for old people with lack of vital heat, or premature old age with debility. It causes DRYNESS of skin and mucous membranes—eyes, throat, rectum, etc., or *irritability* and *relaxation.* Profuse mucus discharges. Discharges are thin, acrid and scanty. Tendency to induration. Functions become sluggish, actions are delayed, e.g., prick of needle will be felt late, impressions reach consciousness slowly. Patient is *thin, inactive, wants to lie down,* but it increases the fatigue. It is useful in delicate children, products of artificial baby foods. Pulsations are felt in various parts; and pains go upwards. Patient gets better entirely for some time, then without apparent cause gets worse. Chronicity. Exhaustion:

after talking; after menses. Degeneration of spinal cord. Unable to walk with closed eyes. Involuntary movement of single parts. Girls dried up and wrinkled, at puberty. Ill effects of disappointment. Sensation of constriction. Trembling, convulsive movement, spasm, with tears and laughter, at times alternately.

WORSE: Warmth of Room, of bed. Food: artificial, potato, starch, salt. *Speaking. Dry weather. Early on awaking.* Sitting. After menses. Periodically, on alternate days. Coition. Tobacco smoke. Lifting. Exertion. Full and new moon.

BETTER: Evening. Open air. Moderate exertion and temperature. Damp weather, cold washing.

MIND: Illusion; of being larger, *numb, smooth,* heavy. *Hasty but slow of execution,* hence makes mistakes in speaking and writing. Depressive mental states. Timorous. Fears, his own impulses, sight of knife, of blood; fears loss of reason. When he sees or states something, he has the feeling as though another person had said or seen it or as though he was placed in another person and could see only then. Time passes too slowly. Always groaning, moaning, worrying, fretting. Memory bad, variable mood. Depressed on awakening. Peevish. Everything is viewed in sad light. Alternating moods. Sensation as if he would fall forward, which he greatly fears. Things seem unreal. Laughs and talks between paroxysms of spasms. Sneers at everything. Grumbles. Suicidal tendency on seeing knife or blood.

HEAD: Vertigo, < talking, on closing or opening eyes, before breakfast. Vertigo, with white stars before the eyes, when eyes suddenly went out of focus; one has to wait for normal vision, > wiping eyes. Violent stitches in the brain, with nausea. Headache as if one were dragged by the hair. Falling of hair; scalp itches and is numb. Headache > by lying quite in bed. Dry hair.

EYES: White stars before the eyes, with vertigo, Eyelids weak, thickened, dry, burning, smartingptosis. Double squint (Strabismus), < teething. Objects look yellow. Eyes; inflamed burning agglutination at night, lacrimation during day. Eyes feel cold.

EARS: Heat and redness of one ear. Eustachian tube seems plugged. Crackling noises and buzzing in ears when chewing or swallowing.

NOSE: Nostrils sore and red. Point of nose cracked. Scales with thick yellow mucus.

FACE: *Old look;* dusky, wrinkled. Sensation as if white of egg or a cobweb on face. Blood-boils, and pimples. Involuntary spasmodic twitching of the lower jaw. Maxillary joints feel tight while chewing or opening mouth.

MOUTH: Musty bad odor from mouth. Teeth feel long; pain extends to other parts down larynx, neck, shoulders. Mouth feels dry with increased saliva. Tingling, itching on tongue.

THROAT: Dry; feels full of sticks, or *constricted,* food cannot pass. Sore from eating onions. Constant inclination to clear the throat. Uvula hangs down. Swallowing painful, < solids, > empty swallowing, warm drinks. Tightness from pharynx down to stomach as if food could not pass; can swallow but small morsels at a time. Clergyman's sore throat. Feels food whole length of esophagus.

STOMACH: Abnormal craving; for coarse food, chalk, charcoal, dry food, clean white rags, tea or coffee grounds, fruits, vegetables, dry rice and indigestible things. Constriction of esophagus. Pain lasting three hours after meals. Big bellied children. Aversion to potatoes, to meat, which disagree.

ABDOMEN: Left-sided abdominal complaints. Pressing in both groins, towards sexual organs. Pains from rectum to ankle. Inactive rectum, even a soft stool is passed with difficulty, hard stools cause severe cutting. Stools of small balls, hard knots or bright clots of blood. Evacuation is preceded by painful urging, long before stool, then straining at stool. Constipation: of suckling babies, old people and women of sedentary habits. Can pass stool only when standing.

URINARY: Muscles of the bladder paretic, *must strain at stool to urinate.* Renal pain, < dancing. Frequent desire to urinate in old people, slow flow. Fears he will wet bed. Retention, with dribbling. Smarting while urinating. Feeling of weakness in bladder and genitals.

MALE: Sexual desire increased. Voluptuous itching or tickling in genitals. Involuntary emission while straining for stool, followed by old symptoms. Pain in the perineum during coition and while the erection continues. Priapism at night.

FEMALE: Menses too early, short, scanty, pale, followed by great exhaustion. Leukorrhea: acrid profuse, runs to feet, < daytime; before menses, > by washing with cold water. Intolerable bearing-down pains. Tickling and itching in genitals; with strong desire for embrace. Nipples itch, burn, look angry (during pregnancy). It takes a woman all her time to recuperate from one menstrual period to the next.

RESPIRATORY: Cough, constant, dry, hacking, interrupts breathing, with sneezing; < after waking in the morning, from elongated uvula, from condiments or eating irritating things, talking or singing. Sudden loss of voice; on taking cold. Chest feels constricted, < sitting bent or stooping. Soreness of chest on talking; on lifting.

HEART: Palpitation and shocks in heart. Wakes between 4 and 5 a.m., with anxiety at heart, > after rising.

NECK & BACK: Pain in the back, as if a hot irons were thrust through lower spine. Violent stitches in back. Back feels bandaged by a cord.

EXTREMITIES: Pain in the arms and fingers, as if a hot iron penetrated. Arms feel heavy, as if paralyzed; short; go to sleep. Lower limbs heavy. Staggering on walking. Legs feel numb especially when sitting cross-legged. Heels feel numb, when stepping. *Festination*. Locomotor ataxia. Nails brittle or thick. Gnawing under nails. Inability to walk except when eyes are open or in daytime. Totters if eyes were closed. Soles painful on stepping on it, as if they were too soft, and on walking; cramps when crossing legs. Bones feel squeezed.

SKIN: Intolerable itching, when getting warm in bed. Dry, rough, cracked skin. Itching, burning, over seat of pain. Must scratch until it bleeds. Eczema. The slightest injuries of the skin smart and become inflamed. Skin symptoms < winter, fullmoon and new moon.

SLEEP: Anxious, restless, with confused dreams, about thieves, ghosts, of boats foundering.

FEVER: Chilliness, > open air. Heat with itching.

COMPLEMENTARY: Bry.

RELATED: Bry; Plb.

ALUMINA SILICATA

GENERALITIES: It affects spinal cord. Constriction is a marked general symptom. Constriction of orifices. Aching and burning in spine. Formication, numbness and pain in all limbs. Epileptiform convulsions. Coldness during pain.

WORSE: Cold air; after eating; standing.

BETTER: Warmth; fasting; resting in bed.

AMBRA GRISEA

GENERALITIES: It affects the NERVES, causing nervousness, twitches and jerks. It is adapted to hysterical subjects, to thin scrawny women, to patients who are weakened by age and overwork, to the aged with impairment of all functions. Patients *are worn out yet over-impressionable.* Shock due to business failure or due to the death one after another in the family. Weakness of upper part of the body, with trembling of lower parts. Slight or unusual things < the breathing, the heart, start the menses, etc. One sided complaints. *Symptoms suddenly change place.* Sensation of coldness, numbness, in spots or of single parts, fingers, arms, etc., with twitching. Itching, trembling and ebullition. General pulsation. Numbness and torpor of the whole body esp. in the morning. Coldness of the body, with twitching. Effects of domestic shock, business worry. Loss of near relatives. Imaginations. Young modern society girls.

WORSE: *Music. Presence of others.* Embarrassment. Agitation; worry; thinking of it. Overlifting. From any unusual thing. Morning. Warmth. Warm milk.

BETTER: Slow motion, in open air. Lying on painful parts. Cold drinks.

MIND: Memory impaired; slow comprehension. *Dreamy.* Flitting ideas of fixed disagreeable fancies. Imagines diabolic faces, sights. Melancholy; sits for days weeping. Awkward. Flitting, flighty talker, modern society girls. Dread of people. Desire to be alone. Cannot understand what one reads. Sad. *Bashful;* blushes easily. Hearing others talk or talking himself affects him. Time passes slowly. Aversion to laugh. Jumping from one subject to another, never waiting to have first question answered. Music causes weeping and trembling.

HEAD: *Vertigo*, senile, with weakness in head and stomach. Tearing pain in upper part of the brain. Brain feels loose, seems as if it falls to side lain on. Hair fall out. *Confusion* in occiput, also sprained feeling. Headache, < blowing nose.

EYES: Stitching in the eyelids as if a stye were forming. Eyelids heavy, cannot open them though awake. Spots float before the eyes after sewing.

EARS: Hardness of hearing, with cold sensation in abdomen. Deaf in one ear, roaring and whistling in the other.

NOSE: Bleeds while washing the face in the morning. Epistaxis, during menses. Stoppage mostly at night, must breathe through the mouth, with chronic coryza.

FACE: Twitching of the facial muscles. Cramps in lips; lips hot. Left cheek red. Flushes of the face, jaundiced color. Embarrassed look. Lock-jaw in newborn.

MOUTH: Profuse bleeding from the gums; offensive breath. Ranula. Sour mouth, < after milk. Salivation, with cough.

THROAT: Sensation of a plug, with difficulty in swallowing. Sore, raw, from exposure to air, < motion of tongue.

STOMACH: After eating, cough and gaping and a feeling as if food did not go down into the stomach. Eructations, with violent convulsive cough. Heartburn from drinking milk. Distention of stomach, after midnight. Thirstlessness.

ABDOMEN: *Flatulence; cannot have others present during urination and stool:* < during pregnancy. Sensation of coldness in the abdomen. Constipation, during pregnancy, and after delivery. Aching in small spot in the region of liver, > pressure. Much flow of blood with stool. Sweat on abdomen and thighs. Frequent ineffectual urging for stool.

URINARY: Pain in the bladder and rectum at the same time. *Cannot pass urine in presence of others.* Feeling in urethra as if few drops passed out. Urine, turbid even during emission, forming a brown sediment. Urinates more than drinks. Urine smells sour, during whooping cough. Burning, smarting, itching in vulva, during urination.

MALE: Voluptuous excitement. Itching in genitals. Parts externally numb; burn internally. Erection without desire. Impotence.

FEMALE: Itching of pudendum, with soreness and swelling. Itching labia. Discharge of blood between the periods, at every little accident, after hard stool, walking a little longer, etc. Leukorrhea of bluish mucus, profuse, < at night. Sexual desire increased. Lying down < uterine symptoms. Menses too early and too profuse.

RESPIRATORY: Asthmatic breathing; in old people; < by coition. Hollow, spasmodic, barking cough, coming from deep in chest, then eructation. Bluish, white expectoration. Cough, < music; in presence of many people, talking, reading aloud, lifting weight. Loss of breath from cough. Cough with emaciation.

HEART: Palpitation, with pressure in chest as from a lump lodged there, or as if chest is obstructed. Palpitation, with pale face. Anxiety at heart.

EXTREMITIES: Cramps in hands and fingers, < grasping anything. Left leg becomes quite blue during menses. Twitching of limbs, with coldness of body, during sleep. Cramps in legs and calves. Limbs go to sleep easily. Fingernails brittle. Drops what one is carrying. Coldness of hand (L), with headache. Sore and raw between thighs.

SLEEP: Cannot sleep from worry, must get up. Retires tired, wakeful as soon as head touches the pillow.

SKIN: Itching and soreness, esp. around genitals.

FEVER: Frequent flushes of heat at short intervals. Sweat on slightest exertion, esp. on abdomen and thighs.

RELATED: Bar-c., Ign.

AMBROSIA

GENERALITIES: A remedy for hay fever, lacrimation and intolerable itching of the eyelids. Nose-bleed. Stuffed feeling in nose and head.

RELATED: Ars-i., Sabad.

AMMONIUM BROMATUM

GENERALITIES: It is indicated in laryngeal and pharyngeal catarrh. Sudden strangling, suffocating, cough. Suffocating sensation before epilepsy. Irritable feeling in fingernails, > by biting them.

AMMONIUM CARBONICUM

GENERALITIES: It affects HEART, *circulation and blood.* Heart becomes weak, collapse. Circulation becomes sluggish, and under-oxygenation of blood produces LIVIDITY, WEAKNESS *and drowsiness. Vitality becomes low and there is lack of reaction.* It is adapted to fat patients, with weak heart, with wheezing and suffocative feeling.

Stout women who are always tired and sweaty, take cold easily and suffer from cholera-like symptoms before menses; and who lead a sedentary life. *Very sensitive to cold air.* Great aversion to water, cannot bear to touch it. Heaviness in all organs. Uncleanliness in bodily habits. Pains are bruised and sore. There is internal raw burning. Discharges are *hot, acrid,* adherent. *Hemorrhage, dark, thin.* Malignancy. Prostration from trifles. Scorbutic states. Old age. Lies down from debility or soreness of whole body. Ill effects of charcoal fumes. Active but soon exhausted.

WORSE: Cold; Cloudy days. Damp Cold. *Cold open air.* Falling asleep; 3-4 a.m. *During menses.* Motion. Chewing. Pressing teeth. Bending down. New moon.

BETTER: *Pressure;* eating; lying on abdomen. Dry weather. Lying on right side.

MIND: Active but soon exhausted. Forgetful, ill-humored, gloomy, during stormy weather. Heedless and unruly. Depressed, with weakness of intellect. Vacant mind. Loss of memory, < vexation. Hearing others talk or talking himself affects him. Aversion to work. Peevish, fretting, as if crime has been committed. Disposed to weep. Tendency to make mistakes in speaking, writing and calculating.

HEAD: Shocks through head, eyes, ears and nose, on biting. Violent headache; fullness bursting in forehead. Brain seems loose.

EYES: Burning and dry. Prolonged use of eyes causes asthenopia; with appearance of yellow spots on looking at white objects. Flood of tears. Large black spots float after sewing. Pain in the eyes, > afternoon sleep.

EARS: Hardness of hearing. Itching above the ears, spreads over the whole body. Hard swelling of parotid and cervical glands.

NOSE: *Stoppage of nose,* at night, with long-continued coryza, must breathe through mouth. Snuffles of children. Nose bleeds; if hands or face are washed, after eating, or on waking. Continuous urging to sneeze. Profuse watery coryza. Catarrh starting in nose. Boil on tip. Inability to blow the nose in children.

FACE: Boils and pustules, during menses. Corners of the mouth are sore, cracked, and they burn. Cracks and burning in lips. Hard swelling of the cheek.

MOUTH: Tender, bleeding gums. Pressing teeth together sends a shock through head, eyes, ears and nose. Mouth and throat dry. Loose or blunt teeth. Vesicles on tongue. Burning, hindering eating and speech. Toothache during menses. Swelling inside cheek.

THROAT: Enlarged tonsils, and glands of the neck. Gangrenous ulceration of the tonsils. Diphtheria, when nose is stopped, membrane extends to upper lip.

STOMACH: Pain at the pit of stomach, with heartburn, nausea, waterbrash and chilliness. Flatulent dyspepsia. Appetite good, but easy satisfaction.

ABDOMEN: Bleeding piles, < during menses. Discharge of blood before and after stool. Protruding piles, < after stool or without stool, > lying; cannot walk. Dark acrid diarrhea. Colic with pain between the scapulae. Constipation—stools hard, dry.

URINARY: Frequent desire. Urine white, bloody, sandy, copious, turbid and fetid. Involuntary urination towards morning.

MALE: Persistent erection without desire or violent sexual desire without erection. Seminal emission frequent, after coition.

FEMALE: Cholera-like symptoms, with menses. Menses too frequent, profuse, early, clotted, black, with colicky pain and hard difficult stool, with fatigue, esp. of thighs, yawning and chilliness. Menses flow more at night, then dyspnea or weakness. Copious leukorrhea, burning, acrid, watery. Irritation of clitoris.

RESPIRATORY: *Increasing difficulty in breathing,* it wakes him, > cool air. Much oppression in breathing, < every effort, entering a warm room. Emphysema. *Rattling in chest but gets up little.* Hoarseness. Pulmonary edema. Cough after influenza. Hypostatic congestion of lungs. Expectoration of pure blood, after cough.

HEART: WEAK. Wakes with difficult breathing and palpitation. Palpitation audible, with fear, cold sweat and lacrimation, inability to speak and trembling hands. Angina pectoris. Weak heart causes stasis.

EXTREMITIES: Parts lain on become numb. Cramps in calves and soles. Finger and hands swell when arms are hanging down. Inclination to stretch limbs. Whitlow. Tearing pain, > by heat of bed. Right foot numb. Ganglion. Aching in bones, > change of weather. Right arm heavy and weak.

SKIN: Red or mottled skin. Erysipelas, in aged. Malignant scarlatina.

SLEEP: Sleepiness during day. Wakes up with strangling. The sooner one goes to bed the better one sleeps.

FEVER: *Coldness.* Burning heat with thirst.

RELATED: Ant-t., Carb-v., Glon., Lach., Mur-ac.

AMMONIUM MURIATICUM

GENERALITIES: It affects MUCOUS MEMBRANES increasing the secretion and retaining them, esp. in CHEST and *gall ducts.* It causes *irregular circulation,* blood seems to be in constant turmoil, causing *ebullitions, burning* and *localized throbbing.* Many symptoms are accompanied by cough or PROFUSE GLAIRY *mucus* discharges, with liver trouble. Tension and *tightness, as if the muscles* or *tendons are too short,* in groins, hamstrings, lumbar region, etc. It causes ulceration and ulcerative or festering pain. Neuralgic pain in the stumps of amputated limbs. Hemorrhage. Boiling sensation. It is adapted to patients who are fat, puffy and sluggish, with thin limbs, who always feel tired and sore. Effects of grief.

WORSE: Morning — head and chest symptoms. Afternoon—abdominal symptoms; Evening - skin, fever and limb symptoms. Chronic sprain. Walking erect. Periodically. Night 2 to 4 a.m.

BETTER: Open air. Rapid motion. Walking crooked.

MIND: Desire to cry, but cannot. Involuntary aversion to certain persons. Melancholy and apprehensive, as from internal grief.

HEAD: Heaviness in the forehead; pressive pain towards the root of the nose, with a sensation as if brain were torn. Hair fall out, with itching and dandruff. Brain paralysis.

EYES: Mist before eyes in bright light. Flying spots, yellow spots, before the eyes. Incipient cataract, capsular cataract.

NOSE: Free acrid, hot, watery coryza, closing one nostril. Loss of smell. Obstructed stuffy feeling, with a desire to blow it out. As of a rough body obstructing upper nares. Nose sore to touch. Sneezing aroused her from sleep with shooting pain in the nape of the neck as far as the shoulders. Coryza in children, with bluish discharge.

FACE: Pale. Lips burning like fire, dry, shrivelled, cracked, must moisten them with tongue. Burning eruptions, > cold application.

MOUTH: Slimy. Burning blisters on tip of tongue.

THROAT: *Slimy.* Throbbing and swelling of the tonsils. Internal and external swelling of the throat, with sticky mucus. Stricture of esophagus.

STOMACH: Thirst for lemonade. Nausea, with bitter waterbrash, < eating, with shuddering. Gnawing, burning, stitching in stomach, extending to right axilla and upper arm. Cancer of stomach. Empty sensation, but no desire to eat. Diarrhea and vomiting, during menses.

ABDOMEN: Stitches in spleen while eating, with difficult breathing. Cough with liver symptoms. Excessive fatty deposits around abdomen. Scanty, hard, crumbling stools, changing color and consistency. Blood from anus or diarrhea during menses. Hemorrhoids, after suppressed leukorrhea. Burning in the rectum, during and for hours after stool. Tense, sprained feeling in groins, must walk bent. Groins feel swollen and sore.

URINARY: Profuse and frequent urination. Urging, yet a few drops pass until next stool when it flows freely. Profuse ammoniacal smelling urine.

FEMALE: Menses too early, with pain in abdomen and small of the back; flow more at night. Prolapse of uterus. Leukorrhea, like white of an egg, with pain about the navel, < after every urination.

RESPIRATION: Hoarseness and burning in larynx. Cough with profuse salivation or with liver symptoms. Cannot breathe from coughing. *Noisy, rattling, tenacious mucus in chest.* Pulsation, burning spots in chest. Cough, < lying on back or right side.

NECK & BACK: *Swollen cervical glands. Sore sprain* or *icy coldness between scapulae,* not relieved by warmth.

Lumbago. Bruised pain in coccyx when sitting. Fatty swelling on nape, extending from ear to ear.

EXTREMITIES: Tense sprained feeling in groin, must walk bent. Contraction of hamstring tendons. Sciatica (L), < sitting, > lying. Ulcerative pain in fingertips. Pain in or ulcer on heel. Pain in feet during menses. Shooting pain in scapulae, < breathing. Buttocks large. Hamstrings feels as if too short, pain on walking.

SLEEP: Erotic dreams. Anxious, fearful dreams. Starts in sleep.

SKIN: Bleeding eruptions. Peeling of skin between fingers and wrists. Itching in various parts of the body, esp. of the evening.

FEVER: Chilly as often as he wakes. Sense of heat, > open air, alternating with chill. Chilly in the evening after lying down. Profuse night sweat. Sweats by every motion.

RELATED: Calc., Caust., Seneg.

AMYL NITROSUM

GENERALITIES: Vaso-motor nerves are affected by *Amyl nit,* causing dilatation of all arterioles and capillaries, flushing of face, heat and *throbbing in the head. Flushing heat, followed by drenching sweat* (unilateral) is a marked symptom. Cerebral vessels dilate. Exophthalmic goitre, from grief. Unconsciousness, with inability to swallow. Throbbing, esp. in head. Weak, emaciated, walking with tottering gait, inclined to go to one side when walking. Cannot sit still.

WORSE: CLIMAXIS. SLIGHT CAUSES. *Emotions.* Heat. Close room.

BETTER: Exercise in open air. Cold water.

MIND: Anxiety as if something might happen; must have fresh air.

HEAD: *Surging of blood to the head;* with fiery red face. Migraine, with pallor.

FACE: Easy flushing or blushing of the face, on slightest emotion. Chewing motion of the lower jaw. Smacking of lips as if in act of tasting.

THROAT: Choking feeling in the throat; collar seems too tight.

STOMACH: Hiccough and yawning with stretching.

FEMALE: Hemorrhage, with facial flushing. Neuralgia during menses. Climacteric flushings, with headache, anxiety and palpitation. Convulsion immediately after delivery.

CHEST: Pain and constriction around the heart. Fluttering of heart on least excitement. Tumultuous palpitation. Angina pectoris with great anxiety. Full, soft pulse. Aching backward along the left floating rib.

SLEEP: Repeated yawning in coma. Yawns profoundly and repeatedly. Stretches almost constantly, it is almost impossible to satisfy the desire to stretch. Stretching and yawning with hiccough.

FEVER: Abnormal sweat after influenza.

RELATED: Glon., Lach.

ANACARDIUM

GENERALITIES: *Anac.* subjects are neurasthenic. Mind, nerves, muscles and joints are affected. There is physical and mental LACK OF POWER. *Special senses are weakened*—sight, hearing, touch etc. *Sensation* of a plug in various parts, or of a DULL PRESSURE, which is repeated from time to time. Sensation of a band or hoop. Intermittence of symptoms. Fear of examination in students. *Trembling,* on slight exertion, < knees or arms. Paralytic condition. Wants to lie or sit continually. Eating temporarily relieves all the symptoms. Nervous exhaustion from over-study. Paresis of muscles subject to volition. Wounded tendons. Joints contracted. Old people. Ill-natured children. Nervous hysterical women. Diseases of spinal cord. Heaviness and fullness of the whole body after piano playing.

WORSE: MENTAL EXERTION. EMOTION. *Anger.* Fright. Care. Mortification. *Stepping hard.* Motion. Drafts, open air, cold. Long after eating. Rubbing, scratching. Talking Morning, Evening to midnight. Checked eruption. Strong smell.

BETTER: By eating. Lying on side. Rubbing. Heat—hot bath. In the sun.

MIND: Fixed ideas; thinks he is possessed of two persons or two wills. Illusion of *duality;* others are present behind her etc. Her husband is not her husband, her child is not hers. There is no reality in anything, everything appears like a dream. Apprehends trouble from everything. Senseless talk. Screams loudly, as if to call someone. Religious mania. BAD MEMORY. Suddenly forgets names, those around her, what she has seen. Aversion to work. Lack of self-confidence. Desire to swear and curse. Fear of paralysis. Despairs of getting well. *Contradictory impulses* - laughs at serious things, remaining serious when anything laughable occurs. Cowardly. Vacillating. At odds with himself. Melancholy. *Ill-natured. Profane.* Takes everything in bad part. Absent-minded as if in a dream. Clairaudient - hears voices far away or of the dead. Suicidal tendency, by shooting. Sees everybody's face in the mirror except his own. Hard hearted, cruel. Hesitates, often does nothing. Unsocial. Neurotic. Suspicious. Very easily offended. Senile dementia. Refuses to eat for fear of being poisoned.

HEAD: Vertigo, < walking, stooping and rising from stooping; objects seem too distant. Pressing pain as from a plug in temples, occiput, forehead and vertex, > during meals, falling asleep; < coughing, deep breathing. Itching and little boils on the scalp. Gastric and nervous headache. Headache from strong smell.

EYES: Pressing pain as of a plug on upper orbit. Threads and black spots before the eyes. Objects appear too far off. Vision indistinct. Short-sightedness.

EARS: Hard of hearing. Pressing pain as of a plug. Imagines whispers in the ears.

NOSE: Sense of smell perverted, lost or acute. Illusory smells. Frequent sneezing, followed by coryza and lacrimation. Violent coryza with palpitation, esp. in the aged.

FACE: Pale, *wan* looking. Blue rings around the eyes. Eczema of face and neck. Expressionless, wild, childish.

MOUTH: Bad breath and taste. Painful vesicles in the mouth. Tongue feels swollen and stiff impeding speech and motion, with much saliva in the mouth. Taste lost.

STOMACH: Empty feeling. Weak digestion. Breath stops on eating and drinking. Gastric pain, > by eating, but again < after 2 - 3 hours. Hastily drinks and swallows food. Vomiting >. Loss of appetite, alternating with violent hunger.

ABDOMEN: Pain as if a dull plug was pressed into intestine. Hardness of abdomen. Flatulent colic, with rumbling, pinching and griping. Rectum feels plugged and powerless, cannot evacuate even a soft stool. Ineffectual desire. Itching of anus; moisture from rectum.

URINARY: Frequent emission of clear watery urine; deposit turbid, clay-coloured sediment. Sensation of burning in the glans during and after urination.

MALE: Voluptuous itching of scrotum, exciting sexual desire. Seminal emissions without dreams. Prostatic discharge during stool. Enjoyment absent.

FEMALE: Leukorrhea, with itching and excoriation of the parts. Frequent but scanty menses, with spasmodic pain in abdomen. Nausea during pregnancy, > eating.

RESPIRATORY: Breathing stops on coughing or swallowing. Cough excited by talking, after eating, with vomiting of food, with pain in occiput; in children after a fit of temper. Coughs, then yawns and sleeps. Asthma, hysterical, ends in flow of tears.

HEART: Double stitch (Stitches in paroxysms of two) at the heart, passing into lumbar region. Palpitation with coryza in the aged.

NECK & BACK: Dull pressure or feeling of a heavy load on shoulders. Stiffness of nape and neck down back; pain, < motion.

EXTREMITIES: Neuralgia of the thumb. Knees feel paralyzed or bandaged. Dry hands. Cramp in the calves, < walking or rising from a seat. Pain in ankle as if sprained, < stepping. Painful thumping on the middle upper arm (L). Cramp from toe to instep, from heel up calf. Warts on palms and hands. Writer's cramps.

SLEEP: Spells of sleeplessness, lasting several nights. Anxious dreams.

SKIN: *Skin insensible;* itching, < scratching. Dermatitis. Eczema, neurotic. Yellow vesicles. Urticaria. Promotes expulsion of splinters. Warts on palms and hands.

FEVER: Easily chilled. > Sunshine. Clammy sweat on palms, esp. left. Heat from 4 p.m. till evening, passing off after supper.

RELATED: Ign., *Lyc.,* Plat., Rhus-t.

ANTHRACINUM

GENERALITIES: This nosode is a very valuable remedy in malignant or septic inflammations of connective or cellular tissues. It produces boil or boil-like eruptions; carbuncle; malignant ulcer, abscess, bubo, where there is a purulent focus. Hemorrhage thick, black, tar-like from any orifice. Glands swollen; cellular tissue oedematous and indurated. There is a terrible burning with great prostration. *Black and blue blisters.* Gangrene, dissecting wounds. Bad effects of inhaling foul odor. *Abscess of septum.* Quinsy. Succession of boils. Hard stony swelling at right lower jaw and submaxillary glands.

RELATED: Ars., Tarent-c.

ANTIMONIUM CRUDUM

GENERALITIES: The choice of this remedy is determined by the symptoms which develop in mental and gastric sphere. As the last word of its name implies, the *Ant-c.* patient is crude, mentally and physically. Patient is a *Gross feeder* — a glutton, he eats beyond the capacity of his digestion or without discrimination; therefore the *mental and skin symptoms* are due to the GASTRO-INTESTINAL DISTURBANCE. It produces *lumpy effects*-stools are watery containing lumps, leukorrhea is watery mixed with lumps, lumps appear upon the skin; nails become thick, distorted and lumpy. There is a tendency to formation of CRACKS — in canthi, nostrils, angles of the mouth. Mentally the patient is either sentimental, esp. in moonlight and twilight, during diarrhea and before menses; or cross and touchy. It produces strange *absence of pain,* where it could be expected, e.g. in bed-sore. It is suitable for infants and children; also elderly persons and young persons who have tendency to *grow fat.* When symptom groups recur, they change their locality or go from one side to the other, they recur every five or six or twelve weeks. Gout recedes and stomach is affected. Nervous symptom such as restlessness, twitches in the muscles, and disposition to start on slightest noise are also found. Ill effects of disappointed love and suppressed eruption. Chronic complaints traceable to suppression of eruptions or ulcers. Anasarca. Marasmus. Trouble from swimming or falling into water. Rheumatoid arthritis. He is always *sleepy* and *weary.*

WORSE: COLD BATHING; *Cold dampness;* COLD WATER (on head). *Acids, Sweets.* Moonlight. Rising up. Ascending stairs. Touch. HEAT OF SUMMER, *of Sun.* Radiated heat. OVEREATING. Nightly debauches, after getting drunk. Vinegar. Pork.

BETTER: In open air; during rest; moist warmth. Lying down.

MIND: Great anxiety about his fate; inclination to shoot himself. *Fretful, cross* and *peevish; cries if looked at or touched* or washed, esp. children; adults are sulky, do not wish to speak with anyone. Loathing of life, of food, bathing, etc. *Ecstasy and exalted love. Dreamy, sentimental.* Angry at every little attention. Lovesick. So busy with oneself one forgets to urinate or defecate, eats only when asked. Excitability. Nervous, hysterical girls and women who are overcome by mellow light from stained-glass windows. Talks in rhymes or verses. Taciturn.

HEAD: Aches from bathing in cold water or from disordered stomach, < candy or acid wine, fruits, fat, ascending stairs. Tendency to take cold about head. Heaviness in forehead, with vertigo, nausea and nose-bleed. Itching of the head, with falling of hair. Headache after stopped coryza.

EYES: Canthi raw, cracked, red and moist. Pustules on the margins of the lids, chronic blepharitis. Lids red and inflamed. Looking into the fire causes cough. Chronic sore eyes of children. Photophobia.

EARS: Ringing and deafness. Moist eruption around the ears. Otorrhea. Deafness, as if ear were bandaged or a leaf lying on one.

NOSE: *Nostrils scabby,* sore and cracked. Nose bleed after headache. Eczema of nostrils. Feeling of coldness on inhalation.

FACE: Sallow, haggard or sad. Pimples, pustules and boils on face. Yellow crusted eruption on cheeks and chin. Cracks in the corners of the mouth. Small, sore honey colored granules on chin.

MOUTH: *Tongue* COATED THICK WHITE, AS IF WHITE WASHED. Toothache in hollow teeth, pain extends to head, < touching the tooth with tongue, > walking in open air, Grinding of teeth, when sleeping in sitting position. Canker sores. Toothache before menses. Pimples around the mouth. Aphthae. Gums bleed easily. Taste bitter. Salivation, tastes salty.

THROAT: Much thick yellowish mucus from posterior nares. Rough voice from over use. Hoarseness after cold water bath. Sensation as if a foreign body had lodged, with constant desire to swallow.

STOMACH: Loss of appetite, with disgust for food. No thirst. Desire for acid, pickle. Eructation tasting of the ingesta; food leaves an aftertaste or causes constant belching. DIGESTION DISORDERED easily. Vomiting, < eating or drinking; without nausea or relief. Stomach is painful to pressure. Gouty metastasis to stomach, and bowels. Sweetish waterbrash. Bloating after eating. Child vomits milk in curd after nursing and refuses to nurse afterwards (reverse *Aeth.*). Appetite does not return after severe illness. Vomiting, fearful, with convulsions, which cannot stop. Great desire to eat, but no strength to do it (child). Pork disagrees. Stomach seems to be always overloaded.

ABDOMEN: Diarrhea alternating with constipation, esp. in old persons. Stool, pappy or *watery* mixed with lumps. Mucous piles — prickling and bursting with continuous mucus discharge from anus, staining linen yellow. Catarrhal proctitis. *Fullness in abdomen.* Hemorrhage with solid stools, piles. Stools entirely of mucus. Diarrhea, summer, after nursing.

URINARY: Cutting in urethra while urinating. Urination frequent, profuse, with burning and backache. Involuntary urination on coughing. Foul odor.

MALE: Atrophy of penis and testicle. Biting, itching of scrotum, with eruption. Excited sexual desire, with uneasiness of the whole body.

FEMALE: Menses suppressed from cold bathing, with tenderness of the ovaries, pressure in womb as if something would come out during menses. Nymphomania from checked menses. Leukorrhea watery containing lumps. Nausea, vomiting and diarrhea, during pregnancy. Ovaries painful in lovesick girls.

RESPIRATORY: Cough, < coming in warm room; with burning in chest. First attack of cough is always most severe, the subsequent attacks become weaker and weaker. Looking into fire < cough. Pain in the chest with heat. Voice lacks control, harsh, badly pitched, > using it. Aphonia from overheating. Itching in chest. Expectoration of large quantities of mucus, exhausts the patient.

NECK & BACK: Violent pain in small of back when rising, > when walking. Itching of neck and back. Coccyx heavy.

EXTREMITIES: Arthritic pain in the joints of fingers. Horny or split nails; nails grow slowly, out of shape; horny growth under the nails. Horny warts on hands and soles. Painful inflammation of the tendon of elbows with great redness and curvature of the arms. Shiny elbows. Feet very tender; soles tender while walking. Callosities on soles. Skin on soles is withered on account of foot sweat. Weakness and shaking of hands in writing, followed by offensive flatus. Twitching in muscles. Jerks in arms. Crippled feet. Growth beneath nails.

SKIN: Eczema, with gastric derangement. Tendency to form pimples, vesicles and pustules. Urticaria, white, with red areola, itching fearfully. Measle like eruptions. Warts horny. Dry gangrene. Itching when warm in bed. Callosities from slight pressure.

SLEEP: *Sleepy and weary.* Drowsy old people. Deep unrefreshing sleep.

FEVER: Great heat from little exercise, esp. in the sun. Heat and thirst after sweat. Disturbances of stomach during apyrexia, in intermittent fever.

RELATED: Sulph.

COMPLEMENTARY: Squil.

ANTIMONIUM TARTARICUM

GENERALITIES: There is some similarity of symptoms between Ant-c and Ant-t esp. in mental and digestive spheres. Ant-t., affects the MUCOUS MEMBRANES, esp. of *Bronchi and* Lungs, causing GREAT ACCUMULATION OF MUCUS, *with coarse rattling,* thereby *respiration* is impeded and *heart action becomes labored;* defective oxygenation in the circulation of *blood occurs.* All these conditions cause cyanosis, depression of vital power. Patient becomes INCREASINGLY WEAK, SWEATS, BECOMES DROWSY and RELAXED WITH LACK OF REACTION. It is suitable for old people and children; to gouty subjects and drunkards with gastric affections. Trembling of whole body, great prostration and faintness. Sensation of weight or heaviness in many parts—head, occiput, coccyx, limbs. Convulsive twitching. Fretfulness, whining and crying, before the attack of sickness. Chronic trembling of head and hands (as in paralysis agitans). Chill and contracture and pain in muscles. Dropsy of synovial membrane. Convulsions when eruptions fail to appear. Child continuously wishes to be carried erect, unwilling to be looked at or touched. Complaints arising from digestive sphere. Effects of anger and vexation. Prostrated in mind and body. Nursing infants let go the nipple and cry out as if out of breath. Children have convulsions if attention is thrust upon them. Ill effects of vaccination when *Thuja* fails and *Silicea* is not indicated. Sensation of coldness in blood vessels. Bilharziasis. Clings to attendant.

WORSE: WARM: *room, wraps, weather. Anger. Lying.* Morning, Overheating. Cold; dampness. On sitting down, when seated, on rising from it. Motion. Sour things. Milk.

BETTER: *Expectoration.* Sitting erect. Motion. Vomiting. Eructation. Lying on right side.

MIND: Fear of being alone. Bad humor. Despondent, Frightened at every trifle. Muttering delirium. Stupid on awakening. *Apathy* or easily annoyed; wants to be left alone. Peevish; whining and moaning. Despair of recovery. Consciousness wanes on closing eyes. Melancholic; complains of numerous sufferings. Lump in forehead. Vertigo from lifting head from pillow. Fits.

HEAD: Band-like feeling in the forehead. Head hot and sweaty. Trembling of head; while coughing. Vertigo, with dullness and confusion, alternating with drowsiness. Vertigo with sparking before the eyes. Head complaints > in open air, washing with cold water and motion. Head bent back.

EYES: Dim, swimming eyes. Collection of mucus in margins of lids (in pneumonia). One eye closed. Pustular eruptions on the conjunctiva. Flickering, sparks before the eyes. Eyes: staring look.

NOSE: Pointed. Nostrils dilated, *black*. Alae flapping.

FACE: Sickly, sunken. *Pale, bluish or twitching,* with cough. Covered with cold sweat. Incessant quivering of chin and lower jaw. Upper lip drawn up. Anxious, despairing. Pustules, leaving ugly blue-red scars.

MOUTH: Flow of saliva during pregnancy. Tongue thick, white, pasty; very red or red streaks; dry in the middle; papillae show through white coat. Mouth remains open after yawning. Taste bitter, flat. Tongue flaccid, dry. Imprints of teeth on border of the tongue.

THROAT: Much mucus in throat with short breathing. Swallowing painful or impossible.

STOMACH: Craves apples, fruits and *acids* which disagree. NAUSEA comes in waves, with weakness and cold sweat; *Loathing*, anxiety or fear, followed by headache, with yawning and lacrimation and vomiting. *Vomiting forcible,* then exhaustion and sleep. Violent retching. Sinking in stomach. Vomits with great effort. Thirst for cold water, little and often. Eructation like bad egg. Vomiting > lying on right side. Aversion to milk, to all kinds of nourishment. Thirstless.

ABDOMEN: Feels as if full of stones. Violent colic with drowsiness. *Diarrhea*, of eruptive diseases. Stools — mucous, grass green. Pain in the groins and creeping cold before menses. Palpitation during stools.

URINARY: Burning in urethra during and after urination. Last drop bloody, with pain in the bladder.

MALE: Pain in testicles after checked gonorrhea. Orchitis. Warts on glans penis.

FEMALE: Leukorrhea, of watery blood, < sitting. Puerperal convulsions, > after the child is born.

RESPIRATORY: *Unequal breathing; abdominal breathing*; SUFFOCATIVE SHORTNESS OF BREATH, before cough or alternating with cough. A leaflet seem to close the trachea. COARSE, LOOSE, RATTLING COUGH. CHEST SEEMS FULL, YET LESS AND LESS IS RAISED. Cough followed by vomiting or sleep, < anger. Must sit up to breathe or cough. Coughs and yawns alternately. Expectoration thick. Asphyxia neonatorum, child breathless and pale when born. Paralysis of lungs, with edema. Cough and dyspnea, > lying on right side, by eructations, < warm drinks. Capillary bronchitis; pleuropneumonia; Emphysema. Velvety feeling in chest. Child bends backwards, with cough.

HEART: Great precordial anxiety, with vomiting of mucus and bile. Palpitation with uncomfortable hot feeling. Paralytic depression of heart. Weak, quick pulse. Sensation of coldness in blood vessels. Palpitation with loose stool.

NECK & BACK: *Violent pain in sacro-lumbar region,* slightest effort to move may cause retching and cold clammy sweat, < lifting. Sensation as if a heavy load was hanging on end of coccyx, dragging downward all time. Vertebrae seem to rub against one another.

EXTREMITIES: Trembling of the hands. Fingertips icy cold or dead, numb, dry and hard. Restless arms. Feet go to sleep on sitting. *Dropsy* of the legs, of knee joint (left). Tension in hamstring when walking. Synovitis. Joints swollen. Jerking up of limbs during sleep, with loose stool.

SKIN: Pustular eruption leaving a bluish red mark. Thick eruptions like pocks. Sycosis barbae. Smallpox. Impetigo. Delayed or receding eruption. Blue eruptions.

SLEEP: GREAT DROWSINESS with all complaints, or from warmth. *Yawning* with many complaints. Shocks on dropping to sleep. Cries during sleep with fixed eyes and trembling. Lies on back with left hand pressed under head.

FEVER: COPIOUS COLD CLAMMY SWEAT. Coldness, trembling and chilliness. Burning sensation. Heat coming from heart. Coldness creeping before menses.

COMPLEMENTARY: Bar-c., Ip., Op.

RELATED: Aesc., Am-c., Ip., Lob., Op.

APIS MELLIFICA

GENERALITIES: The well-known effects of a bee-sting; *burning, stinging, smarting, prickling,* lancinating pain, with excessive swelling are the leading symptoms for the selection of this remedy. It acts on CELLULAR TISSUE, esp. of eyes, face, throat, ovaries, causing edema of skin and mucous membranes. In the SEROUS MEMBRANES of heart, brain, pleura etc. it produces inflammation with effusion. Various parts are swollen, PUFFED UP; become edematous and *of a shiny, red, rosy color.* The burning is like hot needles. There is great debility, as if he had worked hard; is compelled to lie down. *Symptoms develop rapidly. The pains are sudden* that extort cries. SUDDEN SHRILL CRIES in hydrocephalus and meningitis. Extreme sensitiveness to touch. General *bruised* SORENESS is marked, of brain, ABDOMEN, ovaries, bladder. Sensation of constriction. Sensation of stiffness and of something torn off in the interior part of the body. Great restlessness and fidgetiness. Trembling, jerking and twitching. One half of the body twitches, the other lame or paralyzed. Neuralgia of lips, tongue, gums. Great prostration even to faintness. Infections. Ill effects of grief, fright, rage, jealousy, hearing bad news, mental shock, suppressed eruption. *Right side* is affected more. Symptoms go from right to left. Numbness. Thrombosis. Lymphangitis. Inflammation of kidneys, bladder. Edema; of eyelids, lips; red, saccular. BURNING-*itching*. Paralysis after diphtheria and other severe diseases.

WORSE: HEAT of *room*, of weather, of fire; *hot drinks,* bath, bed. *Touch,* even of hair. Pressure. After sleep. Lying down. Suppressed eruption. 4 p.m.

BETTER: COOL AIR; cool bathing; uncovering. Slight expectoration. Motion. Sitting erect.

MIND: *Jealous,* with lewd talk. *Fussy* and fidgety; hard to please. *Awkward* — drops things and laughs either due to nervousness or absent-mindedness. Foolishly suspicious. Childish, silly behavior in women, after delivery. Irritable, excitable. Fruitless activity. Frivolous, cheerful. Constant whining in children. Great tearfulness, cannot help crying, weeps day and night without any cause. Sexual mania alternating with stupor (in women). *Indifference,* says nothing ails him.

Cannot concentrate mind on attempting to read and write (hysterical girls at puberty). Cannot bear to be left alone. Nothing seems to satisfy, everything seems to be wrong and out of place. Premonition of death. Borrows trouble about everything. Fear of being poisoned.

HEAD: Brain feels very tired. Vertigo, with sneezing, < lying or closing eyes. Sudden stabbing in head, or as of a blow, < occiput, with occasional SHARP SHRIEKS. Numb, tired headache, > pressure. Flow of tears, with headache. ROLLING OF THE HEAD from side to side in hydrocephalus; *boring of the head backward in pillow* in meningitis. Fontanelles sunken. *Painful hair.* Musty head sweat. Inability to hold the head in meningitis. Head feels swollen. Hair fall out; bald spots.

EYES: *Puffy*; lids or conjunctiva red; edematous, like waterbags, red. Hot lacrimation. Eyes brilliant. Burning, stinging, shooting pain. Staphyloma of cornea. Bag-like swelling under eyes. Photophobia, yet covering intolerable. Blindness, > stool. Squint. Myopia. Puffy or red about eyes. Cannot look fixedly at any object; or cannot read in artificial light. Cornea opaque. Styes — prevents their recurrence. Perforating corneal ulcer.

EARS: External ear red and inflamed. Raises the hands to the back of ear with each scream. Scarlatinal otitis.

NOSE: Swollen, red and edematous. Nose and tip cold. Boils in nostril, > cold. Coryza, with feeling of swelling in nose.

FACE: Expression happy, terror stricken or apathetic. Face red, hot, swollen and edematous with piercing pain; or *waxy pale* and edematous. Lips; bluish, oedematous; upper. Jaws stiff, with stiffness of tongue. Paralysis of right side, with right eye closed. Desire for washing face with cold water. Formication and prickling in face.

MOUTH: *Tongue* red or vesicles on edge; swollen, raw; feels, as if burnt, as if wooden; sore; stiff. *Grinding of the teeth.* Mouth glossy as if varnished. Tongue hangs out, or cannot be protruded. Sudden involuntary biting teeth together.

THROAT: Sandy, glossy or translucent, > cold; swollen inside and outside. Throat purple. Tonsils swollen, fiery red, stinging pain while swallowing, > cold drink. Angina. Diphtheria with early prostration, dirty membrane, edema of uvula. Throat sore, swallowing painful, < solid, sour or hot substances.

STOMACH: THIRSTLESS, with dropsy. Craving; for sour things, for milk, which >. Child nurses by day, refuses at night. Nausea. *Vomiting.* Soreness in the pit of stomach when touched. Neither eats nor drinks for weeks. Eructation tasting of ingesta, < drinking water; flow of water.

ABDOMEN: Feels *tight,* as if about to break, on straining at stool. Sore, bruised on pressure, when sneezing. Dropsy. Peritonitis. Diarrhea watery, yellow-orange, yellow or tomato sauce-like stool. Stools odorless, or offensive, involuntary, < motion. Anus; sore, swollen, profuse hemorrhage from, remains open, prolapsus ani. Electric shocks in rectum before urging to stool. Burning, pain and tenderness in epigastrium. Pain from below ribs going upwards. Burning or soreness below ribs.

URINARY: Burning urination. Dysuria with stinging pain. Urine; scanty, foul, high colored; last drops burn and smart; milky in hydrocephalus. Albuminuria. Urine profuse, more than he drinks. Coffee-ground sediment. Incontinence of urine, < night, coughing. Cannot urinate without a stool. Nephritis. Cystitis. Retention of urine in newborn. Difficult, frequent or slow urination, must press to pass urine, in prostatic affections.

MALE: Dropsy of the scrotum. Hydrocele, in multilocular cysts. Affections of prostate gland.

FEMALE: Amenorrhea of puberty. Ovaries numb, or congested, with suppressed menses. Ovarian cysts. Edema of labia. Burning, stinging pain in ovaries or uterus. Dysmenorrhea, with scanty discharge of slimy blood or with ovarian pain. Menorrhagia, with abortion. Leukorrhea profuse, acrid, green. Stinging burning pain in mammae. Tumor or open cancer of mammae. Abortion, during early months. Dropsy in later parts of pregnancy, with puerperal convulsions. Mania in women from sexual excesses or suppressed menses. Pain in ovaries, < coition. Menses last a day or appear at intervals of one day. Ulceration of navel in newborn.

HEART: Beats shake the whole body. Stitching backward from apex. Palpitation of heart from scanty secretion of urine. Pulse hard, small, intermittent, and quick, weak. Insufficiency of mitral valves. Organic heart disease.

RESPIRATORY: *Panting breathing, feels every breath would be his last.* Air hunger. Edema of larynx. Burning, stinging pain throughout entire front of the chest. Hydrothorax, after pleurisy. Chest feels beaten or bruised. Painful shock in head and chest from every cough. Asthma, from hives, > small quantity of expectoration. Larynx drawn in. Hoarseness. Expectoration sweetish.

NECK & BACK: Back of the neck stiff. Rheumatic pain in back. Burning, pressing in coccyx, < when sitting down. Back tired and bruised. Vascular goitre.

EXTREMITIES: Numbness of hands and tips of fingers. Palms hot. Edema of hands. Felon, in the beginning, with burning, stinging, throbbing pain. Limbs immovable, heavy, numb. Feet numb and stiff. Legs and feet waxy, pale, swollen, edematous. Trembling of hands and feet. Nails feel loose. Hemiplegia from severe mental shock. Staggers when eyes are shut.

SKIN: Rosy red, sensitive, sore. Rough eruptions or stinging spots on skin. Large urticaria. Skin dry, hot, alternating with gushes of sweat. Oedematous swelling. Erysipelas. Scarlatina. Carbuncle.

SLEEP: GREAT INCLINATION TO SLEEP; but cannot sleep from nervous restlessness. Drowsiness during fever. Screams during sleep and suddenly starts from sleep. Kicks off covers during sleep. Dreams full of care and toil.

FEVER: Chill, anticipating, with dyspnea, urticaria, desire to uncover; alternate with heat. BURNING HEAT, but chilly when moved. *Thirstless* during fever. *Heat of one part with coldness of another.* Sweat in gushes, partial. Sweat breaks out and dries frequently. Thirst during chill.

COMPLEMENTARY: Arn., Ars., Hell., Merc-cy., Nat-m., Puls.

RELATED: Ars., Canth., Graph., Iod., Lyc., Puls., Stram., Sulph., Urt-u.

APOCYNUM CANNABINUM

GENERALITIES: This remedy acts upon URINARY ORGANS producing diuresis and removing the dropsical effusion. Heart's action is depressed. *Digestion is disturbed.* It is a useful remedy for general dropsy, with or without organic disease. Swelling of every part of the body, with scanty urine and sweat, feels if he could only sweat he would get well. Dropsies are usually accompanied by digestive disturbances — nausea, vomiting, and great thirst; drowsiness and difficult breathing may accompany these symptoms. In acute hydrocephalus the child lies in stupor, with automatic motion of one arm and leg. Paralysis of left side; one eye motionless, other rolling. Weakness is marked. Dropsy after hemorrhage, quinine. Uterine hemorrhage. Scanty discharges.

WORSE: COLD weather; *cold drinks*. Uncovering. Lying. After sleep.

BETTER: Warmth.

MIND: Low-spirited, nervous and bewildered. Cannot think. Faints when raised from pillow.

HEAD: Dull ache. Hydrocephalus, with loss of vision and projecting forehead.

EYES: Hot and red; sensation of sand. One eye motionless and other rolling.

NOSE: Filled with thick yellow mucus in morning, Snuffles of infants. Takes cold easily.

FACE: Bloated, < lying down, passes off after sitting up. Face pale, covered with cold sweat, in diarrhea, Dry lips, mouth.

STOMACH: Nausea, with drowsiness. Thirst but water disagrees, vomits every drink or food at once (dropsy). Sensation of *sinking in the pit of stomach,* after profuse urination - diabetes insipidus. Uremic vomiting.

ABDOMEN: Ascites. Diarrhea, with dropsy, yellow, painless, noisy, gushing stool. Feeling as if anus is open and stool runs through.

URINARY: Retention of urine, with paralysis of lower limbs. Urine copious, *scanty.* Bed wetting in old men.

MALE: Penis and scrotum dropsical. Prostate gland enlarged.

FEMALE: Amenorrhoea of young girls, with bloating of abdomen and legs. Uterine hemorrhage, blood expelled in large clots or sometimes in fluid state, at climaxis. Ovarian tumor. Cough during pregnancy.

RESPIRATORY: Breathing short and unsatisfactory, difficult. Oppression of the chest. Short, dry cough. Sighing. Hydrothorax.

HEART: Pulse slow, fluttering, irregular or intermittent. Mitral and tricuspid regurgitation.

SKIN: Rough, *dry*. Cannot sweat.

SLEEP: Sleepy. Great restlessness with little sleep.

RELATED: Chinin-ar., Nux-v.

ARALIA RACEMOSA

GENERALITIES: This remedy affects respiration causing asthmatic condition with coughing, < lying down. Patient is weak, relaxed and exhausted. Biliousness. Mucus secretions acrid.

WORSE: After a short nap. Drafts. 11 p.m. (cough).

BETTER: Lying, with head high. Sitting up.

MIND: Fear of lung disease; cannot be shaken off.

NOSE: Sneezing, < least draft, with copious watery excoriating nasal discharge. Hay fever, with frequent sneezing.

MOUTH: Aphthae. Sensation of foreign body in throat. Nausea in throat.

ABDOMEN: Pain from liver to right scapula.

RESPIRATORY: Dyspnea or violent cough after first sleep, > slight expectoration. Raw, burning feeling behind the sternum. Salty expectoration; feels warm in mouth.

COMPLEMENTARY: Lob.

ARANEA DIADEMA

GENERALITIES: This spider poison is the remedy for the constitution susceptible to malarial poisoning. Patient feels cold to the very bones, cannot get warm enough. There is an abnormal susceptibility to damp and cold, Inability to live near fresh water, rivers, lakes, etc. or in damp chilly places. It affects the nerves, causing neuralgic pains which are violent and sudden and appear at the same hour every day, every other day, week, month or at regular period. SENSATION OF ENORMOUS ENLARGEMENT, or *numbness of parts,* < on waking or he wakes with such a feeling. It is a hemorrhagic remedy. It affects bone causing periostitis. Punctured wounds. Many symptoms appear on right side. Pains are like electric shock. Great desire to lie down. Creeping as of ants all over the body. EXACT PERIODICITY.

WORSE: *Cold.* DAMPNESS. *Cold bathing.* During rain.

BETTER: Tobacco smoking. In open air. Pressure. Summer.

MIND: Nervous. Despondent; longs for death.

HEAD: Ache, > smoking and going out in open air. Vertigo, with flickering before the eyes.

EYES: Heat and glittering before eyes; before headache.

FACE: Trigeminal neuralgia. Cheeks feel as if swollen during toothache.

MOUTH: Violent pain in all upper teeth at once on retiring. Taste bitter, > smoking.

STOMACH: Epigastrium painful to pressure. Cramps after eating a little.

ABDOMEN: Spleen enlarged. Colic occurring at the same hour. Pain > by rubbing.

FEMALE: Menses too early, too copious. Lumbo-abdominal neuralgia, with vomiting and yawning, during menstrual cycle.

RESPIRATORY: Hemoptysis, bright red. Inter-costal neuralgia extending to spine.

EXTREMITIES: Bones painful. Pain in *os calcis,* > continued motion. Numbness of parts supplied by ulnar nerve. Arms and legs feel numb. Bones cold as if made of ice. Ulcer on heel. Limbs feel heavy.

SLEEP: Restless. Waking with feeling as if hands and forearms were swollen and heavy.

FEVER: Chilliness, with pain in long bones, and feeling of a stone in abdomen. No sweat.

COMPLEMENTARY: Cedr.

ARGENTUM METALLICUM

GENERALITIES: Silver affects NERVES causing convulsive and spasmodic effects. It acts upon joints and their component elements — bones, condyles, *cartilages* and ligaments. Secretion of mucous membranes are THICK, *gray* or *tenacious*, or like boiled starch. It THICKENS the tissues, esp. cartilages, tarsi. LARYNX is also prominently affected. Symptoms appear insidiously; slowly, lingering but progressing, deeply penetrating. Pains gradually increase, become violent then suddenly cease, < by touch. Pains are accompanied by polyuria. Painless twitching or electric-like shock. *Loss of control over* MIND *and body.* Cramps in muscles; limbs *feel powerless.* In epilepsy the attacks are followed by delirious rage, jumping about and striking those near. Arthralgia. Bones painful, tender. It is adapted to tall, thin, irritable people. Exostosis of skull. Ill-effects of onanism and sunstroke. *Sore rawness.* Lies down on account of tiredness and weakness. Emaciation. Caries.

WORSE: *Using voice*—speaking, singing. *Mental strain.* Noon. Cold damp. 3 to 6 p.m. Touch, pressure. Riding in carriage. Lying on back. Sitting. Stooping. Entering warm room. Sun.

BETTER: Motion. Coffee. Wrapping up.

MIND: *Loss of mental power. Forgetful.* Hasty. Deceitful. Talkative, or disinclined to talk in society; changes subjects. Restless anxiety which drives him from place to place. Time passes slowly. Bars out all sympathy for friends. Takes on all sorts of whims, often does strange and unaccountable things. Anxiety about his health.

HEAD: Vertigo, whirling, < looking at running water, or entering warm room. Crawling and emptiness in head. Scalp very tender to touch.

EYES: Itching in eyelids and canthi. Abundant purulent discharge. Lacrimal stricture. Eyelids and tarsi become thick.

EARS: Itching of earlobes. Itching, has to scratch until it bleeds.

NOSE: Violent fluent coryza, with frequent sneezing, causing exhaustion. Nose-bleed, with tickling; < blowing nose.

FACE: *Pale, sallow*, with *weakness*. Red. Sudden heat, with palpitation.

THROAT: Feels raw and sore during expiration or when swallowing or coughing. Viscid, gray-jelly like mucus easily hawked up in the morning. Tension in throat, < yawning. Hawks. Fauces numb.

STOMACH: Burning in stomach, ascending to the chest. Anxiety and pressure in the pit of stomach. Appetite increased or repugnance to all food. Hiccough on smoking. Nausea in dreams.

ABDOMEN: Loud croaking, with hunger. Painful soreness of abdomen, < riding in a carriage. Vomiting during stool.

URINARY: Copious and frequent urination. In diabetes if there is swelling of the ankles. Urine, like whey, of sweet odor. Chronic urethritis.

MALE: Crushing pain in right testicle. Clothing increases pain when walking. Seminal emission without sexual excitement and erection. Yellowish green discharge.

FEMALE: Pain in left ovary. Ovaries feel too large. Prolapsus uteri, with pain in left ovary and small of the back, extending front and downwards. Eroded spongy cervix. Scirrhus of uterus. Climacteric hemorrhage. Leukorrhea, foul, bloody water, excoriating. Ovarian cysts, tumors. Palpitation during pregnancy.

RESPIRATORY: Hoarseness and aphonia, < using voice. Total loss of voice in professional singers. Larynx feels sore and raw. Cough, < laughing. *Easy expectoration of gray, gelatinous* or *starchy* mucus. Feeling of raw spot near suprasternal fossa. Great weakness in the chest (left), stitches in chest impeding breathing, while reading aloud or talking. Boil near the last rib. Neuralgic pain along the entire border of left lower rib.

HEART: Stops, then trembles, then throbs, > inspiration. Palpitation with cardiac unrest, > by lying on left side. Palpitation during pregnancy, > deep inhalation. Pulse intermittent and very irregular during palpitation.

NECK & BACK: Severe backache must walk bent. Icy cold feeling near sacrum.

EXTREMITIES: Upper limbs feel powerless. Legs weak and trembling, < descending stairs. Calves feel too short on going downstairs. Swelling of ankles (diabetes) Contraction of the fingers, with partial paralysis of the forearm. Writer's cramp. Limbs feel numb or stiff. Burning in corns.

SKIN: Nervous itching, crawling, tickling on various parts.

SLEEP: Electric shock on dropping to sleep. Nausea in dream.

FEVER: Hectic fever at noon. Sweat only on abdomen and chest.

RELATED: Calc., Puls., Selen., Sep., Stann., Zinc.

ARGENTUM NITRICUM

GENERALITIES: This drug affects the MIND causing neurotic effects. By its action on *Cerebro-Spinal nerves,* it produces incoordination, loss of control, and loss of balance, mentally and physically. Mucous membranes are inflamed and ulcerated causing muco-purulent discharge and SPLINTER-LIKE PAIN. It is a useful remedy for those persons *who are dried, withered up and prematurely old,* with *trembling* and weakness. Hysterical, nervous persons. Emaciation is progressive. *Ascending paralysis.* Parts seem ENLARGED or *bound up.* VIOLENT PAIN, LIKE DEEPLY STICKING SPLINTER; or *sharp, shooting like lightning, grinding* or radiating; cause starting; extending down back or legs. Pains increase and decrease gradually. *Ulceration,* with much bloody yellow pus. It is a convulsive remedy; attacks of epilepsy; from fright, < during menses, at night; pupils are always dilated for a day or two before the attack, and followed by restlessness and trembling of hands. Periodical trembling of the body. Loss of voluntary motion. Paraplegia. Sinking downward from head. Myelitis. Disseminated sclerosis of brain and cord. Sensation of a sudden pinch. Ill-effects of eating ice, onanism and venery. Tobacco. Symptoms appear on the left side. Conjoined mental and digestive symptoms. Unable to walk with closed eyes. Pains cause starting. Suitable for businessmen, students, brain workers. Examination funk. Desire to talk. Anemia. Errors of perception. Perversion of senses.

WORSE: EMOTION, ANXIETY, apprehension, fear or fright, suspense. *In room,* in shut place. Mental strain and worry. *Sugar. Lying on right side.* Looking down. Drinking. Crowd. Warmth in any form. Cold food, ice cream. Before and during menses. Riding. Thinking intently.

BETTER: COOL AIR, *open air.* Cold bath. Hard pressure. Motion. Eructations. Bending double.

MIND: Tormented by strange ideas and emotions. *Nervous, impulsive and hurried,* yet timid and anxious. Fearsome. *Dreads ordeal.* Fear of impending evil, of crowds, passing a certain point, of high building, of dark. *Hesitates. Falters in speech,* in gait, erection etc. Loss of ambition. Believes that he is despised by his family; that all his undertakings will fail. Despondent. Melancholy. Impulse to jump when crossing a bridge, or from a window. Brain fag. Loss of memory. Time passes slowly; time seems short, wants to do things in a hurry, must walk fast, etc. Weeps, says he is lost beyond hope. Everything seems changed. Irrational, does strange things and comes to strange conclusions; does foolish things. Incoherence. Childish talk. Talks about his sufferings. Remains in bed, with trifle indisposition.

HEAD: Nervous headache, with coldness and trembling, < mental exertion, dancing, > tight bandaging. Head as if in a vise. Compressive or deep head pain. Loses his senses. Boring in left frontal eminence. Migraine. Head feels much enlarged. Vertigo, before epilepsy, < night, with transient blindness, < closing eyes. Itching, crawling sensation on the scalp, as if skull bones were separated. Headache ends in vomiting. Headache of hysterical young women, of delicate literary persons.

EYES: Balls feel big. Violent purulent ophthalmia; ophthalmia neonatorum. Blepharitis, thick crusts on eyelids. Pupils dilated. *Caruncluae swollen;* photophobia. Ulceration of cornea. Chemosis. Acute granular conjunctivitis. Eye symptoms, < with abdominal symptoms. Opacity of cornea. Pterygium of pink color.

EARS: Buzzing in ears, with vertigo. Ringing with deafness.

NOSE: Loss of smell. Violent itching. Coryza with chilliness, lacrimation and headache. Violent itching, rubs it.

FACE: Sickly, sunken, grayish, of muddy color. Old man's look. Lips tremble while speaking. Lips blue.

MOUTH: Tip of the tongue is red and painful. Papillae erect and prominent. Tongue furred with clean edges. Aphthae on edges of the tongue. Astringent, sour or bitter-sour taste. Toothache, < chewing, cold things; sour things. Food escapes from mouth during chewing. Cannot talk, spasm of muscles of tongue and throat. Stammers.

THROAT: Thick tenacious mucus in the throat, causes hawking. Uvula and Fauces dark red. Sensation of a splinter lodged in the throat when swallowing, breathing or moving the neck, > cold drinks. Food lodges in pharynx. Smoker's catarrh, with sensation of a hair in throat. Strangulated feeling.

STOMACH: Craves sugar, which disagrees. Desire for cheese. Loss of appetite. Appetite good, but every kind of food disagrees. Astringent, sour or bitter-sour vomiting. Alcoholic gastritis. Vomited substance tinges the bedding black. Gastralgia; pain occurring in small spot, radiates in all directions, < slightest pressure. Painful swelling in the epigastrium. Ulceration of the stomach, < cold food. Eating > nausea but < stomach pain. Sour things > nausea. Eructates ingesta. Wind presses upward but the esophagus seems spasmodically closed. Trembling and throbbing in the stomach.

ABDOMEN: FLATULENCE, causing distention and *bursting* of abdomen. *Loud, explosive belchings* discharged upwards and downwards. *Diarrhea, emotional, noisy,* < immediately after eating and drinking, after sweets. Fluids go right through him. *Stools shreddy, mucous,* turning green like chopped spinach. Itching of anus. Shivering through bowels, extending up the back. Diarrhea; nervous, after sugar candy; of children, after weaning. Constipation, < every complaint, alternates with diarrhea.

URINARY: Violent pain from kidney to bladder (nephralgia), < touch, motion, deep inspiration. Incontinence of urine day and night. Urging to urinate, urine passes less easily and freely. Cutting in urethra, with painful erection. Divided stream. Yellow, bloody gonorrhea, early stage. Urine highly colored, dark red, with albumin. Retention of urine.

MALE: Impotence; erection fails when coition is attempted. Coition painful, urethra as if put on stretch or sensitive at orifice. Chancre-like ulcer, on the prepuce. Testes drawn up high.

FEMALE: Coition painful, followed by bleeding. Prolapsus, with ulceration of os or cervix uteri. Metrorrhagia, with nervous erethism at the change of life; also of young widows and childless women. Ovaries painful, with pain radiating to sacrum and thighs. Menses irregular, too soon, too late or last for a day only. Pain in stomach and spasmodic contraction in chest before menses. Menses scanty, with dyspnea. Infants die early after delivery. Leukorrhea profuse, with erosion of cervix.

RESPIRATORY: Chronic laryngitis of singers, raising voice causes cough, high notes cause cough. Rawness, soreness, high up in trachea, < coughing. Crowd, in room, take away his breath. Desire to take deep breath which < dyspnea. Dyspnea, nervous or flatulent, < gastric pain. Cough; < laughing, stooping, smoking, ascending stairs, before menses. Chest feels as if a bar were around it, as if weight of stone in middle of the sternum. Craves fresh air. Loss of voice. Pain in the chest putting on boots. Asthma, < in summer, in cold weather or taking cold.

HEART: Palpitation, with nausea, < lying on right side, riding in car; > pressing by hand. Unpleasant sensation of fullness about the heart, > fresh open air. Pulse, irregular intermittent. Anxiety, with palpitation and throbbing throughout the whole body.

NECK & BACK: Pain in the small of the back, < rising from sitting, Standing or walking. Glands of the neck indurated. Throbbing in spine or weak spine.

EXTREMITIES: Trembling of hands, cannot write. Numbness of finger-tips, ring and little fingers. Fingers half clenched, cannot be separated. Lassitude and weariness of forearm and legs, with trembling. Weakness, rigidity or twisting in calves. Paralysis, with mental and abdominal symptoms. Cannot walk with eyes closed. Walks and stands unsteadily, < when unobserved. As if a weight hanging from the coccyx. Chorea-like convulsions, legs drawn up, arms jerked outwards and upwards. Peripheral neuralgias. Oedema of legs. Legs feel as if made of wood or padded. Paraplegia, after debilitating causes.

SKIN: Brown, tense and hard. Ulcer angry, deep, with hard edges. Warty granulations. Adherent crusts.

SLEEP: Horrible dream of snakes and sexual gratification.

FEVER: Chilly when uncovered yet smothers when covered. Chilly with nausea.

COMPLEMENTARY: Calc., Nat-m., Puls., Sep.

RELATED: Lyc., Puls.

ARNICA MONTANA

GENERALITIES: It is a traumatic remedy par excellence. Trauma in all its varieties - mental or physical, and their effects recent or remote are met with in this remedy. It affects BLOOD, causing putrid and septic condition. BLOOD VESSELS are relaxed, causing ecchymosis, blue-black spots, with TENDENCY TO HEMORRHAGE, *epistaxis,* etc. It acts upon nerves causing neuralgia. *Muscles feel* VERY SORE, PAINFUL, BRUISED all over. Part becomes sore after the pain, or after bleeding. It is a prophylactic for pus formation. Burrowing pus. Has absorbent action. Progressive emaciation. Great prostration; tired feeling. Discharges are FOUL; *breath,* taste, flatus, stool etc. Crushing pain. BED FEELS HARD or full of lumps. Involuntary evacuation. Abscesses that do not mature. Pains are paralytic; sudden shifting pain from joint to joint. It acts best in plethoric, dark-haired persons of rigid muscles; nervous, sanguine nature. It acts but feebly on persons who are positively debilitated, with impoverished blood and soft flesh. Compound fracture. Twitching in tendons, muscles. Osteomyelitis. Ill-effects of fright, financial loss, anger, repentance; excessive use of any organ, vaginitis in females and impotence in males from excessive sexual indulgence, *exertion* of any kind. Mind and uterine symptoms alternate. Complaints when over hurried. Apoplexy. Typhoid, septic fever. Recurring boils. Surgical operations. Insect sting. Splinters. Thrombosis.

WORSE: INJURIES - *falls, blows,* BRUISES; *shock, jarring; after labor;* over-exertion; sprain. TOUCH. After sleep. Motion. Old age. Alcohol. Damp cold. Coal gas. Lying on left side.

BETTER: Lying down and lying with head low or out-stretched.

MIND: Fear: of being *struck or touched,* or approached; of sickness; of instant death; with cardiac distress at night; of space; on awakening; of crowds, public places. Morose, repentant mood. Mentally prostrate and apathetic, but *physically restless; says nothing ails him.* When spoken to, answers slowly with effort. Feels well in serious cases. Forgetful, what he reads quickly escapes his mind. After rage, sheds tears and makes exclamations. Hopeless; indifferent. Violent attacks of anguish. Angina pectoris. Delirium tremens. A sudden fear that rouses one from sleep at night, esp. after an accident. Great desire to scratch, will scratch, wall, bed, head, etc. *Coma.* Muttering delirium. Feels good for nothing. Easily frightened, unexpected trifles cause him to start. Sits as if in thought.

HEAD: Brain feels tired, burning. Vertigo: chronic, of the aged, with nausea, vomiting and diarrhea; objects whirl < walking. Vertigo, sitting erect, closing eyes. Headache as from a nail. Head hot with cold body. Cold spot on the forehead, hot spots on vertex. Meningitis from injury to head. Head thrown backwards while walking.

EYES: *Bloodshot.* Retinal hemorrhage. Photophobia. Feel tired and heavy, after sight-seeing, moving pictures. Tall objects appear to lean forward and about to fall. Right eye protrudes, looks larger than left.

EARS: Hardness of hearing; noises in ears. Blood from ears. Bruised pain in external ears. Hearing impaired from injury to the head. Sensitive to shrill noise.

NOSE: Bleeding: after every fit of coughing, after washing face. Violent sneezing from over-lifting. Nose, feels sore, cold. Post-nasal dropping. Catarrh of antrum. Burning in typhoid fever.

FACE: *Ruddy*, congested, bluish red in apoplexy, fever. Sunken, pale. Lips burn, are swollen and cracked. Lower lip trembles, while eating. Lower jaw hangs down, paralysis. Painful acne. Cheeks puffed; red.

MOUTH: Fetid breath. Dry, with much thirst. Taste as of bad egg, after operation - plugging etc. Bright red, puffy fauces. Tongue dry, almost black. Swallowing is prevented by a sort of nausea as if food would not go down.

STOMACH: *Eructation: tasting of bad egg*, after coughing. Loss of appetite by day, but canine hunger before midnight. Nausea. Vomiting of dark red coagulated blood. Feeling as if stomach were pressing against the spine. Fetid vomiting. Sensation of a lump at the back of stomach. Aversion to milk and meat. Longing for vinegar. Constant desire to drink, but all drinks seem offensive.

ABDOMEN: Cramps from epigastrium down over the bowels, then foul stool. Sharp pain from side to side. Stool bloody, foamy, purulent, acrid; involuntary during sleep. Dysentery, with dysuria, all through summer and autumn. Cramps in rectum while standing. Flatus smelling of rotten egg. Must lie down after every stool. Prolapsus ani, < after walking only for few minutes, > washing the whole body.

URINARY: Cutting pain in kidneys. Retention of urine in bladder, from over exertion, after labor. Involuntary dribbling, with constant urging. Has to wait for a long time for urine to pass. The bladder feels full and sore; the pressure of urine hurts him.

MALE: Impotence from excess or abuse. Phimosis, from friction. Seminal emission during caress. Hematocele.

FEMALE: After-pain, < suckling. Soreness of the parts after labor. Feeling as if fetus were lying crosswise. Cannot bear fetal movements, cause nausea and vomiting. Hemorrhage after coition. Nipples sore. Children lose their breath when angry. Mastitis. Threatened abortion from fall etc. Labor, weak and ceasing. Menses early, hot, profuse. Soreness of the whole body during pregnancy. Tumor of mammae from injury. Puerperal fever.

RESPIRATORY: Hoarseness, < exertion, cold or getting wet. Cough in sleep without waking. Cough produced by yawning, weeping or lamenting. Child cries before paroxysm of whooping cough. Cough causes bloodshot eyes or epistaxis. Cardiac cough. Dyspnea, with hemoptysis. Violent spasmodic cough, with facial herpes. Bones and cartilages of chest are painful, < motion, breathing or coughing. Heavy lower chest. Stitching pain in chest taking the breath away, > pressure. Hoarse voice from overuse.

HEART: Beats shake the whole body. Sudden pain as if the heart is squeezed or has got a shock, pain felt in left elbow (angina pectoris). Strain of heart from violent running. Cardiac dropsy. Hypertrophy of heart. Fatty heart. Heart pain, left to right. Pulse feeble and irregular. Weakened heart muscles. Horror of constant death, with cardiac distress at night. Palpitation after any exertion.

NECK & BACK: Muscles of neck weak, head falls backward, or any side. Back sore. Cervical vertebrae tender.

EXTREMITIES: Limbs ache as if beaten. Pain in arms, > hanging down. Want of strength in the hands on grasping. Cramps in the fingers - writer's cramp. Veins of hands distended. Cannot walk erect on account of bruised pain in pelvic region. Hygroma patellae. Gout. Knee joints suddenly bend when standing. Feet numb.

SKIN: Dusky, mottled. Every little hurt makes a black and blue spot. *Very sore acne or crops of small boils. Symmetrical eruptions.* Petechiae. Erysipelas. Bed sores. Tingling and itching which moves from place to place; after scratching, itching begins somewhere else. Carbuncle; of thigh.

SLEEP: *Comatose drowsiness*, drops to sleep as he answers. Dreams of death, mutilated bodies, anxious and terrible, awakes in terror, then sleepless. Severe fatigue causes restlessness and sleeplessness.

FEVER: Chilly with heat and redness of one cheek. Head or face hot, body cold. Coldness of part lain on. Thirst during chill. Must uncover but it chills him. Intermittent, typhoid, septic, traumatic fevers.

COMPLEMENTARY: Acon., Calc., Nat-s., Psor; Rhus-t; Sul-ac.

RELATED: Bell-p., Echi., Hyper., Rhus-t.

ARSENICUM ALBUM

GENERALITIS: A very deep-acting remedy, affecting every organ and tissue. MENTALLY the patient is extremely nervous, restless and anxious. Discharges of MUCOUS MEMBRANES are ACRID, THIN and SCANTY—coryza, saliva, sweat, etc. *Blood is disorganized* causing pernicious type of anemia and severe septic conditions. Hemorrhage, black, offensive. *Weakness, and emaciation is rapid.* Prostration seems to be out of proportion to his illness. *Pains are maddening;* BURNING LIKE FIRE, *hot needles or wires,* > heat. Pain is even felt during sleep, awakes the patient. Pain cause *shortness of breath* or chilliness. Pains alternating between head, stomach or body. It acts on the nerves producing inveterate neuralgia and multiple neuritis, > heat. Frequent fainting. Trembling, jerking, convulsions and choreic twitching. *Sudden intense effects;* SUDDEN GREAT WEAKNESS from trivial causes. VERY RESTLESS, restlessness even of affected part; even stupor is interrupted by fits of restlessness, with anxious moaning. Low vitality. Gradual loss of weight. PUTRID CADAVERIC ODORS. Emaciation. Paralysis. Destructive process - carbuncle, gangrene, cancer, malignancy. Dropsy; pale, puffy, baggy SWELLING. Spleen is enlarged in malarial fever, kala-azar. Child > when carried about quickly. Ill effects; of eating ice, poor diet, fruits esp. watery, tobacco, quinine, sea bathing and travelling, mountain climbing; care, grief, fright; ptomaine poisoning, dissecting wound. It is a prophylactic for Yellow fever. Acute and chronic burns. Epilepsy; suddenly becomes unconscious with convulsions, restlessness, then becomes drowsy.

WORSE: PERIODICALLY; MIDNIGHT; after midnight; *After* 2 a.m.; 14 days; yearly. COLD; Ice, DRINK; COLD FOOD; *Cold air; cold and damp.* VEGETABLES. Watery fruits. DRINKING LIQUIDS, ALCOHOLISM. Infection. Bad meat, food. Eruption undeveloped or suppressed. *Quinine.* Lying on affected part. EXERTION. Tobacco chewing. Sea shore.

BETTER: HOT; APPLICATION (dry); FOOD; *drinks*. Warm wraps. Motion. Walking about. LYING with head elevated. Sitting erect. Company. Sweating. Open air.

MIND: *Oversensitive.* Anxious. *Fastidious. Fault finding.* ANGUISH; *despair of recovery.* EXACTING. AGONISING FEAR OF DEATH, yet tired of living, < night. Fear of death from starvation, of financial loss. VIOLENCE, self-torture, pulls her hair, bites her nails, tears his own body. *Suicidal;*

impulses, mania. Restless, changes place continually, wants to go from one bed to another; children are capricious, want to be carried, want to go from father to mother to nurse. Melancholy. Sees vermin, throws away bugs by handful. *Suspicious.* Fear of being left alone, lest he do himself bodily harm. Fears he has murdered somebody. Miserly, malicious, selfish. Lacks courage. *Irritable increasingly.* Sensitive to disorder. Delirium tremens. Dotage. Fixed ideas, hallucination. Imagines house full of thieves, jumps and hides. Hasty. Sees ghosts day and night. Groans, moans and weeps during menses. Her desire exceeds her needs. Does not want to meet his acquaintances, thinks he has offended them.

HEAD: Ache, congestive, > cold. *Restless head,* it is in constant motion. Pain over left eye. Hemicrania, with icy feeling. Vertigo; with loss of consciousness, during coughing fits, in asthmatics, before epilepsy. Scalp very sensitive, cannot brush hair. Hair becomes gray early; falling of hair. Dandruff. Chronic eruptions filled with pus. Pain alternates between head or stomach or body, < by people's talks. Walks with head thrown backward.

EYES: Sunken or protruding. Burning in eyes, with acrid lacrimation. Edema around eyes. Intense photophobia. Lids granulated. Spasms of the eyelids. Everything appears green; sees as through a white gauze. Conjunctiva injected, yellow. Scrofulous ophthalmia. Eyelids red and ulcerated. Falling of lashes. Eyelids edematous.

EARS: Thin, offensive, excoriating discharge. Roaring in ears, during pain. Hard of hearing to human voice.

NOSE: *Thin, watery, excoriating discharge.* Nose feels stopped up, with fluent coryza. Nose colds descend to chest. *Cold sore,* in nose. *Sneezing,* without relief. Cannot bear the sight or smell of food. Hay fever. Knotty swelling of the nose. Nose-pointed. Acne of nose.

Epistaxis, after fit of passion or vomiting. Dyspnea felt in nose. *Sneezing, with biting watery coryza.*

FACE: PALE, *anxious, sunken*, haggard or *distorted*, hippocratic, covered with cold sweat. Old look in children. Edematous swelling of face. Burning, stinging pain as from red hot needles. Lips black, livid. Eruptions on lips. Cancer of lips. Black dots, acne.

MOUTH: Tongue dry, clean and red, *bluish* white. Edge of tongue red, takes imprint of the teeth. Burning pain in tongue. Tongue burning, trembling, stiff; coated white, yellowish, brown, black. Swelling about the root of the tongue. Neuralgia of teeth, feel long, > heat, < night. Swollen bleeding gums, painful to touch. Grinding of the teeth in sleep. Bites tumbler while drinking. Dryness of mouth. Aphthae in mouth. Fetor oris. Gulping up of burning water. Taste; bitter, to water; after eating and drinking; sour, foul, saltish, sweet in morning. Bloody saliva. Speech rapid. Lisping.

THROAT: Swollen, edematous, constricted, burning, unable to swallow. Everything swallowed seems to lodge in esophagus.

STOMACH: *Cannot bear the sight, smell or thought of food.* INTENSE, UNQUENCHABLE, BURNING THIRST; DRINKS LITTLE AND OFTEN; CRAVES ICE COLD WATER, WHICH DISTRESSES THE STOMACH AND IS VOMITED IMMEDIATELY. Loss of appetite; with thirst; with nausea. Nausea, retching and vomiting after eating and drinking. Anxiety felt in the pit of stomach. Burning pain in stomach > by sweet milk. Heart burn, gulping of burning water. *Vomiting and purging.* Hiccough; frequent; also when fever ought to have come; with eructations. Aversion to sweets, butter, fats; meat. Gastritis. Drinks LITTLE and OFTEN, eats seldom and much. Qualmishness. Desire for sour things, brandy, coffee, milk. Gastralgia, from slightest food or drink. Black vomit.

ABDOMEN: Induration and enlargement of spleen and liver. Violent pain in abdomen, with anguish. *Has no rest* anywhere, rolls about on floor and despairs of life. Epigastrium sore, tender. Stools; rice water, foul, small, involuntary, acrid, *burning,* black, mucous, lienteric, < cold drink, with much prostration. Ulcer above navel. Dysentery, cholera, in children. Anus; red and sore, *burning.* Acute prolapse of anus. Prolapse of piles, with burning, > hot applications. Itching and eczematous eruption around anus. Peritonitis. Ascites.

URINARY: Urine scanty, burning, involuntary. Feeling of weakness in abdomen after urination. Atony of bladder, in old persons. Uremia. Albuminuria. Diabetes. Retention of urine, as if the bladder were paralyzed, after parturition. Urine black as if mixed with dung. Dysuria.

MALE: Scrotum edematous. Emission during diarrheic stool. Erysipelatous inflammation of scrotum. Syphilitic ulcers, with burning, stitching.

FEMALE: Profuse acrid, yellowish, thick leukorrhea, < standing, passing flatus. Cancer of uterus. Burning in ovarian region. Pressive, stitching pain in ovary, goes into the thigh, which feels numb and lame, < motion or bending. Menorrhagia, with black blood. Burning in mammae, > motion. Increased sexual desire at menses. Menses suppressed in weak, tired careworn women. Stitching in rectum during menses. Dysmenorrhea, > heat.

RESPIRATORY: SHORTNESS OF BREATH, unable to lie down, must sit up, < odors, laughing, ascending, turning in bed or during receding eruption, > coffee or sweet water. Whistling, wheezing breathing. Asthma, < taking cold, in midsummer. Cough alternately dry and loose, dry at night, > sitting up, < drinking. Expectoration scanty, frothy. Great dyspnea, in nose; face cyanotic, covered with cold sweat, great anxiety. Aphonia. Emphysema.

Pulmonary edema. Burning or coldness in chest. Cough excited by smoking. Sensation of vapor of sulphur in larynx. Cough with bloody sputum. Hemoptysis with burning all over or with pain between scapulae in drunkards after suppressed menses. Gangrene of the lungs. Darting pain through upper third of the right lung. Yellowish spots on chest.

HEART: Weak, trembles. Palpitation with anguish, < lying on back, ascending stairs, slight causes. Heart pain goes into neck and occiput, with anxiety, difficult breathing, fainting spells. Angina pectoris. Pulse more rapid in the morning. Hydro-pericardium. Palpitation with tremulous weakness after stool. Beats audible. Visible pulsation.

NECK & BACK: Stiffness of the back ascends from coccyx to nape. Cold creeps on back. As if warm air streaming up spine to the head. Bruised pain in small of back. Weak lumbar region.

EXTREMITIES: Twitching, trembling, violent starting, during sleep. Drawing pain from elbow to axilla. Weariness of limbs. Trembling of hands, of limbs. Tingling in fingers. Fingers cannot be extended. Nails blue, discolored. Ulcer on fingertips, with burning pain. Feet weak, weary and numb; edematous. Ulcers on soles and toes. Wooden feeling in soles. Sore pain in ball of toes while walking. Uneasiness in lower limbs, must move feet constantly or walk about. Toes bend downwards. Peripheral neuritis. Cramps in calves. Swelling of feet. Limbs heavy. Restless feet. Sciatica, > walking and hot application. Paraplegia, with atrophy. Paralysis, with contraction of limbs.

SKIN: Dry, rough, scaly, dirty, shrivelled. *Looks seared.* Eczema. Acuminate eruptions. Free desquamation. Hives, < eating shell fish. Ulcer, chronic, with burning, with cutting pain and bloody discharge. Gangrene.

Phagedena. Carbuncle. Psoriasis. Skin like parchment. Skin symptoms alternate with internal affections. Spots; blue, black, white. Pimples, vesicles, burning violently.

SLEEP: Disturbed, anxious, *restless.* Shocks on dropping to sleep. Dreams of death, full of care, sorrow and fear. Sleeps with hands over head. Yawning, with stretching of limbs. Sleeping sickness. Talks in sleep. Awakened by pain.

FEVER: Externally COLD, with internal burning heat. COLDNESS in spots. Sensitive to cold, yet > in open air. Chill irregular, shaking; craves hot drink during chill; dyspnea during chill. Sensation of hot water in veins; or they burn like lines of fire. High fever, hectic fever. Sweat, with great thirst, dyspnoea or exhaustion. Sweat cold. Waves of icy coldness in blood vessels or intense boiling heat. Intermittent fever, yellow fever.

COMPLEMENTARY: All-s., Carb-v., Lach., Nat-s., Phos., Puls., Sulph., Thuj.

RELATED: Sul-ac., Verat.

ARSENICUM IODATUM

GENERALITIES: This remedy should be thought of when the discharges of MUCOUS MEMBRANES are persistently *acrid, profuse,* thick, gluey, yellow like honey, in chronic affections, and thin in acute conditions. Discharges cause BURNING of the part on which they flow. Its symptoms are very similar to the symptoms of an early stage of tuberculosis, with afternoon rise of temperature. In chronic inflammatory state of the lungs and bronchial tubes the expectoration is greenish-yellow, pus-like, with short breath. There is a profound prostration, emaciation, recurring fever and sweat, and tendency to diarrhea. It is a remedy for senile heart, and myocarditis and fatty degeneration of the heart. Heart weakened by chronic lung affection. Sensation of *heaviness* occurs in many parts. Axillary tumors. Erethistic weakness; debility.

WORSE: Dry, *cold weather.* Windy, foggy weather. Exertion. In room. Apples. Tobacco smoke.

BETTER: Open air.

MIND: Unable to study, study causes headache.

HEAD: Vertigo with tremulous feeling, esp. in aged. Dull, heavy headache across forehead or occiput. Study causes headache. Pain over the root of nose, driving her crazy.

EYES: Eye-balls feel heavy.

EAR: Foul otorrhoea. Tympanum thickened. Hypertrophy of eustachian tube; deafness.

NOSE: Drips water, which is *hot, green, acrid, reddens upper lip.* Persistent but unsatisfactory sneezing. Tingling in the nose and constant desire to sneeze. *Coryza* with dyspnea. Post-nasal catarrh. Hay fever. Influenza. Cold with hunger.

FACE: *Aching in malar bones.* Cancer of lips.

THROAT: Raw burning, tonsils swollen. Chronic follicular pharyngitis. Goiter.

STOMACH: Intense thirst, with desire for cold water which is ejected at once. Vomiting an hour after food. Uncomfortable nausea.

ABDOMEN: Diarrhea and dysentery; stools scalding, glass-white. Enlarged mesenteric glands. Painful swelling in right groin on extending leg.

FEMALE: Lump in mammae, < touch. Nipple retracted. Foul, bloody, yellow irritating leukorrhea, with swelling of labia. Emaciation of mammae.

RESPIRATORY: *Short of breath; air hunger.* Hacking cough. *Expectoration yellow-green, foul.* Asthma, in phthisis. *Pneumonia that fails to clear up.* Burning heat in chest. Tubercular pleurisy. Hoarseness. Aphonia.

HEART: Weak, irritable. Pulse rapid, irritable.

NECK & BACK: Burning heat in lumbar region, as if clothes were on fire.

EXTREMITIES: Pain in humerus, < writing. Clothes feel cold, > walking.

SKIN: Dry, harsh, dusky. Psoriasis. Icthyosis. Marked exfoliation of skin in large scales leaving a exudating surface beneath. Acne hard, shotty. Venereal bubo. Eczema of beard, < washing.

FEVER: Recurrent fever with sweat. Drenching night sweat, with weakness. Chilly, cannot endure cold.

COMPLEMENTARY: Kali-i.

RELATED: Kali-bi.

ARSENICUM SULPHURATUM FLAVUM

GENERALITIES: Leukoderma is supposed to be favorably influenced by this remedy. There is amelioration by steam or hot water.

ARTEMISIA VULGARIS

GENERALITIES: It has a prominent place in convulsive diseases of childhood and girls at puberty. The patient is irritable and excitable before the attack of epilepsy. Epilepsy; without aura, after fright or grief, after a blow on the head, with menstrual disturbance. Attacks are accompanied or followed by profuse offensive sweat of garlicky odor and seminal emission. Somnambulism. Gets up at night and works, but remembers nothing in the morning. Chorea, with inability to swallow. Right side convulsed, left paralyzed. Colored light produces dizziness. *Petit mal.* Walks in the street, suddenly stops, stares into space, often mumbles a few words, becomes normal and remembers nothing. Inclination to steal.

ARUM TRIPHYLLUM

GENERALITIES: It is an irritant poison causing excitability of mind and irritability of body. *Mucous membranes* of *mouth,* THROAT and *larynx* are affected prominently. DISCHARGES ARE ACRID, causing PAINFUL, SORE, RAWNESS AND BURNING OF PARTS. Rawness, with itching. Jerking, shooting pain. Children lose their appetite, do not want to play, lose flesh, have *headache.*

WORSE: Overuse of voice. TALKING, singing. Cold, wet, cold wind. Heat. Lying down.

MIND: Excessively cross and stubborn. Nervous. PERSISTENTLY BORES INTO NOSE, or *picks at lips,* fingers, at one spot, until it is sore or bleeds, esp. in children.

HEAD: Bores into pillow. Child puts hand on back of head and cries during headache. Headache, < warm clothes, and hot coffee.

EYES: *Acrid fluent coryza.* Nose obstructed, must breathe through the mouth. Obstruction, with fetid discharge, sneezing < at night.

FACE: Lips dry, swollen, burning, cracked; corner of the mouth sore.

MOUTH: Raw feeling at roof and palate. Mouth painfully raw, sore, inflamed. Aphthae. Saliva profuse, acrid. Tongue cracked and bleeding. Strawberry tongue.

THROAT: Raw, sore, *painful on clearing or coughing,* yet grasps and wants to scratch it. Swelling of glands on throat and neck.

ABDOMEN: Diarrhea. Stools like corn meal. Thin stool escaping from anus and leaving parts raw and burning.

URINARY: Very scanty secretion of urine. Uremia.

RESPIRATORY: Voice hoarse, squeaky or breaks. Clergyman's sore throat. Raw feeling in chest. Hay asthma.

SKIN: Itching of fingers and toes. Eruptions leave a brilliant red stain. Pemphigus. Impetigo contagiosa.

COMPLEMENTARY: Nit-ac.

RELATED: Ars., Merc-c.

ASAFOETIDA

GENERALITIES: Hysterical and hypochondriacal manifestations are covered by this remedy. Though the patient is of *full habit*, and *stout aspect yet he is intolerably nervous* and OVERSENSITIVE. In the digestive tract it produces flatulence and spasmodic contraction of stomach and esophagus, with reverse peristalsis, everything comes up, nothing goes down. It affects bones and periosteum; caries of bones and deep ulcerations are favourably influenced by it. *Fits of hard, violent throbbing.* Pains are pressive, sharp, stitching, *extending outwards,* associated with numbness; they change place and are > by touch. Aching, boring in bones. Easy relapse. Blueness. Foul, thin, acrid secretions. As if a nail or plug driven in. Twitching and jerking in muscles. Fistulae with foul pus. Glands all over the body throb and are hot. Pains jerk and shoot. Clumsy children. Obesity. Left-sided symptoms. Undulating, twitching of muscles. Ill-effects of checked skin eruption or suppressed discharges. Neuralgia of stump, after operation. Nervous disorder from suppressed skin eruptions.

WORSE: *Night*. In room. Rest. Eating. Suppression. Mercury. Noise. *Sitting*. Warm wraps.

BETTER: Motion in open air. Pressure; touch. Scratching.

MIND: Fickle, cannot persevere in anything. Wants now one thing, then another, walks hither and thither. Magnifies her symptoms, craves sympathy. Hysteria from suddenly suppressed discharges. Fainting during pain. Faints when he thinks that he has taken medicine. Faints almost without cause, in a closed room, from excitement or disturbance, after emission. Hysteria, with much trouble about throat or esophagus, clutches throat. Dissatisfied with oneself. Complains of her troubles. Changing mood; fit of joy with burst of laughter.

HEAD: Aches in occipital region, > stool.

EYES: Throbbing pain in and around the eye, < at night. Orbital neuralgia, > pressure and rest. Eyelids stick to balls. Numbness about eyes; ulceration of cornea. Syphilitic iritis.

EARS: Offensive purulent otorrhea, with hardness of hearing. Pain in mastoid with pushing out sensation.

NOSE: Offensive discharge from the nose. Ozena. Caries of nasal bones. Tension over nasal bones, with numbness.

FACE: Puffy, purple, as if heated. Small tubercles in the cheek. Swelling of the lower lip. Numbness of bones.

MOUTH: Greasy, rancid taste. Constant chewing, with frothy saliva from mouth; chorea.

THROAT: *Everything presses towards throat.* Globus hystericus — sensation of a ball rising in the throat. Spasm of gullet and stomach.

STOMACH: *Explosive eructations* smelling like garlic and rancid in taste. Regurgitation of liquids. Pulsation in the pit of stomach perceptible to the hand or even visible. Disgust for all food.

ABDOMEN: *Flatulence*, sudden, pushing upward, hysterical, wind colic with abdominal pulsations. Bowels seem knotted. Diarrhea, stools dark, watery, with disgusting odor. Only mucus is passed. Flatus passing upwards, none downwards. Heat in spleen and abdomen.

URINARY: Urine brown and of pungent odor. Spasm in bladder during and after urination.

MALE: Needle-like stitches in penis. Fainting after seminal emission.

FEMALE: Mammae turgid with milk when not pregnant. Deficient milk with over-sensitiveness. Bearing down in the genitals, esp. while riding in a carriage. Menses too early, too scanty, last for a short time. Leukorrhea profuse, greenish, thin offensive.

RESPIRATORY: Spasmodic tightness of chest, as if lungs could not be fully expanded. Asthmatic attacks at least once in a day, < bodily exertion, coition, satisfying meals. Spasm of the glottis, alternating with contraction of fingers and toes.

HEART: Palpitation more like a tremor. Heart seems full, distended. Reflex heart symptom of nervous origin.

EXTREMITIES: Pain and tenderness in tibia, intolerable, < night. Cannot work on account of backache. Cold swelling around ankles. Convulsive tremors > by holding.

SKIN: Eruptions of air vesicles. Bluish ulcer, with highly sensitive edges. Itching, > scratching. Old cicatrices turn purple and ulcerate. Foul burrowing pus.

COMPLEMENTARY: Caust; *Puls.*

RELATED: Aur; Chin; Lach; Merc; Sumb; Valer.

ASARUM EUROPAEUM

GENERALITIES: *Asarum* produces a remarkable state of OVERSENSITIVENESS OF NERVES; *scratching on silk or linen, rattle of paper are unbearable,* even the thought that someone might scratch with nails produces a disagreeable thrill through his body. Cold *shivers* from any emotion is also a marked symptom. Pressure, tension and *contractive sensation* are also leading features; patient thinks that his whole body or single parts were being pressed together. It is suitable to literary men of sedentary habit who shrink from cold or always feel cold. MUCOUS discharges are glairy. *Lightness as if floating.* Drunkards.

WORSE: PENETRATING NOISE. *Cold dry weather.* Emotion. Retching (except head).

BETTER: *Cold bathing;* of face. Damp, wet weather.

MIND: Gradual vanishing of thought. Stupid feeling in the head, > retching. Feeling of *lightness* as if floating when walking in the open air.

HEAD: Compressive headache. Tension of whole scalp; cannot bear combing.

EYES: Watering and burning of the eyes. Asthenopia. Darting pain in the eye, after operation.

EARS: *Painfully sensitive hearing.* Plugged up sensation, with coryza. Sensation as if skin were stretched over external ear (R).

NOSE: Coryza with sneezing.

FACE: Warm feeling in face, > cold washing.

MOUTH: Accumulation of cold watery saliva in the mouth, with nausea. Tobacco tastes bitter when smoking. Clean tongue. Disgusting taste.

STOMACH: Violent empty retching which < all the symptoms (except head). Violent vomiting, with diarrhea and violent colic. Desire for alcoholic drinks. Horrible feeling at epigastrium on waking in the morning: drunkards.

ABDOMEN: Strings of odorless, yellow mucus pass from bowels. Undigested stool. Dysentery, < after eating and drinking. Gelatinous or shreddy mucus in stool; mucous colitis.

FEMALE: Violent pain in small of back at the appearance of menses, scarcely permitting her to breathe, < motion. Tenacious yellow leukorrhea. Threatened abortion from excessive sensibility of nerves. Menses too early and long lasting, blood black.

RESPIRATORY: Nervous hacking cough. Asthmatic breathing, < odors and cold. Both lungs feel constricted by wire. Stitches in larynx, > cough.

EXTREMITIES: Lightness of all the limbs. Gurgling sensation in patella. Weakness, with staggering.

SLEEP: Frequent yawning; great drowsiness.

FEVER: Chilliness, single parts get icy cold. Cold feeling not > by covering or heat of room. Sweat sour, easily excited.

COMPLEMENTARY: Caust., Puls., Sil.

RELATED: Arg-n., Castm., Ther.

ASCLEPIAS TUBEROSA

GENERALITIES: It increases the SECRETIONS OF SKIN, *serous* and mucous membranes, causing *profuse perspiration* in *pleuro-pneumonia, diarrhea* or rheumatic conditions — colliquative states. It causes sharp, stitching, pricking pain, < motion. Excessive weakness, walking seems impossible. Numbness of the whole body. Influenza with pleurisy. Sensitive to tobacco. Weak and languid as if he had been sick a long time. Unfit for business from pain in bowels and frequent stools.

WORSE: Motion. Deep breathing. Lying. Tobacco. Rising. Coughing.

MIND: Memory weak.

HEAD: Ache, > after foot-bath.

NOSE: Sticky yellow nasal discharge. Snuffles of children.

MOUTH: Tough yellow coating on tongue. Taste putrid, of blood.

ABDOMEN: *Stools smell like rotten egg,* or *burn like fire.* Catarrhal dysentery, with rheumatic pain all over. Stool evacuted with a feeling as if a stream of fire were passing through abdomen.

MALE: Flabby genitals.

RESPIRATORY: Dry cough, with constriction of throat. Chest pain, > bending forward, < lying, breathing. Short of breath and weak on walking. Pleurodynia. Pericardial effusion. Pleurisy. Pain beneath left nipple, with palpitation.

RELATED: Ant-t.

ASTACUS FLUVIATILIS

(See Cancer Fluviatilis)

ASTERIAS RUBENS (RED STARFISH)

GENERALITIES: This remedy produces disturbance of the circulation, with *pulsations* and congestion in head, womb, chest, etc. *Nervous affections* include neuralgia, chorea, hysteria and epilepsy. It has a decided action on female organs. Epilepsy is preceded by twitching over whole body. Drawn back feeling in eyes, nipples, etc. Cancer of mammae. Flabby lymphatic constitution. Chorea, ceasing only when the hands are in the pockets. Left-sided symptoms.

WORSE: Heat. Menses. Contradiction. Cold wet weather. Coffee. Night.

MIND: Easily excited by any emotion, esp. contradiction. Epilepsy. Weeps from least emotion. Hallucinations, of hearing voices; being away; among strangers. Sense of impending misfortune. Fears bad news.

HEAD: Rush of blood to head, with throbbing. Head feels as if surrounded by hot air. Shock in brain.

EYES: Drawn backwards. Winking of eyelids.

FACE: Red, flushed face. Pimples on side of nose, chin and mouth. Acne.

ABDOMEN: Obstinate constipation. Diarrhea; watery, brown stool gushing out with force in jet.

MALE: Sexual desire increased.

FEMALE: Violent and constant sexual desire, not > by

coition, with nervous agitation, with disposition to weep. Left breast feels as if pulled inwards. Dull, aching neuralgia in mammae. Nodes and induration of mammary glands; nipples retracted; cancer, in ulcerative stage; acute lancinating pain; axillary glands swollen, hard, and knotted. Vagina moist with feeling of ease. Jerking or distress in uterus.

EXTREMITIES: Numbness of hand and fingers — left side. Pain from mammae extends over inner arm to end of little finger. Gait unsteady, muscles refuse to obey the will.

SKIN: Acne, black tipped puncta, small red base. Psoriasis. Herpes zoster.

RELATED: Murx., Sep.

AURUM METALLICUM

GENERALITIES: Gold makes a profound impression on the MIND, producing acute mental depression, hopelessness and loss of love of life. CIRCULATION IS DISTURBED; all the blood seems to rush from head to lower limbs. Orgasm, as if blood were boiling in all the veins. *Erratic ebullitions. Venous congestion* - more to head and chest. Caries of *bones,* esp. of nose, palatine and mastoid. Bone pains are boring and cutting. Pains wander, impelling motion, finally attack heart. Induration and glandular swelling. Exostosis, osteitis. Sclerosis of arteries—coronary, liver, brain. Extremely violent symptoms. Mercuric-syphilitic dyscrasia. Chronicity of complaints. Heart feels loose on walking. As if air blowing on part. It is adapted to nervous, hysterical women; girls at puberty; pining boys; old people with *heart disease;* persons who are low-spirited, lifeless, a weak memory; sensitive to pain, which drives them to despair. Ill- effects of grief, fright, anger, disappointed love, contradiction, reserved displeasure, prolonged anxiety, unusual responsibility, loss of property. Hopeless with heart disease, hopeful with lung disease. Cancerous ulcer. Necrosis. Dropsy.

WORSE: *Emotion.* Depressing affection. *Mental exertion. Cold,* weather. *Night* — sunset to sunrise. Mercury. Alcohol. Potassium iodide. Cloudy weather. Winter.

BETTER: Cool, open air. Cold *bathing.* Becoming warm. Music. Walking. Moonlight.

MIND: *Intense hopeless depression, and disgust of life.* Talks of committing suicide. *Suicidal anguish.* Peevish and vehement on least contradiction, or cheerful alternately. *Brooding* melancholy, alternating with irritability or moroseness. Feeling of condemnation and utter worthlessness. Weeping, praying and self reproaching from heart disease. Loquacity. Rapid questioning, without waiting for a reply. Fears the least noise. Weak memory. Vexed mood. Violent hysteria, with desperate action, thrashes oneself about, etc. Changing mood. She does everything wrong, thinks she has neglected something—her friends, her duty. Indisposed to talk. Hateful and quarrelsome. Future looks dark. Grumbling.

HEAD: Violent pain in head causing confusion. Headache of students, with precordial anxiety and flushes of heat to the head. Head hot, full. Exostosis with boring pain. Boils on scalp. Lump under scalp. Baldness from syphilis. Sensation as if air passed over the brain.

EYES: Photophobia. Hemiopia; upper half of object invisible. Orbits feel sore. Glaucoma. Pupil irregular. Yellow crescent bodies floating obliquely upward. Black spots, flames, sparks before the eyes. Everything looks blue.

EARS: Caries of the mastoid. Obstinate fetid otorrhea. Nerve deafness, with embarrassed speech. Oversensitive to noise, but > music.

NOSE: Ulcerated, painful, swollen — caries; fetid discharge, purulent, bloody. Red, knobby tip of nose. Ozena. Snubbed.

FACE: Congested, bluish-red. Parotids swollen, painful to touch. Pain in zygoma. Fine eruption on lips, face or forehead.

MOUTH: Offensive odor, in girls at puberty. Tongue leathery, hard. Milky or sweetish taste, foul even to water. Warts on tongue. Caries of teeth. Ulcers on palate. Gums swollen, dark red, bleeding.

THROAT: Stitches on swallowing. Caries of *palate*. Drinks come out through nose.

STOMACH: Burning in stomach, with hot risings. Desire for milk and coffee. Loss of appetite in pining boys. Thirst. Voracious appetite.

ABDOMEN: Liver region hot and painful. Hepatitis. Jaundice, of pregnancy. Liver problem with heart symptoms. Ascites, with heart affections. Constipation > during menses. Stools, knotty, hard, large. Warts around the anus. Rumbling. Inguinal hernia of children.

URINARY: Urine turbid like buttermilk. Painful paralytic retention.

MALE: Pain and swelling of testicles — orchitis. Atrophy of testicles in boys. Hydrocele, of children. Chronic induration of testicles. Sarcocele. Epididymitis.

FEMALE: Syphilitic sterility; also of those women who are mentally depressed on account of their barrenness. Uterus enlarged and prolapsed. Constant oozing from the vulva. Vaginismus. Labor pains make her desperate. Uterine troubles, < reaching high with arms. Induration and ulceration of the womb from repeated abortion. Leukorrhea, < walking. Amenorrhea with great sadness. Menses late, scanty.

RESPIRATORY: Crushing weight under sternum, < ascending. Dyspnea, < laughing, at night. Dry, nervous spasmodic cough, peculiar to women, from sunset to sunrise. Always takes a deep breath, cannot get enough air.

HEART: Sensation as if the heart heart stopped beating, immediately followed by hard re-bound. Oppression at the heart. *Violent palpitation,* at puberty. Cardiac hypertrophy. Angina pectoris. Aortic disease. Carotids and temporal arteries throb visibly. Pulse, rapid, feeble, irregular. High blood pressure. Heart feels loose on walking. Palpitation compels him to stop. Heart bruised, sore, < suppressed foot-sweat.

NECK & BACK: Swollen cervical glands, like knotted cord. Sensation as if lower spine bulged backwards. Lumbar muscles painfully stiff, thigh cannot be raised. Pott's disease.

EXTREMITIES: Nightly leg pains. Holds the left arm during attack of palpitation. Knees weak. Paralytic feeling in legs. Nails turn blue. Pain in both the knees as if tightly bandaged. Trembling feet. Hot bruised soles, at night. *Cold foul foot-sweat.*

SLEEP: Restless, with anxious, frightful dreams. Sobs aloud in sleep. Disturbed by sexual excitement.

SKIN: Lipoma. Warts. Acne.

FEVER: Painfully sensitive to cold, shivering in bed. Cold and damp all over. Sweat about genitals.

RELATED: Merc.

AURUM MURIATICUM

GENERALITIES: It is a sycotic remedy, causing suppressed discharges to reappear. Catarrhal and glandular affections are marked. Sclerotic and exudative degeneration of nervous system. Valuable in hemorrhage from the uterus at climacteric. Warts appear on various parts, on tongue, on genitals. Cancer of the tongue. Tongue as hard as leather. Desires company, if left alone thinks of nothing but of one's ailments and becomes more out of humor. Hypertrophy of all the fingers. Ill-effects of chagrin, fright, vexation.

WORSE: Ascending stairs. Warmth.

BETTER: Cold washing; cold weather.

AVENA SATIVA

GENERALITIES: *Avena sativa* (Common Oat) improves the nutrition of brain and nervous system. It is useful therefore in nervous exhaustion, sexual debility, debility after exhausting disease. Nervous tremors of the aged, paralysis agitans, chorea and epilepsy. Inability to keep the mind fixed on any one subject, especially when due to masturbation. Bad effects of morphine habit. Insomnia.

DOSE: Tincture 10 to 30 drops in hot water.

BACILLINUM

GENERALITIES: This nosode is prepared from tuberculous sputum. It is indicated in chronic catarrhal condition of the lungs when bronchorrhea and dyspnea are present. Constant disposition to take cold. Tubercular meningitis. Eczema of eyelids. Ringworm, pityriasis. Glands of the neck are enlarged and tender. Useful as an intercurrent remedy.

WORSE: Night and early morning. Cold air.

COMPLEMENTARY: Calc-p., Kali-c., Lach.

BADIAGA

GENERALITIES: *Badiaga* is the Russian name for the River Sponge. It makes the muscles and skin sore, < motion, and friction of the clothes. Glands are swollen. General paresis. Bubo; chancre. Carcinoma of breast. Infantile syphilis.

WORSE: Cold air. Stormy weather. Pressure. Touch.

BETTER: Heat; warm room.

MIND: After pleasurable emotions—palpitation.

HEAD: As if enlarged and full. Pain in forehead and temples extending to eyeballs. Scalp sore. Dandruff. Headache, with inflammation of eyes.

EYES: Neuralgia of eyeballs extending to temples. Twitching of eyelids (left).

EARS: Slight sounds are greatly accentuated.

NOSE: Coryza, sneezing, watery discharge, with asthmatic breathing and suffocative cough.

MOUTH: Hot. Much thirst. Breath hot.

THROAT: Tonsils inflamed, swollen, < swallowing solids.

STOMACH: Lancinating pain in pit of stomach extending to vertebrae, and scapula.

MALE: Syphilis of infants. Chancre. Bubo.

FEMALE: Carcinoma of mammae. Metrorrhagia, < night, with a feeling of enlargement of head.

RESPIRATORY: Cough, < after noon, > warm room; cough excited by sweets, candy, etc; EXPECTORATION *flies from mouth and nostrils.*

HEART: Tremulous palpitation. Heartbeats are felt from chest to neck < lying on right side. Discomfort, soreness, pain about the heart, stitches flying all over.

SKIN: Sore to touch. Freckles. Rhagades. Raised and discolored scars.

COMPLEMENTARY: Iod., Merc., Sulph.

BAPTISIA TINCTORIA

GENERALITIES: Wild Indigo of America is a reputed remedy for typhoid fever. It affects the BLOOD, causing septic conditions, low fever and malaria poisoning. Feeling of SORENESS, HEAVINESS, and ACHING OF MUSCLES is very marked. PROSTRATION IS RAPID; *bed feels too hard* on account of soreness of muscles, yet *he feels too weak to move. Mucous membranes become dark.* Discharges, stools, hemorrhage etc. are dark in color. Dark spots appear upon the body. FOUL odor of the body, breath, EXCRETIONS, stool, sweat, urine, etc. *Brown;* sordes, stools, menses. Bedsore. Influenza. Chronic intestinal toxaemia of children, with fetid stool and eructations. Lifeless body but restless mind. Insensitive to pain. Parts feel numb or too large. Restless, always rubs the hands, hysterical. In low potency it increases the resistant power of the body against typhoid. Ill- effects of anti-typhoid serum injection.

WORSE: *Humid heat.* Fog. In room. Pressure. On waking. Walking. Open air. Cold wind. Autumn. Hot weather.

MIND: Sense of DUALITY. Aversion to mental and bodily exertion. Thinks he is broken or double. PARTS FEEL SEPARATED or *scattered*. Tosses about in bed trying to get pieces together. Hopeless of recovery, and certain of death. *Dull and confused*. Falls asleep while answering or does not complete his sentence. Wandering, muttering delirium. Perfect indifference. Bewildered. Imagines his limbs are talking to each other.

HEAD: Feels too large, heavy, numb. Pain as from a blow, or heavy pain in occiput. Vertigo, with weak feeling esp. of lower limbs and knees. Vertex feels as if would fly off. Brain feels sore.

EYES: Eyelids heavy. Eyes feel swollen. Half closed.

EARS: Early deafness in typhoid-like conditions.

NOSE: Pain at the root. Epistaxis of dark blood. Illusion of smell of burnt feathers.

FACE: Dusky, SODDEN, BESOTTED, stupid. Muscles of the jaw rigid. Cracked, bleeding lips.

MOUTH: *Brown strip* down centre of the tongue. Tongue feels burnt. Breath fetid. Thick speech. Ulcer in the mouth. Taste flat, bitter. *Dark, red, tumid* (swollen) mouth. Tongue cracked, bleeds, feels thick or is heavily coated. Lower jaw drops. Saliva viscid. Sore mouth of suckling children. Tonsils and soft palate swollen.

THROAT: *Dark, red, tumid.* Numb inside but sensitive outside. Can swallow liquids only, least solid food gags. Constriction of esophagus at cardiac orifice. Ragged ulcer in the throat. Spasm of gullet.

STOMACH: Sinking feeling at stomach. Easy vomiting. Pain in epigastric region. Feeling of a hard substance. Sudden attack of vomiting and diarrhea, with fever. Gastric fever. All symptoms are < by beer.

ABDOMEN: Right iliac region sensitive. Soreness of the gall bladder, with diarrhea. *Diarrhea* — sudden, horribly foul, mushy, painless, dark, slaty or bloody stools. Dysentery — of the old people, with pain in limbs, small of back and rigor. Painless dysentery, with fever. Intestinal toxemia of children, with fetid stools and eructations. Stricture from piles.

URINARY: Urine scanty, dark red, alkaline, fetid, light green. Uremia.

MALE: Orchitis. Pressing pain in testes as if squeezed.

FEMALE: Threatened abortion, from mental shock, depression, low fever. Menses; too early, too profuse. Lochia acrid, foul. Puerperal fever. Stomatitis of nursing mothers.

RESPIRATORY: Breathing difficult from weakness of chest, < on waking, > standing. *Craves air.* Bronchial asthma. Lungs feel tight and compressed. Afraid to go to sleep on account of suffocation and nightmares.

HEART: Pulse first accelerated, then slow and faint.

NECK & BACK: Neck tired, cannot hold it easy in any position. Pain in sacrum around hips and legs. Back sore and bruised. Bed sores. Feels as if lying on a board. Symptoms radiate from small of back.

EXTREMITIES: Stiffness and pain, aching and drawing in arms and legs.

SLEEP: *Drowsy, stupid* and *languid;* slides down in bed. Nightmare, and frightful dreams. Lies curled up like a dog on one side.

SKIN: Livid spot all over the body and limbs.

FEVER: Hyperpyrexia. Adynamic fever, typhoid, shipboard fever. Sweat relieves. Gastric influenza.

RELATED: Arn., Gels., Hyos., Lach., Mur-ac., *Op.,* Rhus-t.

BARYTA CARBONICA

GENERALITIES: It has a marked influence on GROWTH, esp. of children and old people who become childish. In children the growth is retarded, they become *dwarfish* mentally and physically; children are late coming into usefulness, to take on their responsibilities and do their work. *Dull, apathetic,* or marasmic. There is a tendency to enlargement of the glands, with induration, esp. of tonsils, cervical and prostate. Prostration, weariness; constant inclination to lie down, sit or lean on something. Upper half of the body feels stiff and numb. Too tired even to eat. It is a remedy for early *senility* and when degenerative changes in old men begin in heart, brain and vascular system. *Tendency to take cold* and everytime tonsils are swollen. *Paralytic effects.* Symptoms occur in single parts, such as paralysis, numbness, burning. Sensation *as if forced through a narrow place* is peculiar. *Vascular softening and dilatation,* aneurism, rupture, apoplexy. Ill-effects of checked foot-sweat. Cyst. Sarcoma, with burning. Lipoma. Emaciation of persons who were well nourished. Sleepiness and weariness on slightest exertion.

WORSE: *Company.* Thinking of symptoms. *Cold damp.* Cold to feet and head. *Lying on painful part,* left side. Odors. Heat of sun, of stove. Raising arms. Eating.

BETTER: Cold food. Warm wraps. When alone.

MIND: SLOW GRASP; SILLY; *absurd and backward.* Childish and thoughtless behaviour. Timid. *Cowardly.* Groans from every little thing. Whining mood. Increasing *mental weakness. Beclouded mind. Bad memory.* Forgets her errand or word in her mouth. Irresolute. *Mistrust ful. Shy of strangers.* Thinks his legs are cut off and he is walking on his knees. Child does not want to play but sits in the corner doing nothing. Children cannot remember and learn. Grief over trifles. Thinks one is being laughed at and made fun of. Hides behind the furniture and keeps the hands over the face, peeping through the fingers. Always borrows trouble. Loss of self- confidence. Talking mania; during menses, in young girls. Idiocy.

HEAD: Vertigo, of old people, with nausea, < stooping, when lifting arms up. Brain feels loose, > cold air. Baldness of vertex. Wen on scalp. Heavy pressure over eyes. Dry eruptions or moist crusts on the scalp. Stitching pain when standing in sun.

EYES: Pupils dilate and contract quickly. Pressure deep in eyes, > looking downward. Light dazzles. Opaque cornea. Lids granular, thickened. Fiery sparks before eyes, in dark.

EARS: Crackling noises, < swallowing, walking. Glands around ear painful and swollen. Eruptions on lobes of ears. Hardness of hearing. Sound on sneezing.

NOSE: Dry, < blowing it. Coryza, with swelling of upper lip and nose (children with large abdomen). Sensation of smoke in nose. Discharge of thick yellow mucus, scabs around wings of nose. Epistaxis.

FACE: Pale, puffed; sensation of a cobweb. Upper lip swollen. Lips pendulous.

MOUTH: Tongue weak, paralyzed, hard in old people, cannot speak. Burning soreness or vesicles on tip or under the tongue. Toothache, < before menses. Mouth feels numb. Whole mouth filled with vesicles, esp. inside the cheek. Saliva runs out, while asleep. Fetor oris, unnoticed by himself. Frequent and considerable bleeding from gums.

THROAT: *Tonsils are affected by every cold,* or < during menses. *Chronic quinsy. Enlarged tonsils.* Spasms of oesophagus, as soon as food enters esophagus, causing gagging and choking. Pain in throat, < empty swallowing. Can swallow liquids only. Waterbrash, sudden. Submaxillary gland swollen. Much burning in throat. Throat trouble from overuse of voice.

STOMACH: Sore spot in stomach. Hungry but refuses food. Aversion to sweet things, fruits, esp. plums. Sudden disgust while eating. Dyspepsia of young masturbators or with seminal emission. Pain while fasting and after eating. Weak digestion of old people with possible malignancy, > cold food.

ABDOMEN: Hard and tense, tender, distended, with emaciation of body. Diarrhea with lumbar ache. Sensation as if intestines fell from one side to other on turning in bed. Stools hard, knotty. Piles protrude, while urinating. Crawling in the rectum. Oozing at anus. Habitual colic of children who do not thrive, and though apparently hungry refuse food. Mesenteric glands hard and swollen.

URINARY: Urging to urinate, cannot retain the urine. Burning in urethra, while urinating. Frequent urination. Urine dark brown, scanty.

MALE: Genitals flabby. Enlarged prostate gland. Testicles indurated. Impotency. Premature emission. Erection when riding. Falling asleep during coition. Genitals feel numb. Painful nodes in mammae in old fat men.

FEMALE: Menses scanty, last only one day. Before menses pain in stomach and lumbar back. Genitals feel numb. Dwindling of ovary and mammary gland. Amenorrhea. Leukorrhea immediately before menses.

RESPIRATORY: Paralytic aphonia. Asthma of old people, < wet, warm air. Larynx feels as if smoke were inhaled. Lungs feel full of smoke. Cough, < in the presence of strangers, eating warm food. Chronic bronchitis. Dry suffocative cough in old people, full of mucus but lacking strength to expectorate.

HEART: Cardiac symptoms after suppressed foot sweat or after masturbation. Heart feels bruised, sore. Palpitation and distress in region of heart lying on left side. Palpitation felt in head. Aneurism. Pulse slow, small. High blood pressure. Arteriosclerosis.

NECK & BACK: Glands swollen in nape and occiput. Chronic torticollis. Spine weak. Pulsation in back; after mental emotion. Fatty tumors upon the neck.

EXTREMITIES: Fingers numb. Limbs feel numb. Trembling of feet, and of hands while writing. Soles feel hot or bruised at night, during sleep. Numbness from knees to scrotum, > when sitting. *Cold, foul foot sweat.* Pain in deltoid, < raising arm. Pain in the knees, while kneeling.

SKIN: Warts. Acne. Lipoma. Cyst. Burning sarcoma.

SLEEP: Talks in sleep (old man). Awakes frequently; feels hot. Twitching during sleep.

FEVER: Flushes of heat, more at night. Sweat on single parts—one hand, one foot, one side of body, face; stinking; of feet, < in presence of stranger.

COMPLEMENTARY: Ant-t; Dulc; Psor; Sil.

RELATED: Kali-p; Lyc; Med; Puls; Sep; Sil; Tub.

BARYTA IODATA

GENERALITIES: This remedy is used clinically for enlarged and indurated glands, esp. tonsils and breasts. Leukocytosis.

WORSE: Walking.

BETTER: Cold open air.

BARYTA MURIATICA

GENERALITIES: Like *Bar-c.*, this salt is also useful in old age and childhood, when mental and physical dwarfishness is present. It causes vascular degeneration causing hypertension when high systolic pressure with comparatively low diastolic tension is present, with cerebral and cardiac symptoms. It is a convulsive remedy. Convulsive attacks occur periodically, with starting and excessive tossing about. Electric shocks with convulsions. Mania in every form when sexual desire is increased. Enlargement of the glands and induration—tonsils, pancreas. Multiple sclerosis of brain and cord. Icy coldness of the body, with paralysis. Voluntary muscular power gone, but perfectly sensible. Children who go around with their mouth open and who talk through the nose. Great weakness, wants to lie down. Leukocytosis. Child lies on the abdomen all the time, to shun the light. Stupid appearance. Hard of hearing.

MIND: Idiocy. Sexual mania.

HEAD: Vertigo due to cerebral anemia and noises in the ears. Heaviness of head (old people).

EARS: Noise on chewing and swallowing, sneezing. Earache, > sipping cold water. Offensive otorrhea.

NOSE: Sneezing in sleep; without waking.

THROAT: Uvula elongated. Tonsils enlarged. Feels too wide open. Swallowing difficult. Spasm of gullet at the cardiac end, pain immediately after eating, with tenesmus in epigastrium.

STOMACH: Gone feeling in epigastrium. Sensation of heat ascending to head.

ABDOMEN: Distressing throbbing in abdomen, aneurism. Induration of pancreas.

URINARY: Great increase in uric acid.

FEMALE: Nymphomania. Tumor, or atrophy of ovaries. Sterility.

RESPIRATORY: Bronchial affections of old people, with cardiac dilatation; expectoration becomes easy.

EXTREMITIES: Toes cramped, better drawing up the limbs. Fatigue of legs as from long walk, with stiffness of joints.

BELLADONNA

GENERALITIES: Belladonna acts upon *nerve centres* producing twitching, convulsion and pain. Its action upon the *brain* causes furious excitement and perversion of special senses. Circulation in blood vessels and capillaries becomes active causing congestion, throbbing, and dilatation of arteries. Mucous membranes become dry. Its effects are *sudden and violent.* BURNING HEAT, BRIGHT REDNESS and DRYNESS are very marked. HOT body, part, discharges, etc. Redness occurs in streaks. SEVERE NEURALGIC PAIN, that comes and goes suddenly. FULLNESS; CONGESTION, esp. to head and SWELLING are other characteristic features. PAINS ARE THROBBING, SHARP, CUTTING, SHOOTING, or *clawing,* of maddening severity; *coming and going in repeated attacks. Discharges are hot and scanty.* SPASMS, SHOCKS, JERKS and TWITCHINGS. CONSTRICTION occurs in parts of the body like throat, vagina, etc. or in whole body. Sensitive *to Light, Noise, Jarring.* Epileptic attacks are followed by nausea and vomiting. Convulsion commences in the arm. Spasms are followed by prolonged unconsciousness. Throws body forward and backward; chorea. Acts as a prophylactic in scarlet fever. Exophthalmic goiter, with extreme thyroid toxemia. Hydrophobia. Useful in airsickness. Its influence is felt more in intelligent and plethoric persons who are jovial and entertaining when well, but violent when sick, therefore, a great children's remedy. Ill effects of hair cutting, head getting wet, sausages, sun, walking in wind or draft. Hemorrhage, hot. Heat in body; parts are hot, swollen, and dry. *Right sided symptoms.*

WORSE: Heat of Sun, if heated. DRAFTS *on head;* haircut; washing head. After taking cold. Light; noise; jarring. CHECKED SWEAT. *Touch.* Company. Pressure. *Motion. Hanging down affected part.* Afternoon. Lying down. Looking at shining object or running water.

BETTER: Light covering. *Bending backward,* semi-erect position. Rest in bed. Standing. Leaning head against something. Bending or turning the affected part.

MIND: Acuteness of senses. WILDLY DELIRIOUS. *Excited, ferocious, noisy, cries out.* Talks fast. VERY RESTLESS. Biting, striking, tearing mania. Spits on face of other persons. Sees monsters, hideous faces. Fear of imaginary things. Desire to escape or hide himself. Perversity, with tears (children). Excitable, easily weeps. Quarrelsome. Tendency to dance, laugh, sing, whistle. Starts in fright at the approach of others. Constant moaning. Craving for snuff. An angel when well and a devil when sick. Sits and breaks pins. Mental symptoms > taking light food. Patient lives in his own world.

HEAD: THROBBING, HAMMERING HEADACHE, < *temples;* < motion, > letting hair down, laying the hand on head, bending head backward. Feeling in the brain like swashing of water. It rises and falls in waves. Cold sensation at the middle of the forehead. Vertigo, < stooping and rising from stooping. Hydrocephalus, with boring head in the pillow. Hair split, get dry and come out. *Rolls head.* Pulls her hair. Meningitis. Sunstroke. Pains go downward from head. *Head sensitive to drafts and cold, or washing hair.*

EYES: PUPILS DILATED. Eyes *sparkling, prominent, staring. Red conjunctiva.* Fiery, red, vivid hallucination, even on closing the eyes. *Attacks of blindness,* then yellow vision. Sees red flashes in vision. Photophobia. Diplopia. Triplopia. Moonlight blindness. Sensation as if eyes were half closed. Eyelids feel sore, congested and swollen. Exophthalmus. Lacrimation like brine. Lines appear crooked when reading.

EARS: Pain causes delirium; child cries out in sleep. Otitis media. Autophony - hearing one's own voice in the ear. Hematoma. Noise in ears.

NOSE: Red; swollen. Imaginary odors, odor of tobacco intolerable. Bleeding from nose, with flushed face.

FACE: Fiery, RED, *turgid* and *hot;* or becomes pale and red alternately. Semilateral swelling of the face. Spasmodic distortion of mouth (risus sardonicus). Convulsive motion of muscles of face. Facial neuralgia, with twitching of muscles and flushed face. Lower jaw felt as if drawn backwards.

MOUTH: Dry Hot. Tongue red, hot, swollen. Edges of tongue red. Strawberry tongue. Red streak in middle of tongue, wider at tip. Grinding of the teeth. Tongue hangs out of the mouth (children). Forepart of the tongue cold and dry. Toothache, > biting. Chewing motion of the mouth. Stammering speech. Lock-jaw. Hot breath.

THROAT: DRY and HOT. Tonsils enlarged. *Tonsillitis,* < right side. Urging to swallow, with choking. Throat feels constricted. Swallowing difficult; Drinks in sips. Must take a drink to swallow solid food. When swallowing, bends the head forward and lifts up knees. Clutches at throat, during epilepsy.

STOMACH: Desire for lemonade or lemons (which agree). Distaste for meat, acid, coffee, milk, beer. Vomits everything, with paleness and weakness. Great thirst for cold water. Dread of drinking. Spasmodic hiccough, with sweat and convulsion. Pain in stomach extending to shoulder and throat, < pressure.

ABDOMEN: Distended, hot < touch of bedclothes. Cutting pain in epigastrium, > bending backwards. Transverse colon distends and protrudes, like a pad, during abdominal colic. Cramp and colic, as if a hand has clutched some part. Acute pain in liver region, extending to shoulder and neck, < lying on it. Clawing pain around the navel. Downward forcing in abdomen as if all the viscera would protrude through genitals. Acute prolapsus ani. Stools green, dysenteric or contain chalky lumps. Involuntary stool. Piles with back pain as if breaking. Pain in splenic region, < sneezing, coughing, touch.

URINARY: Involuntary urination, on lying down when standing, when sleepy. Retention of urine, with paralysis of bladder; post partum. Fiery red urine; frequent and profuse urination. *Hematuria without pathological condition.* Sensation in bladder as if a worm were turning in, without desire to micturate.

MALE: Testicles hard, drawn up, inflamed. Sweat on genitals. Soft painless tumor on glans.

FEMALE: Menses bright, red, with clots, too early, too profuse, hot, gushing, offensive. Metritis. Rigidity of the os. Violent bearing down towards genitals, as if everything would fall out, > standing and sitting erect, < lying down. Mastitis; pain throbbing, redness, streaks radiate from the nipples. Breast; heavy, hard and red. Lochia diminished, hot, offensive. Useful in confinement of women who have children late in life. Leukorrhea, with colic. Labor pains come and go suddenly, or cease.

RESPIRATORY: Tickling, short, dry cough, < night. Larynx very painful, feels as if foreign body were in it, with cough. Cough, < fine dust in air. Child cries before cough. Cough, < yawning. High piping voice. Barking cough or voice. Whooping cough, with pain in stomach before attack, with hemoptysis. Cheyne-stokes respiration. Moaning at every breath. Difficult, short, quick respiration. Asthma in hot damp weather.

HEART: Throbbing in carotid and temporal arteries. Pulse full, hard, tense. Violent palpitation, with labored breathing. Bubbling at the region of the heart.

NECK & BACK: Stiff neck and shoulder (right). Swelling of glands in the nape of the neck. Back feels broken. Lumbago, with pain in hips and thighs.

EXTREMITIES: Jerks or spasms in limbs. Joints swollen, red, shining, with red streaks radiating. Heaviness and paralytic feeling in limbs. *Cold extremities.* Involuntary limping. Phlegmasia alba dolens. Trembling of limbs. Weakness and tottering gait. Lies or sits with feet crossed, cannot uncross them.

SKIN: BRIGHT, RED, *glossy*. Dry and hot. Alternate paleness and redness of skin. Intense dermatitis. Scarlatina. Erysipelas. Boils, returning every spring.

SLEEP: *Sleepy but cannot sleep.* Moans and tosses about in sleep. JERKS DURING SLEEP. Frightful dreams of quarrel, fire, robber, assassin. Sees frightful visions on closing eyes. Sleeps with hands under the head. Heavy sleep with hot skin.

FEVER: High fever with comparative absence of toxemia. Internal coldness, with external *pungent, burning, steam-*

ing heat. HOT HEAD *with cold limbs.* Skin hot but moist and dry alternately No thirst with fever.

COMPLEMENTARY: Borx., Calc., Hep., Merc., Nat-m.

RELATED: Glon., Hyos., Stram.

BELLIS PERENNIS

GENERALITIES: Bellis is known commonly as wound wort, therefore, like *Arnica* it is a great traumatic remedy. It is especially useful in *deep trauma* or septic wounds of abdominal and pelvic organs; after major surgical operation. It removes the ill effects of auto-traumatism — excess of masturbation. It affects BLOOD VESSELS causing venous stasis, and varicose veins. Injury to the *nerves,* with intense soreness, > by cold bathing. *Muscles* become SORE AND BRUISED. Pains are hard, aching, squeezing or throbbing. It removes the exudation of swelling of many kinds due to injury. It is a suitable remedy for old laborers, and commercial travellers. Patients feel tired and fagged, desire to lie down. Boils all over. *Near and remote effect;* of blow, fall, accident, railway spine. Ill-effects of cold drinks when overheated, wetting or getting chilled when overheated. Hemorrhage. Pus acrid, destroying hair. Unbearable pain that drives to distraction, < heat, > cold. Sprains and bruises. Tumors from injury.

WORSE: INJURY; *sprain.* TOUCH. *Cold bath* or drink. *Becoming chilled when hot.* Hot bath; warmth of bed. Before storm. *Surgical operation.*

BETTER: Continued motion. Cold (locally).

MIND: Impulse to move.

HEAD: Vertigo, in elderly persons (cerebral stasis). Headache from occiput to vertex, or sinciput. Shooting pain.

STOMACH: Effect of cold or iced drink when heated.

ABDOMEN: Soreness of abdominal walls. *Fullness about the spleen,* and stitches. Foul, painless yellow diarrhea, < at night.

FEMALE: Breasts and uterus engorged; uterus feels squeezed, sore. Inability to walk during pregnancy. Varicose veins during pregnancy.

BACK: Effects of fall on coccyx.

EXTREMITIES: Pain down anterior of thigh. Wrists, feel contracted as if from elastic band.

SKIN: Boils all over. Ecchymoses. Swelling sensitive to touch.

SLEEP: Wakes too early, at 3 a.m. and cannot get to sleep again.

RELATED: Arn.

BENZINUM

GENERALITIES: Benzol affects the blood causing decrease of red cells and increase of white cells, so it ought to be of use in leukemia. Patients are tired and nervous. Hallucination of a large white hand appearing to him in darkness. Pains travels from below upwards. Sensation of falling through bed and floor. Epileptiform attacks, coma and anesthesia.

WORSE: Night. Right side.

BENZINUM NITRICUM

GENERALITIES: It produces faintness, sinking, convulsion, twitching and sopor. Blueness of lips, face and fingernails. Head drawn backwards and to the left in spasm. *Rolling of the eyeballs in their vertical axis* is a prominent feature. *Pupils dilated.* Nystagmus. Respiration slow, difficult, sighing. Involuntary evacuation. Paralysis of all limbs. Secretions smell strongly of bitter almond.

BENZOICUM ACIDUM

GENERALITIES: It is a remedy for uric acid diathesis. The urine is highly colored, very offensive, with gouty symptoms. Urination profuse and scanty alternately. Patient gives out a very strong urinous odor. *Pains suddenly change their locality but are mostly felt in the region of the heart, or alternate with urinary symptoms.* Pain alternates with heart symptoms. Renal insufficiency. Gouty and asthmatic. Hygroma, bunion. Menier's disease. Painful gouty nodes. Highly intensified odor of urine as a concomitant to any diseased condition. Symptoms fluctuate according to the fluctuation of urine.

WORSE: Open air. Cold. Changing weather. Motion. Uncovering.

BETTER: Heat. Profuse urination.

MIND: Inclined to dwell on unpleasant things. Omits words in writing. Child cross, wants to be nursed in arms, will not be laid down. Shudders if he sees anyone deformed.

HEAD: Aches when urine becomes scanty. Vertigo, with inclination to fall sideways.

EARS: Noise, of confused voices in ear, < swallowing or walking in open air.

NOSE: Seems to smell cabbage, dust, or something stinking. Itching of septum.

FACE: Copper-colored spots on face. Involuntary biting of lower lip while eating.

MOUTH: Tongue; spongy on surface, with deep cracks and spreading ulcer. Mouth and throat symptoms are > by eating. Toothache, < lying down.

THROAT: Sensation of a lump, swelling and constriction, > eating.

STOMACH: Vomiting of salty or bitter substance. Sweat while eating.

ABDOMEN: Cutting about navel, > stool. Stitching in liver region. *Copious grayish stools,* like soap-suds, of a pungent urinous odor, very foul, white.

URINARY: URINE; HOT, DARK BROWN; STRONG, *of foul ammoniacal; or odor of horse urine.* Enuresis; dribbling of offensive urine in old men. Gravel. Sheets are unusually stained brown in enuresis. Retention of urine in infants.

FEMALE: Prolapse of uterus, with foul urine.

RESPIRATORY: Hard, dry cough, followed by expectoration of green mucus. Asthma, with rheumatic complaints. Cannot tolerate pressure of clothes on chest. Cough, < night, lying on right side.

HEART: Pains change place, but are constant about the heart. Awakes after midnight, with violent pulsation or burning at heart.

BACK: Coldness in sacrum. Dull pain in region of kidney; stiffness in loins. Trembling in lumbar region.

EXTREMITIES: *Cracking in joints,* in knee. Ganglion of the wrist. Bunion of great toe. Pain in tendo-achilles, at the os calcis, with pain in heart, when stepping on foot.

SKIN: Red spots. Itching with agreeable sensation on being scratched, but leaving a burning sensation.

FEVER: Profuse sweat, without relief. Night-sweat. Hands, feet, back, knees cold, as from a cold wind. Sweat, with aromatic odor.

RELATED: Calc.

BERBERIS AQUIFOLIUM

GENERALITIES: It affects the skin which becomes dry, rough, scaly, pimply. Eruptions on scalp extending to face and neck. Acne. Psoriasis. Dry eczema. Clears the complexion. It should be given in mother tincture in rather material doses.

BERBERIS VULGARIS

GENERALITIES: It acts upon urinary organs, when there is tendency to the formation of calculi and lithemia. It affects the liver markedly — promotes the flow of bile, therefore it is a useful remedy for fleshy persons with good liver, but with little endurance. Often useful in arthritic and hepatic affections with urinary, hemorrhoidal, or menstrual complaints. Venous stasis occurs in pelvic region, causing hemorrhoids. Patient is mentally and physically tired, not inclined to do anything.

Prematurely old and worn out men and women. *Pains rapidly change their locality and character.* Symptoms *rapidly alternate,* thirst alternates with thirstlessness; hunger alternating with loss of appetite etc. *Pains* are RADIATING *from one point, shooting* outward or all over, *sticking, burning, smarting*; soreness. Numbness; insensible to extreme heat and cold. GURGLING or bubbling sensation. *Mucous membranes become dry* — mouth, vagina, etc. Discharges or skin is *dirty gray*. Cold feeling in the bones, eyes, ears, etc. Chest affected after operation for piles, fistula, etc. Sees things in twilight.

WORSE: *Motion; jarring; stepping hard.* Rising from sitting. Standing. Fatigue. Urinating. Twilight.

MIND: Mental labor, requiring close thinking very *difficult;* the least interruption breaks the chain of thought. Apathetic. Indifferent. Objects seem twice as large as natural. Sees terrifying apparitions in twilight, esp. children.

HEAD: Sensation as if the head were becoming larger. Cold temples. Vertigo, with attacks of fainting. Sensation as of a tight cap on head.

EYES: Dry. Feeling of sand between the lids, and in eyes. Eyes feel cold as from a cool wind, with lacrimation on closing the eyes. Quivering of the eyelids when reading. Eyes sunken, with dark-bluish circles around.

EARS: Stopped up feeling, with pressure. Nodes on auricle. Tumor behind the ear. Sensation of coldness or bubbling in ears.

NOSE: Dry. Crawling, itching in nostrils.

FACE: Dirty gray, sickly. Bilious. Suppurating acne. Sensation as if cold drops were spurted onto the face when in the open air.

MOUTH: Sticky. Viscid, foamy, cottony saliva. Tongue

feels scalded; painful pimple on tip. Gums dirty gray. Small white nodes in the gums. Teeth feel too long or too large. Taste bitter.

THROAT: Sensation of plug in the side of the throat with dryness.

STOMACH: Nausea, before breakfast, after dinner. Pain from stomach to back or the reverse. Nausea before breakfast, > after.

ABDOMEN: Torn, loose feeling in the epigastrium. Colic, pain from gall-bladder to stomach, < pressure. Biliary calculi. Stools dirty gray, smarting, tough, watery, with jaundice. Fistula in ano, with itching, with chest complaint. Colic, biliary or urinary, arresting breathing.

URINARY: Pain from kidney, extending along ureter, or to liver, stomach, spleen, arresting breathing. Renal colic. Burning, soreness, or bubbling in kidney region. Clear discharge from meatus before urinating. *Urine,* thick, *turbid,* yellow; red, mealy, *sandy* or *slimy sediment.* Sensation as if some urine remained after urination. Urethra burns when not urinating. Pain in thighs and hips on urinating. Prostate gland enlarged, with pressure in perineum. Dysuria.

MALE: Neuralgia of testes and spermatic cord. Testicles drawn up. Pain changes sides. Genitals cold and sweaty. Prepuce and glans cold and numb. Penis hard and contracted, bends upwards.

FEMALE: Menses too slight, watery blood or brown or gray mucus, replaces menses. Vagina sensitive; cutting pain during coition; vaginismus. Enjoyment absent during coition. Neuralgia of ovaries and vagina. Pain changes sides. Prostration after coition. Dysmenorrhea, with blood looking like gray serum. Urinary symptoms with menses and leukorrhea.

RESPIRATORY: Hoarseness; polypus of larynx. Obstruction of breath when raising arms. Short dry cough, with stitches in chest.

HEART: Stitches about the heart. Pulse becomes very slow.

NECK & BACK: Stitches in neck and back, < respiration. *Backache, with severe prostration,* < sitting or lying. Sore spot under (R) scapula. Crushing, stitching, paralysing pain in lumbar region. Pain from *iliac crests down front of thighs,* when urinating. Post-operative pain in lumbar region.

EXTREMITIES: Neuralgia under fingernails, with swelling of finger-joints. Outer side of the thighs cold, ulcerative pain in heels. Pain in balls of feet on stepping. Intense weariness and lameness of legs after walking a short distance. Stitches between metatarsal bones as from a nail, < standing.

SKIN: Flat warts. Itching, burning and smarting, < scratching, > cold application. Eczema of anus and hands. Eruptions leave a brown stain.

FEVER: Chilly. Sensation of coldness in various parts as if spattered with cold water. Lower parts of the back, hips, thighs, warm. Everything excites sweat.

COMPLEMENTARY: Mag-m.

RELATED: Benz-ac., Coc-c., Kali-bi., Lyc., Puls.

BISMUTHUM

GENERALITIES: Bism. exerts its chief action on *stomach and alimentary canal,* causing catarrhal inflammation. *Pains are tearing, pinching, burning, screwing.* Sensation of heaviness in internal parts. Prostration. Affections after abdominal operation.

WORSE: *Eating;* overeating.

BETTER: Cold drink; cold application. Bending backward. Motion.

MIND: Apathetic. Discontended; complains about his condition. Desire for company; children hold on to mother's hand. Anguish. Never long in one place or position. Fickle minded.

HEAD: Cutting or pressure above (Rt.) orbit extending to occiput, < eating, > cold; alternating with gastric pain. Headache returns in winter.

EYES: Eyeballs ache. Thickened mucus in both canthi.

NOSE: Bleed, dark blood. Heaviness at the root of the nose.

FACE: Earthy; blue around the eyes. Pain in cheek bones, > running about and holding cold water in mouth. Face pale and cold. Face pain alternating, with gastric pain.

MOUTH: Gums swollen. Toothache, > cold water in the mouth, < when becomes warm. Taste sweetish, sour or metallic. Black gangrenous looking wedges on dorsum and sides of tongue.

THROAT: Difficult swallowing of fluid, which returns through nose.

STOMACH: *Craves cold drink,* which is vomited *at once, or in great quantities when stomach becomes full;* at interval of days. Vomits fluids only. Burning, cramping, feeling of a load in stomach. Slow digestion, with fetid eructations. Bilious vomiting, after eating. Food presses like a load in one spot. Stomach pain, > bending backwards. Cancer of stomach, vomiting of brownish water. Gastralgia, not associated with any catarrh or any symptom of indigestion. Cold water >. Atrophy of stomach. Stomach hangs down; hard lumps are felt below navel.

ABDOMEN: Flatulence. Prostration, after stool. Painless diarrhea, with thirst and frequent vomiting, and micturition. Painless discharge of blood from rectum. Cholera infantum, when the body remains warm.

URINARY: Urine frequent, copious; pale; suppression of urine.

HEART: Violent beating of heart.

EXTREMITIES: *Dry palms and soles.* Tearing under nails. Limbs cold. Blue color of forearm and thigh.

SKIN: Ulcer, gangrenous, black, bluish.

SLEEP: Restless on account of voluptuous dreams; with emission or without.

RELATED: Ars; Cadm-s.

BORICUM ACIDUM

GENERALITIES: It affects the skin causing extensive exfoliative dermatitis. Edema around the eyes. It is useful in climacteric flushing. Vagina cold as if packed with ice. Coldness, of saliva, vagina. Diabetes, tongue dry, red and cracked. Pain along ureter with frequent urination.

BETTER: Walking in open air.

BORAX

GENERALITIES: It affects the MUCOUS MEMBRANES causing *aphthous, catarrhal condition. Discharges are thick, hot, biting.* Excessively nervous, easily frightened, sensitive to sudden noises. Heat in single parts-mouth, vagina, palms, etc. Sticking or drawing pain-*internal, intercostal,* soles, etc. Poorly nourished, soft and flabby children. Parts which are usually red turn white. Sensation of cobweb on hands, face. Tousy (untidy) persons. Skin and mucous membranes shrivelled. Restlessness in afternoon. General emaciation. Marasmus. Eructation when painful parts are pressed. Favors easy conception. Infants cyanotic from birth. Valuable in epilepsy.

WORSE: DOWNWARD OR UPWARD MOTION. *Sudden noise.* Cold; wet; least uncovering. Fruit. Nurslings; children. Smoking. Warm weather. After menses. Rocking; being dangled up and down.

BETTER: 11 p.m. Pressure. Evening. Cold weather.

MIND: *Nervous, anxious, fidgety,* fickle. *Fears downward motion. Starts* or is frightened at every noise or *sudden noise,* or at trifles. Irritable before stool, cheerful and happy after. Babies cry and *scream when nursing, or before passing stool or urine.* Fear of thunder. Children awake, suddenly scream, hold the sides of cradle, without any apparent cause. Fault-finding. Does not wish to do anything. All the mental symptoms are > at 11 p.m. Changes from one business to another, from one room to another. Fear of being infected by some contagious disease.

HEAD: Vertigo, < ascending stairs or any elevation. Headache, with nausea and trembling of the whole body. Hot head of babies. Hair entangled at tips, stick together, cannot be separated.

EYES: Gummy, crusty, sticky eyelids. Redness about eyes. Entropion. Raw tarsi. Granular eyelids.

EARS: Sensitive to slightest noise, not so much disturbed by loud ones. Sensation as if ear opened and closed.

NOSE: Acrid coryza. Dry crusts in nose. Red nose of young women. Red, shining swelling of the nose, with throbbing and tensive sensation. Stoppage of nostrils alternately; with lacrimation.

FACE: Pale, dirty. Puffy face; bluish in infants. Anxious, during downward motion. Cobweb sensation, as if a bug crawling over lip.

MOUTH: Dry, hot, tender, *aphthous*, after taking sour or salty food. Cracked or puffy, indented tongue. Toothache, < wet weather, > by smoking. Palate hard and wrinkled, feels burnt, pain when chewing, while nursing, in children. Painful gumboil. Taste bitter, even of saliva. Thrush. Ulcer, bleeds on eating or by touch.

STOMACH: Eructation, on pressing painful part. Nausea, when thinking hard, with trembling of body and weakness of knees. Desire for sour things. Pain in the region of stomach, after heavy lifting; stitching,extending to small of back. Sweat on stomach. Vomiting after drinking, of sour mucus. Gastralgia, reflex from uterine trouble.

ABDOMEN: Belly soft, flabby, sunken. Flatulent distention after every meal. Pain as if diarrhea would set in. Stool turning green, or persistently green stool ; like boiled starch. Mucous diarrhea, then weakness. Loose, pappy, foul smelling stools. Stools slender. Catch in groin on coughing. Pulling from spleen to chest. Stitching pain in the groins before or during menses. Burning in rectum during stool.

URINARY: Hot, acrid, smarting urine, of pungent smell. Child screams before the passage. Frequent, every 10 to 15 minutes. Small red particles on diaper. Nephritis. Cystitis.

MALE: Indifference to coition.

FEMALE: Indifference to coition. Menses too early, too profuse; attended with colic and nausea. Leukorrhea — albuminous, clear, hot, pasty, with sensation as if warm water was flowing down legs. Membranous dysmenorrhea. Empty feeling in mammae, after child nurses, with stitches, > compressing. When nursing, pain in opposite breast. Labor pain with frequent eructation. Mother's milk is thick and tastes bad. Sensation of distention in clitoris, with sticking. Sterility. Favors easy conception.

RESPIRATORY: Sticking pain in chest (intercostal), < coughing, inspiration, yawning or any physical exertion. Shortness of breath, < ascending stairs; stitches on speaking. Hacking and violent cough; expectoration blood-streaked or mouldy. Pain in chest, > lying on back, washing with cold water, or pressure. Arrest of breath when lying down, must jump up and catch for breath.

HEART: Feels *as if on right side,* and being squeezed. Infant cyanotic from birth. Violent palpitation.

NECK & BACK: Pain in back, inability to stoop.

EXTREMITIES: Limbs tremble at 10 a.m. Feeling of cobweb on hands. Stitches in soles. Weakness in calves. Pain in heel. Eczema of fingers and toes with loss of nails. Sensation as if warm water running down thighs. Palms hot. Itching on back of hands. Want of strength, esp. in joints.

SKIN: DRY; *festers easily,* won't heal. Psoriasis. Trade eruptions (occupational hazards involving the contact of skin with irritant substances) on fingers and hands; itching and stinging eczema. Wilted, wrinkled skin. Whitish pimples, with areola. Ulceration of feet from rubbing of shoes.

SLEEP: Voluptuous dreams, dreams of coition. Cries out in sleep, as if frightened (children). Cannot sleep on account of excessive heat, esp. of head. Starts from sleep, as if falling.

FEVER: Flushes of heat.

RELATED: Bell; Bry; Calc; Nux-v; Sul-ac.

BOTHROPS LANCIOLATUS

GENERALITIES: The venom of this snake is most coagulative, therefore, it is expected to be useful in thrombosis and thrombotic affections such as hemiplegia. Aphasia, without the affection of tongue. Nervous trembling. Great lassitude and sluggishness. Blindness from hemorrhage into retina. Day blindness - can scarcely see her way after sunrise. Paralysis of one arm or one leg only. Slight shivering, followed by profuse sweat. Intolerable pain in the big toe. Bone becomes bare from gangrene and becomes necrotic.

WORSE: Right side.

BOVISTA

GENERALITIES: This fungus commonly known as puff-ball, exerts its influence on CIRCULATION, causing relaxation of capillary system, thereby producing *hemorrhagic diathesis.* On *skin* it causes *herpetic* eruption. There is a *general puffiness,* bloated condition of body surface, which produces *easy indentation by blunt* instrument (scissors etc.). *Laxity,* esp. felt in joints which seem loose. *Enlarged or swollen feeling in head,* heart, etc. It is adapted to old maids with palpitations and stammering children. Multiple neuritis, with numbness and tingling. Asphyxia due to charcoal fume. Effect of over-exertion, and contact of tar locally. Nervous and weak-jointed.

WORSE: *Menses.* Full moon. Hot weather. *Getting* warm. Cold food. Wine. Coffee.

BETTER: Bending double. Hot food. Eating.

MIND: *Awkward in speech and action;* drops things, stutters, etc. Ineffective. Absent minded. Weak memory. Irritable, takes everything amiss. Laughs and cries alternately. Stares vacantly into space. Sad when alone. Quarrelsome.

HEAD: Confusion on awakening. Sensation as if head were enlarging, as if wedge were pressed in occiput. Staggering, confusion and numbness in head after coition. Itching of the scalp, < warmth.

EYES: Objects seem to be nearer than they really are. Staring at one point. Loss of vision from paralysis of optic nerve.

EARS: Boil in right ear, with pain, < swallowing. Discharge of fetid pus. Hearing indistinct, misunderstands much that is spoken.

NOSE: Stringy, tough discharge from nose. Nose stopped up, cannot breathe, < lying down. Scurfs and crusts about nostrils. Bleeding early in the morning (during sleep); few drops escape on sneezing.

FACE: Cheeks and lips swollen. Crusts about corners of mouth. Acne, < in summer or by use of cosmetics. Twitching of muscles before asthma. Lips cracked, crusty.

MOUTH: Numb. Increases saliva. Gums bleed easily on sucking them. Cutting pain in tongue before asthma.

STOMACH: Sensation of a lump of ice. Nausea, > breakfast. Vomits watery fluid.

ABDOMEN: Colic, with bright red urine, > eating and bending double. *Diarrhea, < during and before menses.* Cannot bear tight clothing around the waist. Stitches through perineum towards rectum and genitals. Chronic diarrhea of old people, < night, early morning. First portion of stool is hard, latter part thin and watery.

URINARY: Frequent desire to urinate, even immediately after urination (diabetes mellitus).

MALE: After coition, reeling and confusion in head. Sexual desire increased.

FEMALE: Voluptuous sensation. *Menses early,* oozing, every two weeks, *more at night, less while moving.* Occasional show between the periods. Parovarian (near the ovary) cyst. Thick, acrid, yellow-green leukorrhea, leaving green spots on linen, < while walking, after menses. Jaundice of newborn.

RESPIRATORY: Shortness of breath on moving the arms. Viscid expectoration. Spasmodic laughing and crying, with asthma.

HEART: Visible palpitation of heart, of old maids. Palpitation as if heart were working in water. Palpitation, with tremor of hands, < bathing, excitement.

NECK & BACK: Pain in the back with heaviness, after stooping. *Itching coccyx.*

EXTREMITIES: Great weakness of all joints. Weakness; clumsiness working with her hands. Heavy, painful legs. Edematous swelling of (right) foot even years after a sprain. Sweat in axilla, onion-like smell. Edema of joints after fracture. Weak hands.

SKIN: Blunt instruments leave a deep impression. *Itching* eruption, oozing, forming *thick crust or scabs* with pus beneath. Shooting pain in corns and warts. Urticaria covering whole body, with diarrhea or metrorrhagia. Pellagra. Eczema.

FEVER: Chill with pain.

RELATED: Apis; Calc; Rhus-t; Sep; Ust.

BROMIUM

GENERALITIES: Marked effects of bromine are seen on the RESPIRATORY TRACT, esp. LARYNX and *trachea*. It is useful in scrofulous children, with enlarged glands; *parotid*, thyroid, ovarian and mammary glands are esp. affected, which are swollen and indurated; but seldom suppurate. Constriction and membranous formation occur in larynx, spreading upwards. Patient is *weak and easily overheated, then sweaty and sensitive to drafts.* Blondes. Tremulous all over. Fainting. Emaciation. Boring pain in bones. Cancer.

WORSE: WARMTH; DAMP WARM; *overheating;* warm room. Chilled when hot. Sea-bathing. Dust. Draft. Evening, until midnight, Lying on left side.

BETTER: Nose-bleed > (vertigo, head, chest). At sea. Motion. Shaving. Riding.

MIND: Feels that strange persons are looking over patient's shoulders, or that he would see one on turning, as if someone were at the back of him. Takes no interest in household duties. Cheerful mood; desire for mental labor. Sad. Indifferent. Low-spirited; inconsolable. Does not feel normal but cannot tell why. Sits alone in her room without doing anything, looks constantly in one direction without saying anything.

HEAD: Vertigo, < on bridge, at the sight of running water. Head congested, fears a stroke. Headache, < drinking milk, stooping. Headache in sun, passes off in shade. Headache deep in vertex, with palpitation.

EYES: Lacrimation, with swelling of tear glands. Pupils dilated. Protruding eyes. Flashes before eyes.

EARS: Hard swelling of the parotid gland, warm to touch; after eruptive fever.

NOSE: *Acrid, burning coryza,* with violent sneezing and soreness of the nose. Tickling, smarting as from cobweb. Nosebleed. Fan-like motion of alae. Long continued obstinate coryza.

FACE: Sensation of cobweb. Seems drawn to a point at nose. Ashy gray. Pale and red, alternating.

MOUTH : Dry and parched. Aphthae, with affection of eyes. Water tastes saltish.

THROAT: Tonsils swollen, deep red, with network of dilated blood vessels. Pain < swallowing fluid than solid. Even a small goiter oppresses. Stony hard, swollen glands. Diphtheria.

STOMACH: Sharp burning from tongue to stomach. Pressure like from a stone. Gastralgia, > eating. Sour things disagree. Vomiting; like coffee-ground, bloody mucus. Aversion to customary tobacco smoking.

ABDOMEN: Tympanitic, distended. Diarrhea, after eating oysters and sour things. Piles bleed, intensely painful, < application of cold or warm water. Spleen enlarged, indurated.

URINARY: Urine high colored.

MALE: Swelling and induration of testes, < slight jar.

FEMALE: Flatus from vagina, noisy. Dysmenorrhea. Swelling of ovaries. Queer ill feeling few days before menses. Tumor in breast, stitching pain from breast to axilla. Menses with membranous shreds. Itching in vagina. Suppression of menses, in scirrhous mammae.

RESPIRATORY: Inhaled air seems smoky, cold or raw. Dry cough, with hoarseness and burning pain behind sternum. *Wants to take a deep breath,* but it excites cough. *Suffocative fits;* he starts up with *choked* or *croupy* or *wheezing* cough or with palpitation. Asthma. Spasms of glottis. Asthma of sailors going ashore. Deep hoarseness if heated. Lungs feel coated with down. *Larynx cold.* Cold starts in larynx, goes *upward and downward.* Thick white expectoration. Dyspnea, with great swelling.

HEART: Hypertrophy, from gymnastics, with palpitation. Cutting pain running upwards in heart disease. Violent palpitation, < lying on left side. Nervous palpitation, with nausea, with headache.

NECK & BACK: Glands enlarged, cystic tumors on both sides of neck.

EXTREMITIES: Icy cold forearms or only cold hands. Boring pain in one or both tibiae. Left arm lame, in cardiac affection.

SKIN: Boils on arms and face. Acne, pimples and pustules.

SLEEP: Continued yawning, with respiratory trouble, with drowsiness. Great drowsiness when reading.

RELATED: Lach; Samb.

BRYONIA ALBA

GENERALITIES: Bryonia develops a marked action on all SEROUS MEMBRANES and the viscera they contain, causing INFLAMMATION *and exudation.* It disorders *circulation*, producing congestion; alters the blood, giving rise to typhoid, bilious, rheumatic and remittent fevers. AVERSION TO LEAST MOTION, even distant parts, is due to its action on nerves and *muscles. Mucous membranes become dry,* hence discharges are scanty and adherent. Complaints develop slowly, but forcibly. Pains are BURSTING, STITCHING or *heavy,* sore, going backward. *Effects are very painful;* on coughing holds sides, chest, head. Joints painful. Streaks of red-lymphangitis.

Gastro-bilious-rheumatic constitution. Every spot in the body is painful to pressure. Dropsical swelling gradually increases as the day progresses and disappears during the night. Children dislike to be carried or raised. Physical weakness, on slightest exertion; all pervading apathy. Ill-effects of anger, fright, chagrin. Suppressed eruptions and discharges. Alcohol. Gluttony. Wound. Complaint from taking cold drink in hot weather. Often indicated in injury of the joint when *Arnica* fails. Muscles become hard, after neuralgia. Dryness everywhere, of mouth, throat etc. It is adapted to nervous, dry, slender people. Right sided-effects. Vicarious bleeding.

WORSE: LEAST MOTION; RAISING UP; STOOPING; COUGHING; EXERTION; DEEP BREATHING. Dry cold or heat. BECOMING HOT; IN ROOM. *Hot weather.* Drinking while hot. EATING. Vegetables. Acids, Calomel. VEXATION. TOUCH. Suppression. Taking cold. Early a.m.

BETTER: PRESSURE; LYING ON PAINFUL PART. Bandaging. COOL OPEN AIR. QUIET. Cloudy, damp days. *Drawing knees up.* Heat to inflamed part. Descending. Sitting up. Cold food, drink.

MIND: Very irritable and ugly in behavior. Determined. Taciturn. Delirium, *wants to go home* thinking he is not there. Talks of business. Wants to be let alone. Desire for things which are rejected when offered. Dull. Apprehension and dread for future. Despair of being cured, with fear of death.

HEAD: DIZZY OR FAINT ON RISING UP. Vertigo felt in occiput. BURSTING, SPLITTING OR HEAVY, *crushing fronto-occipital* headache < moving eyes, coughing, straining at stool, etc. Vertigo as though all objects are whirling, or as if sinking deep down in the bed, > cold. Pain over left eye, pressive, going to occiput, thence spreading over whole body. Scalp very sensitive, cannot bear even a soft brush, every part of the scalp touched pains. Oily hair. Headache from ironing, when constipated.

EYES: Eyeballs sore; *pains behind the eyeballs.* Glaucoma. Lacrimation, during day, esp. in the sun. Lids swollen and puffed.

EARS: Aural vertigo. Ringing, humming in ears. Vicarious bleeding from ears.

NOSE: Epistaxis, vicarious, when menses should appear, in pregnancy. Swelling of tip of the nose, feels as if it would ulcerate when touched. Boils. Descending colds.

FACE: Dark red, hot, bloated.

MOUTH: *Dry.* Tongue, very dry, rough, coated along centre; red at base. Taste BITTER, cannot swallow food, > cold drinks. Toothache > cold water, < brushing teeth. Jerking toothache when smoking or chewing tobacco. Collection of soapy, frothy saliva. Chewing motions, in brain affections, of children. Lips; dry, as if burnt, parched, cracked, wants to moisten them. Burning of lower lip in old smokers. Picking of lips. Infant has sore mouth; child does not want to take hold of breast, but after mouth becomes moist it nurses well.

THROAT: Hawks brown lumps, with effort. Throat; dry, scraping roughness in. Back of throat seems swollen. Aphthous patches; recurring.

STOMACH: THIRST FOR LARGE QUANTITY OF COLD WATER; also for warm drinks which >. Craves what he cannot relish. Loathing for food. Nausea, < rising up, lying on right side. Bitter vomiting, of bile and water, immediately after eating. Vomits solid food only. *Heavy load in stomach,* < eating. Stomach sensitive to touch. Great desire for coffee, wine and acid drink. Aversion to milk, but when he takes it he relishes it. Tasteless eructations. Vomits warm drink. Drinks hastily and eagerly.

ABDOMEN: Epigastrium tender, throbbing. Liver heavy, sore, swollen, > lying on it. Abdominal wall very tender. Appendicitis. Peritonitis. Stool; LARGE, DRY, VERY HARD, as if burnt; loose, painless, undigested, involuntary, during sleep. Constipation. Diarrhea, gushing, < in the morning, on rising, eating cabbage. Diarrhoea; in hot weather, after cold drink. Lumps of tough mucus after stool. Burning in anus with stool. Yellow, mushy stool. Jaundice. Groins sore before menses. Complaint from over lifting, concussion.

URINARY: Urine red, brown like beer; scanty, hot. Inclination to make water, with suspended respiration on lifting load. Involuntary urination during exertion. Burning in urethra when not urinating.

FEMALE: Menses suppressed with vicarious discharge or splitting headache. Pain in breast at menstrual period. Breast hot and painful, hard. Milk fever. Intermenstrual pain, with great abdominal and pelvic soreness. Mastitis, stony hard mammae. Abscess of mammae. Ovaritis. Menses dark, foul. Stitches in the ovaries on taking deep breath. Frequent nosebleed at the appearance of menses.

RESPIRATORY: Cough DRY, HARD, VERY PAINFUL, at night as if from stomach, must sit up, < eating and drinking. Wants to take deep breath, but cannot because it excites cough. Expectoration rusty, blood streaked or tough. Bronchitis. Asthma. Pneumonia. SHARP STITCHES IN CHEST or at right *scapula*, < deep breathing and coughing. Pleurisy. Coming into warm room excites cough. Holds chest, or presses the sternum when coughing. Dry friction sound (Pleural rub on auscultation). Cough, with sneezing.

HEART: Stitches in cardiac region. Pulse FULL, QUICK, *harsh*.

NECK & BACK: Intrascapular numbness or pain going to epigastrium or from left scapula to heart. Painful stiffness of neck. Pain in the small of back, < walking or turning. Stitches and stiffness in small of back. Lumbago, < stooping.

EXTREMITIES: Joints red, swollen, hot. Pins and needles in soles, preventing walking. Constant motion of left arm and leg, with sighing. Swelling of elbow. Knees totter and bend under him when walking. Tendency to run backwards. Sciatica, > lying quietly and on painful side.

SKIN: *Slow development or sudden receding of rash,* in eruptive fevers. *Undeveloped measles.* Skin yellow, pale, swollen, dropsical.

SLEEP: Dreams; of hard work, about household affairs, about business of the day, in delirium. Drowsy. Starting when falling asleep. Walks in sleep.

FEVER : Chill with hot head and red face, < warm room. Dry burning heat, with < of all the symptoms. Blood seems hot. Painful continued fever. Sweat sour or oily.

COMPLEMENTARY: Abrot; Alum; Kali-c; Lyc; Nat-m; *Rhus-t; Sep; Sulph.*

RELATED: Phyt; Rhus-t.

BUFO

GENERALITIES: The poison of this toad has a remarkable action on nervous system, and sexual organs. It arouses lowest passions; patient is not only *low-minded but develops a low type of disease* also. It is a remedy for *depravities, due to bad inheritance.* Early broken down, prematurely senile person. It affects circulation, causing ebullition of heat, flushing; *burnings* in different parts. Bloody oozing; from nipples, bloody saliva, etc. Trembling like paralysis agitans. Electric like shocks are felt throughout the body. Feels as if whole body swollen, in a.m. festering sensation. Falls down unconscious, with a blood-curdling scream. Obesity. Epileptic seizures; occur during night; connected with sexual sphere; at the time of menses; in women when sexual desire is excited; in young due to onanism or during coition; attacks are followed by headache. Sensation as of a peg in joint. Dropsy. Paralysis. Cancer. Carbuncle. Bubo. Septic lymphangitis due to injuries, when pain runs up in streaks. Spasms in children, after nursing angry or frightened mother. Anesthetic spots on skin. Aversion to the sight of brilliant objects. Variety of symptoms occur before epileptic spasm. The mind remains childish, only the body grows. Fetid discharges, and exhalation. Convulsions from suppurative condition.

WORSE: Warm room. Sexual excitement. Masturbation. Least motion. Injury.

BETTER: Bleeding. Cool air. Cold bathing. Feet in hot water.

MIND: Moral depravity. Idiocy; childish, silly, tittering. Feeble minded. Fears animals, strangers. Talks nonsense, then angry if not understood. Walks the floor and wrings the hands. Desire for solitude, to practice masturbation. Inclination to bite. Deceitfulness. Music is unbearable.

HEAD: Sensation as if hot vapor were rising to the top of head. Brain numb. Pillow hurts occiput.

EYES: Sight of brilliant objects intolerable. Objects appear crooked. Left lid paralyzed. Pupils dilated. Eyes sunken.

EARS: Least noise distresses. Music is intolerable.

NOSE: Epistaxis, with flushed face and pain in forehead.

FACE: Bloated and distorted. Bathed in sweat (in spasms). Lips black.

MOUTH: Paralysis of tongue, lapping motions of tongue. Bloody saliva. Stammering. Desire for sweet drinks. Tongue cracked, bluish black. Convulsions after extracting teeth.

ABDOMEN: Feels a cold ball running through bowels. Bubo in groins. Convulsive movement in abdomen after spasm. Vomiting after drinking. Yellow fluid in vomit. Vomiting of blood and bile.

MALE: Spasm during coition. Disposition to handle organ, and to masturbation. Impotency.

FEMALE: Epilepsy at the time of menses. Menses too early and too copious. Milk bloody. Cancer of mammary gland. Tumors and polyp of uterus; ulcers of cervix. Burning in ovaries and uterus. Cord like swelling from groin to knee, milk-leg. Violent pain in mammae, < at night. Hydatids in ovaries. Offensive purulent leukorrhea.

RESPIRATORY: Burning like fire in lungs. Suffocative cough. Asthma.

HEART: *Seems to float in water* or air. Rapid heart action, in exophthalmos. Feels too large. Palpitation, with headache, during menses.

NECK & BACK: Jerk in nape of neck, before spasm. Lumbago, < rising up or least motion.

EXTREMITIES: Trembling of limbs. Cramp. Staggering gait. Feeling as if a peg were driven in joint. Limbs become stiff, numb.

SKIN: *Red streaks under skin.* Lymphangitis. Panaris. Yellow bullae. Yellowish, corrosive fluid oozes out. Horripilation (goose-skin).

SLEEP: Comatose, after spasm.

COMPLEMENTARY: Calc.

RELATED: Bar-c., Graph., Tarent.

BURSA PASTORIS

GENERALITIES: It is remedy for hemorrhagic and uric acid diathesis. It removes the ill-effect of suppression of hemorrhage or vaginal discharges from uterus.

WORSE: Every other month.

BETTER: Bathing. Dampness. Rapid motion.

MIND: Impulse to walk far.

HEAD: *Pain from above eyes up over head to nape.*

NOSE: Bleeding in nasal operation.

FACE: Eyes and face puffy.

MOUTH: Taste like bad egg.

STOMACH: Craves butter milk. Flatulence. Blood or mucopurulent discharge after stool.

URINARY: Hematuria. Copious discharge of urinary sand. Dysuria: of old persons, with dribbling; after forceps delivery. Renal colic. Urine runs away in little jets. Brick dust sediment. Albuminuria during pregnancy.

FEMALE: Metrorrhagia, with violent uterine colic; every alternate period very profuse. Uterine fibroid, with cramp and expulsion of clots. Sore pain in womb, < on rising. *Menses and leukorrhea leave a fast stain.* Leukorrhea excites itching. Milky water runs from right nipple. Scarcely recovers from one period when another begins.

BACK: Weakness between scapulae.

RELATED: Sep.

CACTUS GRANDIFLORUS

GENERALITIES: Chief action of *Cactus* centers around the HEART and CIRCULATION. It affects the *circular muscles*, thereby producing CONSTRICTION of the HEART, throat, chest, bladder, rectum, vagina, neck. *Circulation becomes irregular, causing violent congestion or localised pulsation* behind stomach, at odd places. It is a HEMORRHAGIC remedy, favors formation of clots speedily. Constrictive or spasmodic pain that extort cries. *Periodicity is marked, and neuralgic pain* occurs periodically. *Body feels tight* or wrapped. Hot gushing into chest. Toxic goiter, with cardiac symptoms. General weakness and prostration. Fainting. Dropsical affections. Ill-effect of sun, damp, disappointment in love. Many complaints are associated with heart affection. Pulseless, panting and prostrated. Low blood pressure, from weakness of heart.

WORSE: *Lying,* on left side, on occiput. Periodically. Exertion. 10-11 a.m. or 11 p.m. Night. Walking. Going upstairs. Noise. Light. Sun heat.

BETTER: Open air. Pressure on vertex.

MIND: Taciturn. Weeps, knows not why, < consolation. Believes that his disease in incurable. Sad. Ill humored. Easily frightened. Cheerful. Fear; of death, something will happen.

HEAD: Heavy pain, as of a load on vertex, > pressure, < talking, strong light. Headache, < by seeing opera, missing of meals, noise, light, periodic, compressive, pulsating. Vertigo, < deep breathing, exertion.

EYES: Dimness of sight. Eyes bloodshot. Exophthalmic goiter.

EARS: Pulsation in ears. Singing, ringing in ears.

NOSE: Profuse epistaxis, but soon ceases.

FACE: Right-sided prosopalgia, < missing of meals. *Face; red, bloated*, pale, emaciated.

THROAT: Constriction of esophagus, must drink to swallow. Suffocative constriction, with full throbbing carotids.

STOMACH: Pulsation in celiac artery behind the stomach. Vomiting of blood. Nausea in the morning—continues all day. Loss of appetite. Aversion to meat of which he was previously fond.

ABDOMEN: Intense burning in abdomen. Feeling of a weight in anus. Pricking in anus, > slight friction. Fistula-in-ano, with violent palpitation of heart. Engorgement of liver due to heart disease. Sharp pain shooting through diaphragm and up into chest; as if a cord were tied tighter and tighter around attachment of diaphragm, taking his breath away.

URINARY: Constriction of neck of bladder, causing retention of urine. Urine suppressed in fever. Hematuria; urination prevented by clot in vagina in females.

FEMALE: Menses lumpy, *black*, too soon, cease on lying. Constriction of vagina preventing coition; vaginismus. Painful menses, extorting loud cries. Menstrual disorder, with heart symptoms. Pulsation in ovarian region. Cyanotic infants.

RESPIRATORY: Oppressed breathing, going upstairs. Cough, from heart affection. Continuous rattling of mucus in chest. Constriction in chest, as if bound, hindering breathing. Periodical suffocation, with fainting, sweat on face and loss of pulse. Hemoptysis, with convulsive cough. Inflammation of diaphragm, with difficulty in breathing.

HEART: FEELS CLUTCHED AND RELEASED ALTERNATELY BY AN IRON BAND, or feels it expand and contract, seems to turn over. Endocarditis, with mitral insufficiency. Palpitation, < lying on left side, at the approach of menses, during the day while walking, from disappointed love. Stitches in heart. Endocardial murmur. Hypertrophy. Low blood pressure. Pulse; irritable, intermittent, feeble. Irregular and intermittent action, after forceps delivery. Heart disease, with edema of left hand. Seems heart would fly to pieces on holding the breath. Pulsations increase on holding the breath. Aneurism of large arteries and heart. Tobacco heart.

EXTREMITIES: Left arm numb. Fingers tingle. Icy cold hands. Edema of hand (left) in heart disease, and of feet extending to knee. Hands soft, feet enlarged. Pain in left arm down to fingers.

SLEEP: Sleeplessness, on account of strong pulsation in different places. Dreams of falling, frightful, lascivious. Awakes in fright.

FEVER: Chill, not < by covering. Persistent subnormal temperature.

RELATED: Acon; Coc-c; Dig; Lach; Nux-v; Sulph.

CADMIUM SULPHURATUM

GENERALITIES: Its chief action centers on stomach and respiration. There is extreme exhaustion and prostration, with vomiting. Patient must keep quiet. Icy coldness even near a fire. Low form of disease, runs deathward. Weakness remaining after epileptic attacks, of one arm and one leg. Formication between the skin and deep tissue. Numbness, of parts, nose, head etc. Paralyzed part painful, or crawling in it.

WORSE: Raising up. Least motion. Carrying burden. After sleep. Stimulant. Open air. Cold. Sunshine. Walking. Ascending stairs. Vexation. Swallowing.

BETTER: Eating. Rest.

MIND: Horror of solitude and work.

HEAD: *Faintness* on rising. Vertigo; room and bed seem to spin around.

EYES: Opacity of cornea, from injury or inflammation. Night blindness. Tears hot. Cannot read small type.

NOSE: Ozena. Polypus. Boils on nose. Nose numb.

FACE: Distortion of mouth, from facial paralysis. Trembling of lower jaw. Facial paralysis, left side, < cold air; cannot close eyes, difficult talking and swallowing.

STOMACH: Craves little drinks of cold water which are vomited at once. Burning and cutting pain; intense retching and gagging. Intense nausea and vomiting, > quiet. Black vomit. Coffee ground vomit. Cancer of stomach. Least thing touching lips will excite nausea and vomiting. Dysphagia. Stomach symptoms < carrying burden.

URINARY: Urine mixed with pus and blood.

RESPIRATORY: Suffocation on dropping to sleep. Chest contracted with asthma. Chest symptoms < squatting.

SKIN: Blue, yellow, scaly. Horripilation (goose-flesh), after drinking, with hot hands, with heartburn. Chloasma, < exposure to sun.

SLEEP: Breathing stops on going to sleep. Fears to go to sleep again. Protracted sleeplessness. Sleeps with open eyes.

FEVER: Yellow fever. Body icy cold.

RELATED: Zinc.

CALADIUM SEGUINUM

GENERALITIES: It has a special action on the GENITAL ORGANS of both sexes. Masturbation, and its results in men; pruritus vulvae in females, which may sometimes be due to threadworms finding their way into vagina, inducing masturbation and even nymphomania. There is a great desire to lie down and aversion to motion, but if he makes the effort he is strong enough. Attacks like fainting after writing and thinking, when lying down or when rising. DRYNESS of parts which are usually moist. *Dry feeling.* Modifies craving for tobacco. Tobacco heart. Asthma, alternating with itching rash. Lascivious; ogles women on the street, but impotent. Unable to walk with closed eyes. Mosquito bites that itches and burns intensely.

WORSE: *Sexual excess.* Motion. Sudden noise. On falling asleep. Tobacco.

BETTER: Cold air. Short sleep. Sweating.

MIND: Very careful about his health. Restless, cannot control himself after smoking. Refuses to take medicine. Forgetfulness. *Nervous excitation.* Fear of catching disease. Afraid of his own shadow. Foolish boldness.

HEAD: Vertigo, as if rocked, < closing eyes and lying down. Numbness in side of head.

EYES: Close even while walking in open air.

EARS: Sensitive to noise, slightest noise startles from sleep.

NOSE: Discharge of bloody mucus on blowing nose.

FACE: Sensation of a cobweb or crawling.

MOUTH: Food seems too dry, must drink to swallow. *Red, dry stripe down centre of tongue widening towards tip.* Saliva like white of an egg. Milk tastes sour.

STOMACH: Feels full of dry food (with asthma). Burning, < deep breathing, taking tea or chocolate. Fluttering sensation. Tolerates only warm drink. Eats without hunger and drinks without thirst. Thirstless for days.

ABDOMEN: Sensation as of a long worm writhing in transverse colon.

URINARY: Urine offensive, scanty.

MALE: Flaccid, sweaty, cold genitals. Impotence. Pruritus. Impotence after gonorrhea, with mental depression. Organs seem larger, as if puffed. Glans like a rag. Atonic pollution. Prepuce retracted after coition.

FEMALE: PRURITUS VULVAE, inducing masturbation, with burning, from pinworms, during pregnancy. Violent sexual erethism or neurasthenia.

RESPIRATORY: Catarrhal asthma, mucus not readily raised, by > expectoration. Hard cough, with asthma. Sighing respiration.

EXTREMITIES: Weak, cannot get out of bed. Hands numb. Cannot walk or stand, with closed eyes.

SLEEP: Groans and moans anxiously, loudly in sleep. Vivid dreams.

SKIN: Feels rough and dry. Burning in spots, must touch the parts, but cannot scratch them.

FEVER: Cold single parts—feet. Sweat of sweetish odor, attracting flies. Low fever. Falls asleep during fever, wakes up when it stops.

COMPLEMENTARY: Nit-ac.

RELATED: Caps.

CALCAREA ARSENICOSA

GENERALITIES: This remedy was found useful clinically in complaints of fat women around climacteric, when slightest emotion causes palpitation; in children with enlarged liver and spleen; in complaints of drunkards after abstaining. Nephritis, albuminuria and dropsy. Epilepsy with rush of blood to the head; aura felt in the region of heart; with heart disease. Flying sensation or swimming sensation, as if feet did not touch the ground.

WORSE: Slight exertion. Error in diet. Cold air.

MIND: Depression and anxiety. Desire for company.

HEAD: Rush of blood to the head, with vertigo. Weekly headache, > lying on painful side. Headache with palpitation, increase and decrease together.

ABDOMEN: Enlarged liver and spleen in chronic malaria, in children. Pancreatic disease. *Relieves burning pain in cancer.* Diarrhea, < sweet potato or yam. Swollen inguinal glands, with tearing pain in legs.

URINARY: Kidney region sensitive to pressure. Passes urine every hour.

FEMALE: Offensive bloody leukorrhea. Cancer of the uterus. Burning in uterus and vagina.

RESPIRATORY: Burning heat in chest. Feeling as if he would suffocate, with palpitation. Drawing as with a thread from larynx backward.

HEART: Palpitation and heart pain before epileptic attack. Pulse intermits every 4th beat regularly.

NECK & BACK: Pain and stiffness near nape of neck. Violent throbbing pain, drives out of bed.

EXTREMITIES: Weariness and lameness of lower limbs. Removes inflammatory products in veins of lower limbs.

FEVER: Marked malaria. Chilly.

CALCAREA CARBONICA

GENERALITIES: Calc-carb is the chief representative of calcium compounds. Calcium metabolism is active during childhood and becomes defective after middle age. Improper assimilation of calcium gives rise to defective NUTRITION of GLANDS (cervical and mesenteric in children); BONES and SKIN. It alters the BLOOD causing anemia. GLANDULAR SWELLING below the jaw and in the neck; *faulty development of bones*. OPEN FONTANELLES. Curvature; exostosis; rickets. Muscles and skin become *lax* or *flabby;* patient grows FAT, but not strong. SWEATING IS EASY; partial—on HEAD; CHEST; SWEAT DURING SLEEP. DISCHARGES ARE PROFUSE, OFTEN SOUR—stool, *sweat,* saliva etc. Sour odor of body. It is suitable to *Blondes of soft and sluggish* habit. Complaints of teething—convulsion, sour diarrhoea; *tardy teething* and *late walking*—child does not put his feet down on the ground. Emaciated children, with big head and big belly. Patient is susceptible to COLD; *Cold moist air chills through and through; takes cold easily,* esp. in chest. Tendency to sprain the muscles easily. Parts lain on become numb. Tendency to the formation of calculi. Malnutrition. Muscular atrophy. Early stage of tuberculosis of lungs, with tickling cough, fleeting chest pain, nausea acidity and dislike for fat. A jaded mental and physical stage due to overwork. Cramp in muscles which draws limbs. Abscess deep in muscle. Polypi nasal, uterine etc. Cyst. In short, Calc patient can be described as *fat, flabby, fair, forty, perspiring, cold and damp.* In epilepsy the aura spreads up from solar plexus or like a mouse running up the arm or down epigastrium to uterus or limbs. Twitching, trembling, chorea; neuralgia; horrible fantasies; paralyses are among the *Calc.* effects. Varicose veins; burning in veins. Osteomyelitis. Ill-effect of alcohol, loss of vital fluid, excessive venery (sexual intercourse), masturbation; strain, overlifting; suppressed sweat, eruption, menses; fright, egotism. Affections of stone-cutters. Dull lethargic children who do not want to play. Pituitary and thyroid dysfunction. Diarrhea, tremors, after burns.

WORSE: COLD; RAW AIR; BATHING. Cooling off. Change of weather to cold. EXERTION—*physical,* mental, *ASCENDING.* Eye strain. DENTITION. Puberty. PRESSURE OF CLOTHES. MILK. Anxiety. Awakening. Full moon. Standing. Looking up. Climaxis. Turning head.

BETTER: Dry climate and weather. Lying on painful side, on back. Sneezing (headache). Rubbing, scratching. Wiping or soothing with hand. After breakfast. Dark.

MIND: Forgetful; learns poorly. *Depressed. Melancholic* or *Doubting Mood.* Fears; disease, misery, disaster, insanity, of being observed. Fear excited by report of cruelty. Cautious. Confused, misplaces words and expresses himself wrongly. Sad. Apathetic. Taciturn. Indolent, suddenly. Visions, of fire, murder, rats and mice in delirium. Melancholy; desire to weep, to go home. Hopeless of ever getting well. Suspicious, thinks people look at him suspiciously, and he looks at them suspiciously. Inability to apply himself. Sits and thinks about little affairs that amount to nothing. Sits and breaks sticks etc. all day long. Imagines someone walking behind her. Feels as if she would run up and down and scream. Easily frightened or offended. Children are self-willed. Child is afraid of everything it sees. Mischievous. Obstinate. Irritable, cries about trifles; borrows trouble.

HEAD: Vertigo with many conditions, < ascending or turning head, scratching head; vertigo after epilepsy. Rush of blood to the head. *Icy cold* in, and *on the head;* much perspiration, < occiput, wets the pillow. *Scratches head,* on waking. Deep head pain, beating, shattering, < wind, > dark, closing eyes, pressure; with eructations.

Headache from overlifting or other muscular strain. *Thick, foul, milk crust,* with swollen cervical glands. BIG HEAD WITH LARGE HARD ABDOMEN. VERTEX ICY COLD. Head hot with mental exertion. Cold spot on head. Hydrocephalus, chronic. Burning in vertex, after grief. Sweat, with palpitation. Falling of hair.

EYES: DILATATION OF PUPILS. Sees; visions on closing eyes besides field of vision. Spots and ulcer on cornea. Suppurating fistula. Lacrimation. *Great photophobia.* Itching. Cannot read in gaslight. Feels as if she squinted. Ophthalmia in newborn, after taking cold. Vision dim by constant reading, writing etc. Easy fatigue of eyes. Ulcer of cornea. Opacity of cornea.

EARS: Deafness, from working in water or quinine. Perversion of hearing. Easily bleeding polyp. Aching when blowing nose and coughing. Purulent offensive discharge, and enlarged glands. Illusory noises on swallowing, chewing. Throbbing pain, with sensation of something coming out.

NOSE: Nostrils dry, sore, ulcerated. Coryza, with polyuria. Offensive odor in nose; offensive yellow discharge. *Swelling* of the nose and UPPER LIP, in children. Polyp with loss of smell. Senile catarrh. Sneezes frequently, without a cold. Epistaxis in children inclined to be fat. Obstruction in nose.

FACE: Pale, puffy, pasty. Old, wrinkled. *Swelling of upper lip,* in the morning, with cracks and bleeding. Submaxillary glands swollen. Chewing and swallowing in sleep, in children. Itching eruptions on chin.

MOUTH: Sour taste. Mouth fills with sour water. Ranula under the tongue. Epulis, soft, painless. Tongue dry, at night, does not like to talk. Tip of tongue feels scalded, < warm food. Toothache, < cold air or hot thing.

THROAT: Swelling of tonsils. Goiter. Parotid fistula. Stitching pain on swallowing. Small ulcers spreading up to palate. Uvula swollen, edematous. Hawks salty mucus.

STOMACH: Anorexia from over work. Craving for indigestible things—chalk, coal, slates pencil. Craves eggs, ice-cream, salt and sweets. Aversion to meat, milk, boiled things, fat. Sour eructation, sour vomiting of curdled milk. Loss of appetite, but when he begins to eat he relishes it. Thirst for cold water at night. *Swelling over pit of stomach like an inverted saucer.* Hyper-chlorhydria. Water drunk, if ever so little, causes nausea, but not if iced. Milk disagrees. Sensations as if something rising to head.

ABDOMEN: LARGE AND HARD. Colic, with coldness of thighs, after stopped coryza, or with cold feeling in abdomen. Incarcerated flatulence. Distended, > slightest pressure. Liver region painful < stooping. Gall-stone colic. Peritonitis, when pain > by cold application. Twisting or cramps about umbilical region. Navel sore, excrescences like proud flesh in infant. Mesenteric and inguinal glands swollen and painful. Chalky, gray or green watery stools. Children's diarrhea with ravenous appetite. Stool at first hard, then pasty then liquid. Prolapsus ani, crawling in rectum. Hemorrhoids painful when walking, > sitting. Stool, < eating and drinking. Undigested stools—food eaten is passed without any change. Feels best when constipated. Persistent tenesmus after dysentery. Worms—tape, round. Diarrhea, chronic, after burn.

URINARY: Urine dark, brown, sour, foul or of *strong odor.* White urinary sediment, with milky urine. Urine bloody. Polyp of the bladder. Renal colic. Enuresis, in bed, when walking.

MALE: Increased sexual desire, with retarded erection. Frequent emission. Burning, with seminal emission.

Coition followed by profound weakness, vertigo, irritability, lameness of back and knees, headache and sweat. Itching and burning in genitals. Impotence, from sexual abuse or indulgence. Seminal discharge premature. Hydrocele, of children.

FEMALE: Menses too early (in girls), too profuse, too long; with vertigo, toothache and damp cold feet. Thick, milky, gushing or yellow leukorrhea, < during urination, with itching and burning. Breast tender and swollen, before menses. Abundant milk, but disagreeable to the child. Deficient milk. Sterility, with copious menses. Uterine polyp. Nipples cracked, ulcerated, very tender. Mental excitement brings on dysmenorrhea or causes menses to return. Cramps in toes, or soles, during pregnancy. Menses late in fat, flabby girls, with palpitation, dyspnea and headache. Coition followed by sweat and prostration. Itching and burning in genitals. Absence of menses in plethoric women, from fright. Clumsy, awkward and tired, during pregnancy. Severe stitches in mammae, when nursing.

RESPIRATORY: Painless hoarseness, < morning. Everything makes him *short of breath*. Emphysema. Tickling cough as from dust or feather in throat. Cough, < inspiration, playing on piano, eating. Sharp pains in chest going backward. Purulent, loose, sweet expectoration. Chest very sensitive to touch, percussion or pressure. Suffocative spells. Weak feeling in chest, cannot even speak. Ulcer or abscess in the lung. Habit cough.

HEART: *Weak*. Palpitation, with feeling of coldness, with restless oppression of the chest.

NECK & BACK: Neck pain, < lifting. Pain in back as if sprained, can scarcely rise from his seat. Pain between shoulder blades impeding breathing. Nape of neck stiff and rigid. Cannot sit upright in the chair from weakness of back. Vertebrae feel loose; painful on pressure.

EXTREMITIES: COLD DAMP FEET, feels as if damp stockings were worn. Cold, clammy, hands; cold knees. Cramps in calves when stretching out leg at night. Burning of soles. Soles raw. Arms weak, lame. Hands numb when grasping. Want of mobility of fingers. Creeping on the limbs like from a mouse. Chapped hands. Clumsy, awkward, easily falls. Weakness of ankles in children, turn inward, while walking. Tired from short walk. Swelling of joints esp. knee. Weakness and trembling of limbs. Arthritic; nodosities; deformans.

SKIN: Cold, like snake; flaccid; unhealthy. Small wound does not heal readily. Psoriasis. Urticaria, > in cool air. Visible quivering of skin from head to foot, followed by giddiness. Blood boil, recurring. Milk white spots. Petechial eruption. Chilblain. COLDNESS, ICY, on *vertex*. Cold spot on head or *coldness* of head, hands, knees, feet, affected part.

SLEEP: Sleepless from rush of ideas; some disagreeable idea always arouses from light slumber. *Nightmare;* children scream after midnight and cannot be pacified. Fearful and fantastic dreams. Horrible vision on closing eyes.

FEVER: Chill with thirst. *Coldness, icy,* in different parts of the body, of affected part. Internal heat with external coldness and sweat. Fever with sweat. Sweat cold, partial. Heat, at night, during menses.

COMPLEMENTARY: Bar-c; Lyc; Sil.

CALCAREA FLUORICA

GENERALITIES: This tissue salt relaxes the *Elastic* Fibers; esp. of veins and glands. *Glands enlarge and* BECOME STONY HARD. *Veins dilate and become varicose,* inflamed. It disperses bony growths, osteo-sarcoma, exostosis, after injury. Cephalic-hematoma. *Deficient enamel of teeth.* Removes the tendency to adhesion after operation. *Induration of stony hardness*—tonsils, tumor, in neck, after injury; margins of ulcer etc. Aneurysm. Induration threatening suppuration. Arteriosclerosis. *Fistula. Cataract. Discharges turn grass green.* General stiffness. Weakness, in the morning. Feeling of fatigue all day. Numbness, in different parts. Threatened apoplexy. Sluggish temperament. Nails hypertrophied. X-Ray burn. Stinking pus. Periosteitis of lower jaw, ribs, etc. Congenital syphilis manifesting itself in ulceration of mouth and throat. Nodes in breast.

WORSE: *Beginning of motion.* Cold; wet. Drafts; changing weather. Sprain.

BETTER: Continued motion. Warm application. Heat. Rubbing.

MIND: Indecision. Groundless fear of financial loss. Fear of poverty.

HEAD: Cracking noise in head, disturbing sleep. Cephalic-hematoma, of newborn.

EYES: Aching in eyes, > closing and pressure. Sparks and flickering before the eyes. Phlyctenular keratitis. Subcutaneous palpebral cyst. Cataract. Cornea opaque, in spots.

EARS: Chronic otorrhea. Calcareous deposit on tympanum.

NOSE: Copious, yellowish, thick, lumpy, offensive discharge. Ozena.

FACE: Hard swelling on jaw bone. Hard swelling on the cheek, with pain or toothache. Small, hard, cold sore on lips.

MOUTH: Gumboil, with hard swelling of the jaw. Teeth loose. Tongue indurated, hard. Toothache, if any food touches the tooth. Periosteitis of lower jaw.

THROAT: Tonsils *rough and ragged,* forming plugs of mucus. Pain and burning, > warm drink.

STOMACH: Vomiting of infants, of undigested food. Acute indigestion from fatigue and brain-fag, in overtaxed children. Hiccough, when one hawks off mucus.

ABDOMEN: Flatulence, of pregnancy. Stool gushing, watery, of fetid odor. Bleeding piles, with pain in sacrum. Fissure. Fistula.

MALE: Hydrocele. Testes indurated.

FEMALE: Hard knots in mammae. Favors parturition.

RESPIRATORY: Cough, with expectoration of tiny, tough, yellow lumps. Hoarseness, after laughing or reading aloud. Difficulty in breathing as if epiglottis is nearly closed.

HEART: Fibroid deposits about the endocardium. Valvular disease.

NECK & BACK: Goiter. Lumbago, from strain, > motion and warmth. Backache after a long ride. Rachitic enlargement of femur in infant.

EXTREMITIES: Encysted tumor at the back of wrist. Bursitis. Chronic synovitis; of knee-joint. Cold wrists and ankles. Swelling and induration around tendons and joints. Recurrent fibroid in the hollow of the knee. Hip joint disease. Rice bodies in joints.

SKIN: Cracked, dry, hard, and of alabaster whiteness. Birth mark. Ulcer with hard edges. Warty growths.

SLEEP: Vivid dream, with weeping. Jumps out of bed in a dream.

COMPLEMENTARY: Rhus-t.

RELATED: Graph; Hecla.

CALCAREA HYPOPHOSPHOROSA

GENERALITIES: Hypophosphate of calcium is indicated in those persons who become pale, weak, with violent drenching sweat, rapidly emaciate, with extreme debility, on account of vital loss or continued abscesses having reduced the vitality. Emaciation of children.

WORSE: Vital loss.

MIND: Excitable, nervous and sleepless. Talks rapidly, and easily angered.

EAR: Frying or sizzling in ears.

STOMACH: Ravenous hunger, < 2 hours after meals, > when stomach is full. Loss of appetite.

ABDOMEN: Sore throbbing in spleen. Mesenteric tuberculosis. Diarrhea; of phthisis.

RESPIRATORY: Acute pain in chest. Cough; of phthisis. Bleeding from the lung. Asthma. Bronchitis.

HEART: Angina pectoris. Veins stand out like whip-cord.

EXTREMITIES: Habitually *cold extremities.*

SLEEP: Starts in sleep.

SKIN: Exhausting night-sweat. Acne pustulosa all over the body.

RELATED: Chin.

CALCAREA IODATA

GENERALITIES: It is usually used for induration of glands, suggested by its two components. It can be given in enlarged tonsils filled with little crypts. Thyroid enlargement about the time of puberty. Adenoids. Flabby children subject to cold. Discharges profuse and yellow. Indolent ulcer accompanying varicose veins. Headache while riding in cold wind. Indurated growth in mammae, movable, painful on pressure, and on movement of arm. Profuse sweat.

CALCAREA PHOSPHORICA

GENERALITIES: This tissue remedy, though resembles in many aspects *Calc-carb,* has its own characteristic symptoms. It affects the NUTRITION of bones and glands; bones become *soft, thin and brittle;* it promotes ossification of bones in nonunion of fracture. *Glands are swollen.* It has a special affinity where bones form sutures or symphysis; pain, burning, along sutures. Patient, esp. children are delicate, *tall, thin* or scrawny, with dirty brownish skin. Anaemia, after acute disease or chronic wasting disease. Trembling, or trembling hands, with pain or other complaints. *Coldness or soreness in spot—vertex,* eyeballs, tip of nose, finger etc. Sensation of *crawling and numbness,* after bad news. Anemic children who are peevish, flabby, have cold extremities and weak digestion; they start convulsively when lying on back, > lying on side. They lose breath when they are lifted. Discharges are albuminous. Shifting pain. Arthritis. Rheumatism. Malassimilation. Rickets. Addison's disease. Ill effects of over-growth, lifting, overstudy, sexual excess or irregularities, grief, disappointed love, unpleasant news, operations for fistula, getting wet, girls slow in maturing. Effects of taking cold during 1st menses. Slow ossification, non-union of bones. Idiocy of children. Diabetes. With lung affection.

WORSE: *Exposure to weather* changes. Drafts. Cold; *melting snow. Dentition.* Mental exertion. *Loss of fluid.* Puberty. Fruits, cider. Motion. Thinking of symptoms. Lifting. Ascending.

BETTER: In summer. Warm dry weather. *Lying down.*

MIND: *Peevish, restless and fretful.* Forgetful. Always wants to go somewhere; when away from home wants to go there and when there wants to go to some other place. Idiocy, agile cretinism.

HEAD: Ache; in occiput down spine, > cool bathing, or sneezing. Headache of *school children,* with diarrhea. Burning, < near the *region of sutures.* Feels as if brain was pressed against skull. Delayed closure or reopening of fontanelles. Skull soft and thin, cracking like paper, < at occiput. *Cold or sore vertex.* Head hot, with smarting at the root of hair. Feels as if ice were placed in occiput. Depression on occipital bone. Hydrocephalus. Cannot hold the head up, it wobbles.

EYES: Cool feeling behind the eyes, as if something in there < thinking of it. Diffused opacity of cornea. Cannot use the eyes in gaslight.

EARS: Sudden swelling of external ear. Cold feeling in; noises in; after stools.

NOSE: Tip icy cold. Polyp, large, pedunculated. Coryza, with salivation.

FACE: Pale, yellowish, earthy; full of pimples. Cold sweat on face. Upper lip swollen.

MOUTH: Retarded *dentition.* Teeth, soft, decay easily. Complaints during teething; convulsion without fever.

Teeth sensitive to chewing. Disgusting taste, < in morning on awakening; bitter, with headache.

THROAT: Sore aching in throat; feels hollow. Pain on opening the mouth. Tonsils enlarged. Adenoid growth.

STOMACH: Infant wants to nurse all the time and vomits easily. Craving for raw, salty, piquant food, ham, salted or smoked meat or bacon. Weak digestion, every bite hurts the stomach. Persistently vomits milk, of breast or other. Desire for tobacco smoke which > headache. Vomiting, while hawking mucus, with trembling hands.

ABDOMEN: Colic, at every attempt to eat; by taking ice cream, cold water or fruit. FLABBY, SUNKEN abdomen. Oozing of bloody fluid from navel of infant. *Festering navel.* Tendency to diarrhea, from juicy fruits; during dentition. Stools; foul, hot, lienteric, spluttering, watery, green, slimy, undigested, with fetid flatus. As if something alive in andomen. Fistula in ano, alternating with chest symptom. Fissure of anus in tall, slim children. Hemorrhoids; watery fluid oozing all the time.

URINARY: Urine increased, with sensation of weakness. Pain in region of kidneys, < blowing nose or lifting. Pain in bladder, < when empty.

MALE: Stitching in perineum extending to penis. Erection while riding in carriage, without desire. Weak feeling in sexual organs, after stool.

FEMALE: Menses early, scanty, every two weeks; excessive, bright; in girls too late, with dark blood. Sexual desire increased, before menses, during lactation. Abnormal craving during pregnancy. Burning leukorrhea, albuminous, from one term to another, follows pain in abdomen. Crawling; voluptuous in genitals. Prolapsus; in debilitated women, < while passing urine or stool, during menses, with rheumatic pain. Child refuses breast, milk tastes salty. Uterus heavy, weak, or aching.

Eruption < during menses. Late menses, with violent backache. Tumors in mammae (left), painful on pressure. Mammae sore, feel large.

RESPIRATORY: Child loses breath on being lifted up. Cough, > lying; cough during dentition. Involuntary sighing. Phthisis; with cavities, with night-sweat, yellow expectoration. *Pain in chest from draft.* Must scrape mucus from larynx before one can sing or talk. Whooping cough, obstinate.

HEART: Dropsy from heart disease. Palpitation, with trembling weakness in calf.

NECK & BACK: *Neck painful from drafts.* Neck *weak, thin,* head bobs about. Curvature of the spine to the left. Violent pain, < least effort, screams, with pain. Sacrum numb and lame. Lumbar vertebrae bend to the left. Spina bifida. Pott's disease.

EXTREMITIES: Rheumatism in cold season. Fingertips sore. Sensation as of a splinter under the nail. Buttocks numb. Weakness through the hips. Hipjoint disease. Cold limbs with digestive trouble. Pain, burning, along edges of nails. Hard bluish lumps in axillae. Trembling of arms and hands, with many complaints. Fistulous ulcer on ankle joint.

SLEEP: Constant stretching and yawning. Children cry in sleep. Cannot awaken in early morning.

SKIN: Dark, brown, yellow. Scars from amputation, ulcerate. Ulceration from mustard poultice.

FEVER: Easily chilled. Chilly with pain. Chills up the back, but heat down the back. Sticky sickly sweat, < head and throat; at night.

COMPLEMENTARY: Hep; Ruta.

RELATED: Carb-an; Chin; Ferr-p; Nat-m.

CALCAREA SULPHURICA

GENERALITIES: It is Schuessler's CONNECTIVE TISSUE remedy. Affects *glands, mucous membranes,* bones and skin. Torpid glandular swelling. Cystic tumor. Fibroid. *Tendency to suppuration,* after pus has found its vent, comes within the range of this remedy. *Pus is thick, yellow,* lumpy, bloody. *Mucous discharges are yellow, thick and lumpy.* Recurrent or running *Abscess.* Ulcer malignant, corneal, deep. Fistula. Pains are cutting. Poor reaction. Infant with bloody coryza, diarrhea or eczema. Burn and scald, after suppuration starts. Malignant growth after ulceration has set in.

WORSE: *Draft*; Touch; Cold; wet. Heat of room.

BETTER: *Open air. Bathing.* Eating. Heat (local). Uncovering.

MIND: Hurried. Despises those who do not agree with him. Grumbling that his value is not understood by others. Sits and meditates over imaginary misfortune.

HEAD: Scald head of children, with purulent yellow discharge.

EYES: Conjunctivitis, with discharge of thick yellow matter. Red, itching tarsi.

EARS: Flow of dark wax. Pimples around the ear. Otitis after a slap.

NOSE: Bloody coryza of infants. Sneezing, > open air.

FACE: Pimples and pustules on the face.

MOUTH: Tongue flabby. Taste soapy.

ABDOMEN: Diarrhea of children, with discharge of pus or bloody pus. Stool, coated white. Painful abscess about anus in case of fistula. Diarrhea after maple sugar.

URINARY: Pyelitis. Chronic nephritis.

FEMALE: Thick white leukorrhea. Cutting pain in (right) ovary. Menses late, long-lasting.

RESPIRATORY: Choking croup. Empyema.

EXTREMITIES: Foot-sweat foul, cold. Burning, itching, in soles.

SKIN: *Unhealthy*; cuts, wounds, etc. *would not heal.* Dry eczema, < in infants.

SLEEP: Starts from sleep, as if wanting air.

FEVER: Hectic fever caused by formation of pus. Averse to cover when cold. Dry heat at night. Easy sweating, < coughing.

RELATED: Hep; Sil.

CALENDULA

GENERALITIES: It acts on MUSCLES, *spine*, liver, and is a remarkable healing agent in open, torn, *cut, lacerated, ragged or suppurating* wound; *pain is excessive, and out of proportion* to the injury. Hemorrhage; in scalp wound, after tooth extraction. Disposition to take cold. *Prevents pyemia.* Sensitive to damp or open air. Cancer, as an intercurrent remedy. Application of sponge saturated with hot solution of Calendula after delivery gives the greatest comfort to the patient. Paralysis after apoplexy. Promotes healthy granulation and rapid healing by first instance. Prevents gangrene.

WORSE: Damp, cloudy weather. During chill.

BETTER: Walking about or lying perfectly still.

MIND: Extremely nervous, easily frightened, starts with fright.

HEAD: Weight on brain.

EYES: Blenorrhea of lacrimal sac; yellow vision.

EARS: Hears best in a train, and distant sounds. Hearing acute.

NOSE: Coryza in one nostril, with much green discharge.

THROAT: Painful swelling of submaxillary gland, < on moving head.

STOMACH: Heartburn, with horripilation (goose-flesh). Nausea in chest. Hiccough when smoking.

ABDOMEN: Epigastric distention. Stools curdy. Jaundice. Stretching and dragging in groins.

MALE: Excoriation of prepuce after coition.

FEMALE: Warts at os cervix; os lower than normal. Hypertrophied uterus. Menorrhagia. Profuse offensive discharge after forceps delivery.

BACK: Bruised pain at angle of right scapula. Cold hands.

SKIN: Yellow. Horripilation.

FEVER: Coldness. Great sensitiveness to open air. Shuddering in back, with warm skin. Heat in evening.

RELATED: Arn; Bell-p.

CAMPHORA

GENERALITIES: Coldness, cramps and convulsions, with mental anguish are the marked features of Camphor indications. Convulsion with blue lips, froth at mouth and lockjaw. It is a remedy for sudden collapse, from over-powering influence acting on nerve centres. Patient becomes ICY COLD; YET HE IS AVERSE TO COVER, or wants it off and on, with *internal burning heat and anxiousness. Sudden weakness*, fainting spells growing worse. Dry collapse, little vomiting and purging, in cholera. *Tetanic* spasm with showing of the teeth, with retraction of the lips, followed by stupor with coldness. Trismus of newborn. Chilly at the start of cold. *Scanty or retained discharges. Very sensitive to cold air or easy taking of cold.* Suppressed eruption. Awkwardness. Soft parts drawn in. Ill-effects, of shock from injury, operation, sunstroke. Vexation. Corrects spoiled cases and antidotes most medicines (specially vegetable ones). DIGESTIVE TRACT, Cerebro-Spinal nerves, urinary organs and nose are prominently affected. Feeling of hot waves during pain, with restlessness.

WORSE: *Cold, draft. When half-asleep.* Mental exertion. Shock. Suppression. Inattention. Motion. Night.

BETTER: *Free discharge. Sweat. Thinking of it.* Drinking cold water.

MIND: *Insensibility*, vanishing of all senses or anxiety. Awkwardness. Loss of memory. Delirium. Mania—religious, puerperal. Wants to jump out of bed or window. Does not like anyone near him. Nothing satisfies him. Excited, talks constantly, scolds in indecent language. Feeling that she is going to die, relieved, when she finds herself alive. Attacks of anguish at night. State of frenzy, hysterical—scratches, spits, bites, tears her clothes. Screams and calls for help. Closes her eyes and answers no question.

HEAD: Feels knotted up. Occiput throbbing, synchronous with the pulse, > standing; when deprived of sexual intercourse. Fleeting stitches in temples and orbits. Head is drawn to one side (in spasm). Pain runs from head to tip of fingers.

EYES: Objects appear too bright, or move to one side with a jerk. Fixed, staring, turned upwards or outwards. Pupils dilated. Eyes protrude, with mania. Eyes deeply sunken.

EARS: Ear lobes hot and red.

NOSE: Cold and pinched. *Coryza*; in old age. Inhaled air seems cold. Persistent epistaxis, with goose-flesh state of the skin.

FACE: Haggard, pale, bluish, old, pinched. Pale and red by turn. Cold sweat. Upper lip retracted. Lockjaw. Distorted. Grimace. Froth or foam at the mouth.

MOUTH: Tongue bluish, cold, trembling. Speech broken, feeble, hoarse. Cold breath. Boiling hot tea seems cold. Toothache, > beer.

STOMACH: Burning thirst. Burning in stomach, in abdomen. Asiatic cholera. Little vomiting or purging, with dry collapse. Rice water stools. Vomiting in morning, bilious, sour.

URINARY: Strangury. Hematuria. Retention.

MALE: Sexual excitement. Satyriasis. Priapism, during dreams. Impotence.

FEMALE: Sexual desire increased. Hot flushes with coldness of abdomen and limbs, at climaxis. Constantly bares her breasts; mania.

RESPIRATORY: Asphyxia neonatorum. Hoarse, squeaking voice. Cold breath. Suspended respiration. Violent attacks of dry cough.

HEART: Pulse weak, not perceptible, frequent, small. Palpitation after eating.

EXTREMITIES: Thumbs drawn backward. Cramps in calves. Cracking in joints. Cold, numb, tingling. Feet cold, pain as if sprained.

SKIN: Dry; livid. Blue, *cold*, cannot bear to be covered. *Erysipelas*. All sequelae of measles.

SLEEP: Insomnia with cold limbs. Very restless. Comatose sleep.

FEVER: Shaking chill with *cold skin;* wants covers during the hot stage only. Sudden inflammatory fevers, with rapid alternation of heat and cold, followed by rapid prostration. Heat or sweat, > covering. Chilly, below scapula, before colds. Sweats when covered, body becomes cold when uncovered.

COMPLEMENTARY: Canth.

RELATED: Carb-v; Cupr; Op; Sec.

CANCER FLUVIATILIS (Astacus fluviatilis)

GENERALITIES: Commonly known as river crab or crawfish. The tincture is prepared from the whole animal. It markedly affects the liver and lymphatic glands. It produces URTICARIA, with *liver* complaints; jaundice of children. Itching in various parts. Crusta lactea, with enlarged lymphatic glands. Enlarged glands of neck in children and old people. *Stinging pains* are felt in various parts. Inward chilliness or shivering. Nervous crawl over the body. *Erysipelas,* with nettlerash. Cramp in liver region, liver inflamed, < pressure. Cough, > when walking but returns as soon as he sits down. Violent fever, with headache; red glowing face. It constricts and may completely close both duodenum and esp. the opening of the gall duct into the duodenum.

WORSE: Air. Uncovering.

RELATED: Calc; Rhus-t.

CANNABIS INDICA & SATIVA

GENERALITIES: *Cannabis indica* is used as an intoxicant. It produces most marked effects on MIND and EMOTION, which are EXALTED INTENSELY, and in which CONCEPTIONS AND PERCEPTIONS ARE EXAGGERATED to the utmost degree. Patient experiences the most *wonderful hallucinations and imaginations,* feels very happy and contented, or sometimes the hallucinations may be of agonizing terror and pain. Sense of proportion or sense of time and space is lost. Mania of grandeur. Levitation. Gaiety; uncontrollable laughter. Violence. Delirium tremens. Feels weak and all gone to nothing. Exophthalmic goiter. Catalepsy. When URINARY AND SYMPTOMS *of acute gonorrhea* are most marked *Cann-s.* should be used in preference to Cann-i. *Trickling* sensation as if hot water were poured over him or *as if drops of cold water were falling*—on head, from the anus, *from the heart,* is found in Cann-s. Paralysis, with tingling of the affected part.

WORSE: URINATING (*Cann-s.*). DARKNESS. *Exertion.* Talking. Walking. Coffee. Liquor. Tobacco. Lying down and going upstairs (*Cann-s.*).

BETTER: Fresh air. Cold water. Rest.

MIND: *Loquacity.* Very forgetful cannot finish the sentence. Time seems too long. Distance seems immense. Craves light. Lectophobia (*Cann-s.*), fear of going to bed. Laughs immoderately, at serious remark, or at mere trifle. Laughs and weeps. Ecstatic, heavenly. Hears; voices, bells, music. Fixed idea, *extreme psychic mobility.* Thinks everything is unreal. Clairvoyance. When he speaks it seems as though someone else is speaking. Moaning and crying.

HEAD: Violent headache; with hallucination. *Vertex seems to open and shut,* < noise. Head seems separated from the body. Involuntary shaking of the head. Shocks through brain.

EYES: Fixed gaze. Letters run together while reading. Weak vision. Sees objects outside of visual field. Opacity of cornea (*Cann-s.*).

EAR: Noise like boiling water.

FACE: Skin of the face seems tight. Dejected and careworn. Lips glued together. Chin drawn to sternum.

MOUTH: *Grinding* of teeth in sleep. Saliva white, thick, frothy. Stammering and stuttering. Every article of food is extremely palatable. Aversion to meat of which she was previously fond (*Cann-s.*).

ABDOMEN: Feels something alive in abdomen. Sensation in anus as if sitting on a ball. Throbbing here and there.

URINARY: Pain in kidney, while laughing. Must strain to urinate; has to wait for some time before the urine flows; urine dribbles after flow ceases. SCANTY BURNING URINE PASSED DROP BY DROP, with pain going backwards (to bladder). Acute stage of gonorrhea, urethra sensitive, walks with legs apart (*Cann-s.*). Nephritic colic. Urethral caruncle.

MALE: Swollen prepuce. Sexual desire increased. Priapism. Erection without amorous thought.

FEMALE: Profuse menses, with violent uterine colic, with dysuria. Sexual desire increased in sterile women or with dysmenorrhea. Threatened abortion, from too frequent sexual intercourse, or complicated with gonorrhea. (*Cann-s.*). Infantile leukorrhea (*Cann-s.*).

RESPIRATORY: Humid asthma. Difficulty in breathing with palpitation, > standing up (*Cann-s.*). Cannot control voice. Suffocative attacks.

HEART: Palpitation wakes him. Pulse slow. Sensation as if drops were falling from the heart (*Cann-s.*).

BACK: Pain across shoulder and spine, must stoop, cannot walk erect. Torticollis, chin drawn to the sternum.

EXTREMITIES: Pain in the limbs, < deep breathing. Paralysis of lower limbs. Contraction of fingers, after sprain (Cann-s.). Feels very exhausted after a short walk. Feels as if bird's claws were clasping the knees. Dislocation of patella on going upstairs (*Cann-s.*).

SLEEP: Dreams erotic, of the dead. Sleepy but cannot sleep.

ANTIDOTE: Ap. is.

CANTHARIS

GENERALITIES: Commonly known as Spanish fly, it attacks THE URINARY AND SEXUAL ORGANS, perverting their function, and setting violent inflammation, causing frenzied delirium. Its action is *rapid and intense.* INFLAMMATIONS ARE VIOLENTLY ACUTE, or *rapidly destructive*, in the mucous and serous membranes. PAINS ARE CUTTING, SMARTING OR BURNING BITING, or *as if raw,* causing mental excitement. Discharges are bloody, acrid, watery, tenacious. Sudden attack of weakness that takes the voice away. Serous effusion. Nephritis, acute parenchymatous. Expels moles, dead fetus, placenta; promotes fecundity. Hemiplegia of (R) side with aphasia. In any condition when the urine is scanty, with cutting and burning, *Canth* should be considered. Convulsions, with dysuria and hydrophobic symptoms. Excitement during pain. Valuable remedy for *burn and scald.* Painful urination, as a concomitant in any diseased condition.

WORSE: URINATING. *Drinking. Cold. Bright objects. Sound of water.* Touch, esp. in larynx. Coffee.

BETTER: Warmth. Rest. Rubbing.

MIND: Amorous frenzy. Acute mania, of sexual type. Excessive sexual desire, not > by coition. Paroxysm of rage with crying, barking, biting, < by bright object, by touching the larynx, drinking cold water. Sudden loss of consciousness, with red face (dentition). Constantly attempts to do something but accomplishes nothing. Sings lewd songs. Prattles about genitals, urine, feces. Insolent, contradictory mood.

HEAD: Sensation of burning or boiling water in brain. Head heavy; aches from bathing or washing. Hairfall when combing.

EYES: Objects look yellow. Fiery, sparkling, staring look.

EARS: Sensation as if wind were coming from ear, or hot air.

FACE: Pale, wretched, death-like pallor. Expression of extreme suffering, terror or despair. Hot and red. Itching vesicles on face. Jaws tightly closed; acute mania.

MOUTH: Grinding of the teeth, with lock-jaw. Burning in mouth, pharynx and throat. Swollen, *tremulous tongue;* edges raw. Saliva disgustingly sweet.

THROAT: As if on *fire.* Painfully constricted; great difficulty in swallowing liquids. Full of blisters.

STOMACH: *Burning thirst,* but aversion to all fluids. Violent retching and vomiting. Sensitiveness over stomach; slightest pressure produces convulsion. Aggravation from drinking coffee, even in small quantity. Aversion to everything.

ABDOMEN: Violent burning pain throughout the whole intestinal tract, with painful sensitiveness to touch.

SHREDDY BURNING STOOL, *with tenesmus of rectum and bladder,* shuddering after stools. Dysentery or diarrhea with dysuria. Cutting in rectum, partially > by flatus, entirely by stool. Constipation, with retention of urine. Desire for stool while urinating.

URINARY: Kidney region *very sensitive.* URINE BURNING, SCALDING; WITH CUTTING, INTOLERABLE URGING, AND FEARFUL TENESMUS OR DRIBBLING. STRANGURY. Dysuria. Bloody urine. Griping in bladder. Acute nephritis; nephritic colic; cystitis. Dropsy. Renal colic, > somewhat by pressure on glans penis. Atony of bladder, from long retention of urine.

MALE: Painful swelling of genitals. Priapism. Pulls at penis. *Sexual desire increased,* not > by coitus. Bloody semen. Pollution. Gonorrhea. Burning in urethra, after coition.

FEMALE: Nymphomania. Cutting, burning, in ovaries; ovaritis. Menses too early, too profuse, blood black or scanty. Breasts painful, with dysuria. Expels moles, dead fetus and placenta. Pruritus, with strong sexual desire; at climaxis. Leukorrhea, with sexual excitement, causing itching and masturbation.

RESPIRATORY: Voice hoarse, feeble. Tenacious mucus in air passages. Short, dry coughing spells. Pleurisy with exudation. Chest pain, > eructation. Burning in chest. Stitches at sternum.

HEART: Tendency to syncope. Pericarditis with effusion. Pulse; feeble, irregular.

BACK: Emprosthotonos and opisthotonos. Pain in loins with frequent desire to urinate.

EXTREMITIES: Knees totter when ascending steps. Ulcerative pain in soles, cannot step.

SKIN: Vesicular eruption, turning black, with burning and itching. Erysipelas, vesicular. Burns and scalds, > cold water. Tendency to gangrene. Eruptions burn when touched.

FEVER: Chilly, as if cold water poured over him, during stool. Hands and feet cold. Urinous sweat, on genitals.

COMPLEMENTARY: Apis.

RELATED: Apis; Ars; Merc-c.

CAPSICUM

GENERALITIES: It acts with great intensity on the *Mucous membranes,* and also on the bones, esp. *Mastoid.* Mucous membranes become dark, red, spongy or ooze bloody mucus. Pains are BURNING SMARTING, pungent or *strangling, threadlike,* < by cold water. Sensation of SORENESS and constriction. It seems suitable to those persons who are of *lax fibres,* weak, *lazy,* indolent, *fat, red, clumsy, awkward* and of *unclean habits.* Such persons are opposed to physical exertion, averse to go outside of their routine and get *home sick* easily. Old people who have exhausted their vitality, esp. by mental work and poor living. Patients *react poorly and are afraid of cold.* Abstainers from accustomed *alcohol.* Discharges are foul. Myalgia. Neuralgia. Deep abscess. The circulation is sluggish and the parts pinched remain in raised position for a long time. *Shuddering,* during pain or drinking.

WORSE: SLIGHT DRAFT, *even warm.* COLD AIR; water. Uncovering. Dampness. Bathing. Empty swallowing. *Drinking,* < throat or excites urination. After eating. Drunkards.

BETTER: Continued motion. Heat. While eating.

MIND : Capricious and changeable mood. *Homesick,* with red face and sleeplessness, and disposition to suicide. Peevish, irritable, angry, easily offended. Clumsy. Awkward; runs into everything. Refractory, esp. children. Dipsomania. Jocular and singing, yet at slightest cause gets angry. Always on the lookout for insult. If she wants from sometime a certain thing, she will oppose it if proposed by someone else. Laughs and weeps alternately.

HEAD: Bursting headache, < coughing, > heat, movement, lying with head high.

EYES: Objects appear black. Eyes prominent, with burning and lacrimation, during cough.

EARS: Affected alternately. Swelling and pain behind the ears. Mastoiditis. Tenderness over petrous bones. Hot ears. Otalgia, then deafness. Affection of ears during pregnancy. Tympanum perforated.

NOSE: RED BUT COLD; tip very hot. Nose-bleed in the morning; in bed.

FACE: RED, BUT COLD or pale and red alternately. Pain in fine line coursing along the nerve. Lips swollen, cracked, burning.

MOUTH: Vesicles or flat painful aphthae. Stomatitis. Fetid odor from the mouth. TONGUE GREENISH AT BASE. Gums hot, spongy, retracted. *Burning-smarting at the tip of tongue.* Saliva increased. Taste foul like putrid water, sour to food.

THROAT: *Burning-smarting in throat.* Constriction of throat with urging to swallow. Sore throat of smokers and drinkers. Pain and dryness extending to ears. *Uvula swollen,* elongated, with sensation as if it were pressing on something hard. Hot pungent air comes up from the throat, tasting foul when coughing. Pain when coughing. Paralytic dysphagia.

STOMACH: Craves stimulating, pungent things; wants a bracer. Much thirst but drinking causes shuddering. Waterbrash. *Acid dyspepsia;* burning or trembling in stomach, or icy coldness, or as if filled with cold water. Desire for coffee, but it nauseates. Vegetables cause flatulence.

ABDOMEN: Flatulent colic. Colic about umbilicus with mucous stool. Small, hot, burning, bloody mucous stool, with tenesmus of rectum and bladder, then thirst < *drinking. Burning piles;* bleeding, with soreness in anus. Dysentery. Violent pulsation of arteries in abdomen. Mucous diarrhea.

URINARY: Frequent, almost ineffectual urging to urinate. Strangury. Burning orifice. Urine comes first in drops, then in spurts. Thick white creamy discharge from urethra; gonorrhea. Drinking excites urination and stool. Meatus everted.

MALE: Scrotum cold, and shrivelled. Atrophy, softening of testes, with loss of sensibility; spermatic cord shrivelled. Excessive burning pain in prostate; gonorrhea. Trembling of the whole body during amorous caress. Prepuce swollen. Cramp in testes, after emission.

FEMALE: Climacteric disturbances, with burning of tip of tongue. Pushing or sticking sensation in left ovarian region, with disorders of menses. Menorrhagia, with nausea.

RESPIRATORY: Wants to take deep breath, thinking that it would relieve all her symptoms. *Cough causes distant pain;* in bladder, ear, leg etc. or raises foul air, > drinking cold water. Too weak to cough out phlegm. Constriction of chest arrests breathing. Hoarseness, in singers and preachers. Asthma with redness of face, < ascending. Ribs seem dislocated. Gangrene, of lung.

BACK: Lumbar pain after stool. Pain in sacrum with piles and dysentery. Pain in the back while drinking water. Sensation as if cold water were dropping down back.

EXTREMITIES: Joints crack, are stiff, painful on beginning to move; pain as if paralysed. Pain from hips to heel, < *coughing*. Sciatica, < bending backwards and coughing. Leg (left) atrophied, with violent pain. Staggers when walking.

SLEEP: Sleeplessness, from emotion, from homesickness, or from cough. Sleepy after meal. Sensation as if falling from a height during sleep. Yawning by day.

SKIN: Burning. Bloated, flabby.

FEVER: *Chilly, with the pain.* Chill begins in back with violent thirst, but *shivers from every drink,* with excruciating backache. Chill alternating with heat mounting to head, then sweat. Coldness of affected part. Sweats easily. Cold sweat on thighs. Fever; after emotions, with; homesickness.

COMPLEMENTARY: Nat-m.

RELATED: Canth.

CARBO ANIMALIS

GENERALITIES: Carb-an or animal charcoal is made from charred ox-hide; it contains Calcium phosphate in small quantity. It is suitable for *old persons of feeble constitution* or those whose vitality becomes low on account of some serious, or deep seated diseased condition, or loss of fluid. *Patient is susceptible to cold and gets sprained easily. They are over-affected by small vital losses.* On account of venous stasis, *the skin becomes blue. Glands enlarge,* slowly and *painfully,* and *become indurated.* Burning like fire. Tendency to malignancy.

Ulceration, decomposition. *Discharges are acrid and foul.* Sensation of looseness, crawling as of bugs. Gumma. Neglected bubo. Weakness of nursing women, they weep while eating, unable to walk even across the room. Stitch remaining after pleurisy. Hemorrhage. Copper coloured eruption. Slow, *hard, painful* processes. More deep-acting than *Carbo-v.* Ill- effects of eating spoiled fish or decayed vegetable.

WORSE: *Slight causes;* small loss of vital fluids; sprain, lifting. Taking cold. *Dry, cold air.* After menses. Shaving. While EATING.

BETTER: Laying hand on affected part.

MIND: *Whining.* Desire to be alone. Sad and reflective. Avoids conversation. Weeps during meal. Easily frightened. Homesick. Fear of the dark, < closing eyes.

HEAD: Brain feels loose , < motion and coughing. Feels as if skull had been split or blown to pieces; must press it with both hands, > eating. Throbbing headache, after menses. Vertigo followed by nosebleed. Vertigo, after shaving, > reeling.

EYES: Pain moves down through (R) eyeball. Sensation as if something lay above eyes, so that she could not look up. Eye- ball feels loose in the socket. Objects seem to be far off. Dimness of vision when reading, > rubbing eyes. Senile cataract.

EARS: Does not know from what direction the sound comes. Ringing in ears, when blowing the nose. Parotid gland swollen. Lancinating pain. Otorrhea, with swelling of mastoid.

NOSE: Hard, red, swollen, hot, with itching pimples and desquamation. Brown stripe across the nose. Hard, bluish tumor on tip of nose. Fluent coryza, with loss of smell, with yawning and sneezing.

FACE: Bluish cheeks and lips. Copper colored eruption. Acne. Large number of pimples.

MOUTH: Knotty induration in the tongue. Bites cheeks while eating. Teeth loose, < chewing and least cold. Toothache, > eating salty things.

THROAT: Raw feeling like heartburn > eating.

STOMACH: Eating causes fatigue. Saltish water runs from the mouth. Retching, vomiting; hiccough; cancer. Faint, gone feeling in stomach not > by eating, in suckling women. All food distresses the stomach. Nausea, from smoking, which causes aversion to tobacco. Digestion weak. Nausea, < at night; nausea of pregnancy. Sensation of coldness around the stomach, > rubbing and pressure.

ABDOMEN: Great distension; after operation. Feels as if a hard body is in groin (left), < sitting, > pressure and passing flatus. Neglected bubo. Anus sore. Moisture oozing from anus, and on perineum. Feeling of coldness rising into the throat. Induration of pancreas.

MALE: Syphilis. Bubo.

FEMALE: Menses; dark, clotted, putrid; flow in morning only, followed by great exhaustion, so weak can hardly speak. Right ovary seems a heavy ball. Leukorrhea watery; burning, biting, < walking or standing; stains linen yellow. Cancer uteri; burning pain down thighs; pelvic bones pain on sitting. Indurated os, with burning. Darting pain in mammae, while nursing, arresting breathing. Painful induration in breast (right). Hard painful nodes in breast. Uterine hemorrhage, with affections of glands. Lochia; long lasting, thin, offensive, with numb limbs.

RESPIRATORY: Suffocation on closing eyes. Nervous dyspnea. Ulceration of lung, with feeling of coldness in lungs. Cough with discharge of greenish pus. Stitch remaining after pleurisy. Sputum dark, brown, tough, syrup-like.

HEART: Palpitation when hearing singing in church, or in public places. Coldness in precordial region, with horripilation (goose-flesh).

BACK: Coccyx feels bruised, burns when touched, < sitting or lying. Coldness and aching in lumbar region, with cough.

EXTREMITIES: Axillary glands swollen, indurated. Ankles turn easily. Hands numb, with chest affection. Joints weak, easy dislocation.

SKIN: *Bluish* affected part. Spongy ulcer. Copper-colored eruptions. Unsightly scars from eruptions.

SLEEP: Full of vivid fancies. Talks, groans, sheds tears in sleep.

FEVER: Surgings or hot flushes. Sweat; foul, exhausting, at night, *staining yellow.*

COMPLEMENTARY: Calc-p.

RELATED: Calc-fl; Graph.

CARBO VEGETABILIS

GENERALITIES: *Carbo-veg,* or charcoal, is itself a product of imperfect oxidation. Therefore imperfect oxidation and disintegration is the key-note of this remedy. It contains small quantity of Potassium carbonate. Its deodorant, disi tant and antiseptic properties are more enhanced in potencies. It acts upon the VENOUS CIRCULATION, esp. capillaries, where blood seems to stagnate, causing blueness, coldness and ecchymoses. *Vital power becomes low* from loss of vital fluid, *from grave or serious diseases, from effect of drug and disease* or from obstinate complications. It is suitable to atonic conditions where *there is lack of reaction.* The typical Carbo-veg. patient is fat, sluggish, lazy and has a tendency to chronicity of complaints. Complaints of old people. Persons who have never fully recovered from the effect of some previous illness. State of collapse, in cholera, typhoid, or other grave diseases, when the patient is almost lifeless, with cold body, breath cold, pulse imperceptible, respiration quickened, must be fanned very hard, *but head remains hot.* HEMORRHAGE; blood dark, oozing; from shock, after surgical operation, persistent for hours or days. Numbness, of parts lain on. *Burning; sense of weight or heavy aching* in bones, ulcer etc. WEAKNESS, FLATULENCE, *Fetor, or Air Hunger,* are present with most of the complaints. *Tremulous.* Always WEAK, SICK AND EXHAUSTED, but these states may occur suddenly. Fainting fits. *Thick acrid discharges. Cold, but wants to be fanned,* or thirst for cold water. BLUENESS and *decomposition.* Septic condition. *Sensation* of *overfulness. Venous stasis. Ulceration,* aphthous. General bruised soreness, old catarrh. Schoolgirls and boys are sluggish, slow to learn, suffer from night terror, will not sleep alone or go to bed in the dark. Lack of reaction, after some violent attack, violent shock, violent suffering. Never well since. Lymphatic glands swollen, indurated or suppurating. Gangrene, humid, senile.

WORSE: WARMTH. DEPLETION. *Cooling off.* EXHAUSTING DISEASE. HIGH LIVING; RICH FOOD; decayed food; poultry. DISSIPATION. Over-lifting. Walking in open air. Pressure of clothes. Extremes of temperature; cold night air; frosty, humid wind on head. Suppression. Old age. Reading.

BETTER: ERUCTATIONS. *Cool air. From fanning.* Elevating feet. Singing loud. Icy drink.

MIND: Slow thinking. *Indolent.* Anxious. *Irritable.* Dejected. Unhappy. Indifference, hears everything without pleasure or pain. Aversion to darkness. Fear of ghosts. Sudden loss of memory. Sluggish, stupid, lazy. Easily frightened or startled.

HEAD: Dull, compressive, heavy headache, < occiput; < overheating, lying or pressure of hat, over-indulgence. Vertigo, with nausea and tinnitus. Scalp itches when warm in bed. Hair sore, falls off easily, in handfuls, after severe illness, after parturition. Cold sweat on forehead. Head hot; with cold extremities. Takes cold in head easily.

EYES: Sensation of heavy weight on eyes. Hemorrhage from eyes with congestion to head. Vision of floating black spots. Burning in eyes. Muscles of eyes pain when looking up. Pupils do not react to light.

EARS: Something heavy seems to lie before the ears. Deafness or otorrhea, following exanthemata. Deficient or badly smelling yellow wax. Mumps, with metastasis.

NOSE: Sneezing from irritation in larynx, < blowing nose. Ineffectual effort to sneeze. Epistaxis in daily attacks, with pale face. Descending cold. Red. Rose cold; hay asthma. Frequent sneezing, much coryza. Sneezing < sneezing.

FACE: PINCHED, HIPPOCRATIC or *dusky*. Face cold, with cold sweat. *Twitching upper lip.* Brown or blackish looking, cracked lips. Great paleness of face.

MOUTH: Breath cold. Tongue cold, black swollen, covered with white yellow-brown mucus. Aphthae; bluish, blackish ulcer, with burning. Loose teeth. Scorbutic gums. Blood oozes from gums when cleaning teeth. Pyorrhea. Taste bitter, sour. Bad smell. Increased saliva. Gums painful while chewing. Gums black. Teeth pain while eating hot or cold things.

THROAT: Sensation as if closed. Aphthous, sore. Hawking of bloody black mucus. Painful on swallowing food.

STOMACH: Digestion slow, food turns into gas. Aversion to meat, fat, to milk which causes flatulence. Loathes even the thought of food. Desire for salty-sour or sweet things, coffee. Nausea in the morning. ERUCTATIONS RANCID, *Loud; without* >; with cough. Heaviness, fullness and sleepiness after food. Contractive pain extending to chest. Burning in stomach extending to back along spine, with coldness. Gastralgia of nursing women. Dyspepsia. Aversion to most digestible and the best kind of food. Vomiting of blood; ulcer, cancer.

ABDOMEN: EXCESSIVE FLATULENCE, greatly distending the abdomen, esp. *Upper part,* < lying down. Obstructed flatus, with complaints arising from it. The simplest or smallest amount of food < the suffering in abdomen. Colic forcing the patient to bend double. Epigastric region very tender. Pain in the liver. Cannot bear tight clothing around the waist. Abdomen feels as if hanging down, walks bent. Burning in rectum. Itching in anus. Flatus hot, moist, offensive. Acrid moisture from rectum. Moisture on perineum. Bluish, white, burning piles, pain after stool. Colic brought on by riding in car, > passing flatus. Painful diarrhea of old people. Stool putrid; ineffectual urging; even soft stool passed with difficulty. Feces escape with flatus. Jaundice; from overeating or eating too rich food.

URINARY: Albumin in the urine. Nephritis, septic or from alcohol. Urine copious, of clear yellow color or thickish and whitish. Diabetes. Wetting the bed at night. Urine; suppressed in cholera; retained from standing on cold pavement.

MALE: Seminal discharge too soon during coitus, followed by roaring in head. Discharge of prostatic fluid, while straining at stool. Itching and moisture at thighs near scrotum. Swelling of testes from metastasis of mumps.

FEMALE: Menorrhagia, burning across sacrum, passive flow. Sore, hot, itching, swollen vulva. Leukorrhea thick, greenish, milky, causing itching and burning, < before menses. Lumps in mammae, with induration of axillary glands. Mammae; hard, swollen, with impending abscess. Feels at her best when she has a free leukorrhea. Menses too early. Varices on pudendum and vulva, with burning, bluish ulcer. Prostration after suckling. Vaginal fistula, burning pains.

RESPIRATORY: Voice hoarse in the evening. Cough, with itching in larynx. Attacks of tormenting hollow or choking cough, with headache and vomiting, and burning in chest, < cold drink and in bed. Roughness in larynx, with deep rough voice. Expectoration with retching. Whooping cough, with bluish face and its complications. Heavy, sore or weak chest, on awakening. Breathing laborious, quick and short, < walking. Asthma in aged with blue skin, > summer. Cheyne-Stokes breathing in organic heart disease. Wants to take a deep breath. Burning in chest, with hemoptysis. Brown yellow spots on chest. Destructive lung disease. Sore ribs. Expectoration thick, sticky, yellowish and profuse.

HEART: Continuous anxious palpitation; < eating, sitting. Pulse; thread like, weak and small, intermittent. Burning around the heart. Pulsation throughout the body.

BACK: Severe pain in small of back, with sensation of a plug, unable to sit down, had to put a pillow under it when lying. Burning behind shoulder.

EXTREMITIES: Heavy, stiff, feels paralyzed. Numb when lying on them. Paralytic weakness of the wrists and fingers, when seizing anything. Arms weary when writing. Cramp in soles. Feet numb and sweaty. Cold from knees down. Senile gangrene of fingers and toes, with fiery burning vesicles, oozing bloody water. Foul foot sweat, < walking.

SKIN: Raw, mottled, blue, cold, ecchymosed. Ulcers; foul, burning and bleeding. Varicose ulcers. Carbuncle. Senile gangrene beginning in toes. Bed sores, bleed easily. Varicose veins during pregnancy. Wounds heal and break out again. Burning in various places. Blue color. Fine moist rash with burning. Ulcers; varicose, easily bleeding, pus smelling like asafoetida, heal and break out again.

SLEEP: Horror during sleep. Awakes often, from cold limbs, esp. cold knees. Unrefreshing. Comatose sleep, with rattling in throat. Frequent yawning and stretching which seems to >.

FEVER: Alternate chill and heat. ICY COLDNESS, unilateral, of tongue, *knees*, legs, feet, at night. Warm head and cold limbs. *Internal burning heat,* at heart, chest, with cold icy skin and cold sweat. Sweats easily. Sweat sour, cold, < coughing; sweat on face. Yellow fever.

COMPLEMENTARY: *Ars; Chin; Kali-c;* Lach; Phos.

RELATED: Am-c; Ars; Colch; Graph; Lyc.

CARBOLICUM ACIDUM

GENERALITIES: *Carbolic acid* is a powerful antiseptic, irritant and anesthetic. It affects the *mucous membranes, heart, blood* and *respiration.* It is a *languid, painless, foul* and *destructive* remedy. PROSTRATION *is very marked;* paralytic prostration, with loss of sensation and motion. Discharges are *foul, burning.* Terrible pain coming and going suddenly. Acuteness of smell is a strong guiding symptom. Pricking, burning sensation.

Malignant and *septic conditions*. Physical exertion brings on abscess somewhere. In cholera when *Verat-alb* is indicated but fails. Collapse. Bloody exudation. Unfit for study, as reading < all symptoms. Trembling; uncertain, staggering walk.

WORSE: Jar. Reading. Pregnancy. Combing hair.

MIND: Mental and bodily languor, disinclination to study or to do any physical work.

HEAD: Tight feeling as if compressed by a rubber band, > green tea and smoking. Hot ball sensation in forehead. Scalp tender. Headache appearing at the time of menses.

EYES: Severe orbital neuralgia over right eye.

NOSE: Smell very acute. Ozena with great fetor and ulceration.

FACE: PALE ABOUT NOSE AND MOUTH. Dusky face.

MOUTH: *Intensely foul breath,* with constipation. Burning in mouth through stomach.

THROAT: Glazed. Uvula whitened and shrivelled. Diphtheria, fetid breath, regurgitation on swallowing liquids, but little pain.

STOMACH: Nausea and vomiting, of pregnancy. Seasickness. Cancer. Vomitus is dark olive-green. Heartburn. Sore stomach. Fermentative dyspepsia with bad breath and taste. Craving for stimulant or for smoking.

ABDOMEN: Flatulence. Constipation with retraction of abdomen. *Shreddy stools.* Passes mucus from anus while urinating. Diarrhea, rice water, stool, fetid.

URINARY: Urine scanty, green or dark, almost black. Frequent urination at night in old men. Diabetes. Albuminuria.

FEMALE: Leukorrhea thick, causing itching. Severe backache across loins, with dragging down thighs; uterine displacement. Fetid acrid discharge; erosion of cervix.

HEART: *Thready pulse.*

BACK: Aching between scapulae.

SKIN: Burning, itching vesicles and pustules. Burns tend to ulcerate. Erysipelas. Bloody vesicles or pustules.

SLEEP: *Very sleepy.*

FEVER: Profuse cold sweat.

RELATED: Kreos.

CARBONEUM SULPHURATUM

GENERALITIES: It has a specific affinity for eyes. It is useful for loss of vision, progressive, with central scotoma. Color-blindness for red and green, not for white. Ill effect of coal gas.

CARCINOSIN

GENERALITIES: A nosode prepared from carcinoma is claimed to act favorably, modifying the cases in which there is a history of carcinoma or the disease itself exists. Can be used as an intercurrent remedy along with the indicated one.

CARDUUS MARIANUS

GENERALITIES: It is primarily a *liver* and spleen remedy and for hemorrhage due to the affection of these organs, which gives relief. It acts on veins causing vascular stasis, varicose veins and ulcers. Diseases of miners associated with difficult breathing. Dropsical conditions depending upon portal congestion and congestion of pelvic organs. Abuse of beer. Debility, fatigue, < eating and riding, with frequent yawning. Stitching, drawing, burning pains. Liver affections associated with lung affection.

WORSE: Lying on left side. *Beer.* Eating. Touch. Motion. Cellar.

BETTER: Bleeding.

MIND: Forgets what he has just intended to do. Hypochondriacal. Despondent. Joyless.

HEAD: Dull frontal headache. Vertigo with tendency to fall forward, > by nosebleed.

EYES: Burning and pressure in eyeballs.

NOSE: Epistaxis, habitual in psoric young persons.

MOUTH: Tongue has white centre, with red indented edges. Tongue weak. Taste bitter.

STOMACH: Poor appetite. Nausea, retching and *vomiting of green acid fluid,* or blood. Aversion to salted meat.

ABDOMEN: *Liver engorged,* swollen laterally, painful to pressure. Jaundice. Stitches near splenic region, < on inspiration, on stooping. Stitches in liver, < lying on left side. Liver affections causes lung disease, producing hemoptysis. Gall-stones. Cirrhosis, with dropsy. Distension of abdomen with rumbling. Diaphragm high. Hard, difficult, knotty, clayey stools. Hemorrhagic piles. Profuse diarrhea due to rectal cancer. Melena. Sensation of motion in intestines on expiration, around navel.

URINARY: Urine turbid; *golden yellow.*

FEMALE: Chronic uterine hemorrhage, with portal derangement.

RESPIRATION: *Pain in chest* going to shoulders, back, loins and abdomen, with urging to urinate. Asthmatic respiration. Cough; with stitches in sides of chest, with bloody sputum.

EXTREMITIES: Pain in hip-joint spreading through buttocks down the thighs, < stooping, with difficulty in rising. Feet weak, on sitting. Drawing pain in entire back.

SKIN: *Broken or hard thrombosed veins.* Varicose ulcer.

FEVER: Chill and fever, with jaundice.

RELATED: Calc; Sang.

CASTOR EQUI

GENERALITIES: Trituration is made from the scales of rudimentary thumbnail of the horse. It acts on skin causing its thickening, on nails which become brittle and fall off. Bones esp. tibia and coccyx, are painful. It is a highly useful remedy in cracked and ulcerated nipples of nursing women, excessively tender, cannot bear touch of clothing. Breasts swollen, sensitive, < descending stairs. Itching in breast, areola reddened. Nipples almost hanging. Warts on forehead and mammae. Psoriasis of tongue.

CASTOREUM

GENERALITIES: Tincture is prepared from the secretion found in preputial sacs of beaver. It is suitable for nervous, hysterical women, with cramps, pains, weakness after severe illness. Nervous women who do not recover fully, but are continually irritable, and suffer from debilitating sweats. *Weakness and lack of reaction.* Reflex uterine effects; nervous and spasmodic. Fibrillar twitching. Heaviness of the whole body. Yawning continuous. Chorea. Epilepsy. Nervous palpitation.

WORSE: Emotion. Cold. During menses. Debilitating disease.

BETTER: Pressure.

MIND: *Irritability*. Easily sheds tears. Melancholic and full of anxious longings.

EYES: Day-blindness. Cannot endure the light.

MOUTH: Tongue swollen; twitching. Round pea-like elevation in centre of tongue, with redness around. Tongue sensitive to touch or food, with drawing pain towards hyoid bone.

ABDOMEN: Colic or other abdominal complaints are accompanied with yawning. *Colic with weakness,* > pressure. Summer diarrhea with green mucous stools. Violent thirst, could not drink enough.

FEMALE: Violent cutting, dysmenorrheal colic, with few drops of blood, then cold sweat. Amenorrhea, with painful tympanites.

SLEEP: Constant yawning as accompanied symptom. Restless sleep with frightful dreams and starts. Yawns in sleep.

FEVER: Chilliness with icy coldness in back. Exhausting sweat, after fever.

RELATED: Mosch; Valer.

CAULOPHYLLUM

GENERALITIES: It is a woman's as well as rheumatic remedy esp. acting on small joints. It causes ERRATIC PAINS flying from place to place, *drawing*, cramping, shooting, *rheumatic* in character, ending in neck which gets stiff. Many of the complaints are due to uterine disorders. *Internal tremors,* with weakness. Want of tonicity in womb. Hysterical or epileptiform spasm at puberty, during dysmenorrhea. Paraplegia, after childbirth. *Exhaustion*. General debility. Chorea at puberty.

WORSE: *Pregnancy*. Suppressed menses. Open air. Coffee.

MIND: Fretful and fearsome. *Nervous*. Excitable. Easily displeased.

HEAD: Aches from uterine or spinal trouble, with pressure behind the eyes, < stooping, from light, from noon to night.

FACE: Moth spots; on forehead, with leukorrhea. Heavy upper lid, has to raise it with fingers.

MOUTH ; Aphthae. Thrush (locally and internally).

STOMACH: Frequent gulping of sour, bitter fluid, with vertigo. Vomiting of uterine origin.

FEMALE: Violent, intermittent, cramping pain with little flow; dysmenorrhea - uterus retroverted. LABOR LIKE PAINS, FLY to breast. In labor the pains are WEAK OR IRREGULAR, they cease from exhaustion or they are too painful; *false labor pains. Eases labor;* when the patient is exhausted from a long continuance of labor. *Habitual abortion,* from want of tonicity of uterus. Afterpain; after protracted and exhausting labor. Os rigid, needle-like pain in cervix. Profuse acrid leukorrhea, often in little girls. Menses late. Irritable vagina, spasmodic intense pain. Menorrhagia, after hasty labor, flow very profuse. Lochia, profuse and prolonged.

NECK: Stiff. Head drawn to left.

EXTREMITIES: *Sore nodes on finger joints. Rheumatism of small joints.* Cutting pain in finger joints on closing hands. Aching sore lower limbs, before menses. Paraplegia after childbirth.

SKIN: *Chloasma* on neck.

FEVER: Feels as if overfull of blood. High fever.

RELATED: Cimic; *Puls; Sep.*

CAUSTICUM

GENERALITIES: The chemical composition of Causticum is still uncertain though it is considered to be potassium hydrate or Caustic potash. It is a great polychrest remedy, acting upon NERVES, *motor and sensory,* and on MUSCLES, voluntary and involuntary; of BLADDER, *larynx* and limbs. Weakness, progressive; loss of muscular strength, causing increasing uncertainty of control over the muscles, finally ending in PARALYSIS *of single organ* or *part.* Paralysis from exposure to cold, post-diphtheritic, from lead. Chronic rheumatic affections cause contraction of tendons and deformities about the joints. Pain is tearing, drawing, *burning,* of the part grasped by hand. *Soreness, rawness. Trembling,* convulsion, chorea, in nervous girls, < during menses. Sympathetic jerking, twitching, starting and restlessness are other characteristic symptoms. Cramps here and there. Emaciation due to disease, fright, worry, grief, and with long-lasting illness. Children are slow in learning to talk and walk. Anesthesia. Epilepsy, runs in circle, then falls down, at puberty. Patient is susceptible to both cold and heat. Joints stiff. It is adapted to broken down, worn out senile persons or to dark complexioned, rigid fibered persons. Restlessness at night, esp. the legs are constantly on the go. Ill-effects of burns and scalds, fright, grief, worry, sorrow, night-watching. Ulcer maltreated with lead. Warts. Cold water tones the paralysis. Fissure; from least provocation, about wings of nose, lips, anus, etc. Motion as of coition; chorea. Awkward at talking, chewing, walking. Mental-effects; convulsions, from suppressed eruptions. Sensation of cold water running from clavicle down to toes.

WORSE: DRY COLD or raw air. *Wind.* Drafts. Extremes of temperature. Stooping. Suppressed eruptions. Coffee. Fat. 3-4 a.m. or evening. Exertion. Change of weather. After stool. Motion of carriage. Twilight. Darkness. Taking hold of anything. Sour things. Bathing in river in summer.

BETTER: COLD DRINKS (even chill). Damp wet weather. Washing. *Warmth, of bed.* Gentle motion.

MIND: Hopeless, despondent, wants to die. Ambitionless. *Mental fatigue. Anxious foreboding,* < in twilight. Reticent. Oversympathetic. Child does not want to go to bed alone; least thing makes him cry. Thinking of complaints < them, esp. hemorrhoids. Weeps, laughs; chorea. Laughs before, with or after spasm. Conscious-struck as if she had committed some crime. Sadness. Whining mood. Suspicious, mistrustful; absent-minded. Looks on the dark side. Lacks control, balance. Spoonerism, confounds letters and syllables. Vexed with business worries.

HEAD: Painless commotion in the whole head. Sensation as of an empty space between the forehead and brain, > hot application. Too and fro or nodding motion, or turning to right. Tight scalp. Stitches in temples on mental exertion. Nausea and vomiting or blindness during headache, then paralysis. Vertigo, during sleep, at night, in the morning, while lying down, on stooping, at menstruation, looking up. Small soft round nodes on scalp or glabella.

EYES: Sparks and dark spots before the eyes. Paralysis of one eyelid (R). Heavy drooping eyelids. Ptosis. Weakness of recti muscles - diplopia, > looking to right. Continuous eye pain with inclination to touch and rub the eyes which seems to relieve the pressure in it. Vision obscured as from gauze, on blowing nose. Objects look large. Profuse acrid tears. Cataract. Rolling of eyes in epilepsy. Eyelids quiver. Warts on eyebrows. Fissures in canthi. Eyes remain open, without winking; paralysis.

EARS: Ringing, roaring, pulsating, with deafness. Words and steps re-echo in ears. Burning in ears, they become red. Much foul ear-wax, brown. Meniere's disease. Thick, gluey, purulent discharge.

NOSE: Coryza with hoarseness. Pimples on tip of nose. Old warts. Sneezing in the morning. Thick yellow or greenish yellow discharge. Nose-bleed, during spasm.

FACE: *Prosopalgia,* > cold water. *Facial paralysis* (R), < opening mouth. Pain in jaw, cannot open the mouth. Face yellow, sickly looking. Cramp in lips. Feels furry. Eruptions on face.

MOUTH: Bites inside of cheek while chewing. Paralysis of tongue, with indistinct speech, words seem to jerk out. Swelling at root of tongue. Gums, bleed easily. Recurrent abscess in gums-dental fistula. Fatty taste. Gums spongy, receding. Teeth, feel loose, elongated; ache, < from cold or warmth. Swelling of inner side of cheek, or induration. Tongue; red in middle, sides coated. Painful vesicles on tip.

THROAT: Urging to swallow continuously as if the throat were too narrow. Swallows the wrong way, or food comes through nose. Throat symptoms < stooping. Difficulty in swallowing, from paralysis of throat; unable to hawk out mucus, swallows it. Scraping, burning, rawness in throat.

STOMACH: Greasy taste, eructations. Waterbrash, salty. Aversion to sweets. Feels as if lime were burning in stomach. Pain in stomach from ice water. Sensation of a ball rising in the throat. Sour vomiting followed by sour eructations. Fresh meat causes nausea, smoked meat agrees. Feels hungry but appetite vanishes at the sight of food, or thought or smell, during pregnancy. Vomiting of blood at night. Acid dyspepsia.

ABDOMEN: Enlarged in children. Colic, spasmodic. Pain radiates to back and chest, > bending double, < least food. Stool hard, tough, covered with mucus, shines like grease, soft and small, size of goose squill. Stool passes easily when standing. Cramps in rectum on stooping, with desire for urination. Anus prolapses on coughing. Itching in anus, > cold water. Small hard pustules around anus. Large piles impeding the stool, < walking, standing and when thinking of it. Fistula, with pulsation and pain in perineum. Rectum insensible to solid stool. Diarrhea from cold. Painful swelling of the navel. Constipation, with frequent ineffectual urging.

URINARY: Paralysis of bladder, from long retention of urine, and consequent incontinence (as in sleep or in schoolgirls). INVOLUNTARY PASSAGE OF URINE; ON COUGHING, walking, blowing nose, sneezing. *Retention of urine after labor,* after surgical operations. Burning in urethra when urinating, < after coition. Urine dribbles or passes slowly. Insensibility of urethra while passing urine. Urine is passed better sitting. Bed wetting, during first sleep at night. Urine; black, cloudy, white. Itching of meatus.

MALE: Increase of smegma about the glans. Semen bloody during coition. Red spots on penis. Bruised soreness in testes.

FEMALE: Aversion to coition. Menses; flow only during day, with clots, scanty, with prosopalgia. Leukorrhea profuse, flow during night, with great weakness. Uterine inertia during labor. Smarting in the pudendum after urination. Nipples sore, cracked, surrounded by herpes. Leukorrhea smelling like the menses. Disappearance of milk, from fatigue, night-watching, or anxiety. Dysmenorrhea, with tearing pains in back and thighs. Anxiety, sadness and weakness during menses. Dreams during menses. Menses late and profuse. Sticking pain below left mammae; dysmenorrhea. Violent itching about mammae in nursing women.

RESPIRATORY: Aphonia, or *hoarseness,* with pain in chest, < a.m., of speakers, singers, < stooping, > talking. Cough hollow, hard, dry, during pregnancy, from tickling in throat pit or larynx; incessant; dry, night and morning, < stooping, heat of bed, cold air, > sips of cold water. Cannot cough deep enough; *expectoration slips back,* scanty; greasy, ropy, like soapsud, must be swallowed. Sore streak in larynx. Chest tight, sore, vest seems tight. Short breath, before coughing. Purring in chest. Wandering chest pain, > pressure, < sneezing. Pain in the larynx, < blowing nose. Oppressive breathing while talking and walking. Tightness or scraping in chest.

HEART: Palpitation, with pain in chest, burning and languor.

NECK & BACK: Stiffness of neck, or back, on rising from a chair, could scarcely move the head. Back pain goes forward or to the thighs. Pain in spine, < swallowing. Pain in hips, < coughing. Torticollis. Bruised, darting pain around coccyx. Cramp in lumbar region and buttock.

EXTREMITIES: Paralytic feeling in the right hand, with paralysis of tongue. Paralysis of deltoid, cannot raise hand to head. Trembling of hands. Writer's cramp. Numbness of hands. Fullness of hands while grasping anything. Bursting in fingertips; warts. Cramp in calves, feet, toes and tendo-achillis. Unsteady walking and easy falling, of children. Weak ankles. Tearing rheumatic pain in limbs, > warmth, of bed. Cracking and tension in the knees. Disposition to stretch, bend or crack the joints. Stiffness in the hollow of the knees, < sitting, > continued walking. Burning in joints. Tendons contracted. Twisting and jerking in limbs; chorea. Arthritis deformans. Cracking in knees, < walking and descending. Restless legs at night. Pain like electric shock in legs. Cannot stand on heels. Whitlow of great toes.

SKIN: Cracks, ulcers. Soreness in folds of skin. Warts, seedy, large, jagged, bleeding easily, ulcerating; on tip of fingers, nose, lids, brows. *Itching. Deep burns and their effects.* Cicatrix reopens. Skin prone to intertrigo during dentition.

SLEEP: Frequent movement of arms and legs during sleep. Laughs and cries during sleep. Very drowsy, can hardly keep awake. Yawning and stretching. Nocturnal sleeplessness with dry heat, inquietude. Wakes with slightest noise. Yawning when listening or paying attention to others.

FEVER: Coldness not > by warmth. Sweat about 4 a.m., profuse, on slight exertion, in open air. Heat from 6 to 8 p.m. Coldness; left sided, of diseased part, with pain. Flushes of heat followed by chill.

COMPLEMENTARY: Carb-v; Graph; *Lach; Stann;* Staph.

RELATED: Gels; Kali-bi; Phos; Rhus-t; Sep.

CEANOTHUS

GENERALITIES: This remedy has a special affinity to the spleen, which enlarges enormously. Pain in left hypochondria, with dyspnea, diarrhea, profuse or suppressed menses, leukorrhea. Menses every two weeks. Anemic patient whose liver and spleen are at fault. Leukaemia. Enlargement of liver. Urine green, frothy. Periodical neuralgia.

WORSE: Cold weather. Lying on left side. Motion.

RELATED: Chin.

CEDRON

GENERALITIES: Neuralgias occurring with EXACT PERIODICITY is the most marked feature of this remedy. It is adapted to persons of voluptuous disposition, and of an excitable nervous temperament. Antidotes the effect of snakebite and sting of insects. Complaints after coition—chorea in women, neuralgia in men. Trembling. Numbness of the whole body. Malarial affection of damp, warm, marshy countries. Convulsion during menses. Lectophobia.

WORSE: *Periodically*; at the same hour. Open air. Lying down. Before storm. After sleep.

BETTER: Standing erect.

HEAD: Orbital neuralgia. Crazy feeling from pain across forehead. Whole body feels numb, during headache. Stammers after coition. Head feels as if swollen.

EYES: *Burn like fire.* Severe pain in eyeballs, with radiating pain around the eye; scalding lacrimation. Iritis.

Choroiditis. Eyes red. Pain over the eye, < coition. Objects appear red at night and yellow by day.

EXTREMITIES: Sudden acute pain in ball of right thumb moves up to shoulder, same in right foot to knee, causing her to drop to the floor.

FEVER: Excitement before chill. Malaria.

RELATED: Aran.

CHAMOMILLA

GENERALITIES: It is a highly EMOTIONAL, TEMPERAMENTAL AND OVERSENSITIVE remedy. Oversensitiveness from abuse of coffee and narcotics. It is particularly suited to *diseases of pregnant women, nurses and little* CHILDREN. *Bad temper; frantic irritability and snappish. Pain is intolerable becomes mad with pain,* or magnifies her *pain, prostrated* with pain. Very cross, cannot be appeased. Tosses about. Cries out or walks the floor. Demands instant relief for his suffering, he would rather die than suffer. Mental and physical symptoms appear in paroxysm—*irritability, restlessness,* COLIC, cough, etc. *Numbness, after pain;* on awakening. Repeated spasms; of face, arms, legs, etc. Colic, diarrhea, jaundice, twitching and convulsion after anger. Neuralgic gouty, rheumatic diathesis. *Cramps;* with bilious vomiting; of muscles. Convulsions during dentition. *Hot and thirsty. Hot sweat with pains.* Opium of homeopathy. Bad effects of ill temper. During convulsion body becomes stiff, with opisthotonos, eyes roll about, face becomes wry, thumbs turn inward.

WORSE: ANGER. NIGHT. DENTITION. Cold air, damp air. Wind. Taking cold. COFFEE. *Narcotics.* Alcohol. Lying in bed. Music. Eructation. Heat. Warm food and covering. Touch. Looked at.

BETTER: BEING CARRIED. Mild weather. Heat. Sweating. Cold application.

MIND: UGLY *behavior;* CROSS and UNCIVIL. QUARRELSOME. *Vexed at every trifle.* Abrupt. *Averse to being spoken to, touched* or being looked at. Children WANT TO BE CARRIED, and petted. *Want many things, but refuse them when given.* Piteous moaning because he cannot have what he wants. Aversion to talking. Omits words while writing and speaking. Women become suddenly capricious, quarrelsome, obstinate, before menses. Hasty, hurried. Cannot bear anyone near him.

HEAD: Throbbing headache in one half of the brain; inclination to bend head backwards. Feels as if hair stood on end, with shivering. Hot clammy sweat on forehead and scalp, during sleep, wetting the hair. Headache of delicate over fatigued women. Headache > when mind is engaged. Headache < morning and 9 p.m.

EYES: Yellow conjunctiva. Spasmodic closing of lids. Bloody water from the eyes of newborn babies.

EARS: Sensitive to cold wind about ears, or noise. Earache, sticking, > warmth. Ears feel stopped. Hears voices of absent persons, at night. Ringing after hemorrhage. Roaring in the ears as of rushing water. Music is insupportable. Sensation of hot water running out.

NOSE: Extremely sensitive to all smells. Hot coryza, with obstruction of nose; inability to sleep. Skin wrinkled. Crawling until eyes water.

FACE: *Swelling* or REDNESS OF THE CHEEK. One cheek red and hot, other pale and cold. Face pale, sunken, distorted by pain. Neuralgia of the face, with hot sweat about the head; pain extending into ear. Jerking of facial muscles. Jaws feel tired. Sweats after eating or drinking.

MOUTH: Toothache, < after warm drink, during pregnancy, by coffee. Jerking in tongue. Thick white or yellow fur on tongue. Nightly salivation, of sweetish taste. Bad, sour breath. Bitter taste. Teeth feel elongated.

THROAT: Inability to swallow solid food when lying. Constricted or plugged feeling.

STOMACH: Eructation like bad egg. Severe bitter bilious vomiting, With griping. Vomiting after morphia. Gastralgia as from a stone in stomach. Sweats after eating and drinking. Thirst for cold water, sour drink. Aversion to coffee. Violent retching before vomiting.

ABDOMEN: Distended. SPELLS OF COLIC. Pain from side to side or going upwards, after anger. *Cutting* wind colic, < night, urinating, > warm, application. STOOL *hot,* SOUR, GRASS GREEN, SLIMY, HACKED, *yellow green,* or LIENTERIC, smelling like bad eggs. Haemorrhoids, with painful fissure. Diarrhoea, during dentition, from cold, from anger. Jaundice, after anger. Cheek becomes red during colic, with hot sweat. Anus swollen and pouting, as if bowels were knotted and abdomen empty.

URINARY: Urine hot and yellowish. Stitches in urethra.

FEMALE: Irregular labor-like pain, going up, down inner thighs; with profuse discharge of clotted, dark blood. Puerperal convulsions, after anger. Distressing after pains. Breasts sore, nipples inflamed and very tender. Infants' breasts tender. Cramps, when child nurses. Yellow, dark, lumpy, acrid leukorrhea. Membranous dysmenorrhoea, specially at puberty. Milk is spoiled, baby won't suck. Dysmenorrhea, from anger or emotions with sexual desire. Oozing of dark foul blood, with occasional gush of bright red blood. Menorrhagia, with black clots, profuse, with coldness of extremities and much thirst. Intolerable labor pain sends the doctor and nurse away, then calls again. Lochia too profuse and bloody or suppressed.

RESPIRATORY: Spells of dry tickling cough. Asthma, from anger, < dry weather, > bending head back. Rattling of mucus in child's chest. Anger provokes the cough, in children. Whooping cough, suffocating, then vomits. Cough, < 9 to 12 p.m., during sleep, does not wake up the child.

BACK: Severe pain in loins and hips, in side opposite to that on which patient is lying. Lumbago.

EXTREMITIES: Numbness and stiffness of hands, when grasping objects. Cramp in calves. Violent rheumatic pain driving him out of bed at night, compelled to walk about. Burning of soles at night. Ankles give way in the afternoon, as if she is walking on the ends of bones of her legs. Feet feel paralyzed, cannot step on them, at night. Palms dry.

SLEEP: Drowsiness, with moaning, weeping and wailing in sleep. Pain disturbs sleep. Sleepless from abuse of narcotics. Sleeps with thighs separated. Drowsy but cannot sleep.

SKIN: Rash of infants and nursing mothers. Jaundice. Burning, smarting in ulcers at night. Skin unhealthy, every injury suppurates.

FEVER: Chilly yet easily overheated, hence takes cold. Coldness of one part, with heat of another, < uncovering. Alternate chill and heat. Feverish from suppressed discharge. Sweat on head. Thirst during fever.

COMPLEMENTARY: *Bell;* Mag-c.; Sanic.

RELATED: Nux-v; Staph.

CHELIDONIUM

GENERALITIES: It is predominantly a *right sided* remedy. It acts upon the *liver, portal system, right side of abdomen* and right lower lung. It is closely allied to *Lyc;* when *Lyc.* seems indicated but fails to act, *Chel* should be given. YELLOWNESS *and bilious disturbances* are its marked features. Constant pain at the inferior angle of the right scapula is its chief indication. Pains shoot *backwards* or in all directions. Stitching pain due to serous effusion. *Heavy, stiff,* sore, paralyzed, dislocative or broken feeling. Numbness. There is great general lethargy and indisposition to make any effort. Horror of motion. Feels tired on little exertion. Bilious complication, during gestation, in lung affections. Jaundice.

WORSE: *Motion. Cough.* Touch. *Change of weather.* North east wind. 4 a.m. and 4 p.m. Looking up.

BETTER: *Hot food.* Eating. Dinner. Milk. Pressure. Hot bath. Bending backward. Lying on abdomen.

MIND: Aversion to mental exertion or conversation. Despondent. Anxiety as if she had committed a crime; fear of going crazy. Feels like crying with ill humour or without any reason. Restless, hence agile.

HEAD: Vertigo; felt in vertex, < closing eyes, with bilious vomiting and pain in liver. Headache extends backwards. Occiput feels heavy as lead, *icy coldness of occiput from nape* of neck. Neuralgia over right eye, right cheek bone and right ear, with excessive lacrimation. Cranium feels too small.

EYES: Dirty yellow color of whites. Soreness of eyes, < looking up. Dazzling spot before the eyes. Lacrimation when looking intently, with pain in eyes, or from tickling in larynx. Mucus in eyes. Could not open eyes with prosopalgia.

EARS: Sensation in both the ears as if wind were rushing out, or something crawling out. Loss of hearing during cough.

NOSE: Red. *Flapping of the alae nasi.* Obstruction, with liver complaint. Tip of nose swollen and red. Dryness.

FACE: Dark red or *sallow, sunken.* Yellow, esp. forehead, nose and cheeks. Right cheek bone feels as if swollen, with tearing pain. Flushes of heat. Nodular eruption.

MOUTH: Taste bitter. *Tongue yellow,* with imprint of teeth, large, flabby, Offensive breath. Tongue narrow, pointed. Salivation with nausea, giddiness. Bitter water collects in mouth.

THROAT: Choking, < breathing. Choking, as from hasty swallowing or as if too large a morsel had been swallowed. Left-sided goitre.

STOMACH: Craves milk, piquant or hot food and drink. Nausea, > drinking milk. Vomiting, > very hot water. Gastric pain, gnawing, scraping, > eating. Sensation of a plug in stomach. Aversion to meat, coffee, cheese. Loss of appetite.

ABDOMEN: Epigastric region tender. LIVER PAIN GOING BACKWARD, or fixed at angle of right scapula. Liver enlarged; tender. Gall-stones. Constriction across abdomen, as by a string. Stool pasty, pale, bright yellow, clayey, or hard balls. Alternation of diarrhea and constipation. Ascites, with yellow palms. Crawling and itching in rectum. Feels an animal wriggling in epigastrium. Navel drawn in during colic.

URINARY: Profuse foaming, yellow urine like beer. Spasmodic pain in right kidney and liver. Urine stains the diaper dark yellow.

MALE: Frequent erection, even during day. Pain in glans. Itching, creeping on scrotum and glans.

FEMALE: Menses too late and too profuse. Longing for unusual food during pregnancy. Leukorrhea white, stains linen yellow. Burning in vagina, recurs at the same hour during day.

RESPIRATION: Short breath and tight chest, clothing seems too tight, > deep breathing. Dyspnea, < urinating. Pain pressive in chest on deep inspiration. *Cough, as from dust with much rattling; but little expectoration, or it flies from mouth.* Deep seated pain or *nailing sensation, deep in right chest.* Bilious pneumonia. Respiratory symptoms with liver symptoms. Pressure in larynx as if air could not pass through. Stitches in chest.

HEART: Violent palpitation, with tightness in chest. Periodic palpitation.

NECK & BACK: Fixed pain under inner and lower angle of the right scapula; which may extend into chest and stomach causing nausea or vomiting. Pain from neck to temple. (R); pressing pain in vertebrae, < bending backwards and forward. Occiput heavy with pain in right side of back. String sensation around the neck. Cervico-brachial neuralgia.

EXTREMITIES: Very sore to touch. *Cold fingertips.* Pain in heels as if pinched by too narrow a shoe. Burning and stiffness in right knee, < moving. Limbs feel paralyzed. Heavy lower limbs. Ankles stiff. Edema around ankles and feet. Paresis of lower limbs, with rigidity of muscles. One foot cold, other hot.

SKIN: Yellow. Itching, > eating. Painful pimples and pustules. Skin wrinkled.

SLEEP: *Lethargic.* DROWSY and *chilly.* Dreams of corpses and funerals. Sleepiness, without being able to sleep. Falls asleep while speaking.

FEVER: Burning heat spreads from hands over the body. Sweaty, with aversion to uncover and without relief.

Sweat during sleep, after midnight, from slight exertion. Fluctuating temperature. High fever.

COMPLEMENTARY: *Lyc;* Merc-d.

RELATED: Bry; Kali-bi; Merc; Op.

CHENOPODIUM ANTHELMINTICUM

GENERALITIES: Just like *Chel* it causes dull pain below the right angle of right scapula, but nearer to spine. It causes apoplexy and consequent right hemiplegia with aphasia. Stertorous breathing with a rattle as of a ball rolling loose in trachea. Heavy breathing with flapping of cheeks. Repeats the same action over and over again. Deafness progressive for human voice but great sensitiveness to sound of a passing vehicle, or to distant sounds. Paralysis; with spasm of forearms and hands in flexion; contraction of limbs. Jaundice. Aural vertigo. Meniere's disease. Urine profuse, foamy, yellow, burning.

CHIMAPHILA UMBELLATA

GENERALITIES: It acts principally on kidneys and bladder, producing gravel in kidneys, and acute and chronic catarrh in the bladder (cystitis). Also acts on the glands—mesenteric, *prostate,* mammary and liver. Useful in hepatic and renal dropsy. Women with large breasts, or plethoric women, with dysuria. Incipient and progressive cataract.

WORSE: Cold damp. Standing. Sitting; on cold stones. Beginning urination.

BETTER: Walking.

HEAD: Pain in frontal eminence.

EYES: Halo around the light. Stabbing pain in left eye, with lacrimation.

MOUTH: Jaws feel stiff, cannot close mouth at night; sleeps with the mouth open. Toothache as if being gently pulled ,< after eating and exertion, > cold water.

URINARY: Urine; ROPY or *muco-purulent, foul, scanty, thick, turbid.* Must strain before urine flows. Acute prostatitis with retention and dysuria, and *feeling in perineum* as if sitting on a ball. Gonorrheal prostatitis. Fluttering in kidney region. Vesical tenesmus, < sitting, > walking. Cannot pass urine without standing with feet apart and body inclined forward. Acute inflammation of urinary tract. Suppressed urine in infants. Clots of blood pass with urine.

FEMALE: Painful tumour in mammae; with undue secretion of milk; in women of large breasts, sharp pain through mammae. Rapid atrophy of the breasts.

COMPLEMENTARY: Kali-m.

RELATED: Berb; Coc-c; Sabal.

CHINA OFFICINALIS

GENERALITIES: This was the first remedy proved by Dr. Hahnemann. It affects the *blood,* making it thinner, and impoverished. It weakens the heart and impairs the CIRCULATION, producing congestion and HEMORRHAGE, anemia, complete relaxation and collapse. The *debility* in China, is due to PROFUSE EXHAUSTING DISCHARGES, loss of vital fluid, excessive suppuration, diarrhea, hemorrhages, etc. INTERMITTENT periodicity is very marked in fever and neuralgia. Patient becomes *weak, oversensitive and nervous;* everything upsets him—*light, noise,* *odor, pain, etc. Bursting pain.* Neuralgia. Dropsy, after loss of fluids, hemorrhage. Emaciation esp. of children. Anaemia. Hard swelling. Rheumatism. Sepsis. Inflammation of bleeding organ, after hemorrhages, and the part rapidly turns black. Convulsion during hemorrhage. Hemorrhage, profuse, with loss of sight, faintness, and ringing in ears. Post-operative gas pain not > from passing it. Ill-effect of masturbation, vexation, cold, stopped coryza, tea, mercury, alcohol. Psoas abscess. It is suited to persons of thin, dry, bilious constitution. Wounds become black and gangrenous. Epilepsy; chorea; paralysis; from loss of fluids.

WORSE: VITAL LOSS. TOUCH. *Jar. Noise.* PERIODICITY; *alternate days. Cold. Winds, drafts.* Open air. Eating. *Fruits.* Milk. Impure water. Spoiled fish, meat. Tea. Mental exertion. During and after, stool. Smoking. Autumn, summer.

BETTER: *Hard pressure.* Loose clothes. Bending double. In room; warmth.

MIND: Disobedient, stubborn, contempt for everything. Fixed idea, that he is unhappy, persecuted by enemies. Disposition to hurt other people's feelings. Fear of dogs and other animals, at night. Sudden crying and tossing about, when cheerful. Ill-humor, < petting and caressing. Dislike for all mental and physical work. Builds air castles. Indifference, sad, no desire to live. Wants to commit suicide but lacks courage. Reluctant to speak. Mistakes in speech and writing. Spoonerism. Loss of control over mind.

HEAD: Bursting, throbbing pain, with throbbing of carotids. Sensation as if brain were swashing to and fro, causing pain; bruised pain in brain, < temples. Vertigo, falls backward while walking. Stitches from temple to temple. *Sore sensitive* scalp, < touching or combing hair. Headache, < in sun, > by moving head up and down, hard pressure, rubbing. Sweats when walking in open air. Head heavy.

EYES: Blue color around the eyes. Night blindness, due to anemic retina. Scalding tears. Pressure in eyes as from drowsiness. Black spots before the eyes. Pupils dilated. Intermittent ciliary neuralgia. Smart as from salt. Stitching as from sand. Eyes painful on reading and writing.

EARS: Red, hot. Ringing in ears, with headache. *Tinnitus,* then vertigo. Stitches in ears. Hardness of hearing. Foul, purulent, bloody discharge.

NOSE: Ill-effect of suppressed coryza—headache. Habitual easy bleeding from the nose, esp. morning on rising. Smell too acute. Cold sweat about nose. Nose hot, red. Violent dry sneezing.

FACE : Earthy, sickly, pale; hippocratic, bluish around the eyes. Face bloated; red. Lips dry, blackish and shrivelled. Swelling of veins. Red hot face, with cold hands. Flushed, after hemorrhage, sexual excess, loss of vital fluid, in coma.

MOUTH: Toothache while infant sucks the breast, > by pressing teeth firmly together and by warmth. Toothache with sweat. *Food tastes bitter,* even water, or too salty. Tongue; thick, dirty-coated; tip burns, followed by salivation. *Taste bitter,* salty or acute. Gums swollen.

STOMACH: *Bitter* or sour eructations, after milk. Craving; for dainty; sour or sweet things, highly seasoned food, desires various things without knowing what (children). Quick satiety. *Anorexia,* feels satiated all the time, aversion, to all food, to bread, butter, coffee. Voracious appetite in emaciation of children. *Loud belching without relief.* Digestion slow. Milk disagrees. Weight, after eating small quantity of food. Ill effects of tea. Cold feeling in stomach. Thirst for cold water that < diarrhoea. Pulsations and rumbling, in epigastrium. Frequent vomiting. Hiccough. Hematemesis. Stomach sore. Fermentation after eating fruits. Thirst; during apyrexia; before chill. Hungry and yet want of appetite; only while eating, some appetite and natural taste for food return.

ABDOMEN: Liver and spleen enlarged. *Flatulent bloating;* > motion. Colic > by bending double. Post operative gas pains, no relief from passing it. Heat in abdomen as if hot water running down. Periodical liver symptoms. Pain from rectum to genitals. Gall stone colic. Jaundice; after leukorrhea, masturbation, sexual excess, diarrhoea. Stools; Lienteric; *dark, foul; watery;* Bloody; painless; < eating; at night, from fruits; milk, beer, during hot weather. Diarrhea; after weaning, in children; chronic in children, who become drowsy, pupils dilated, body becomes cold esp. chin, nose and rapid respiration. Involuntary stools.

URINARY: Frequent urination. Burning at meatus < rubbing of clothes. Urine turbid, dark, scanty. Pinkish sediment. Hematuria. Enuresis of weakly children.

MALE: Impotence, or morbid sexual desire, with lascivious fancies. Frequent emissions followed by great weakness. Swelling of testes and spermatic cord — after gonorrhea. Orchitis. Sexual desire, with craving for dainties.

FEMALE: Ovaritis from sexual excess. Desire too strong in lying-in women. Menses; too early, dark, profuse, clotted, with abdominal distention. Bloody leukorrhea; seems to take blood dark, with fainting, convulsions. Asphyxia of new born due to great loss of blood by the mother. Painful induration in the vagina.

RESPIRATORY: *Hemoptysis.* Puffy, rattling, breathing suffocative catarrh; cannot breath with head low.

Asthma; < damp weather, autumn or after depletion. Every motion excites palpitation and takes his breath. *Painfully sore chest*, with a soreness between scapulae, cannot bear percussion or auscultation. Suppurative phthisis. Paroxysms of cough after eating or laughing < evening, night. Want to be fanned but not too hard, for it takes her breath.

HEART: Every movement excites palpitation.

NECK & BACK: Pressure as of a stone between scapulae. *Inter-scapular spine painful.* Sharp pains across kidneys < movement, at night. Knife like pains around the back. Heavy pressure on sacrum. backache as from sitting bent for long time. Lumbago < slight motion.

EXTREMITIES: As if heavy load on shoulders. Spasmodic stretching of arms, with clenched fingers. Hands tremble, (while writing). Twitching in knees. Sensation as of a band about legs, or arms. One hand is icy cold other is warm. Swelling of veins of the hands. Nails blue. Pain in limbs and joints feel as if sprained < slight touch; > hard pressure. Weariness of joints < morning, sitting. Pain in marrow. Caries of bones with profuse sweat.

SKIN: Extreme sensitiveness to touch; hard pressure relieves. Dermatitis. Humid gangrene. Yellow colour.

SLEEP: Drowsiness. Heavy, snoring sleep; esp. in children/ Anxious frightful dreams; fear of dreams remains. Sleeplessness as a prodrome.

FEVER: *Marked prodrome.* Stages of chill, heat and sweat well marked. Chill, then thirst, then heat, then thirst. Chill begins in the breast. Red hot face, with cold hands. *Hectic fever.* DRENCHING SWEATS; AT NIGHT; < *least motion;* from weakness; from depletions etc. Tropical fevers. Sepsis.

COMPLEMENTARY: Carb-v., Ferr., Kali-c.

RELATED: Carb-v.

CHININUM ARSENICOSUM

GENERALITIES: Weakness, weariness, prostration and disinclination for mental work are marked symptoms of this remedy. Irritability precedes headache. Sudden attacks of vertigo < looking up. Hemicrania (L), from fright. Anorexia. Eggs and fish produce diarrhea. Short breath on ascending. Cardiac dyspnea; early myocardial degeneration, after acute infections. Palpitation. Sensation as if heart had stopped. Periodic asthmatic attacks, with great prostration. Sleeplessness due to nervous causes. Coldness; of hands and feet; knees and limbs. Continuous fever; with oscillating temperature. Sweat; profuse, exhaustive; at night. Ill effects of tobacco. Pressure in the solar plexus with tenderness. Hyperacidity alternating with decrease of acidity.

WORSE: Rest. In the a.m. When stomach is empty.

BETTER: Motion.

CHININUM SULPHURICUM

GENERALITIES: Quinine sulphate acts on the NERVES causing great *sensitiveness to external influences* and periodical neuralgia. In blood it causes rapid decrease of red blood cells and reduction of hemoglobin; with tendency to leukocytosis. Weak and nervous, little exertion causes palpitation Retro-bulbar neuritis, with sudden loss of sight. Inability to remain standing. Falling in street Wants to lie down. Deathly sick and faint; felt as if she would sink through bed.

WORSE: EXACT PERIODICITY. Cold. 100-11 a.m. Touch.

BETTER: Yawning. Pressure. Bending forward.

MIND: Nervous. Lost power of naming object.

HEAD: Pain of malarial origin increasing gradually at noon < at left side. *Vertigo with tinnitus;* with twitching of the eyelids; with throbbing headache. Orbital neuralgia.

EYES: A net, fog or smoke before the eyes. Can see objects only when looking sideways. Squint on alternating days (children).

EARS: Tinnitus. Deafness. Menier's disease.

FACE: Neuralgia pains return with great regularity > by pressure. Bro ague. Pale anxious face.

URINARY: Deposit of straw yellow, granular or brick red sediment. Urine bloody.

BACK: *Cervico-dorsal spine aches or is very tender;* with oppression of breath.

EXTREMITIES: Acute articular rheumatism. Joints very sensitive.

SKIN: Itching. Petechiae. Urticaria.

FEVER: Anticipating chills. Thirst in all stages. Delirium during heat. Increasing fever and prostration, with profuse night sweats. Profuse sweat > but exhausts. Clear apyrexia. Typical malaria. Subnormal temperature.

RELATED: Chin.

CHIONANTHUS

GENERALITIES: It has a powerful action on LIVER, and on head, where it is useful for neurasthenia; periodical sick, menstrual or bilious headache. *Bruised soreness* is felt in various organs—*liver,* eyeballs, etc. Pains ascend from forehead, stomach, etc. Jaundice occurring every summer.

WORSE: *Jarring.* Motion cold.

BETTER: *Lying on abdomen.*

MIND: Feels played out. No desire to do anything; wants to be left alone.

HEAD: Severe *bilious sick headache,* < stooping, motion, jarring.

EYES: Eyeballs feel bruised. Yellow conjunctiva.

NOSE: Pressing at the root of nose, or squeezing on bridge.

MOUTH: Dry, not relieved by water. Tongue broad, with thick greenish-yellow fur; feels drawn up. Salivation.

STOMACH: Bitter-sour, hot, bilious, ropy, gushing vomiting; sets the teeth on edge. Vomiting with colic and *cold sweat* on forehead and *back of hands.*

ABDOMEN: Liver enlarged enormously with uneasy ache and jaundice. Griping at navel. Feels as if a string were tied or a stop-knot around the intestines which was suddenly drawn tight and gradually loosened. Cholecystitis. Gall-stone. Jaundice, with arrest of menses. Weakness in hypogastrium. Stool tarry, clay colored or undigested. Cold sweat on forehead and back of hand during stool. Affection of pancreas.

URINARY: Urine of orange-yellow color, thick, black, syrupy. Bile and sugar in urine. Diabetes mellitus. High specific gravity.

RESPIRATORY: Astringent expectoration.

SKIN: Yellow all over. Jaundice, chronic, recurring every summer, caused by drinking too much cider.

FEVER: Heat with aversion to uncover. Cold sweat on back of hands.

RELATED: Bry; Iris; Lept; Merc.

CHLORAL HYDRATE

GENERALITIES: This drug affects the *brain* causing cerebral excitement with hallucination, and night terror in children. Heart is dilated or weakened with peculiar fullness and lightness in chest and sense of emptiness in stomach. Muscular prostration. Chorea, long standing, obstinate; patient could neither lie nor stand.

WORSE: *Alcohol*. Night. Exertion. Lying down. Hot drink. Stimulant.

BETTER: Open air. Being fanned.

MIND: Melancholia, idiocy and insanity. Hurried and excited, walks up and down the room, conversing with imaginary being, or with himself.

HEAD: Hot band feeling from temple to temple.

EYES: Eyeballs feel too large, blood shot and watery. Objects look white, color blindness. Eyelids heavy, can hardly lift them.

EARS: Hears voices.

FACE: Face and eyelids are swollen, could hardly see, urticaria.

STOOL: Bileless.

URINARY: Bed-wetting; passes water in bed copiously without knowing it, during later part of night.

RESPIRATORY: Dyspnea, as from a weight on chest. Inspires through the nose, expires through the mouth, when lying on back.

HEART: Weak or dilated.

SKIN: Urticaria, < by night, disappears by day, suddenly appears from chill, > by warmth, < alcohol. Skin stone cold.

SLEEP: Sleepless from fatigue. Horrid dreams.

RELATED: Apis; Calc-fl.

CHLORUM

GENERALITIES: This gas is proved in the form of chlorine water. It has marked action on *respiratory organs* producing spasm of the glottis. Sensation of *constriction* is another marked feature. Patient rapidly emaciate. *Mucous membranes* are inflamed and ulcerated.

WORSE: *Expiration*. After midnight. Lying.

BETTER: Open air. Motion.

MIND: Fears insanity or losing senses. Forgets names and persons.

EYES: *Protruding.*

NOSE: Smoky or sooty. *Coryza acrid,* with headache, suddenly running in drops, with lacrimation.

FACE: Swollen, with protruding eyes.

MOUTH: Putrid odor from mouth. Putrid aphthae. *Tongue dry,* black.

THROAT: Choking sensation, inability to swallow. Aching, tickling or whistling in throat pit.

RESPIRATORY: Sudden DYSPNEA from spasm of the vocal cord, with protruding eyes, blue face, cold sweat. Inspiration free but CANNOT EXHALE. Laryngitis. Laryngismus stridulus. Hay asthma. Feels air being forced into upper chest.

SKIN: Sensitive, dry, yellow, shrivelled.

FEVER: Easy sweat.

RELATED: Ars-i; Iod; Meph; Merc.

CHOLESTERINUM

GENERALITIES: This substance is abundantly present in bile and biliary calculi. It is a useful remedy for obstinate hepatic engorgement, for cancer of the liver, for obstinate gall stone, for vitreous opacity and obstinate jaundice.

WORSE: Touch or jar. Lying on side. Bending or sudden motion.

CICUTA VIROSA

GENERALITIES: Commonly known as water hemlock, it exerts its chief influence on BRAIN AND NERVOUS SYSTEM, producing *violent spasmodic effects.* Convulsion, trismus, tetanus, hiccough. JERK of head, and twitching of various parts, of arms and fingers. *Frightful contortions. Spasms move downwards with terrific violence,* with sudden shocks through body or head, then *rigidity* or shrieks; then prolonged unconsciousness; OPISTHOTONOS, and *frightful facial distortion,* with bloody foam from the mouth, then *utter prostration;* spasm is renewed by touch, by noise, loud talking. Epilepsy. Spasm of diaphragm, hiccough; spasm of gullet. Muscles become rigid. Cerebro-spinal meningitis. Concussion of brain. Trouble arising from shaving. Catalepsy. Does not remember what has happened, does not recognize anybody but answers well.

WORSE: INJURY TO THE BRAIN, to esophagus from splinter in flesh. Jar. Noise. Touch. Cold. Dentition. Suppressed eruption. Draught. Tobacco smoke. Turning the head.

BETTER: Thinking of pain. Warmth.

MIND: Childish behavior. Sings, dances, shouts. Moaning, howling, and weeping. Excessively affected by sad stories. Mistrust and shunning of man. Despises others. Confounds present with the past. Mania, with dancing, laughing and ridiculous gesture. Feels as if he was in a strange place. Everything appears strange and terrible. Violent. Rash. Delirium. Sad when seeing others happy. Memory blank, for hours or days. Falls to ground and rolls about with or without convulsion. Feels herself unsteady; over-estimation of himself. Does not remember what has happened, does not recognize anybody but answers well.

HEAD: Twisted or turned to one side (spasm). *Jerks the head.* Congestion of head, with vomiting and purging. *Vertigo,* objects move from side to side or approach and recede. Sudden violent shocks through the head. Head symptoms > by thinking of it, sitting erect and passing flatus. Thick yellow scabs on head. Sweat during sleep. Meningitis. Vertigo with gastralgia and muscular spasm. Head retracted, spine rigid.

EYES: Pupils dilated in concussion of the brain, contracted in spasm. Letters go up and down or disappear when reading. When staring at any object, or sitting in apparent sleep, the head inclines forward. Squint - periodic, spasmodic, after a fall or blow. Effect of exposure to snow. Objects appear double and black. *Eyes roll, jerk and stare.* Eyelids twitch.

EARS: Bleeding, in cerebral trouble. Sudden detonation, esp. on swallowing. Ears hot or cold.

NOSE: Slight touch causes it to bleed. Frequent sneezing without coryza.

FACE: Red, or pale and drawn, sweaty; distorted horribly or ridiculously. Lockjaw. Confluent pustules forming thick scabs. Epithelioma of lips.

MOUTH: Foam in and around. Grinding of the teeth, with lockjaw. Swelling of the tongue; speech difficult. Bites the tongue.

THROAT: Feels as if closed or *grown together*. Spasm of esophagus; cannot swallow—from injury, fish bone, etc. Effect of swallowing sharp fish bones. Stricture of oesophagus.

STOMACH: Craves coal, chalk and many other strange articles from inability to distinguish between edible and things unfit to be eaten, etc. *Loud hiccough,* with crying, alternating with thoracic spasm. Vomiting of bile, of blood on stooping, on rising, in pregnancy. Throbbing in pit of the stomach with distention. Waterbrash; saliva flows from mouth, with heat all over.

ABDOMEN: Colic, with convulsion, with vomiting. Flatulence with anxiety and crossness.

URINARY: Involuntary urination, in old men. Urine is passed with great force. Stricture of urethra, after inflammation, gonorrhea. Paralysis of bladder.

MALE: Testes drawn up towards external abdominal rings.

FEMALE: Spasmodic state when menses do not appear. Coccyx painful during menses. Puerperal convulsion.

RESPIRATORY: Chest feels tight, can hardly breathe. Heat or cold sensation in chest.

HEART: Trembling palpitation of the heart. Feels as if the heart has stopped beating, with faint feeling.

NECK & BACK: Spasms and cramps in muscles of neck, head drawn backward. Opisthotonos. Jerks in coccyx during menses.

EXTREMITIES: Jerking and twitching in the arms and fingers. Jerking in left arm all day. Trembling of left leg. Feet tilt inwards while walking. Feet turned inwards and toes turned upwards in spasm. Curved limbs cannot be straightened nor straight ones bent. Swings feet in half circle while walking.

SLEEP: Bites the tongue in sleep. Deep sleep. Dreams vivid, but unremembered.

SKIN: Pustules coalesce into *thick, yellow*, massive scabs, < head and face. Impetigo *Eczema without itching.* Suppressed eruptions causes brain disease. Barber's itch, baker's itch.

RELATED: Cupr; Strych.

CIMICIFUGA (Actea racemosa)

GENERALITIES: This remedy has a wide action on NERVES AND MUSCLES. It causes *depression of mind with low spirit,* and exhaustion along with *oversensitiveness* esp. to pain. It is a great female remedy. Plump, delicate, sensitive, nervous, chilly women who complain of aching in back, neck, here and there; many of the complaints are dependent upon utero-ovarian irritation. *General sick feeling,* with exhaustion. Many of the symptoms are irregular, changeable or they alternate in groups; alternation of physical and mental effects. Alternate mental and rheumatic symptoms. Pain is violent; aching, shooting, wanders *here and there,* shock-like; with cries, *fainting,* etc. go upward or *from side to side, up the neck;* about the throat, from *ovary to ovary.* Belly of the *muscles feels bruised, sore, heavy, aching. Trembling,* twitching in various organs or of part lain on. Compressive pain. Hysterical or epileptic convulsion at the time of menses. Alternating clonic and tonic spasms. Sore and tender along the tract of pain. *Nervous* shuddering. Given before the term it renders labor earlier, cures sickness of pregnancy, prevents the afterpain. It has also ensured live birth in women who have previously borne only dead children without any discoverable cause (should be given in daily doses of 1x potency two months before term). Myalgia. Ovaralgia. Lumbago. Spasm of cerebro-spinal fever. Influenza. Chorea, at puberty, with delayed menses; cardiac chorea. Ill-effect of anxiety, fright, disappointed love, overexertion, business failure, childbearing. Children during dentition.

WORSE: *Menstruation*; when suppressed. During labor. Emotion. *Alcohol.* Night. Change of weather. Heat and cold. Sitting. Puberty and climaxis. Motion. *Damp cold air. Wind.* Draft.

BETTER: *Warm wrap.* Open air. Pressure. Eating. Continued motion. Grasping things.

MIND: Desire to wander from place to place. Melancholy. Agitation. *Nervous, fidgety, excitable* and jerky. Irritable, least thing which goes wrong makes her crazy. Depressed and talkative, with constant change of subject. Suspicious. *Gloomy* forebodings, of death, of insanity, of impending evil, etc. *Thinks she is going crazy.* Feels faint in epigastrium when meeting a friend. Fear of riding in a closed carriage. Fears those in house will kill him. *Deathly fear of rat.* Vision of rats, mouse, various colors and forms. Mania, before menses; alcoholic; tries to injure himself. Puerperal mania, mania following disappearance of neuralgia. Weak will. Takes no interest in housework. Indifferent. Despondent; seems to feel she is under a heavy black cloud. Suspicious, would not take medicine. Sits and mopes, in great sadness; when questioned breaks into tears. Mental symptoms are > by diarrhea or menses, < after rheumatism.

HEAD: Waving or wild sensation in brain. *Head retracted* (meningitis). Shooting, throbbing pain, after worry, over-study or from reflex uterine disease, > open air. Head or brain, feels too large. Opening and shutting sensation in brain. *Vertex feels as if it would fly off,* < going upstairs, or as if it opened and let in cold air. As if cold air were blowing upon the brain, or heat on vertex. Feeling of a blow, or as if a bolt had been driven from *occiput* through vertex up to the eye (left). Headache of students.

EYES: *Intense aching in eyeballs or behind it,* > pressure, < slightest motion. Pain from eyes to vertex. Eyes feel big; wild look. Sees red flashes with dark borders. Cannot tolerate artificial light. Sensation if a needle were run into the eyeballs, < closing eyes. Ciliary neuralgia.

EARS: Tinnitus. Sensitive to least noise, with spasmodic labor pain. Violent noises in ear with deafness.

NOSE: Sensitive to cold air; every inhalation seems to bring the cold air in contact of brain.

FACE: Pale, hot. Neuralgia affecting malar bones, > night, reappears the next day. Forehead cold. Facial blemishes in young women. Forehead feels cold. Wild, fearful expression.

MOUTH: *Saliva thick.* Coppery taste. Hawks up viscid coppery tasting mucus. Trembling of tongue. Thick mucus on teeth. Cannot speak a word though she tries. Tongue and mouth feel warm. Tongue swollen.

THROAT: Burning. Thyroid aches before menses.

STOMACH: *Nausea,* in morning, of pregnancy, of alcoholism, felt in bowels, < pressure on spine and cervical region. Vomits green substance, groans, raves and presses the head with both the hands for relief. Sinking in epigastrium, on meeting a friend. Eructations, with nausea, vomiting and headache (women).

ABDOMEN: Colic, > bending double and after stool. Frequent, thin, dark, offensive stools. Morning diarrhea of children. Sharp pain across hypogastrium. Alternate diarrhea and constipation.

URINARY: Profuse clear urine, causing weakness, with yellow sand. Nervous urination.

FEMALE: Menses, profuse, dark, coagulated, *scanty,* with backache, nervousness; irregular in time and quantity; *more flow more pain.* Great debility between menses. Ovarian neuralgia; pain across pelvis, from *ovary to ovary,* or goes upward or downward along the thighs. Menses suppressed from emotion, from cold. Hysteric or epileptic spasm at the time of menses. Uterine atony. Presses mammae as though in pain. Mania. Burning in mammae. Slow labor pain with nervous shivers. Intolerable afterpain, < in groins. Leukorrhea, with a sensation of weight in the uterus. Cardiac neuralgia in parturition. Inframammary pains, < left side. Lochia suppressed by cold or emotion. Nervous, when coughing and urinating. Shudders.

RESPIRATORY: Tickling, short, dry, constant cough, < at night, speaking. Sharp stitches in left chest, motion extorting cries. Pleurodynia. Nervous cough.

HEART: Sore, swollen, or feels enlarged, . Needle-like pain at heart. Angina pectoris - pain spreads all over the chest and back, and down the left arm which feels numb and bound to the side. Heart action ceases suddenly, impending suffocation. Pulse weak, irregular, trembling; drops every 3rd, or 4th beat.

NECK & BACK: Neckache, throws the head back. Stiff neck, pain < moving the hands. Neck retracted. Spine, cervical and upper dorsal, very sensitive, < pressure, which causes nausea and retching. Soreness of all the muscles. Stiff, contracted neck and back. Pain in the angle of left scapula. Heavy pulsating lumbar pain, through hips and down the thighs.

EXTREMITIES: Uneasy and restless feeling in the limbs. Left arm feels as if bound to the side; constant irregular motion of left arm (chorea). Hands tremble while writing. Cramp in limbs, in calves. Tendo-achilles, stiff and contracted. Soles itching. Cold sweat on hands and feet. Alternation of rheumatic and mental symptoms. Trembling of legs, can scarcely walk. Numbness of limbs.

SLEEP: Comatose, as if drunk. Sleeplessness. Sleeps with arms over-head or yawning.

RELATED: Bapt; Caul; Gels; Ign; Puls.

CINA

GENERALITIES: *Cina* is the source of the alkaloid santonin. NERVOUS mental and bodily symptoms which are produced by this drug may be due to the presence of round worms or reflex from *abdominal irritation,* and affection of the *digestive tract.* It is a children's remedy; children who are big, fat, rosy and scrofulous; they stiffen out when *looked at during cough or when they become cross.* Child is restless, tosses about. Twitching. Spasm due to worms, unilateral. In spasm, children throw arms from side to side. Whole body is painfully sore to motion and touch, bruised soreness. Children are hungry and greater the hunger greater the emaciation. Complaints concomitant to yawning, which comes on whenever someone yawns. Sour smell of body, esp. of children. Shocks as from pain. Patient will jump suddenly as though he felt pain. Trembling, with shivering, when yawning. Convulsion with consciousness. Paraplegia, with unnatural hunger. Chorea.

WORSE: TOUCH. Worms. Vexation. *Looked at.* DURING SLEEP. Staring. Yawning. *Full moon.* In sun, summer. Looking fixedly at any object.

BETTER: *Lying on abdomen.* Wiping eyes. Motion. Shaking head. Rocking.

MIND: Very TOUCHY; *ugly, cross; petulant and dissatisfied. Children* do not want to be touched, or carried, want to be rocked; they desire many things, but reject everything offered; uneasy and distressed all the time. Nervous. Unreal feeling of having done something wrong. Convulsion in children when they are scolded or punished. Children are proof against all caress. Good-natured children become cross.

HEAD: Ache, alternating with pain in abdomen, > stooping. Pain in head when reading or staring. Child leans his head sideways all the time, turns the head from one side to other. Women must let hair down during headache. Children cannot have the hair combed. Headache, before and after epileptic attack.

EYES: *Pupils dilated.* Pulsation in superciliary muscles. Eyebrows twitch when staring at any object, he sees as through gauze, > wiping eyes. Fatigue of eyes. Vision yellow, blue, violet or green. Squint from worms. *Dark ring around the yes.* Weak sight from masturbation.

NOSE: Itching. PICKS AND BORES AT NOSE till it bleeds, wants to rub it. Sneezing, with whooping cough. Nostrils drawn in.

FACE: Pale, with sickly look, during cough. Bluish White about the mouth. Face alternately pale and cold or red and hot. Choreic movements of the face and hands.

MOUTH: *Grinds the teeth* at night during sleep. Chews and swallows in sleep. Clean tongue.

THROAT: Difficult swallowing of liquids; noisy swallowing. Clucking from throat to stomach; after coughing or convulsion. Constant swallowing, involuntary.

STOMACH: *Hunger, voracious, after eating,* after vomiting, with gnawing in stomach, alternating with loss of appetite. Hunger before chill or follows sweat. Hunger in paraplegia. Desires many different things; craving for sweets, bread. Vomiting with a clean tongue. Vomiting and diarrhea immediately after eating and esp. drinking. Aversion to mother's milk.

ABDOMEN: Twisting pain about the navel, > pressure. Distended and hard. Cutting, pinching pain from worms. Stool white, watery. Itching at anus. Unpleasant warm feeling.

URINARY: Bed wetting, < every full moon. Urine; turbid, WHITE, MILKY, or turns milky on standing.

MALE: Bad effect of onanism, with weakness of sight.

FEMALE: Uterine hemorrhage before puberty. Child refuses breast. Menses, too early and profuse.

RESPIRATORY: Recurrent choking cough, with sneezing. Violent cough bringing tears and sternal pain, feels as if something is torn off. Gurgling from throat to stomach after coughing. Child keeps still and does not talk or move because of the fear of cough. Sternum feels too close to back. Cough ends in spasm. Suffocative attacks. Expectoration difficult.

EXTREMITIES: Tosses arms from side to side (children). Sudden inward jerking of fingers of right hand. Stretches out feet spasmodically (children). Twitching and jerking in limbs. Left foot in constant spasmodic motion. Paraplegia, sudden, with unnatural hunger.

SLEEP: Restless. Gets on hands and knees or on abdomen in sleep. Night terrors of children, *cries out,* screams, wakes frightened. Screams and talks in sleep.

FEVER: With pale cold face and warm hands. Much fever, clean tongue during fever. Cold sweat on forehead, nose and hands. Hungry before chill and after sweat.

COMPLEMENTARY: Calc; Dros; Rat.

RELATED: Cham; Nat-p.

CINNABARIS

GENERALITIES: Mercuric sulphide is an anti-sycotic and antisyphilitic remedy. Indolence and indisposition to mental work. General sensitiveness to touch—bones, scalp, etc. While lying on right side feels contents of body were being dragged to that side.

WORSE: Touch. Light. Dampness. Walking.

BETTER: Open air. Sunshine. After dinner.

EYES: *Pain outward along brows,* encircling the eyes or like a saddle at the root of the nose. Redness of the whole eye.

NOSE: *Heavy pressure at the root of the nose,* < pressure of glasses. Discharge from the nose is acrid, foul, burning, watery or dark lumps.

MOUTH: Dry mouth and throat, wakes from sleep, must rinse the mouth. Hawks stringy mucus from throat, or lumpy mucus drops from the posterior nares. Naso-pharyngeal catarrh.

ABDOMEN: Formication in the anus, as from a large worm. Bloody dysentery. Thin white stools. Green mucous diarrhea, which stains the skin about anus and scrotum copper color.

MALE: Jerking in penis during sleep. Foul acrid sweat between scrotum and thighs. Warts on prepuce, esp. fan-shaped. Small red pimples on glans. Old hard chancre. Itching of corona glandis. Redness and swelling of prepuce.

FEMALE: Leukorrheal discharge with a feeling of pressure in vagina.

HEART: Heart flutters, then rush of blood to the head.

EXTREMITIES: Nodes on shin bones. Left leg feels shorter than the right while walking. Cramp in calves after walking. Pain in tendo achilles and os calcis when walking. Cold knees, or joints. Pain from elbow downwards into hands.

SKIN: *Fiery red ulcers* on skin and mucous membranes. Red eruptions. Violent itching and pricking. Sweat on nose. Honeycombed ulcer.

COMPLEMENTARY: Thuj.

RELATED: Merc.

CISTUS CANADENSIS

GENERALITIES: Commonly known as rock rose it is an ancient remedy for scrofulosis. It affects the GLANDS, esp. of *naso-pharynx, neck* and mammae (left). It also produces herpetic eruptions, scorbutic state, chronic swelling and gangrenous ulceration. The patient is *painfully sensitive to cold, to cold inspired* air. *Feeling of coldness in* various parts; of tongue, saliva, in throat; eructations, in stomach, even the discharges. Mucous discharges are *thick, yellow, foul,* leave a painful rawness. *Suppuration.* Internal and external *itching.* Formication through the whole body, with anxious, difficult breathing. Malignant disease of glands of neck. Poisoned wound, bite, phagedenic ulcer. Burning. Induration. Callosities, with cracks.

WORSE: *Cold;* talking; *drafts;* inspired air. Cold water. Mental *exertion;* excitement. Touch. Motion.

BETTER: Eating. Expectoration.

MIND: Bad effect of vexation. Fear.

HEAD: Aches when he misses the meal, > eating. Head drawn to one side by swelling in the neck.

EYES: Feeling as if something moving around the eye. Canthi cracked.

EARS: Fetid watery discharge of pus, after eruptive disease. Tetters on and around the ear extending to external meatus.

NOSE: Cold feeling or burning. Tip painful. Eczema of the nose. Feels a lump in naso-pharynx. Chronic nasal catarrh, frequent violent sneezing. Pressing pain at the root of the nose, with headache.

FACE: Itching, burning and crusts on zygoma. Caries of the lower jaw with suppurating glands of neck. Open bleeding cancer on lower lip. Lips cracked.

MOUTH: Scorbutic, receding gums, easily bleeding, disgustingly putrid. Tongue feels cold. Breath cold. Saliva cold. Hurts when protruding the tongue. Pyorrhea.

THROAT: Cold affects the throat which feels cold. Soft, spongy feeling; itching in the throat. Becomes sore on inhaling least cold air. Dry spot in throat, > by sipping water. Pain when coughing. Glands swollen and suppurating. Goitre, with frequent diarrhea.

STOMACH: Cool feeling, before and after eating. Desire for cheese, for pungent things. Eructations cold.

ABDOMEN: Cool feeling all over. Diarrhea, from coffee and fruits, with goiter, with nausea. Thin hurried stools, < in morning.

MALE: Itching on scrotum.

FEMALE: Induration and inflammation of mammae (left). Sensitive to cold air. Cancer. Bad smelling leukorrhea.

RESPIRATORY: Larynx and trachea feel cool on inhaling cold air. Coldness in chest. Expectoration of quantities of glairy, tenacious mucus, on lying down. Trachea feels narrow and breathing becomes difficult preceded by formication. Chest feels raw, after expectoration.

NECK & BACK: *Hard swollen glands* in the neck. Burning bruised pain in coccyx preventing sitting, < touch.

EXTREMITIES: Cold feet. Cracked finger tips, sensitive to cold. Workmen develop hard place on their hands, with cracks.

SKIN: Hard, thick, dry, *cracked.* Itching, crawling all over, without eruption.

FEVER: Chilliness. Sweats easily; fever at night.

RELATED: Calc; Helo; Hep.

CLEMATIS ERECTA

GENERALITIES: It affects *mucous membranes* of *eyes* and urethra and the GLANDS, esp. TESTES, mammae, ovaries, which become VERY HARD and PAINFULLY *swollen.* Neuralgic pain in various parts. Burning, itching, stinging, crawling. Great debility. Muscles flaccid or twitch. Vibrating sensation through the body after lying down. Emaciation. Aversion to washing. Rheumatic, gonorrheal and syphilitic patients. Organic stricture.

WORSE: GONORRHEA. *Heat of bed.* Night. *Cold washing.* Cold air. Light. Moon < and >. Mercury.

BETTER: Sweating. Open air.

MIND: *Indifference*. Fear of being alone, but disinclined to meet even agreeable company. Ailments from homesickness. Peevish, dissatisfied without any cause. Melancholy.

HEAD: Confused feeling, > open air. Eruptions, on occiput at the base of hair, moist, pustular, sensitive, itching.

EYES: Iritis. Chronic conjunctivitis. Lacrimation. Sensitive to air, must close them. Complaints from bright sun light. Burning, as if fire were streaming out, and smarting, < closing eyes.

EARS: Ringing as from bell.

FACE: Pain in right side of face, eye, ear and temple, > holding cold water in the mouth. Swelling of submaxillary glands, with hard tubercles, throbbing, < touch. Cancer of the lip.

MOUTH: Toothache, < at night and tobacco, > drawing in air, cold water. Breath offensive to others.

STOMACH: Weakness in all the limbs after eating, with pulsation in arteries. Nausea on smoking tobacco, with weakness of legs. Disagreeable sensation of coldness in stomach.

ABDOMEN: Pain from abdomen to chest, < breathing and during urination. *Swelling of inguinal glands* with jerking pain in scirrhus, suppressed gonorrhea, rheumatism of joints.

URINARY: Urine stops and starts, or *dribbles* after urination. Has to strain for passing few drops, then full stream flows. Stricture of urethra. Urethra feels like a large whipcord painful on pressure. Burning in urethra during urination. Inability to evacuate all the urine at once. Last drops of urine cause violent burning.

MALE: Aversion to coition. Testes indurated, with bruised feeling. Orchitis. Testes hang heavy or retracted. Swelling of the spermatic cord, with burning and soreness, extending to abdomen. Burning in penis during seminal discharge in coitus. Swelling of right half of the scrotum. Violent erections, with stitches in urethra.

FEMALE: Full, heavy, sensitive breasts; pain darts outward. Swelling and induration of mammary glands. Cancer of the breast, with stitches in shoulders and uterus. Menses too early. Shooting pain in breast, < urinating.

RESPIRATORY: Respiration impaired, < ascending hill or walking over uneven road. Barking, dry cough, with stitches in chest.

HEART: Sharp stitches at heart, from within outward.

EXTREMITIES: Weakness in limbs after eating; or with nausea on smoking tobacco. Axillary glands swollen.

SKIN: Itches violently with profuse desquamation, < washing in cold water. Vesicles, pustules. Corroding eruptions ending in flat eating ulcer with thick crust and eczema, < occiput and lower legs. Varicose ulcers. Herpes zoster.

SLEEP: *Sleepiness.* Restless dreamy sleep with vibratory sensation throughout the body.

COMPLEMENTARY: Merc.

RELATED: Phos; Rhod; Staph.

COBALTUM

GENERALITIES: This metal affects the spine (lumbar region), genitals, kidneys and bones, and is useful in neurasthenic states of spinal origin, with sexual disturbances. *Discharges frothy.* Soreness. Aching in bones. Sour taste, stomach, foot, sweat, etc. Fatigue.

WORSE: Sexual loss. Sitting. Heat of bed or sun. Morning.

BETTER: Hawking mucus. Continued motion.

MIND: Sense of guilt. Mental excitement < sufferings. Thinks too little of himself.

HEAD: Vertigo, with feeling as if head grows large, < stool. Headache, < stooping, jarring. Sensation as if the brain went up and down on stepping.

EYES: Photophobia in spring. Spring catarrh. Darting pain in the eyes on coming into sunshine.

FACE: Disposition to keep jaws tightly closed.

MOUTH: Teeth feel too long. Tongue coated white; *crack across the middle.* Taste sour.

STOMACH: Sour or bitter water rises up with pain in stomach.

ABDOMEN: Shooting from liver region down into the thighs. Empty feeling at navel. Desire for stool while walking, < on standing, followed by diarrhea. Constant dropping of blood from anus; no blood with stools. Yellow spots on abdomen. Shooting pain in the region of the liver and sharp pain in the region of spleen, < taking deep breath.

URINARY: Albuminuria. Smarting at the meatus at the end of urination. Urine has a strong pungent smell.

MALE: Pain in right testicle, > after urination. *Frequent nocturnal emissions, with lewd dreams, headache and backache.* Yellow-brown spots on genitals. Discharge of semen without erection. Impotency.

RESPIRATORY: Cough with copious frothy, sweetish white mucous lumps in it.

BACK: Aching pain in lumbar region, < coition, sitting, > on rising, walking or lying down, with weak knees, cannot straighten up. Weakness and backache after emission. Pain along the spine, and from the sacrum down through the legs into the feet.

EXTREMITIES: Shooting into thighs from liver. Weak knees. Flushes of heat along legs. Trembling of limbs, esp. legs, aching when sitting. Foot sweat mostly between the toes, smelling sour. Tingling, pricking in feet. Sudden weakness in left hip, < walking.

SLEEP: Wakeful; can do with less sleep. Disturbed by lewd dreams. Drowsy, and can hardly get enough sleep.

SKIN: Pimples about nates, chin, hairy scalp. Itching all over when getting warm in bed.

RELATED: Eup-per.

COCA

GENERALITIES: *Coca* is the source of alkaloid cocaine, is a local anesthetic. It is the remedy for the exhaustion of BRAIN AND NERVOUS SYSTEM from physical and mental strain and for those who suffer from *dizziness, dyspnea and exhaustion* on going to high altitude, mountain climbing, aeroplane flying, etc. A characteristic sensation is as if a worm or small foreign bodies were under the skin, moving away when touched; if this symptom is associated with any diseased condition Coca is indicated. Suitable for old people. Short-breathed people, weakly, nervous, fat, plethoric people. Children with marasmus. Muscle exhaustion.

WORSE: Ascending. High altitude. Cold. Mental exertion. Walking. Sitting. Salty food.

BETTER: *Rapid motion,* riding in *open air.* After sunset. Lying on face.

MIND: Mental prostration alternating with exhilaration.

Timid, bashful, ill-at-ease in society; craves solitude and obscurity. Sense of impending death. Hallucinations of hearing; unpleasant; about himself. Loquacious excitement with blissful visions. Exhilaration before menses. Sense of right and wrong abolished. Personal appearance neglected.

HEAD: Ache, with vertigo, preceded by flashes of light before the eyes Shocks coming from occiput, with vertigo. Migraine, < coughing, > eating, sunset.

EYES: Flickering before the eyes. White, dark and fiery spots before the eyes. Pupils dilated. Diplopia.

EARS: Noises in ears. Tinnitus.

NOSE: Sense of smell greatly diminished.

MOUTH: Caries of teeth. Tongue furred. Peppery sensation in the mouth.

THROAT: Eructation rises with noise and violence, as if it would split the esophagus.

STOMACH: Great satiety for long time. Retards hunger and thirst. Craving for alcohol and tobacco. No appetite but for sweets. Aversion to solid food.

ABDOMEN: Dysentery of high attitude. Abdomen distended.

MALE: Sensation as if penis were absent. Diabetes, with impotency.

FEMALE: Menses flow in gushes, waking her from sleep.

RESPIRATORY: Loss of voice (5 or 6 drops of tincture every half hour before the expected demand on voice). Senile asthma. Emphysema. Want of breadth, short breath, esp. in aged athletes. Hoarseness, < talking.

HEART: Palpitation; with flushing, excessively rapid pulse; with violent sweating.

EXTREMITIES: Crawling numbness of arms. When walking takes involuntary quick steps, head inclined forward with vertigo.

SKIN: Sensation of a worm under the skin moving away when touched.

SLEEP: Sleeplessness. Can find no rest anywhere though sleepy. Awakens with a shock in brain.

RELATED: Cann-i.

COCAINA

GENERALITIES: The symptoms of *Coca* and *Cocaina* are mostly similar. Sensation as if a small foreign body or a worm under the skin, seeing and feeling of bugs on his own person and on his clothes, as if parts of the body were absent, are more pronounced in Cocaina. Moral sense blunted. Frightful persecutory hallucinations. Personal appearance neglected. Thinks he hears unpleasant remarks about himself. Irrational jealousy. Constant desire to do something great, to undertake vast feats of strength. Chorea. Paralysis agitans. Alcoholic or senile trembling.

COCCULUS INDICUS

GENERALITIES: It is a stupefying poison, hence it causes disturbance of the *sensorium* and affection of *cerebrospinal* axis, producing paralytic muscular relaxation, with heaviness. The patient is very susceptible to fear, anger, grief and all mental disturbances. *He is too weak to hold up his head, stand or even speak.* Paralysis - of face; tongue, pharynx; paraplegia, with numbness and tingling. Suitable for light-haired, timid, nervous person; book-worm; unmarried or childless women; sensitive, romantic girls. Hysteria. Numbness. Sensation of HOLLOWNESS or EMPTINESS—head, chest, abdomen. Single parts *feel gone to sleep.* Shuddering. Painful contraction of the limbs and the trunk. *Tremor,* of head, lower jaw; from excitement, exertion, pain. *Cramps,* in muscles, in masseters, in abdomen, in the heart. Spasm through the body like electric shocks. Convulsion from nonappearance or suddenly checked menses. Alternating symptoms. Ill-effect of anger, fright, grief, anxiety, disappointment, night-watching, overstrain, mental and physical, travelling, sun, tea-drinking. *Sensitive to cold.* Falls down suddenly to ground unconscious. Senses acute. *Train and sea sickness.* Slowness, in moving, in answering; wants plenty of time to do everything. Unilateral affections. Twitching of isolated groups of muscles.

WORSE: *Motion,* of BOAT, CAR, *swimming. Loss of sleep.* Touch. Noise. Jar. Emotion. Kneeling. Stooping. Menses. Eating. *Anxiety. Cold.* Open air. Exertion. Pain.

BETTER: Sitting. In room. Lying on side.

MIND: Dazed. Profound sadness. Thought fixed on one unpleasant subject; sits as if absorbed in deep and sad thought and observes nothing about her. Sudden great anxiety. Things seem unreal. Slow grasp. Easily offended, cannot bear contradiction. Extremely sad, taciturn and peevish. Takes everything in bad part. Time passes too quickly. Drunkard; reeling, roaring, quarrelsome, singing. Very anxious about health of others. Talkative, witty, joking, dancing, gesticulating. Sees something alive on wall, floor, chair, etc. Vaccillatory, does not accomplish anything at her work. Fears death and unknown dangers.

HEAD: VERTIGO, with nausea; with palpitation, < in a.m., raising head; felt in forehead. Heavy head. Pain in *occiput* and nape, < lying on it; > bending backwards, < coffee. Cannot lie on back during the headache. *Opening and shutting sensation,* < occiput. Convulsive trembling of head from weakness of muscles of neck. Cramps in left temporal muscles.

EYES: Pain as if torn out of head (with headache). Eyes closed with the balls constantly rolling about; in spasms. Protruding eyes. Pupils contracted or dilated. Objects seem to move up and down. Jerking of eyelids.

EARS: Sensitive to hearing; dreads sudden noise. Feels closed (R). Noises as from rushing water. Hardness of hearing.

NOSE: Sense of smell acute.

FACE: Paralysis, of one side. Cramp in masseter muscles, < opening mouth. Prosopalgia, with radiating pain to fingers. Tremor of lower jaw, and chattering of teeth, when attempting to speak. Bloated, distorted and cold to touch.

MOUTH: Tongue; feels paralyzed, speech difficult, or hasty; pains at the base when protruded. Metallic taste. Food tastes as if salted too little; tobacco bitter. Pain in teeth, > when biting, with empty mouth. Teeth feel chilly.

THROAT: Paralysis preventing swallowing. Tickling in throat, with lacrimation. Esophagus dry, burning. Constriction in throat, with difficult breathing and inclination to cough.

STOMACH: Loathing of all food and drink. Nausea; rising to head or felt in head. Retching. *Vomiting,* with profuse flow of saliva, with headache and pain in bowels, on taking cold, sour, bitter, bad odor. Feels as if a worm is moving. Hiccough and spasmodic yawning. Disgust for smell of food. Vomiting, with syncope. Vomiting from cerebral tumors, from loud talk. Craves beer. Sensation as if one has been a long time without food, until hunger is gone.

ABDOMEN: Bloated. *Seems full of sharp stones,* on every movement, with diarrhea > lying on sides. Colic: wind, twisting, hysterical, nervous, with faintness, with salivation. Cramp in epigastrium, with difficult breathing. Liver more painful after anger, < least jar. Abdominal muscles weak. Pain in abdominal ring as if something were forced through.

URINARY: Frequent desire to urinate, with slight discharge, in pregnant women. Urine watery.

MALE: Drawing sore pain in testes when touched. Genitals sensitive, with desire for coition.

FEMALE: Menses; early, profuse, too often, gushes out in stream when rising on tip toe. Very weak during menses, can scarcely stand. Purulent, gushing leukorrhea between menses, or in place of menses, weakening, can scarcely speak. Dysmenorrhea followed by hemorrhoids. Clutching in uterus. Shivering over mammae. Leukorrhea gushing, when squatting and stooping, during pregnancy, with frequent urging to urinate.

RESPIRATORY: Sensation of emptiness or cramp in chest. Hysterical asthma. Cough from choking in throat. Audible rumbling in chest (L) as from emptiness, < walking.

HEART: Palpitation, < quick motion, mental excitement; palpitation with vertigo and faintness, then stretching of arms, thumbs drawn inward.

NECK & BACK: Weak neck, cannot hold up head. Pain in neck or cracking in cervical vertebrae when moving head, and on yawning. *Spinal weakness; in lumbar region;* < walking. Paralytic pain in small of the back.

EXTREMITIES: Pain in shoulder and arms as if bruised. Hands, numb, or hot and cold alternately; become numb on grasping objects; tremble while eating. Takes hold of things awkwardly and drops them. Limbs go to sleep. Trembling and pain in limbs. Knees weak; crack on motion. Paraplegia. Alternation between arms. Limbs straightened out, painful when flexed or vice versa. Clumsy gait. Edema of feet with paralysis of lower limbs. Humerus feels broken. Soles numb; while sitting. Involuntary motion of right arm and right leg, > during sleep.

SLEEP: Sleepless from mental or physical exhaustion. Constant drowsiness; after night-watching, nursing. Spasmodic yawning, with hiccough. Anxious, frightful dreams.

SKIN: Much itching, < undressing; itching in a feather bed. Ulcer very sensitive to touch.

FEVER: *Chilliness,* with perspiration and heat of skin. Chill alternating with heat. Nervous form of low fever, from fits of anger. Chill with colic, nausea, vertigo. Sweat; from slight exertion, sweat on affected part.

COMPLEMENTARY: Petr.

RELATED: Gels; Ign.

COCCUS CACTI

GENERALITIES: This is an insect infesting the *cactus* plant. The tincture is prepared from the dried bodies of the female insects. It affects the MUCOUS MEMBRANES, causing *catarrhal condition* and irritation of throat, respiratory and genitourinary organs. DISCHARGES ARE STRINGY, including *hemorrhages,* which are generally in large black clots. *Intolerable internal itching,* burning like pepper. *Pulsation* in different organs. Sensation of a fluid forcing its way during pain. *Spasms. Uric acid,* gouty, rheumatic diathesis. Anuria, anasarca. Ascites. General lassitude.

WORSE: *Periodically. Heat. Lying. Cold exposure.* Awakening. Touch. Pressure of clothing. Brushing teeth. Slightest exertion. IRRITATION OF THROAT. Rinsing mouth.

BETTER: Washing in cold water. Walking. Cold drink.

MIND: Sadness, early morning on waking or after noon at 2-3 p.m.

HEAD: Throbbing pain with sensation as if fluid were forcing its way.

EYES: Sensation of a foreign body between the upper lid and the eyeball.

EARS: Cracking in ears, when swallowing.

NOSE: Burning as of pepper in nostrils. Accumulation of thick viscid mucus in nasopharynx.

FACE: Crawling sensation. Becomes purple, red, < coughing.

MOUTH: Loud speaking or brushing of teeth causes cough. Tip of tongue burns like pepper. Sweetish, metallic taste. Salivation, constant desire to spit.

THROAT: Accumulation of much viscid mucus, *hawking* excites cough, retching and vomiting. Sensation of a thread hanging down the back of the throat. Any irritation in throat causes cough, retching and vomiting. Constricted throat; or feeling of a plug lodged in it. Profuse post-nasal discharge. Sensation as if uvula is elongated causing constant hawking.

STOMACH: Irritation of throat, hawking, brushing of the teeth cause retching and vomiting. Thirst; drinks water often and in large quantities.

ABDOMEN: Excruciating pain from left iliac region, extending to the groin half way down the thighs; as if fluid were forcing its way there.

URINARY: Lancinating, violent pain from kidneys to bladder, with dysuria. Nephritic colic. Constant urging to urinate, > after passing blood clots from the vagina. Sticking pain along ureters. Urine; scanty, thick, heavy, sour; sediment *sandy*, dark red, brown or white; bloody mucus. Nephritis.

MALE: Pulsation in glans.

FEMALE: Vulva sensitive, < when urinating. Menses too early, profuse, black and thick, dark clots, with dysuria. Large clots escape from the vagina when passing urine, when quiet or when rising up. Menses; intermittent; flow only in the evening or at night.

RESPIRATORY: REGULAR PAROXYSMS OF VIOLENT TICKLING. RACKING COUGH ENDING IN VOMITING OR RAISING MUCH CLEAR ROPY MUCUS, hanging from mouth, *with purple red face and internal heat.* Chronic bronchitis complicated with gravel. Whooping cough. Cough; periodical, slowly increasing then gradually decreasing in intensity, > cold air or cold drink. Walking against the wind takes the breath away. Soreness or stitches in apices of lungs. Shortness of breath. Cough of drunkards.

HEART: Sensation as if everything were pressed towards the heart.

BACK: Coldness. Regions of kidneys painful to pressure.

EXTREMITIES: Sensation as if a fine splinter were under the nails of fingers.

FEVER: *Burning;* as of pepper.

RELATED: Apis; Berb; Lach; Phos.

COFFEA CRUDA

GENERALITIES: There is no difference between symptoms of roasted coffee and raw coffee. It is believed that coffee antidotes almost all homeopathic medicines, but it is doubtful whether it could do so, esp. when remedies are given in high potency (Clarke). Experience shows that correctly selected homeopathic remedy acts inspite of taking coffee. Coffee increases the sensibility of NERVES, MAKING THEM OVEREXCITABLE AND OVERSENSITIVE; special senses become OVERACUTE; emotions, esp. joy and *pleasurable surprise,* produce dangerous symptoms. *Pain, touch, noise,* odors become intolerable. Unusual activity of mind and body. Convulsion of teething children, with grinding of the teeth and coldness of the limbs. Convulsion from excessive playing or laughing in weakly children. It is suited to tall, lean, stooping persons, with dark complexion; of choleric temperament. Ill effects of fear, fright, disappointed love, *fatigue,* excessive laughing, long journey. Sensation of warmth. Great nervous agitation and restlessness. Hysteria; screaming, weeping. Pains intolerable, drive to despair.

WORSE: *Noise*. Touch. Odor. Air-open, cold, windy. *Mental exertion;* emotion. Overeating. Alcohol. Night. Narcotics. Strong smell.

BETTER: Lying. Sleep. Warmth.

MIND: Ecstasy; full of ideas, quick to act, therefore *wakeful. Weeps, laments and tosses about,* over trifles. Cries and laughs easily; while crying, suddenly laughs quite heartily and finally cries again. Now joyous now gloomy. Resents sympathy. Faints easily. *Irritable* and *wakeful.* Fright from sudden pleasant surprise. Trembles. Throws things about.

HEAD: Seems as if brain were torn to pieces, shattered or crushed or as if a nail were driven into the head. Clavus. Tight pain. Head feels too small. Feels and hears a cracking in vertex. Temples throbbing, with burning in eyes.

EYES: Can read fine print more distinctly. Pupils dilated. Bright eyes.

EARS: Noise is painful. *Hearing is more acute;* hears distant sound. Hardness of hearing, with buzzing as of a swarm of bees.

NOSE: Acute, sensitive smell. Nosebleed, with heaviness of head, and ill humor; nosebleed during straining at stool.

MOUTH: Toothache, > holding ice water in mouth, < as it warms, extends down arms to the fingertips; toothache during menses. Taste delicate. Salivation; during pregnancy.

FACE: Ache, (right), radiating. Dry, hot, with red cheeks.

THROAT: Pain as from a plug, with constant desire to swallow. Uvula too long.

STOMACH: Immoderate hunger; eats and drinks hurriedly. Stomach feels overloaded, during colic.

ABDOMEN: The clothes are oppressive. Abdominal pain, with despair (women). Diarrhea in housewives from too much care about domestic affairs; diarrhea during dentition.

URINARY: Suppression of urine. Frequent, profuse urination, of colorless urine.

MALE: Hot itching genitals.

FEMALE: Menses too early and long-lasting. Dysmenorrhea, large clots of black blood. Voluptuous itching in the vulva, but vagina and vulva are too sensitive to rub or scratch; aversion to coition therefrom. After pains. Severe afterpains or labor pains, with fear of death. Nymphomania.

RESPIRATORY: Short, dry, hacking, constant cough, of measles, in nervous delicate children.

HEART: Nervous palpitation, with trembling of limbs, < sun heat, after excessive joy or surprise. Sudden rise of blood pressure.

EXTREMITIES: Trembling of hands, cannot hold the pen. Sciatic or crural neuralgia, < motion, > pressure. Twitching in the limbs.

SKIN: *Painfully sensitive.* Itching, scratches until it bleeds.

SLEEP: NERVOUS SLEEPLESSNESS, from rush of ideas, mental activity; hears and awakes at every sound; sleepless from pleasurable excitement.

FEVER: Feverish, with pain and weeping. Traumatic fever.

COMPLEMENTARY: Acon.

RELATED: Coca; Ign.

COLCHICUM AUTUMNALE

GENERALITIES: It affects markedly MUSCLES, *fibrous tissue, serous membranes,* JOINTS, esp. small joints. It causes extreme relaxation of muscles, the head falls forward or backward when the patient is raised from the pillow, arms fall helpless. Patient is WEAK, COLD, (internally), BUT SENSITIVE AND RESTLESS. Pains are tearing, digging, drawing. Pain < by mental exertion and emotion, slightest touch and vibration. Many joints are affected at the same time. Small, rapidly shifting areas of severe pain, but little swelling. Tingling, crawling.

Cardio-arthritic affections. Dropsy. Hydropericardium, hydrothorax; ascites, hydrometra. *Tendency to collapse,* moist collapse, due to dehydration after repeated vomiting or purging. Shock as from electricity through one half of the body, < motion. Bad effects of grief, misbehaviour of others, wetting, *checked sweat,* night-watching; hard study. Irritable and sensitive to impressions, strong odors, etc. Rapid sinking. Creeping. Every little hurt pains terribly. Stubbing the toes hurts exceedingly. Paralysis after sudden suppression of sweat, esp. of foot, by getting wet.

WORSE: *Motion. Touch. Night.* Stubbing toes. Vibration. WEATHER, *cold, damp. In damp room.* Changing weather. Autumn. Slight exertion (mental or bodily). Stretching. Checked sweat. Sunset or sunrise. Loss of sleep. Smell of food.

BETTER: *Warmth.* Rest. Doubling up. Sitting. After stool. Stooping.

MIND: *Depressed, irritable and sensitive.* Can read, but cannot understand a short sentence. Memory weak. Extreme impressions such as bright light, strong odors, contact, misdeed of others make him quite besides himself.

HEAD: Creeping in forehead. Pressive headache, > supper, warmth, lying quiet.

EYES: Pupils unequal. Pain in and around the eyeball, goes to occiput. Acrid tears. Variation in visual acuity. Eyes half open, visible contraction in lower lid. Dim vision after reading.

EARS: Hearing very acute. Itching in ears. Feels stopped up.

NOSE: Nostrils dry and black. SMELL MORBIDLY ACUTE; *odors nauseate* even to fainting, etc. Obstinate coryza.

FACE: Pinched. Sunken. Tingling and edematous swelling. Cheek red, hot, sweaty. Pain behind the angle of lower jaw.

MOUTH: Tongue; bright red, heavy, stiff and numb, projected with difficulty. Glossitis. Taste, flat, bitterish. Mouth hangs open. Flow of saliva with a sense of dryness. Heat in the mouth with thirst. Toothache, < cold and warmth.

THROAT: Much greenish, thin mucus in the throat, comes involuntarily in the mouth.

STOMACH: Thirsty, but LOATHES THE SMELL OR SIGHT OF FOOD, > lying quietly. NAUSEA, retching. Burning or *icy coldness in stomach,* with colic. Craving for various things but averse to them when smelling them. Wants aerated water or effervescent drink. Egg disagrees. Nausea and inclination to vomit, caused by swallowing saliva.

ABDOMEN: Distended, contracts when touched, with inability to stretch the legs. Ascites, with fold over the pubic region. Diarrhea, then gouty effects. Stools; very painful, offensive, cholereic; of shreddy, bloody, gelatinous mucus, then tenesmus or spasm of anus. Mucous colitis, after dysentery. Autumnal dysentery. Colicky pain. Agonizing pain remains long after stool.

URINARY: More urging, more discharge of urine. Urine; hot, highly colored, watery, frequent, bloody, black almost like ink; black sediment. Albuminuria, diabetes. Nephritis.

MALE: Edema of scrotum.

FEMALE: Coldness of thighs, after menses. Sensation of swelling in vulva and clitoris. Feverish restlessness in last month of pregnancy.

RESPIRATORY: Chest seems squeezed by a hand. Night cough, with involuntary spurting of urine. Great dyspnea.

HEART: Cutting or stinging at heart; weak heart. Heart disease following rheumatism. Hydropericardium. Cardiac dyspnea. Pericarditis. Pressure and oppression in the region of the heart, > walking. Pulse thready, imperceptible.

BACK: Ache, > pressure and rest. Tension in cervical muscles felt even on swallowing. Violent pain in region of kidneys, > lying on back only.

EXTREMITIES: Limbs cold. Pins and needles in the hands and wrists; fingertips numb. Joints red, hot, swollen; stiff, shifting rheumatism, < at night. Swelling of great toe. Cannot bear to have it touched. Tingling in finger nails. Finger joints distorted, fingers flexed but in constant motion. Knees knock together, can hardly walk. Edematous swelling and coldness of feet and legs. Buttocks hot.

SKIN: Pink spots on back, abdomen and chest. Urticaria. Skin dry; sweat suppressed or profuse.

SLEEP: Falls asleep while reading. Lies on back.

FEVER: Copious sour sweat suddenly coming and going; rheumatism. Body hot, limbs cold. Cold sweat on face. Sour sweat, nightly.

COMPLEMENTARY: Ars; Spig.

RELATED: Ars; Carb-v; Verat.

COLLINSONIA

GENERALITIES: This remedy produces *congestion in pelvic organs, esp. anus, rectum* and uterus, resulting in *hemorrhoids* and constipation, esp. in females. It is useful in affections due to *piles or alternating with piles,* esp. heart. Congestion in portal system; causes chronic nasal, gastric and pharyngeal catarrh. Constipation of children from intestinal atony. Sensation of constriction and *feeling of enlargement* in various parts and organs of the body—limbs, vulva, clitoris, etc. When given before operation on rectal diseases it is apt to reduce complications. Dropsy from cadiac disease.

WORSE: *Piles,* during or suppressed. *Night. Pregnancy.* Cold. Excitement.

BETTER: Heat. Morning.

MIND: Gloomy.

HEAD: Dull frontal headache, with constipation or piles, or from suppressed hemorrhoidal discharge.

MOUTH: Tongue yellow, with bitter taste.

THROAT: Speaker's sore throat.

ABDOMEN: Dull distress in liver region. Heavy digging ache in pelvis. Diarrhea, acrid, destroying hair. Stools light-colored, lumpy, with hard straining. Mucus or black stools. Constipation, or piles of pregnancy. *Rectum* aches, burns, seems dry and full of sticks or sand, with *cardiac pain. Piles* bleeding, chronic; *alternating with heart,* chest or rheumatic symptoms. *Prolapsus ani. Itching of anus.* Alternate constipation and diarrhea. Chronic diarrhea of children. Diarrhea after delivery. Obstinate constipation, with piles, stools hard.

MALE: Varicocele, with rectal symptoms.

FEMALE: Prolapse of uterus, with hemorrhoids. *Itching of vulva,* with piles, during pregnancy. Sensation of swelling of labia and clitoris. Dysmenorrhea, with piles; membranous. Cold feeling in thighs after menses.

RESPIRATORY: Cough from excessive use of voice. Spitting of blood after suppression of hemorrhoids. Chest pain alternating with hemorrhoids.

HEART: Palpitation, in piles subjects. After heart symptoms are relieved, piles or menses return.

EXTREMITIES: Sensation as if limbs were enlarged. Lower limbs seem not to belong to him.

FEVER: *Flushes of heat,* with oppressive breathing, with piles.

RELATED: Lycps; Nux-v; Sulph.

COLOCYNTHIS

GENERALITIES: In ordinary practice *Colocynth* was used as a drastic purgative. In homeopathy it is not only useful in acute affections of DIGESTIVE TRACT AND INTESTINES but also has a long-lasting action on NERVES (large), esp. TRIFACIAL, SCIATIC and *spinal.* In abdomen it produces SUDDEN, ATROCIOUS CRAMPING, *griping, tearing pain* which make the patient TWIST and *turn, cry out,* or wriggle for relief, or bend double; patient presses something hard against the abdomen. Pains are accompanied by nausea and diuresis and the patient vomits from intensity of pain. Neuralgic pains are CUTTING, *pinching, clamping, gnawing or boring,* followed by numbness, > by pressure. Cramp and twitching and shortening of the muscles, or parts seem too short. *Constriction.* It is suitable to easily angered, irritable persons with tendency to corpulency; to women of sedentary habits with copious menstruation. Cystospasm after operation on orifices. Ill effect of anger, indignation, chagrin, grief, catching cold. Excessive venery. Convulsive jerks and constrictions, during pain. Sensation of being encircled with an iron band, screwed up tightly. Throbbing throughout the whole body. Burning. Prostration, as if all his strength was failing.

Faints with pain and with coldness. Formication in affected part.

WORSE: Emotion; Vexation; *chagrin.* Anger. *Lying on painless side. Night, in bed.* Draft. Taking cold. Before and after urination.

BETTER: Hard Pressure; on edge. *Heat. Rest. Gentle motion.* After stool or flatus. Doubling up.

MIND: Greatly affected by the misfortune of others. *Anger, easily vexed during pain.* Want of religious feeling. Screams with pain; wants to walk about, disinclined to talk, to answer. Impatient. Does not want to meet the friend. Morose; becomes offended at everything.

HEAD: Vertigo when quickly turning the head to the left. Head pain, < stooping, lying on back and moving eyelids, with nausea and vomiting. Roots of hair painful. Head hot.

EYES: On stooping feeling as if eyes would fall out. Violent pain before development of glaucoma; eyes become stony hard. Pain and twitching in eyelids. Burning eyelids.

EARS: Sounds re-echo in ears. Crawling, itching, stitching, aching, > by putting finger into ear.

FACE: Prosopalgia, with eye symptoms, or alternating with pain in celiac region, with chilliness. *Face distorted.* Cheeks cold. Pain anywhere is reflected on the face.

MOUTH: Persistent bitter taste. Burning on the tip of the tongue. Scalded sensation of the tongue. Teeth feel too long.

THROAT: Cramp in gullet, with empty eructations and palpitation of the heart.

STOMACH: Vomits from pain. Sensation in stomach as if something would not yield; drawing pain inthe stomach.

Very thirsty. Vomiting of bitter water. Pain in stomach, with pain in teeth and head. Potatoes and starchy food disagree. Coffee > colic.

ABDOMEN: VIOLENT, CUTTING, GRIPING, GRASPING, CLUTCHING OR RADIATING COLICKY PAIN; COMES IN WAVES, > DOUBLING UP, HARD PRESSURE, < *least food;* or drink, except coffee and tobacco smoking. Flatulent colic. *Intestines feel squeezed between stones.* Colic, with cramp in calves, from drinking when overheated. Cutting in bowels at navel. Pressure > the pain in abdomen in acute stage but when pain remains for a long time, parts become tender, then pressure < the pain. *Stools; frothy, watery, shreddy, yellow,* sourish or gelatinous; *with flatulence and pain.* Dysenteric stools, renewed each time by least food or drink. Slippery bubbles escape from anus. During colic, infant lies on abdomen and screams when he is slightly moved. Chronic watery diarrhea < in the morning. Diarrhea from pain, from anger with indignation.

URINARY: Burning along urethra during stool. Pain on urination over the whole abdomen. Renal colic, with diuresis. Cysto-spasm after operation on the orifices. Urine; gelatinous, sticky, stringy. Red hard crystals adhering to the vessels. Urine milky white, coagulates on standing. Diabetes.

MALE: Sensation as if everything were flowing towards genitals, from both sides of the abdomen, causing seminal emission. Para-Phimosis.

FEMALE: Clutching pain in ovarian region, > drawing up double, with restlessness. Dysmenorrhea, < eating and drinking. Ovarian cyst, with pain, > flexing thigh on pelvis. Suppression of menses or lochia from indignation. Menses copious in women with sedentary habits. Painful nodes in mammae. Ovarian tumor, cyst.

RESPIRATORY: Short cough when smoking tobacco. Difficulty of breathing during menses. Ovarian tumor.

HEART: Feels pushed up by a distended stomach. Strong throbbing in all blood vessels.

BACK: Pain under right scapula > pressure. Lumbar ache, > pressure. *Cramp-like pain in the hips,* > lying on the affected side. Neck stiff, < moving head. Feels a heavy weight in lumbo-dorsal region, > lying on left side.

EXTREMITIES: Contraction of muscles. Sciatic pain, shooting, band-like, screwing, > pressure, heat, < least motion, rotation, at night. Limbs drawn up like hedge hog. Cramps in muscles during coition. Pain in deltoid (R). Knees feel stiff, cold. Feet cold, with colic.

SLEEP: Sleeplessness and restlessness, with pain, after anger.

FEVER: Coldness of hands and soles, rest of the body warm. Chill and shivering with pain. Sweat; at night, cold, smelling like urine.

COMPLEMENTARY: Caust.

RELATED: Staph.

COMOCLADIA

GENERALITIES: It is an irritant poison like *Rhus-tox,* causing malignant inflammation of the skin, with enormous swelling or EDEMA, of left leg and foot. Burning, itching of the eyes, which feel too large. Right eye very painful, feels large, protruded than left. Ciliary neuralgia. Burning itching of the nose with violent sneezing. Pain under the left breast or nipple extending to left scapula, when coughing. Wandering rheumatic pain.

Deep ulcer, with hard edges. Leprosy. Skin red all over. Recurrent eczema.

WORSE: Touch. Warmth. Rest. Night.

BETTER: Open air. Motion. Scratching.

CONIUM MACULATUM

GENERALITIES: This is the poison which is supposed to have been given to the Greek philosopher Socrates for killing hm. It affects the NERVES, AND MUSCLES, causing incoordination and paralysis, uncertain gait, difficult speech; patient becomes gradually WEAK. *Irregular action,* development of symptoms. Sudden loss of strength while walking. *Trembling* of all the limbs. *Suddenly sick and weak,* with *numbness.* Useful in old age or for those persons who become old early; for old maids, bachelors, youths who suffer from ill-effects of masturbation. Glands, esp. MAMMARY and ovaries are affected with engorgement, and STONY INDURATION. *Sensation of a lump; in brain;* in epigastrium. Ascending symptoms; paralysis, after diphtheria. Tearing, stabbing pain. New growth. Arteriosclerosis. Multiple neuritis. Cancerous diathesis. Patients who are < when idle. Paroxysms of hysteria and hypochondriasis from sexual abstinence or sexual excess. Hysterical convulsion. Ill-effect of contusions, blows, overstraining, overwork. Grief. Easily intoxicated. Women are broken down, tired of life, discouraged, who feel as if they were to cry, and who swallow and choke as from a lump in the throat. Progressive *debility. Chronicity.* Clothes distress. Faints at stool. Sensation of a hoop or band or something tight around the part.

WORSE: SEEING MOVING OBJECTS. ALCOHOL. *Raising arms. After exertion*—bodily or mental. *Injury.* Sexual abuse or excess. *Continence. Cold; taking cold. Old age.* Lying, with head low. Turning in bed. Pressure of tight clothing. Jar. *Night.* Standing. Before and during menses. Dry, hot air. Spring.

BETTER: Letting affected part hang down. Stooping. Moving, walking. In the sun. Dark. Pressure. Walking bent. On sitting down. Fasting.

MIND: Depressed, timid, averse to society, yet fears being alone. Slow grasp, difficult understanding. Weak memory. No inclination for business or study. Indifferent. Difficulty in understanding what he is reading. Superstitious. Unable to sustain mental effort. Periodical insanity, of alternating type. While walking on the road wants to hold somebody and abuse him. Trifles seem important. Thinks that animals are jumping on his bed. Sad, dissatisfied with herself and surrounding. Cannot think after using eyes. Cares very little for things; makes useless purchases, wastes or ruins them. Likes to wear his best clothes. Sadness, < by sympathy, as if great guilt weighed upon him. Fearful when alone, but dread of strangers or company, during menses.

HEAD: VERTIGO, *whirling, < lying, turning over in bed, least motion of the eyes or head;* of old age. Hot spots on head. Temples compressed, < after meal. Sensation of a lump in right half of brain. Sick headache, with inability to urinate. Pain in head from sinciput to occiput, > stooping and moving the head. Sensation of fullness and bursting in brain during headache. One side numb and cold.

EYES: *Feel crossed. Lids heavy, droop,* < outside. *Photophobia and excessive lacrimation,* without inflammation or from slightest abrasion or ulceration of the eye. Burning in eyes. Vision colored, red. As of fringe falling over eyes. Vision diminished in artificial light. Cataract after eye injury. Ptosis of eyelids. Sweats on closing eyes. Diplopia. Black spots before eyes, with vertigo. Myopia. Vision becomes blurred when vexed.

EARS: Accumulation of earwax like pulp of paper, or blood red hard wax, causing hardness of hearing. Oversensitive to noise. Parotid gland swollen and hard. Ears feel stopped on blowing nose.

NOSE: Smell acute. Easy bleeding. Picks nose constantly. Polypus. Frequent sneezing. Obstinate obstruction of nose.

FACE: Moist and spreading herpes on face. Cancer of the lip (from pressure of pipe). Submaxillary glands are swollen and hard.

MOUTH: Toothache, < cold food, not by cold drink. Speech difficult from paralysis of tongue. Cancer of tongue. Sour saliva. Distortion of tongue and mouth.

THROAT: Sensation as if a round object or a ball were ascending from stomach (globus). Food goes down the wrong way and stops while swallowing. Paresis of esophagus. Constant inclination to swallow as from a lump in the throat < walking in open air. Tonsils enlarged.

STOMACH: Acrid heartburn and acrid eructations, < on going to bed. Distention of stomach after taking milk. Pain in stomach, > eating but < few hours (2 or 3) after eating, > in knee chest position. Nausea and vomiting during pregnancy. Craves coffee, salt, sour things. Aversion to bread. Vomiting, coffee-ground, chocolate-colored lumps or clear sour water. Cancer. Ulcer.

ABDOMEN: Distensions < after taking milk. Cutting pain before passing flatus. Severe aching in and around the liver. Chronic jaundice and pain in right hypochondrium. Trembling of whole abdomen. Abdomen hard and distended. Tremulous weakness, palpitation of heart after every stool. Involuntary stool, during sleep. Cold flatus and stool. Constipation on alternate days. Burning or coldness in rectum. Hypogastric pain goes down legs. Ineffective urging to stool.

URINARY: Interrupted urination, urine stops and starts, > standing. Dribbling in old men. Cutting and burning after urination. Difficulty in passing urine in the beginning even when standing, then it flows freely. Urine feels hot.

MALE: Testes enlarged. Erection imperfect and of too short duration. Seminal discharge provoked by mere presence of a woman or contact. Sexual nervousness, dejection, after coition. Ill-effect of suppressed sexual appetite. Cutting in urethra while semen passes. Dribbling of prostatic fluid, < stool, emotion, etc. Itching in prepuce. Sexual desire without erection. Impotence.

FEMALE: Menses irregular, too late, scanty. Dysmenorrhea, with drawing down thighs. *Breasts enlarged and painful* before and during menses, < at every step. Wants to press breast hard with hand. Mammae lax and shrunken with or without sexual desire. Hard tumor in mammae; with stitches or piercing pain. Cancer. Stitches in mammae, nipples, on taking deep breath or walking. Too much milk before menses. *Leukorrhea;* white, *acrid;* preceded by griping in abdomen leukorrhea after urination. Cutting pain in ovaries and uterus. Ovaries enlarged and indurated; lancinating pain. Ovaritis. Fearful when alone but dread of stranger or company during menses. Ill-effects of suppressed sexual desire, of suppressed menses. Motion of child painful during pregnancy. Prolapse of uterus from straining at hard stool. Itching deep in vagina.

RESPIRATORY: Constant tormenting cough from dry spot in the larynx or tickling in chest and throat pit, < when lying down, laughing, talking and during pregnancy, has to sit up. Cough seems to come from abdomen. Loose cough without expectoration, has to swallow what he coughs up. Caries of the sternum. Want of breath, < least exertion. The clothes lie like weight on chest and shoulders. Cough on taking deep breath. Tightness of chest, > by coughing. Sharp pain from sternum to spine.

HEART: Palpitation, < exertion, drinking, at stool, etc. Pulse unequal, irregular.

BACK: Pain between shoulders. Spinal injuries. Drawing pain in the lumbar vertebrae, < standing. Coccygodynia. Pediculated tumor at the centre of back. Neck cold. Enlargement of neck. Small, flat, wart like growths on buttocks.

EXTREMITIES: Shoulders feel bruised. Clothes lie like a weight on them. Hands weary, heavy, trembling, unsteady. Axillary glands enlarged. Nails yellow. Fingers and toes numb. *Heels feel* as if bone would push through them. Shooting in heels. Perspiration on hands. Weak lower limbs, as if paralyzed. Cracking in knee joint. Can walk straight and steadily with eyes closed, but staggers, becomes giddy, is nauseated, when walking with open eyes.

SLEEP: Drowsiness by day. Sleeps after midnight. Nightmares in sleep.

SKIN: *Greenish,* like an old bruise. Red spots turning yellow or green. Urticaria from violent bodily exertion. Foul or eczematous eruptions. Gangrenous ulcer. Petechiae in old persons. Anesthesia or inactivity of the skin. Pimples small, red, burning, appear with scanty menses and disappear after menses.

FEVER: Coldness of nape, calf, etc. Hot *flushes, or sweat, on dropping to sleep,* or even when closing the eyes. Sweat, under the eyes, on chin, in popliteal fossa; cold sweat on nape and palms; sweat offensive causing smarting of skin.

COMPLEMENTARY: Phos.

RELATED: Arn; Bar-c; Calc-fl; Caust; Gels; Iod.

CONVALLARIA MAJALIS

GENERALITIES: It is useful in heart affections. Dilatation of heart without compensatory hypertrophy, when venous stasis is marked. Increases heart's action, renders it more regular. Soreness of uterine region, with palpitation of heart. Sensation as if heart ceased beating, then starting very suddenly. Movement in abdomen as from fist of a child. Dyspnea; dropsy; anuric tendency. Tobacco heart.

WORSE: Lying on back. Warm room.

BETTER: Open air.

COPAIVA

GENERALITIES: It acts on MUCOUS MEMBRANES *of genitourinary tract,* and bronchial tubes, producing excessive discharge. FOUL; BLENORRHEA; *bronchorrhea,* suppuration.

WORSE: Morning. Taking cold.

MIND: Weeps on hearing a piano.

HEAD: Occipital headache, > gentle hand pressure. Flushes of blood to the head, and face.

EARS: Excessive sensitiveness to sharp sound.

NOSE: Burning and dryness. Epistaxis, lasting several days in small boys. Profuse thick fetid discharge.

FACE: Acne, disfiguring the face. Face red, flushed.

MOUTH: Chronic catarrh of the throat. Teeth cold.

STOMACH & ABDOMEN: Food tastes too salty. Stool of masses of mucus or covered with mucus. Mucous colitis.

URINARY: Pulsation in penis. Urethra feels wide open. Urine acrid, scanty, bloody, has odor of violet. Dysuria. Catarrh of the bladder. Suppuration, ascends urinary tract. Purulent or acrid milky gonorrhea.

RESPIRATORY: Cough with profuse, gray, purulent, greenish, offensive sputum. Bronchiectasis. Painful cough, with heat and oppression of chest. Burning in lungs. Foul bloody expectoration.

SKIN: Hives, with fever and constipation. Chronic urticaria in children.

COMPLEMENTARY: Sep.

RELATED: Ter.

CORALLIUM RUBRUM

GENERALITIES: Red coral contains *calcium carbonate,* and iron oxide. It affects the MUCUS MEMBRANES ESP. OF RESPIRATORY ORGANS, producing ulceration and stringy discharge. Feeling as if cold air were streaming through skull and air passages. Patient is too cold when uncovered and too hot when covered, > by artificial heat. Suited to nervous persons. Syphilis and psora.

WORSE: Inhaling *air;* change of air; eating. Towards morning.

MIND: Peevish, inclined to scold and swear at his pains.

HEAD: Sensation as if forehead were flattened. Headache, with severe pain in back of the eyeballs, < inhaling cold air. Head feels large, empty, hollow. When head is moved quietly or shaken, sensation of cold air blowing through.

EYES: Hot and painful; bathed in tears on closing.

NOSE: Profuse mucus dropping through posterior nares, causing frequent hawking. Postnasal catarrh. Air feels cold. Epistaxis.

FACE: Grows purple and black, with cough.

MOUTH: Food tastes, like sawdust. Bread tastes like straw. Beer tastes sweet. Craves salt.

RESPIRATORY: *Almost continuous paroxysm of violent spasmodic cough,* which begins with gasping for breath, accompanied by purple face, and followed by vomiting of stringy mucus and exhaustion. Reverberating minute-gun cough. Cough as soon as he eats. Continuous hysterical cough; or cough when the patient gives an isolated cough at regular intervals throughout the whole day. Air passages feel cold on deep inspiration. Whooping cough.

SKIN: Very red, flat venereal ulcer, on glans and under surface of prepuce. Psoriasis of palms and soles. Smooth spots of very deep red color; changing to copper color.

SLEEP: Sleeps with head under cover.

COMPLEMENTARY: Sulph.

RELATED: Coc-c.

CORNUS CIRCINATA

GENERALITIES: Remedy for old malaria. The patient is weak and depressed. *Liver symptoms with aching in eyeballs.* Dark foul stool, with burning in anus. Diarrhea dark, bilious, offensive, with sallow complexion. Vesicular eczema of face in infants with nursing sore mouth. Sleepy before chill with heat; sleepy after meal.

WORSE: Taking cold. At night.

CRATAEGUS

GENERALITIES: Acts on muscles of the *heart* and is a heart tonic; does not produce any cumulative action. Patient is weak and exhausted, sometimes suddenly becomes weak. Cardiohemorrhagic or lithemic constitutions. High arterial tension. Arteriosclerosis. Collapse from typhoid. Hemorrhage from bowels. Dyspnea. Dropsy.

WORSE: Warm room.

BETTER: Rest. Quiet. Fresh air.

MIND: Irritability, crossness and melancholy; despairing.

URINARY: Diabetes esp. in children.

RESPIRATORY: Cough with albuminous expectoration.

HEART: Weak, with oppression, stitches and *insomnia.* Cardiac dyspnoea. Myocarditis. Incompetent valves. Cardiac dilatation. Angina Pectoris. Cardiac dropsy. Pulse rapid, irregular and small, intermittent. Pain under left scapula; and under left clavicle.

SKIN: Burning smarting eruptions on back of neck, axillae and chin; < heat and sweating, > washing. Fingers and toes blue.

FEVER: Excessive perspiration. Palms sweaty.

RELATED: Apoc; stroph-h.

CROCUS SATIVA

GENERALITIES: Saffron affects the NERVES and MIND, producing *rapidly changing* or *alternating mental disposition*; opposite to each other; anger with violence rapidly followed by abject repentance; laughter quickly followed by tears. Symptoms rapidly change sides, or mental and physical symptoms alternate. Jerking or spasmodic contraction of single sets of muscles. Chorea and hysteria. Chorea every seven days with hilarity, singing and dancing. Prostration, weariness, fainting, with epistaxis, metrorrhagia. Drowsiness, > by literary occupation. Tingling, crawling, pricking and itching sensations. *Sensation as if something alive were moving* internally, in abdomen, chest, etc., with nausea, faintness and shivering, or *jumping about*, in various parts. HEMORRHAGE dark, viscid, clotting, forming itself into long black strings hanging from the bleeding orifice. Suitable to hysterical persons. Tumor. Lipoma. Encephaloma. Effects of blows.

WORSE: *Motion.* Puberty. Pregnancy. Heat. Fasting. Lying down. Reading. During new and full moon. Looking fixedly.

BETTER: After breakfast. Open air. Yawning

MIND: *Impressionable; affectionate and moody.* Vacillating. Changeable disposition. Laughing mania. Jumping, dancing, laughing, whistling, wants to kiss everybody. Sings on hearing a single note sung. Involuntary laughter, weeping, < music.

HEAD: Throbbing, pulsating headache at climacteric period, during menses or instead of menses; > pressure.

EYES: Dry, burning, as after weeping; sensation as if cold air were rushing through eyes or as if there were smoke in eyes. Must wink and wipe the eyes frequently, as though a film of mucus were over them; must close eyes tightly. Sensation as if looking through sharp spectacles. Electric sparks or jumping spots before the eyes. Lacrimation when reading. Twitching of the upper eyelid.

EARS: Noises in ears with hardness of hearing, < stooping.

NOSE: Nosebleed, strings of dark blood hanging down the nose, with faintness and cold sweat on forehead. Epistaxis at puberty, of young girls.

FACE: Hot, red or alternating with paleness.

MOUTH: Unusual warmth in mouth. Sour taste. Foul odor.

THROAT: Feeling as if uvula were elongated during and when not swallowing, in hysteria. Feeling of nausea in throat and chest.

STOMACH & ABDOMEN: Excessive thirst for cold drink. Sensation as if something living were jumping about in the stomach and abdomen (left side). Stools contain dark stringy blood. Obstinate constipation, of infants. Crawling and stitches in the anus. Gastric troubles, bloatedness, eructations, vomiting, etc. after operation for hemorrhoids.

MALE: Excitement of sexual desire.

FEMALE: *Menses dark, foul and stringy.* Threatened abortion. Uterine hemorrhage, < least movement, < during full or new moon. Metrorrhagia. Jumping pain in left breast, as if drawn towards the back, as if something alive in right breast. False pregnancy. Movements of fetus are violent and painful.

RESPIRATORY: Dry cough, > laying the hand on the pit of the stomach. Expectoration stringy like thread. Heaviness in chest, must take deep breath.

HEART: Sensation of heat ascending to the heart impeding breathing, > yawning. Dull stitches in the left chest. Palpitation anxious, < ascending stairs.

BACK: Sudden feeling of coldness, as if cold water were thrown over him.

EXTREMITIES: Cracking in hip joint and knees, < stooping. Cold as ice in metrorrhagia, epistaxis.

SKIN: Prickling and crawling. Scarlet redness or spots, on the skin; old cicatrices open and suppurate. Disperses tumors. Lipoma. Encephaloma.

SLEEP: Deep sleep. Sings in sleep.

FEVER: Flushes of internal heat, with prickling and crawling in skin. Sweat only on lower half of the body. Continuous foul-smelling sweat, < in debility; hemorrhage after parturition.

RELATED: Ign; Tarent.

CROTALUS HORRIDUS

GENERALITIES: Rattle-snake poison Affects BLOOD, *heart, liver.* It produces profound nervous shock; with *deathly sickness, trembling and prostration.* Easily tired by slight exertion. Paralysis, post-diphtheritic, of the insane. It causes disorganization of blood and tissues. HEMORRHAGES are slow, oozing, of dark thin blood, not clots from all the orifices and surfaces, esp. from *pharynx.* Bloody pus, sweat. Tissues rapidly decompose producing *putrid* and MALIGNANT CONDITIONS. Dark or *bluish parts. Septic conditions*, tonsils, goitre, ulcers, abscesses, *blood* boils. Petechiae. Gangrene. Neuralgia as a sequel to sepsis. Chronic biliousness, climacteric conditions. Fainting. Convulsion, epilepsy, with trembling of the limbs, foaming at the mouth, violent cries, delirium. Plague. Yellow fever. Jaundice. General burning. Mouldy odor of secretions. Sclerosis, multiple, lateral. Progressive muscular atrophy. Suitable in broken down constitutions, and old age nutritional troubles. Ill-effect of fright, sun, lightning, foul water, noxious effluvia. Affects the right side. Edema, general or of affected part.

WORSE: *Lying on right side. Falling to sleep.* Warm weather. *Spring.* Alcohol. Damp and wet. Yearly. Jar. On awakening.

BETTER: Light. Motion.

MIND: Weeping mood. Weak memory; cannot express himself correctly. Plaintive speech. Timid. Fears evil. Mistakes in writing. Delirium, muttering; mumbles, jumbles and stumbles over his words; delirium tremens. Melancholy. Sad. Thoughts dwell on death. Senile dementia, incipient; forgets figures, names and places, or suspicious about his friends or feels as if surrounded by foes or hideous animals. Antipathy to his family. Irritable, cross.

HEAD: Vertigo, with faintness, weakness, trembling. *Pain in occiput*, as from a blow; pain in waves from spine. Severe pain at the centre of forehead. Headache, with pain in the heart on lying on left side. Headache, < jarring, must walk on tiptoe.

EYES: Burning, red, with lacrimation. Yellow color of eye. Neuralgia, as if a cut had been made around the eye. Absorbs the intraocular hemorrhage, esp. non- inflammatory; retinal hemorrhage. Amblyopia, from grief or from overuse of vision.

EAR: Auditory vertigo. Blood oozes from the ear.

NOSE: Epistaxis, esp. during diphtheria, or other septic diseases. Ozena, syphilitic, from exanthemata. Tip of nose blue.

FACE: Distorted on waking. Lips; swollen, stiff and numb. Dark, besotted face. Face yellow; death like pallor. Lock-jaw. Acne, of masturbators, of drunkards; acne with delayed menses.

MOUTH: Mouldy breath. Grinds the teeth at night. Tongue yellow, swollen, protruded to the right. Fills up with saliva. Saliva bloody, frothy. Cancer of the tongue with hemorrhage. Stiff palate. Can not speak on account of sensation of constriction around tongue and throat.

THROAT: Dry with thirst. Tight constriction. Difficulty in swallowing anything solid. Throat gangrenous, swollen.

STOMACH: Craves; pork, stimulants, sugar. Vomiting; bilious, grass-green; cannot retain anything. Cannot bear clothes round the stomach. Vomiting, purging and urination simultaneously. Cancer, ulcer, of the stomach; vomits on lying right side. Vomiting of blood; black. Monthly nausea and vomiting after menses.

ABDOMEN: Swollen, hot, tender. Peritonitis. Inguinal glands enlarged. Bleeding from anus when standing and walking. Stool black, thin, offensive. Perineal abscess. Jaundice hematic, malignant. Coldness in the stomach or abdomen as from a piece of ice. Pain in the liver and top of shoulders. Intestinal hemorrhage.

URINARY: Dark, bloody urine; albuminous, scanty, green yellow. Hematuria, with cancer of bladder or prostate.

FEMALE: Dysmenorrhea, with pain in hypogastrium. Pain runs down the thighs, with aching in the region of the heart. Sensation as if the uterus would drop out. Puerperal fever. Offensive lochia. Phlegmasia alba dolens, < touch.

RESPIRATORY: Anxious, labored breathing. Cough, with bloody sputum of mouldy odor. Oppression in old people.

HEART: Weak, trembles, feels loose, as if it turns over. Palpitation during menses. Heart tender when lying on left side.

EXTREMITIES: Arms and legs become numb, first one and then the other. Pain in top of shoulders. Right-sided paralysis. Paralysis of left hand and leg. When sewing the hands feel dead. Cannot keep legs still.

SKIN: Yellow; jaundice, septicemia. Purpura hemorrhagica. Bloodboil, carbuncle, felon. Old cicatrice breaks open again. Edema about the affected part. Skin cold and dry. Skin shows every tint of color.

SLEEP: Drowsy but can not sleep. Sleepless from nervous agitation. *Horrible dreams*, of dead. Suffocation waking.

FEVER: Malignant fever, high fever, yellow fever, cerebrospinal meningitis, blackwater fever. Sweat cold, bloody.

COMPLEMENTARY: Lycps.

RELATED: Lach; Sul-ac.

CROTON TIGLIUM

GENERALITIES: It is used as a powerful purgative and irritant of the skin in ordinary practice, therefore it affects the *mucous membranes* of the intestines causing watery discharge. Skin esp. of FACE *and scrotum* is more affected. It has a peculiar *feeling as if parts were drawn backwards*—eyes, nipples etc. Skin symptoms alternating with internal symptoms, diarrhea, etc. Skin feels hide-bound.

WORSE: Drinking; *least food*. Washing. Summer. Touch. Motion. Receding eruptions.

BETTER: After sleep. Gentle rubbing.

MIND: Feeling of anxiety, as though some personal misfortune would befall him. Not disposed to work. Can not think outside himself. Feels all spent up. Morose. Dissatisfied.

HEAD: Weight of the hat causes headache. Vertigo, < drinking.

EYES: Purulent ophthalmia, red and raw appearance. Pustules on cornea, with eruptions around eyes. Eyes feel drawn backwards. Tensive pain above the orbit (right).

EARS: Otorrhea, when there is a great itching.

FACE: Pustular eruptions on the face. As though insects were creeping.

MOUTH: Neuralgia of the tongue. Burning in esophagus.

STOMACH: Excessive nausea, with vanishing of sight.

ABDOMEN: Pressure on the navel causes pain in the rectum or urging for stool. Pain in the anus as if a plug were forcing outwards. *Gurgling or swashing of water in bowels.* Then Profuse Sudden Gushing Stool of Yellow Water, < drinking the least quantity or while eating, followed by prostration. Summer diarrhoea. Cholera infantum. Colic, > hot milk.

URINARY: Night urine; foaming, dark orange colored, turbid on standing, greasy particles floating on top. Day urine is pale with white sediment.

MALE: Eczema of scrotum. Vesicular eruptions on scrotum and penis. Left testis retracted, right pendent.

FEMALE: Intense itching of genitals, > by gentle rubbing. Pain from nipple to back as child nurses. Nodes in mammae, with pain from nipple to scapula. Breast hard, swollen. Nipples very sore to touch.

RESPIRATORY: Cough as soon as he touches the pillow, must sit up. *Feels as though he could not inhale deeply enough.* Could not expand the lungs.

EXTREMITIES: Neck and shoulders painful.

SKIN: Feels hide-bound, tense. Violently itching, burning red skin; sore if scratched, > gentle rubbing. *Eruptions, pustular, blisters,* clustered, which burst and form crusts, more in genitals, temples, vertex. Herpes zoster. Eczema.

RELATED: Rhus-t.

CUBEBA

GENERALITIES: It produces catarrh of the *mucous membranes* of URETHRA, bladder, vagina. Burning, rawness is felt in the throat, in stomach, abdomen, rectum, urethra, fossa navicularis. Discharges are thick, acrid, *yellow*, pus-like, green, offensive, after violent inflammation. Suitable to persons of bilious constitution, with tendency to constipation.

WORSE: Night, in bed.

BETTER: Getting up and walking about.

HEAD: Veins of the forehead and temples are distended.

MOUTH: On attempting to smile or speak, his mouth seems to twist to one side.

THROAT: Swallows saliva constantly to relieve burning and dryness of the throat. Catarrh.

STOMACH: Craving for oranges, onions, almonds and nuts.

ABDOMEN: Burning in stomach and abdomen. Stools gelatinous, of transparent mucus mixed with whitish, shining particles like rice, < night, in bed, > getting up and walking about. Stools cold.

URINARY: Cramps, cutting, burning in urethra, after urination. Cystitis. Prostatitis with thick yellow discharge. Stringy gonorrhea.

FEMALE: Urethro-vaginitis, with profuse discharge. Acrid leukorrhea in children.

RESPIRATORY: Catarrh of nose and throat with fetid expectoration.

RELATED: Cist; Cop.

CULEX MUSCA (Mosquito)

GENERALITIES: It produces vertigo on blowing the nose. Sensation as if cold air blowing through a hole in clothes on the chest or back. Menses stain indelibly. Griping over the hips, moves into womb. Edematous swelling.

CUNDURANGO

GENERALITIES: *Condor plant* was introduced as a cancer remedy. Painful crack in the corners of the mouth is a guiding symptom in cancerous or syphilitic condition. Tumor; stricture of the esophagus. Cancer of the stomach, with constant burning and vomiting; food seems to stick behind the sternum. Cancer of the mammae with retraction of the nipples, with lancinating pain emanating from the tumour over the whole breast. Jagged ulcers of the tongue. This remedy is worth trying when other seemingly indicated remedies fail to impress the disease.

RELATED: Ast-r; Con; Hydr.

CUPRUM ACETICUM

GENERALITIES: Head reels when in a high-ceilinged room. Facial neuralgia in cheek bone, upper jaw and behind the ear, > by chewing, pressure and hot application. Chorea; periodical, with melancholy and dread of society. Chronic psoriasis and leprosy-like eruption over whole body, in spots of various sizes, *without itching*. In epilepsy aura begins in the knee and ascends to hypogastrium. Protracted labor.

WORSE: Heat. Motion. Emotion. Touch.

BETTER: Chewing. Pressure. Warmth.

CUPRUM ARSENICUM

GENERALITIES: It produces inflammation of the DIGESTIVE TRACT, with violent colic, vomiting, diarrhea, and *uremia;* with obstinate hiccough and icy cold body. Cholera. *Violent cramps* in chest, fingers, calves, toes etc. Visceral neuralgia - sharp, shooting abdominal pains. Rice water stools; cholera infantum. Weak heart. Cold, clammy intermittent sweat. Convulsions; uremic or preceded by gastro-intestinal symptoms. Leg cramps > pressing foot on the floor. Numb paralyzed feeling in the legs. Chorea after fright. Trembling of the whole body when attempting to walk. Urine of garlicky odor.

WORSE: Touch. Pressure. Dampness. Motion.

CUPRUM METALLICUM

GENERALITIES: Metallic copper is one of the most important remedies, where the diseased conditions 'strike in' on account of non-appearance or suppression of eruptions and discharges. It affects the NERVES of the *cerebrospinal axis and muscles,* causing SPASMODIC EFFECT, convulsion and *cramp of violent form.* Convulsions may be either tonic or clonic; starts in the knees, toes or fingers and radiate over the whole body; with PIERCING CRIES, TWISTING of the head to one side; *trismus,* followed by headache, spasmodic laughter, shivering, deathly exhaustion, cold perspiration, etc. Epilepsy, at night, during menses. In epilepsy the patient falls with a shriek, passes urine and feces; headache follows after spasm or a group of symptoms followed by an appearance as if patient were dead or in a state of ecstasy. Convulsion of children during dentition; children lie on abdomen and jerk the buttock up. Spasms, with blue face and clenched thumbs. Cramp may occur in the chest (angina pectoris) behind the sternum, in toes, fingers, calves, *knotting* the muscles, > stretching the leg out; cramps in soles, etc., *extorting cries. Jerking* during sleep. Pains < touch and motion. Pains are *pressive,* as from a blow, as if being broken; in racking darts through the whole body. Chorea from fright; periodical. Symptoms appear in groups, periodically or recurring at short interval. Complaints begin on left side. Nervous trembling, with acute senses. Continued weakness. Poor reaction. Latency. Ill-effects of mental and bodily exhaustion; loss of sleep. *Blueness. Easy relapses*. The patient is *hypersensitive*; every drug over-reacts without curing. Collapse. Paralysis of isolated muscles. Women who have borne many children (after-pains).

WORSE: Emotions, anger, fright. *Suppression.* Over-worked mentally and bodily. Motion. *Touch.* Loss of sleep. *Hot weather.* Vomiting. Raising arms. Before menses. At new moon.

BETTER: Being mesmerized, laying hand on affected part. *Cold drinks.* Pressure over heart.

MIND: Nervous. *Uneasy*. Says words not intended. *Piercing* shrieks. Weeps violently. Convulsive laughter. Delirium; cold sweat. Fear of society, shuns everybody. Confusion afraid of people who approach him. Loquacious; then melancholy, with spells of fear of death. Sense of losing consciousness. Attacks of rage, wants to bite the by-standers. Sullen; tricky; alternating yielding and head-strong. Malicious. Mania; bites, beats, tears the things. Imitates, mimics.

HEAD: *Vertigo*, with internal tremor, head sinks forward on the chest, > stool, lying down, < looking up. Cannot hold head erect, bores it into the pillow; meningitis. Strange tingling, crawling in the vertex (suppressed menses). Empty feeling, with pain. Headache after epilepsy. Sensation as if water were poured over the head, with headache. Pulls her hair. Shakes the head from side to side.

EYES: Fixed, staring, sunken, glistening, turned upward. Eyeballs rotate quickly behind *closed lids,* or roll from side to side. Bruised pain in the orbits, < moving the eyes. Lids spasmodically closed. Twitching of lids (1) and photophobia. Astigmation.

FACE: *Blue, livid,* pale; or distorted, sunken, pinched. Icy cold. Lips blue. Lockjaw. Chewing motion of lower jaw.

MOUTH: Firmly closed or open, with tongue darting in and out like a snake (in convulsion). Grinds the teeth. Slimy or metallic sweetish taste. Loss of speech; stammering; paralysis of the tongue. Froth from mouth. Food tastes like clear water.

THROAT: Unable to talk on account of spasm of throat. Gurgling noise when swallowing fluid.

STOMACH: Desire for cold drinks. Milk causes water brash. Hiccough; before vomiting; convulsions or asthma. Nausea, more pronounced. Vomiting; violent. tormenting; with *agonizing colic;* diarrhoea; shrieks or convulsions; > cold drinks. Painful crampy pressure in epigastrium < touch and movement. Lies on stomach and jerks the buttocks up in (colic, convulsions). Vomits always on waking up in a.m. Vomits on least motion. Periodical attacks of vomiting. As if something bitter were in stomach.

ABDOMEN: Tense, contracted, hot and tender to touch. *Frightful colic,* with contraction of the abdomen. > pressure; < raising arms. Intussusception; with faecal vomiting Diarrhea; profuse; spurting out; of green water. Cholera; summer diarrhea in children. Round; tape, thread worms. Constipation with great heat of body. Spasmodic movements of abdominal muscles. Cirrhosis of liver.

URINARY: Suppression of urine (in cholera); uremic. Passes clear watery urine during or after spasms.

MALE: Cramps in calves prevents coition, esp. old men or nervous young men.

FEMALE: Menses absent due to suppression of foot sweat. Violent cramps in abdomen extending into the chest before or during menses; or from suppressions of the menses; convulsions before menses. Puerperal convulsions with open mouth and opisthotonos. Most distressing after-pains esp. in women who had borne many children.

RESPIRATORY: Spasms of glottis. Dyspnoea -- cannot bear anything near the mouth < coughing, laughing, bending backwards, before the menses. Asthma; hiccough before; alternating with spasmodic vomiting. Cough, in violent paroxysms; coughs herself out of breath; > *cold drinks;* < deep breathing, bending backwards; with cramps, lacrimation, whooping cough. Painful constriction of the chest (lower). *Loud rattling in chest.* Trembling after coughing. Round balls moving to and fro under the ribs > tight clothing and lying quiet. Hoarseness < breathing cold air. Intermittent aphonia in professional singers.

HEART: Angina, with asthmatic symptoms and cramps. Palpitation, before menses. Pulse slow, hard, full and quick.

NECK & BACK: Paralysis of all muscles upto the neck.

EXTREMITIES: Jerking in hands and feet. Clenching of thumb in palms. Cramps in palms, calves and soles. Joints contracted. Ankles painfully heavy. Knees; aura begins in; feel as if broken. Ankylosis of shoulder joint. Knees double up involuntarily when walking, bringing him down.

SKIN: Suppressed or undeveloped eruptions. Ulcers; itching spots and pimples at the folds of joints. Severe itching without eruptions. Yellow scaly eruptions (bend of elbow). Chronic psoriasis. Leprosy.

SLEEP: Profound sleep; with shocks in the body. Constant rumbling in abdomen during sleep.

FEVER: Icy coldness of skin. Chilly. Sweat; cold, clammy, at night; sour smelling, after convulsions.

COMPREMENTARY: Calc.

RELATED: Verat.

CURARE

GENERALITIES: It is a poison for the muscles, causing paralysis of muscles without impairing sensations and consciousness. Sensation as if the brain were full of fluid. Discharges are fetid. Paralysis—facial, buccal. Threatened paralysis of respiration; pseudo-hypertrophic lungs. Diabetes mellitus. Catalepsy. Leprosy. Feels a heavy weight cling to the parts - arms, legs etc.

WORSE: Motion. Dampness. Cold weather. 2 a.m. Right side.

CYCLAMEN

GENERALITIES: It affects the digestive tract and *female* sexual organs, producing disturbance IN VISION *or vertigo* due to gastric or menstrual disorders. Anemic persons, disinclined to labor and easily fatigued. Dreads open air. Pressive pain in thinly covered bones. Stitching pain. Ill-effect of grief; terror of conscience.

WORSE: Cold. Evening. Sitting. Standing. Fresh air. Fats.

BETTER: Motion. During menses. Rubbing. Warm room. Lemonade. Weeping. Bathing the part.

MIND: Dull, sleepy and morose. Joyous feeling alternating with irritability. Self-reproaches. Sadness as if he had committed a bad act or not done his duty. Silent weeping. The room seems too small. Hallucination as if two persons were lying in her bed. Tearful and broods over imaginary grief. Thinks she is alone and persecuted.

HEAD: Vertigo—objects turn in circles, or look pale, < open air, > in room, and sitting. Brain feels wrapped up in a cloth. Headache, with flickering before eyes, > cold water. *Pain in left temple.* Prolonged migraine. Sensation as if brain wobbled about while walking.

EYES: Dim vision, with headache. *Fluttering, glittering or black spots.* Squint, esp. connected with menstrual irregularities. Convergent squint, after convulsion, left eye drawn inward. Sees countless stars. Diplopia. Hemiopia.

EARS: Itching in the ears, with increased cerumen.

NOSE: Sneezing with itching in the ear. Loss of smell.

FACE: Pale, anemic. Upper lip feels numb or indurated.

MOUTH: Taste lost or salty, which is communicated to all food. Food tastes over-salty. Saliva salty.

STOMACH: Satiety after a few mouthfuls, loathing and nausea from least food afterwards. Loss of appetite after taking tea or a cup of coffee. Hiccoughy eructations. *Hiccough,* < pregnancy; hiccough with yawning. Nausea felt in throat. Hyperemesis of pregnancy. Desire for lemonade, inedible things. Pork disagrees. Craves sardines. Aversion to bread, butter, meat, fat, beer.

ABDOMEN: Diarrhea, < coffee. Running in bowels as if something alive. Pain about anus and perineum as if a spot were suppurating, < walking or sitting.

URINARY: Urine profuse, watery and frequent.

MALE: Prepuce and corona glandis feel sore after slight rubbing. Stitches and pressure in prostate, with urging to stool and urination.

FEMALE: Menses; profuse, black, changeable, membranous, clotted, too early, with labor-like pain from back to pubes, less when moving. Dysmenorrhea. Painful post-partum hemorrhage, > after a gush of blood. Menses suppressed. Swelling of breast, with milky secretion after menses. Air seems to stream from the nipples. Milk in virgin breast, in non-pregnant women. Suppression of menses after excessive dancing or being heated. Leukorrhea, with retarded or scanty menses.

RESPIRATORY: Coughing without waking.

HEART: Frequent palpitation from suppressed menses.

EXTREMITIES: Pain in parts where bones lie near the surface. Burning sore heels, > walking, < sitting, standing. Weakness of knees. Cramp-like slow contraction of the right thumb and index finger; they have to be extended by force. Writer's spasm.

SLEEP: Dreamy, frightful, lascivious.

SKIN: Acne in young women. Pruritus, > scratching and appearance of menses, < at night, in bed.

FEVER: Chilly all over, not > by cover. Offensive sweat.

RELATED: Puls.

DAPHNE INDICA

GENERALITIES: Acts on lower tissues - muscles, bones and skin. Sudden lightening jerk in different parts of the body. Craving for tobacco. Parts of the body feel separated. Bruised pain. *Fetid discharges;* breath, urine, sweat. Exhaustion. Exostoses, with stitching, pressing or dull pain, < at night.

WORSE: Cold air. Waning moon. Evening, in bed.

MIND: Sad. Absence of mind and indecision. Despondent. Agitated.

HEAD: As if separated from the body; feels big. Soft nodular swellings on bones about vertex. Pain, < at night and touch.

MOUTH: *Tongue coated on one side only.* Saliva; hot, foul smelling.

ABDOMEN: Stools scanty, bloody at end.

URINARY: Urine thick, turbid, yellow, foul like rotten egg.

MALE: Prostatorrhea, < tobacco. Erection during toothache. Toothache after coition.

EXTREMITIES: Shooting pains shift rapidly upwards towards the abdomen and heart. Buttocks cold.

SLEEP: Sleepless from *bone-aching.* Dreams of black cats.

FEVER: Clammy sweat, offensive.

RELATED: Rhus-t.

DICTAMNUS

GENERALITIES: It acts on the female organs. Secretions are increased. Sensation of a lump rising in the throat. Frequent emission of copious offensive flatus. Increased secretion of urine. Bearing down with bilious vomiting, < standing. Menses early, of black clots, preceded by blindness. Sensation of milk flowing into mammae. Cramp from anterior thighs going into the uterus before the menses. Profuse corrosive leukorrhea with tenesmus. *Somnambulism.* Dreams of piecing bodies of her children together.

WORSE: Standing.

RELATED: Puls.

DIGITALIS

GENERALITIES: *Digitalis* is a heart remedy. It also affects liver, lung, stomach and genito-urinary organs. It should be considered in all diseases where the heart is chiefly involved, with abnormally SLOW, *irregular* or intermittent pulse, along with indefinite and causeless symptoms. GREAT WEAKNESS, can hardly talk; *sinking of strength, faintness;* coldness of skin and irregular respiration are other symptoms of organic heart trouble. *Hypertrophy of liver,* with induration and jaundice, calls for *Digitalis,* when characteristic pulse is present. Pulse is slow in recumbent posture, quick on motion, irregular and dicrotic on sitting up. Slow pulse after sexual abuse or at puberty. *Must walk about* with precordial anxiety, with urging to urinate. Cyanosis. Dropsy, with suppression of urine. Sensation of an electric shock going through the body. Prostration from slight exertion. Ill-effect of high living. Sexual abuse or excess. Alcohol.

WORSE: *Exertion. Raising up. Lying on left side.* Motion. Smell of food. Cold; drinks, food, weather. Heat. Sexual abuse or excess. Music.

BETTER: Rest. Cool air. Lying flat on back. Empty stomach. Sitting erect.

MIND: Anxious about the future. Sadness; with sleeplessness, from unhappy love, from music. Lascivious thoughts in old men, with enlarged prostate. Fearful. Feels as if he would fly to pieces. Fear of suffocation at night. Wants to be alone. Despondent. Every shock is felt in epigastrium. Great anxiety like from a troubled conscience.

HEAD: Vertigo, when walking or riding, with trembling, < rising up; from cardiac or hepatic affections. Frontal headache extending into nose, intense, after drinking cold drink or eating icecream. *Crashes in head,* on dropping to sleep. Bores head into the pillow, pulls the hair. Spastic hemicrania. Head falls back while sitting or walking.

EYES: Yellowish, red. Lacrimation, < in bright light or cold air. Objects appear either green or yellow. Both the eyes turned to left. Detachment of retina. Pupils irregular. Diplopia. Eyelids blue. Veins distended on eyes.

EARS: Hissing in the ear like boiling water. Veins distended on ears.

NOSE: Pain at the root of the nose, after vomiting.

FACE: Pale, *bluish;* lips blue. Veins distended. Lips dry.

MOUTH: Tongue blue, clean, with nausea and vomiting. Tongue thick, flabby. Bitter taste. Sweetish taste; with salivation, after smoking tobacco. Veins distended on tongue.

STOMACH: Much thirst, but little appetite. *Deathly nausea,* not > by vomiting *or with faint sinking at the pit of stomach.* Persistent nausea and vomiting, with clean tongue. The mere sight or smell of food excites nausea. Epigastric region tender. Neuralgic pain in the stomach unconnected with food. Drinks much and eats little. Desire for bitter things. Nausea before and after urination.

ABDOMEN: Liver, enlarged, sore, hard, painful. White chalk-like, ashy, pasty stools. Diarrhea, during jaundice. Ascites.

URINARY: Feeling of fullness after urination. Continued urging; urine; dribbles (enlarged prostate), hot. Burning with throbbing pain at the neck of bladder, as if a straw were being thrust back and forth. Urine; suppressed; difficult. Uremia; contracted kidneys.

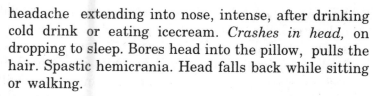

MALE: *Atonic nightly emissions,* after coition. Gonorrhea; balanitis, with edema of prepuce. Prostate enlarged, senile. Dropsical swelling of genitals. Testicles swollen. Hydrocele. Profuse thick yellow white gonorrheal discharge. Early morning erection. Amorous desire without ability. Feels as if something were running out in urethra after emission.

FEMALE: Labor-like pain in the abdomen and back before menses. Vicarious menses from lungs.

RESPIRATORY: Desire to take deep breath, with dyspnea. Breathing slow, < talking, walking, drinking cold things. Cough causes pain in shoulders and arms, or sore, raw feeling in the chest. Expectoration sweetish, like boiled starch, mixed with bloody mucus. Hemoptysis, with weak heart or from chronic bronchitis, before menses. Senile pneumonia. Cannot expectorate without vomiting. Great weakness in the chest, can not bear to talk. Suffocates when he drops to sleep, hence fear of suffocation at night. Cough from suppressed menses.

HEART: *Weak, feels like stopping* if he moved, must hold the breath and keep still. Least movement causes palpitation. Frequent stitch at the heart. Attacks of angina, < raising arms. Heart tired; after sprain. Dilated heart. Hypertrophy with dilatation. Cardiac dropsy. Palpitation, with depression, from grief. Pulse, slow, weak, irregular, intermittent.

EXTREMITIES: Numbness, heaviness or paralytic weakness, < left arm. Fingers become numb easily and frequently. Fingers swell at night. Coldness of hands and feet. Sensation in the legs as if a red hot wire suddenly darted through them. Nails blue. One hand hot, the other cold.

SKIN: Bluish. Dropsical. Cold. Measle like eruptions on back. Creeping all over.

SLEEP: Starts from sleep in alarm that he is falling from a height in a dream. *Drowsy.*

FEVER: Flushes of heat, then great nervous weakness, at climacteric period. Chilliness and shivering of the whole body. Cold clammy sweat.

RELATED: Glon; Spig.

DIOSCOREA

GENERALITIES: It is a remedy for many kinds of pain and colic. It acts on Nerves—*abdominal*, sciatic, and on spinal cord. Pains are Unbearable, Sharp, Cutting, Twisting, griping, Grinding, *that dart about or radiate to distant parts;* they occur *in paroxysms,* suddenly cease in one part, then start in another part. *Nervous shuddering,* from pain. It is suitable to persons of feeble digestive power; excess in eating or error of diet easily affects them. Ill-effect of excessive tea drinking. Fasting, masturbation. Chorea, with seminal emission.

WORSE: Lying; *doubling up*. Tea. Eating. Evening. Night.

BETTER: *Stretching* out; or bending back. Motion; in open air. Hard pressure. Standing erect.

MIND: Calls things by wrong names. Feels cross. Nervous and easily troubled. Depressed, after seminal emission.

HEAD: Dull pain in both temples, or as if squeezed in a vise, > pressure but < afterwards. Sensation as if head were crushed down. Confused, full head.

EYES: Feels a round ball or stick in the eyes. Hot air steaming out of them.

EARS: Pain, < blowing nose or coughing. Nausea felt in ears. Small balls of wax fall out.

NOSE: Any bad smell remains in the nose for a long time.

MOUTH: Bitter, dry, in the morning. Bites the tongue when not eating or drinking. Spasmodic closure of the jaw.

STOMACH: Eructations, with hiccough. Sharp cramping pain in the pit of the stomach, then belching. Hiccough and passing of flatus, > standing erect. Gastrodynia.

ABDOMEN: Sharp pain in the liver extending to the nipples. Gall bladder colic - pain extending to the chest, back and arms. Pains suddenly shift to different parts, appear in remote localities, such as fingers and toes. Renal colic, pain extending to testicles, and the extremities. Flatulence. Piles like a bunch of cherries, with darting pain from anus to liver. Morning diarrhea driving out of bed, causing weakness. Hurried desire for stool. Stool does not relieve the pain in abdomen. Darting from anus to liver. Constant aching, cutting, griping pain in the umbilical region.

MALE: Erection lasting all night. Cold, relaxed sexual organs. Seminal emission without erection, then weakness, esp. in the knees. Strong smelling sweat on scrotum and pubes.

FEMALE: Violent dysmenorrhoea - pain radiates from the uterus, alternating with cramp in fingers and toes.

RESPIRATORY: Chest does not seem to expand on breathing. Chest pain radiates to both arms. Dyspnea from slight exertion.

HEART: Pain back of sternum goes into arms; angina pectoris; with labored breathing and feeble action of the heart.

BACK: Lame, < stooping.

EXTREMITIES: Felon - in the beginning when pricking is felt or when pain is sharp and agonizing. Limbs feel weak, esp. knees; after seminal emission. Sciatic pain (R) shoots down the thighs, with burning and numbness, < motion, sitting up, > standing on toes, lying still. Hamstring seems too short. Nails brittle.

FEVER: Sweats easily when chilly. Sweat; cold, clammy, or of strong odor, on genitals.

RELATED: Coloc; Mag-c.

DIPHTHERINUM

GENERALITIES: The potencies of this nosode are prepared either from the diphtheritic virus or membranes. It is useful as a prophylactic in diphtheria and post-diphtheritic complications, paralysis etc., when *antidiphtheritic toxin* is used. In diphtheria the malignancy is present from the start. Patient *is greatly prostrated, yet restless, without any pain.* Wants to be held. Jerking in single muscles. Internal trembling. Drawing in muscles, then sudden snap. Catarrhal affections of the respiratory passage. Offensive discharge. Carphology. Relapsing diphtheria.

WORSE: Lying.

BETTER: Cold. Drinking milk in sips.

MIND: Carphology. Sees imaginary objects.

HEAD: Moisture at the margin of hair.

EYES: Sees visions.

NOSE: Fanning of the alae with snoring. Thick, yellow nasal discharge. Epistaxis.

FACE: Flushed, center of cheeks purple.

MOUTH: Tongue moist, with red tip, or dark red spot back of tip. Red papillae.

THROAT: Dark. *Thick gray membrane* on tonsil (left). *Painless* diphtheria, swallows without pain but fluids are vomited or returned through the nose. Relapsing diphtheria. Obstinate tonsillitis. Wants cold air down the throat or craves cold drink.

STOMACH: Faintness, > sips of milk.

SKIN: Dry, hot palms; they feel withered. Dry skin.

SLEEP: Talks in sleep, with open eyes.

FEVER: Chilly, then hot. Low temperature.

RELATED: Carb-ac.

DOLICHOS

GENERALITIES: Intense itching of the skin without the appearance of rash or without swelling. Yellow spot all over. Itching excessively at night; jaundice. Neuralgia following herpes zoster. Cold water > itching but it burns the skin and causes trembling.

DROSERA

GENERALITIES: Affects markedly the RESPIRATORY ORGANS, producing spasmodic, catarrhal and hemorrhagic effects. As it raises the resistance against tuberculosis, it is a useful remedy for *tuberculosis* of the lungs, larynx and bones, of joints. Tubercular glands. Constrictive pains in the throat, larynx, stomach, etc. Sticking, lancinating pain. Convulsions, followed by hemoptysis and sleep. Hemorrhage of bright red blood, from nose, mouth, stools, etc.

WORSE: *After midnight. On lying down.* Warmth. Talking. Cold food. Laughing. After measles. Singing. Stooping. Vomiting. Sour things.

BETTER: Pressure. Open air.

MIND: Easily angered; a trifle makes him besides himself. Inclination to drown himself. Cannot concentrate on one subject, must change, to something else. Fears being alone but is suspicious of his friends. Delusion of persecution. Restlessness. Anxiety when alone. Extremely uneasy. Imagines he was being deceived by spiteful, envious people.

HEAD: Heavy, pressing pain. Vertigo when walking in the open air.

EYES: Become prominent from coughing, during measles, in convulsion.

NOSE: Sensitive to sour smell. Painful sneezing. Bleeding from coughing, stooping.

FACE: Left side cold, right side hot, with stinging pain. Face hot with cold hands.

MOUTH: Putrid taste. Bloody saliva. Toothache from hot drink. Small round painless swelling in middle of tongue.

STOMACH: Nausea after fatty food. Aversion to pork and sour food which disagree. Difficulty in swallowing solid food.

ABDOMEN: Painful after sour food.

FEMALE: Leukorrhea, with labor-like pain.

RESPIRATORY: PERIODICAL FIT OF RAPID, DEEP, BARKING OR CHOKING, PROLONGED AND INCESSANT COUGH. Cough seems to come *from the abdomen, takes the breath away; compels holding the sides,* followed by *retching, vomiting,* first of ingesta then of mucus, *nose-bleed; cold* *sweat* and loquacity. Whooping cough. Tickling like a feather or crumb in larynx. *Deep hoarse voice* requires exertion to speak. *Voice hollow, toneless*. Bloody, yellow, purulent expectoration. Constriction of chest, < talking, singing. Asthma when talking, with contraction of throat with every word uttered. Stitches below axillae. Hemoptysis after convulsion. Accompanies cough. Scraping in larynx and cough, after eating. Stitching pain in chest when sneezing or coughing. Harassing cough. As soon as head touches the pillow at night, not during day. Cough < singing, talking.

EXTREMITIES: Fingers contract spasmodically; rigidity when grasping anything. Writer's cramp. Laming pain in right hip joint and thigh with pain in ankle, must limp when walking. Limbs feel sore; bed feels to hard. Pain in the long bones. Pain in humerus at night only.

SKIN: Itching, > by rubbing or wiping with hand, < undressing.

FEVER: Always too cold even in bed. Fever with whooping cough. Shivers when at rest, > moving. Face becomes hot and hands become cold, with shivering. Measles.

COMPLEMENTARY: Sulph.

RELATED: Coc-c; Cor-r.

DULCAMARA

GENERALITIES: This remedy is useful for those persons who are prone to catarrhal, rheumatic and herpetic affections on account of exposure to cold and damp. It affects the MUCOUS MEMBRANES producing *excessive secretion*, esp. of bronchi, bladder and eyes. Stiffness, numbness, aching and soreness of muscles on every exposure to cold, esp. of BACK and LOINS. Skin affections are liable to appear before menses. Paralytic effects of single parts—vocal cords, tongue etc. *Paralyzed parts icy cold.* Tearing pains. *Griping in bowels around the* UMBILICUS; IN TESTES. One-sided spasm with loss of speech. Enlarged glands. Every cold settles in the eyes, throat or affects the bladder, respiration or bowels. Complaints of workers in ice factory. Men who are exposed to constant change of temperature (air condition). Glands; swollen, indurated. Dropsy; anasarca. Exostoses. Haemorrhages; blood watery or bright red.

WORSE: BEING CHILLED WHILE HOT. *Sudden change of temperature.* COLD. WET. Cold drink, ice-cream. Damp ground, cellar, beds. Cold to feet. *Suppressed; discharges, eruptions, sweat, etc.* Autumn. Night. Rest. Injuries. Before storm. Mercury. Uncovering. Hot days and cold nights.

BETTER: Moving about. Warmth. Dry weather.

MIND: *Confusion,* cannot find the right word, can't concentrate his thoughts. *Depression. Scolds* without being angry. Rejects the things asked for. Easily becomes delirious; with pain. Difficult speech.

HEAD: Occiput feels large; cold. Sensation as if a board were pressing against the forehead. Headache, > conversation. Ringworm of scalp. *Scald-head,* thick brown crusts, bleeding when scratching, causing hair to fall out. Feels as if hair stood on end.

EYES: Aching when reading. Ophthalmia from catching cold. Paralysis of upper lid. Thick yellow discharge. Twitching of eyelids in cold air.

EARS: Ache, with nausea, whole night, preventing sleep. Swelling of parotids, after measles. Buzzing in ears.

NOSE: Aching. Dry or profuse coryza. Stuffs up in cold rain. *Summer colds,* with diarrhea. Least cold air stops the nose. Wants to keep it warm, with hot wet clothes. Nosebleed; in place of menses. Coryza of newborn.

FACE: Thick, brown, yellow crusts on face. Tearing in cheeks extending to ear, orbit and jaw, preceded by coldness of parts and attended with canine hunger. Facial neuralgia, < slight exposure to cold. Cold sores on lips. Warts and eruptions on face. Twitching of lips in cold air.

MOUTH: Distorted, drawn to one side. Tongue; swollen; hindering speech; paralyzed; inarticulate or difficult speech. Saliva; tenacious, ropy, with toothache.

THROAT: Pressure as if uvula were too long. Tonsillitis from every cold change.

STOMACH: Aversion to food. Great thirst for cold drink. Nausea, with desire for stool. Shivering while vomiting. Eructations, with shuddering.

ABDOMEN: Cutting pain at navel followed by painful, green, *slimy stools.* Diarrhea. Sour watery stools, < night, summer, damp cold weather. Bowels cold. Eruptions or pain about the navel.

URINARY: Frequent urination. Cystitis. Strangury. Retention of urine, from cold or cold drink. Involuntary urination from paralysis of bladder. Urine; *cloudy, slimy or foul.* Nephritis from cold. Bladder wall thickened.

MALE: Enlarged testes, with griping pain. Impotence. Herpes preputialis.

FEMALE: Menses watery. Rashes appear on the skin before menses. Dysmenorrhea, with blotches all over. Herpes on mammae in nursing women. Menses, milk, lochia suppressed by cold. Mammae; engorged, hard, sore, with absent menses, or leukorrhea. Eruptions on skin after weaning.

RESPIRATORY: Cough caused by tickling in the back of throat, in prolonged fits; with much loose easy expectoration; cough after physical exertion. Winter cough. Pain in left chest as if lung moved in waves.

NECK & BACK: Neck stiff. Pain in small of back as after long stooping. Lumbar region, and sacrum feel cold.

EXTREMITIES: Exostosis in arms after suppressed itch. Palms sweaty. Trembling of arm (r), with urinary difficulty. Rheumatic symptoms alternating with diarrhea or acute eruptions. Warts on hands and fingers. Swelling of calf of leg.

SKIN: *Eruptions* scaly, thick, crusty, moist, bleeding or herpetic, < before menses. Urticaria, > cold, < sour stomach. Warts large, smooth, fleshy, flat. Pruritus. Rash in newborn. Ringworm in the hair in children. Eczema of infant. Small furuncles on places hurt. Thick crusts all over body.

FEVER: *Coldness* in different parts; icy coldness of *paralyzed parts,* with pain. Chill starts in the back, not > by warmth, < evening. Chill with urging to stool and urination. Foul sweat.

COMPLEMENTARY: Bar-c; Nat-s.

RELATED: Rhus-t.

ECHINACEA

GENERALITIES: This remedy corrects the *blood* dyscrasias; hence it is useful in all types of blood poisoning. Auto-infection, septic condition, bite of poisonous animals. Lymphangitis, gangrene, vaccinosis, etc. Symptoms tend to malignancy in acute and subacute disorder. Patient feels *weak* and *tired, aching* in muscles. Slow in every action - speaks slowly, replies slowly, walks slowly. *Weakness* is felt more in stomach, *bowels, heart, knees,* with vertigo. Rheumatism. *Eases the pain of cancer* in the last stage. Foul discharges. Valuable as a local cleansing agent and antiseptic wash.

WORSE: Eating. Injury. Operation. Cold air.

BETTER: Lying. Rest.

MIND: Depressed or crossed. Becomes angry when corrected; does not wish to be contradicted. Out of sorts. Cannot exert mind. Does not wish to think or study.

HEAD: Vertigo, with weakness. Headache, with flushing of face. Sharp pain deep in brain; it seems too large. Throbbing through the temples. Hot burning forehead.

EYES: Brows twitch. Feel hot on closing them.

NOSE: Foul discharge. Feels stuffed up. Bleeding from the right nostril.

FACE: Bluish.

MOUTH: Frothy mucus hawked from throat. Tongue, lips and fauces tingle with sense of fear about heart. Tongue numb; peppery taste. Aphthae. Teeth sensitive to draft of air.

STOMACH: *Nausea, with chilliness.* Sour, bloody vomitus, like coffee-ground.

ABDOMEN: Load felt in back part of the liver. Blood flows after stool.

MALE: Seminal emission.

FEMALE: Puerperal septicemia; discharges suppressed. Abdomen tender and distended.

RESPIRATORY: Pain as if due to a lump under the sternum. Burning under the left scapula.

HEART: Sense of fear about the heart. Increasing but variable pulse.

EXTREMITIES: Aching in the limbs. Hands alternately numb and restless on awakening.

SKIN: Recurring boils. Carbuncle.

SLEEP: Dreams of difficulties; dream laborious or quarrelsome.

FEVER: *Irregular chills; rise of temperature and sweat.* Chill in left occiput. Sweat on upper parts, on forehead.

RELATED: Arn; Pyrog; Rhus-t.

ELAPS CORALLINUS

GENERALITIES: Like all other snake poisons the poison of Coral snake disorganizes the blood, producing black discharge, esp. hemorrhage. Sensation of *internal coldness* in chest, stomach, < after cold drinks. Adynamic sepsis. Spasm, then paralysis. Oscillatory movement Right side feels weak, insensible or paralyzed. Mucous membranes wrinkled. Feels a heavy load or weight on the affected part. Twisting sensation.

WORSE: *Approach of storm.* Cold drink, food, air. Dampness. Night. In room. Touch. Warmth of bed. Fruit.

BETTER: Rest. Walking > nosebleed and pain in abdomen and chest.

MIND: Horror of rain. Fears being left alone, causes chattering of the teeth and trembling. Shuddering from least contradiction, with pricking. Imagines he hears someone talking. Can speak but cannot understand speech. Angry about oneself, does not wish to be spoken to.

HEAD: Vertigo - falls forward. Weight and pain in forehead. Rushes of blood to the head. Faint, with vomiting or on stooping.

EYES: Black rings before eye (left). Large fiery red spots before the eyes.

EARS: Cerumen black and hard. Sudden nightly deafness, with roaring, cracking in ears. Illusions of hearing. Otorrhea, offensive, watery, with deafness, itching.

NOSE: Naso-pharynx stuffed up. Chronic nasal catarrh, with fetid odor and greenish crusts. Pain goes from nose to ears on swallowing. Ozena. Nosebleed, black like ink, after a blow.

FACE: Red spots on face. Bloated. Dull yellowish color.

THROAT: Spasmodic contraction of esophagus and pharynx, food and liquids are suddenly arrested and then fall heavily into the stomach. Sensation of a sponge in esophagus. Painful, difficult swallowing for solids and liquids. Paralysis of esophagus.

STOMACH: Drinks and fruits feel like ice in stomach, and cause coldness in chest. Desire for sweetened buttermilk. Sensation as if food turned like corkscrew on swallowing. Thirst.

ABDOMEN: Bowels feel twisted together in a knot. Stools of black frothy blood.

URINARY: Urine red. Discharge of mucus from urethra.

FEMALE: Dysmenorrhea with black blood. Sensation as if something burst in the womb, then continuous stream of dark-colored blood, > when urinating. Discharge of black blood between menses.

RESPIRATORY: Air-hunger. Coldness in chest after drinking. Stitches in apex of right lung. Cough, with terrible pain through lungs. Lungs seem forcibly separated. Hemoptysis, black like ink and watery.

EXTREMITIES: Arms weak. Arms and hands swollen, bluish. Knee-joints feel sprained. Pricking under the nails. Peeling of skin of palms and fingertips. Icy cold feet.

SLEEP: Dreams of business; of dead persons. Bites hand during sleep.

FEVER: Cold perspiration all over. Skin hot, dry.

RELATED: Crot-h; Helo.

ELATERIUM

GENERALITIES: It is a valuable remedy for certain forms of dropsy, esp. Beriberi. It produces violent vomiting and purging, with copious forceful watery, olive green, bilious or frothy evacuations. Cholera. Infantile diarrhoea. Jaundice of the newborn, with bilious stools, urine staining the diaper. Irresistible desire to wander from home to home. Chilliness with much yawning and stretching. Urticaria, > rubbing.

WORSE: Damp weather. Standing on damp ground.

EPIPHEGUS

GENERALITIES: The use of this remedy is exclusively confined to headache of neurasthenic types, esp. in women, brought on or made worse by any unusual exertion, stooping, nervous strain, etc. Pressive pain, as if fingertips were pressing into the temples inwards, or compressive pain going backwards, < until 4 p.m., then >, with *spitting of viscid saliva* and nausea. Weekly sick headache. Headache preceded by hunger. Tartar on teeth. Neurasthenia. Confusion.

WORSE: Fatigue. Nervous; of shopping. Eyestrain.

BETTER: Sleep

RELATED: Ign; Iris.

EQUISETUM

GENERALITIES: It acts principally on *genito-urinary tract.* Aching, full, tender bladder, not > after urinating. Constant desire to urinate and passes large quantities of clear, light-colored urine without relief. Pricking, burning, cutting pains in urethra while urinating. Cystitis. Dysuria. NOCTURNAL ENURESIS; of children without causes except habit. Retention and dysuria in pregnancy and after delivery. Dribbling urine; in old women, with involuntary stool. *Much mucus in urine.*

WORSE: *At close of urination.* Pressure. Motion. Sitting down.

BETTER: *Afternoon.* Lying.

COMPLEMENTARY: Sil.

RELATED: Canth.

ERIGERON

GENERALITIES: A hemorrhagic remedy esp. when hemorrhage is profuse, *bright red, gushing.* It acts also on the genito-urinary organs; chronic gonorrhea. *Congestions - smarting burning.* Hard aching.

WORSE: Rainy weather. Exertion.

HEAD: Congested, red face. Nose-bleed.

EYES: Smarting, burning. Ecchymosis around, from blow.

STOMACH: Burning in stomach and abdomen. Vomitus or stool of pure blood. Abdomen distended. Anus feels torn. Hemorrhoids.

URINARY: Persistent hemorrhage from the bladder. *Dysuria,* during dentition, crying when urinating. Aching in bladder. Retention of urine. *Vesico-rectal tenesmus,* with metrorrhagia.

MALE: Sticky sweat on genitals. Gonorrhea and gleet. Blue, black spots on genitals.

FEMALE: Metrorrhagia; with vesico-rectal tenesmus; after abortion; with diarrhea or dysentery; after least motion. Leukorrhea, with urinary irritability. Abortion because of exertion.

RESPIRATORY: Cough, bloody expectoration. Incipient phthisis.

EXTREMITIES: Hard aching in all the limbs.

SKIN: Ecchymoses.

RELATED: Canth; Ter.

EUCALYPTUS

GENERALITIES: It is a powerful antiseptic and disinfectant. It affects the *mucous membranes* producing *profuse catarrhal discharges;* which are acrid, and *foul;* with *aching, stiffness and weariness* as from taking cold. Malaria. Influenza. Sticking jerking pains at night. Exhausted with toxaemia and hemorrhage. Rheumatism. Said to be a preventive of influenza.

WORSE: Periodically. Night.

MIND: Mental exhilaration. Desire to move about.

HEAD: Congestive headaches. Migraine. Vertigo during all stages of fever.

EYES: Smart and burn.

EARS: Tinnitus.

NOSE: Watery coryza. Stuffed up sensation. Chronic purulent foetid discharge. Tension across the nose.

MOUTH: Tongue pasty. Aphthae; mouth burns, feels full.

THROAT: Aphthae, with burning. Constant sensation of mucus in throat.

STOMACH: Digestion slow, with putrid gas. Throbbing in stomach. Nausea and vomiting, with chill. Vomiting of blood and sour fluid. Cancer.

ABDOMEN: As of a weight in bowels. Acute diarrhea; stools thin, watery, preceded by sharp pains. Dysentery, with heat in rectum.

URINARY: Acute nephritis, complicating influenza. Diuresis. Catarrh of the bladder. Urethral caruncle. Urine has the odor of violets.

FEMALE: Small nodule below nipple (right) with stabbing darting pains.

RESPIRATORY: *Bronchial asthma.* Profuse offensive expectoration of muco-pus. Bronchorrhoea; senile. Cough of influenza.

EXTREMITIES: Pricking followed by painful aching in the limbs.

FEVER: With aching. Chill then nausea and vomiting. Continued, typhoid like fevers. Vertigo in all stages of malarial fever.

RELATED: Chin; Dulc; Echi.

EUONYMUS

GENERALITIES: Affects the liver and the kidneys. Crawling in back. *Vertigo;* in forehead, as if drawn up and pitched forward. Bilious headaches; pressure over brows;

compressing eyes. Liver engorged. Gall stones. Pain about navel. Profuse stools; varying or of several colors. Albuminuria.

WORSE: Eating; Evening.

BETTER: Cool air. Pressure.

RELATED: Rheum.

EUPATORIUM PERFOLIATUM

GENERALITIES: The leading characteristic is VIOLENT ACHING, BONE BREAKING PAINS. *Muscles of chest, back* and limbs feel *bruised, sore aching.* It affects the liver producing *bilious effects.* Patient is restless, chilly and nauseated. Colds. *Influenza.* Dengue. Sluggishness of all organs and functions. Useful in broken down constitutions of inebriate persons. *Weakness.*

WORSE: COLD AIR. PERIODICALLY; 7 to 9 a.m.; 3rd or 4th day. Lying on part. Coughing. Smell or sight of food. *Motion.*

BETTER: *Vomiting bile.* Sweating. Lying on face. *Conversation.*

MIND: Moans with aching pain.

HEAD: Vertigo; sensation of falling to left; < lying on right side; > vomiting. Sore throbbing pain; in occiput, after lying down, with a sense of weight. Head pains alternating with gouty pains. Sensation as of a metal cap on head. Headaches > by vomiting of bile, by conversation. Sick headaches every 3rd and 7th day. Lifts head with hands, during headache.

EYES: Sore aching eyeballs; with headache. Yellow.

NOSE: Coryza with sneezing, with aching in every bone.

FACE: Sudden severe contraction of muscles of right cheek. Yellow.

MOUTH: Tongue yellow. Taste bitter. Cracks on corners of the mouth.

STOMACH: Thirst for cold water but after drinking, shuddering and *vomiting of bile.* Nausea at smell or sight of food. Craving for icecream, for acid drinks. Hiccough. Distressing pain in the stomach, not > until all is vomited. Tight clothing is oppressive. Retching and vomiting of bile. Thirst before vomiting.

ABDOMEN: Liver sore. Whitish or frequent green watery stools.

URINARY: Urine alternately profuse and scanty.

MALE: Itching of mons veneris.

RESPIRATORY: Hoarseness, < morning. Cough, with soreness of chest, from laryngeal tickling; it hurts head, *must hold the chest,* > lying on knee and hands. Raw, *hot, sore chest and bronchi,* < inspiration.

HEART: Pressure as if heart is in too small a space.

NECK & BACK: Pain in back of neck and between the shoulders. Intense backache, as if beaten; pain ascends. Trembling in back during fever.

EXTREMITIES: Aching of bones and soreness of muscles of the lower limbs. Bruised pain in calves. Dropsy of legs, feet and ankles. Painful gouty *nodes,* associated with headache.

FEVER: *Thirst or nausea, then violent shaking chill* which begins in the small of the back. *Bitter vomiting after chill* or during heat. Burning heat. Sweat relieves all the symptoms except the headache. Sweat scanty.

COMPLEMENTARY: Nat-m; Sep.

RELATED: Bry; Nux-v.

EUPATORIUM PURPUREUM

GENERALITIES: The bone breaking pain and other fever symptoms are similar to *Eup-per,* but less pronounced; it has many other symptoms regarding the urinary and the sexual organs, esp. of females.

WORSE: Motion; changing position.

MIND: Homesick even though at home and in the family. Sighing.

HEAD: Left-sided headache, with vertigo, as if falling to the left side.

STOMACH: Wants lemonade or cold drink during chill. Colic all over the abdomen after voiding urine.

URINARY: Constant desire, even after frequent urination the bladder feels full. Cystitis in pregnant women or after riding on rough road; dysuria. Vesical irritability in women. Urine smells sweet. Urinary stream smaller. Diabetes insipidus.

FEMALE: Quick jerking pain in left ovary. Profuse leukorrhea. Vulva feels wet. Sterility from ovarian atony.

RESPIRATORY: Dyspnea with dropsy.

BACK: Weight and heaviness in back and loins.

EUPHORBIUM

GENERALITIES: It irritates the *mucous membranes* and skin, causing much secretion with a sense of dryness. *Internal burning in bones at night. Pain of cancer.* Slow inflammations. Blisters. Gangrene of old persons. Caries. Paralytic weakness in joints. Everything appears larger than it really is.

WORSE: *Sitting.* Rest. Beginning of motion. Mercury. Touch.

BETTER: Application of oil. Cold application. Motion.

EYES: Sees same person walking in front and behind him. Diplopia.

NOSE: Much abortive sneezing. Coryza, with swelling. Acrid ozena.

FACE: Yellow blisters. Burning in cheeks. Red swelling of cheeks.

MOUTH: Teeth feel screwed together; brittle, crumbling. Caries of teeth. Mouth feels coated with rancid grease. Profuse saliva. Salty.

STOMACH: Thirst for cold water. Burning like fire in abdomen and stomach.

RESPIRATORY: Cough with stitches from the pit of the stomach to side of the chest, day and night; cough with asthma.

BACK: Pain in coccyx < in rising from sitting, < after stool.

SKIN: *Erysipelas; bullosum;* of mucous membranes. Torpid indolent ulcers. Vesicular erysipelas. Vesicles filled with yellow lymph or liquid, as if thin cord lay under skin.

FEVER: *High.*

RELATED: Nit-ac; Sulph.

EUPHRASIA

GENERALITIES: The common name 'Eyebright' gives the indication for the use of this remedy. It affects the MUCOUS MEMBRANES OF EYES, nose, and chest, producing acute catarrh, with *free, acrid, watery secretions.* Tears are acrid; *nasal discharge is bland.* Acrid pus.

WORSE: Sunlight. Warmth. Room. Evening. Wind.

BETTER: *Open air.* Winkimg, wiping eyes.

HEAD: Catarrhal headache with profuse discharge from the nose and eyes. Bursting headache with dazzling of the eyes.

EYES: Watery Eyes; as if swimming in tears. Sees a hair before eyes, ; wants to wipe them. Profuse Hot or Acrid Tears, < open air, lying, coughing; *leaving a varnish-like mark.* Sticky eyegum. Photophobia, with spasms of the lids. Pressive, cutting pain in the eyes. Thick acrid yellow discharge from the eyes. Conjunctivitis, with violent injection, in measles, conjunctivitis instead of menses. Chronic sore eyes. Opacity of cornea, after injury. Red, *burning,* itching tarsi. Cataract, with watery eyes. Pain in the eye, alternating with pain in abdomen.

NOSE: Profuse *bland* fluent coryza, with cough and much expectoration, less when lying down. Flat cancer on the right side of the nose.

FACE: Stiffness of left cheek, tongue. Upper lip stiff as if made of wood.

STOMACH: Vomiting from hawking mucus.

MALE: Prostatitis. Nocturnal irritability of bladder, dribbling of urine.

FEMALE: Menses; painful, flow lasts only one hour or a day. Amenorrhea, with ophthalmia and ulcer on right side of the nose. Stitching pain and itching when walking in open air.

RESPIRATORY: Cough with easy expectoration in daytime only, less on lying down; at night.

SLEEP: Yawning when walking in open air.

RELATED: Cepa.

EUPION

GENERALITIES: It is a lighter volatile oil obtained from distillation of wood tar. It has marked female symptoms, with backache. Menses too early and copious; irritable and disinclined to talk during the menses. Yellow leukorrhea staining the linen yellow, with severe backache, after menses; when pain in the back ceases, leukorrhea gushes out. Burning in right ovary. Sacrum pains as if broken; backache extends to pelvis > leaning against anything for support or bending backwards. Cramp in calves at night. A sensation in the feet as if walking on needles. Uterine displacement. Sensation as if whole body were made of jelly. Profuse sweat from slight exertion.

RELATED: Graph; Kreos; Lach.

FAGOPYRUM

GENERALITIES: Commonly known as Buckwheat, it acts upon the skin and the digestive organs. *Itching* is marked and is felt in different parts of the body—eyes, posterior nares, anus, deep in hands, legs, etc. Visible pulsations of carotids and other arteries. Discharges are offensive. Pain in streaks. Senile pruritus.

WORSE: Scratching. Sunlight. Motion.

BETTER: Cold applications. Pressure. Coffee.

MIND: Inability to study, or remember. Depressed. Irritable. Exceedingly happy.

HEAD: Pain deep in head with upward pressure. Headache with tired neck, > bending backward.

EYES: Itching of the eyes. Feeling as if eyeballs were pushed out. Pain along lacrimal duct. Swollen, red, hot eyes.

EARS: Itching in and around.

NOSE: Sore, red. Fluent coryza, with sneezing.

THROAT: Itching in posterior nares. Post-nasal catarrh.

STOMACH: Scalding, hot, sour eructations. Nausea persistent, > eating.

ABDOMEN: Itching in anus.

FEMALE: Pruritus vulvae with yellow leukorrhea, < rest.

HEART: Pain around the heart extending to the left shoulder, > lying on back.

NECK & BACK: Stiffness and bruised feeling in the muscles of the neck, as if nape would not support the head.

EXTREMITIES: Pain in shoulders, with pain along fingers. Itching in arms and legs. Itching deep in hands. Feet numb, with pricking. Streaking pain in arms and legs.

SKIN: Itching, > cool bathing, < scratching, touch and retiring. Eczema. Erythema. Intertrigo. Blind boil. Skin hot, swollen.

RELATED: Puls.

FERRUM IODATUM

GENERALITIES: This is a useful remedy for glandular enlargements, new growth and uterine displacement, esp. retroversion. Debility following drain upon vital forces.

WORSE: Motion. Night. Touch.

BETTER: Open air.

EYES: Exophthalmic goitre, after suppressed menses.

EARS: Roaring.

NOSE: Thick.

STOMACH: Food seems to push up in the throat.

ABDOMEN: Stuffed feeling, as if she could not lean forward. Crawling in rectum. Feels as if a cord were connecting navel and anus.

URINARY: Crawling in urethra. Urine sweet smelling, dark colored, depositing thick white sediment.

FEMALE: Constant bearing down. Feeling as if something pressed upward in vagina on sitting. Retroversion of uterus. Leukorrhea like boiled starch when bowels move. Menses absent with exophthalmic goitre. Prolapse, difficult to retain the urine.

FERRUM METALLICUM

GENERALITIES: Iron is present in a considerable quantity in blood as also in many articles of daily food. It affects the CIRCULATION, producing irregular distribution of blood, congestion, *irregular surging, etc. and pulsations.* It relaxes the blood vessels causing *hemorrhage* which is bright or with small clots, esp. in rapidly growing youth; or the veins dilate during neuralgia, menses or fever. It is adapted to young; anemic, pseudo-plethoric persons, who, though looking strong, are so weak that they are unable even to speak or walk, want to lie down. Pallor of the skin and mucous membranes, alternating with flush. *Dryness,* of mouth, of food, vagina, etc. *Anemic* young persons, with flushed cheeks but pale lips; delicate girls, who are constipated, and have low spirits. Muscles flabby and relaxed. *Dropsy* or paralysis, after loss of vital fluids. *Red-faced* old men. Rapid emaciation. Nightly pains that *compel motion of the part.* Pressure in chest, stomach, etc. Irritable mind and body. Cachexia. Cracking in joints. Softening of bones. Red parts become pale. Catalepsy. Goitre, exophthalmic, from suppressed menses. Spleen, digestion and left deltoid are also affected.

WORSE: NIGHT. *Emotions; anger. Violent exertion Eating.* Drinking. *Loss of vital fluids, sweating.* Eggs. *Heat and cold.* Sudden motion. Raising arms. Tea.

BETTER: *Gentle motion.* Slight bleeding. Leaning head on something.

MIND: Always in the right; *sensitive* and excitable, < on least contradiction. Weeps and laughs immoderately. Nervous, hysterical. Slight noise intolerable. Anxiety as after committing a crime. Despondent, after menses.

HEAD: Vertigo, < rising suddenly, on crossing a bridge over water. Brain fag. *Throbbing, hammering headache,* starts in the temples, extends to occiput, < coughing, stooping, descending stairs, > letting hair down. Sudden pain over left eye. Head hot, feet cold. Writing causes headache to reappear. Vertigo during headache.

EYES: At night can see in the dark. Blind attacks. Letters run together when reading or writing. Puffy eyelids. Pain over left eye. Exophthalmic goitre, after suppression of menses.

EARS: Oversensitive to noise. Noises in ears, > leaning the head on table. Ringing in the ears, < before menses.

NOSE: *Bleeding* in anemic patients, alternating with hemoptysis.

FACE: Pales; *flushes* or *redness* from least pain, emotions, or exertion. Florid; feels as if bloated. Lips pale. Neuralgia, after cold washing and overheating, < lying down, > sitting up.

MOUTH: Toothache, > ice water. Taste of blood or rotten egg. Mouth dry, food seems too dry.

THROAT: Sensation as if something rolling in the throat and closing it like a valve. Exophthalmic goitre. Sensation of a lump (L), < swallowing empty only.

STOMACH: Increase and loss of appetite alternately. Stomach won't tolerate any food, causes distension and pressure. Aversion to meat; egg, sour fruits, to his accustomed tobacco, beer. Desire for bread, raw tomato. *Spits up food by the mouthful.* Vomiting easy, without nausea, immediately after eating, after midnight, during pregnancy. Burning. Vomits after eating eggs.

ABDOMEN: Hard, distended, sore, bruised when walking. Bowels feel sore to touch. Diarrhea painless, < while eating (attempt to eat brings on diarrhea); nightly diarrhea, gushing, spluttering, stool contains undigested food; diarrhea alternating with constipation, < if nervous or tired. Stool hard, difficult, followed by backache, or cramp in rectum; prolapsus recti. Itching of anus due to ascarides in children. Summer diarrhoea.

URINARY: Albuminuria. Chronic nephritis. Involuntary urination, esp. during day only, when standing, from sudden movement, walking, in children. Copious urination, with nervousness. Urine hot, with menorrhagia.

MALE: Emissions; nightly with backache, after overexertion.

FEMALE: Vagina too dry; pain as if raw, or insensible during coition. Menses pale, watery too early, too profuse and protracted, intermit, with labor-like pains. Leukorrhea milky, acrid, watery, at puberty. Tendency to abortion. Prolapse of vagina. Itching of vulva.

RESPIRATORY: Voice hoarse or changeable. Dry tickling cough, < moving, > lying down. Spitting of blood, of masturbators, in consumption. Surging of blood to the chest. Chest oppressed, constricted, or flying stitches in the chest. Dyspnea, > walking slowly, and talking. Cough, with pain in the occiput. Breath hot. Neglected pleuro-pneumonia, absorbs exudation.

HEART: Palpitation, < least motion, > walking slowly, of masturbators, after loss of fluid. Throbbing in all blood vessels. Pulse full, soft, yielding.

NECK & BACK: Neck and shoulder painful. Lumbago all night, goes off on rising.

EXTREMITIES: Sudden cramp or tearing pain in the limbs, when writing hands tremble, > when writing fast. Irresistible desire to bend the arm, with intense pain. Swollen hands and feet. Heels pain, < lying on back. Cracking in joints. Omodynia. Contraction of limbs.

SKIN: Pale. Flushes easily; pits on pressure. Black or dark violet spots.

SLEEP: Falls asleep; from debility; while sewing, sitting and studying. Sleepless.

FEVER: Chill with red face and thirst. Heat with distended veins. Extremities cold; head and face hot. Sweat; clammy, yellow, cold, acrid or debilitating.

COMPLEMENTARY: Chin.

RELATED: Arn; Mang.

FERRUM PHOSPHORICUM

GENERALITIES: Like *Ferr., Ferr-p* affects venous circulation causing *local passive congestion* and hemorrhages due to hyperemia; so *the discharges are blood streaked* or meat water-like. It is suitable to nervous, sensitive, anemic (blonde) persons. It is a very useful remedy in acute exacerbation of tuberculosis; rheumatism, etc. Emaciation. Takes cold easily. Bruised *soreness*—chest, *shoulders,* muscles. Inflammation of the soft parts. Burning rawness. Ill effects of *checked sweat,* mechanical injuries. Initial stage of fever and inflammation. Great prostration, could hardly move about.

WORSE: *Night.* 4-6 a.m. Motion. Noise. Jar. Cold air. Touch. *Checked sweat.* Cold drinks and sour food. Meat. Herring. Coffee. Cake.

BETTER: Cold application. Bleeding. Lying down.

MIND: Very talkative, hilarious and *excited.* Keeps quiet. Anger. Transient mania from cerebral irritation. Indifferent to pleasurable things. Averse to company. Fear of going into a crowd.

HEAD: Throbbing head with sensitive scalp. Headache, shooting, aching from vertex down over the side of the head, with *earache,* > nosebleed, cold application. Ill-effects of heat of sun. Head often feels pushed forward while walking, with vertigo. Empty sensation in the head, during menses.

EYES: Red, inflamed, with burning sensation. Feeling of a tiny particle in upper eyelid. Encysted tumor of the eyelids. Eyes suffused, cannot see on stooping.

EARS: *Violent earache;* acute otitis media when *Bell* fails. Deafness, from cold, < during menses. Tinnitus, < lying.

NOSE: Epistaxis. Bright red blood, in children. Controls soreness and bleeding after operation.

FACE: Pales and reddens alternately. Hot cheeks with toothache.

MOUTH: Hot. Toothache, > cold.

THROAT: Tonsils red and swollen. Sore throat of singers. Pain < empty swallowing. Soreness after operation.

STOMACH: Vomits ingesta, at irregular times, of undigested food, green matter. Hematemesis. Sour eructations. Aversion to meat and milk. Desires sour things.

ABDOMEN: Distended; intolerance of clothes. Chronic diarrhea. *Stool of bloody water,* of yellow water. Dysentery with fever. Summer diarrhea.

URINARY: Diurnal enuresis, > lying down. Urine spurts, with every cough. Urinates after every drink. Urine retained in children during fever.

FEMALE: Menses early, every three weeks, with heavy pain on vertex. Vagina dry and hot. Pain during coition. Vaginismus.

RESPIRATORY: Laryngitis, with hoarseness, of *singers.* Short, painful, tickling, hacking, tormenting, spasmodic cough, < morning and evening. Hemoptysis, of pure blood, in pneumonia, after concussion or fall. Chest heavy, sore or congested. Pleurisy, stitching pain, < coughing and deep breathing.

HEART: Palpitation; with rapid pulse. FULL, SOFT, FLOWING PULSE.

NECK & BACK: *Crick* in neck and back.

EXTREMITIES: Rheumatism attacking one joint after another, < slightest motion. Sore bruised pain in *shoulders* extending to chest and wrist. Wrists ache with loss of power to grasp. Palms hot, in children. Jerking in limbs. Omodynia. Sprain of the elbows. Hands swollen and painful.

SKIN: Measles. Acne.

SLEEP: Drowsiness. Restless and sleepless.

FEVER: Chill, with desire to stretch, at 1 p.m. Heat with sweaty hands. *Fever* continued, infectious, in *pneumonia,* intermittent, in measles, hemorrhagic.

COMPLEMENTARY: Kali-m.

RELATED: Gels.

FERRUM PICRICUM

GENERALITIES: It is a very useful remedy for senile hypertrophy of the prostate gland, with frequent urination at night, with full feeling and pressure in rectum. Smarting at neck of the bladder and penis. Retention of urine.

FLUORIC ACID

GENERALITIES: Destructiveness is the keynote of this acid. It produces slow, deeply destructive effects, such as, caries of bones, esp. long bones, ulceration, *bedsore*; varicose vein. It is suitable to complaints of old age or prematurely aged. Pale, miserable, *cachectic, flabby* and broken down patients. *Always feel too hot; want to bathe in cold water*. Tissues are *puffy*, indurated and *fistulous*. Discharge are *thin; foul, acrid* or salty, causing itching. Edema. Felon. Secondary syphilis. Increased ability to exercise his muscles, without fatigue, regardless of most excessive heat of summer or coldest winter. Numbness of the part not lain on in brain disease, spinal affection. Calcareous degeneration. Nevus, flat. Suffering if the call for evacuation is not immediately attended to. Dropsy, with numbness or without. Goitre.

WORSE: HEAT, of room. Night. Alcohol (red wine). Sour food.

BETTER: Cool Bathing. *Rapid motion*. Short sleep. Bending head back. Eating.

MIND: *Impulse to walk fast;* necessity to be always on the move. Aversion to his own family, to those loved best; becomes interested and converses pleasantly with strangers. Inability to realize responsibility. Depression of mind. Stands on the street ogling the women as they pass by, so great is his lust. Elated and gay. Sits silently, does not utter a single word, does not answer when questioned.

HEAD: Stunning headache, > urinating. Pressure in occiput. Pain along the sutures. *Puffy glabella.* Falling out of hair, after fever. Brittle, untidy hair.

EYES: Sensation of cold wind blowing through the eyes. Fistula lacrimalis. Sensation of something in the eyes that could not be rubbed off; must wink. Left eye smaller than right.

EARS: Deafness, > bending head back.

NOSE: Fluent coryza, during sleep. Sneezing with salivation.

FACE: Heat in face, wants to wash it with cold water.

MOUTH: Teeth decay rapidly, < at roots; teeth feel warm. Thin enamel. Dental fistula. Tongue; fissured in all directions; painful when talking. Late dentition. Ulcer on and under tongue.

STOMACH: Desire for pungent, spicy, highly seasoned food, cold water; warm drinks produce diarrhea. Gnawing hunger, always eating which temporarily relieves. Stale eructations. Bilious vomiting on slightest error in diet. Stomach symptoms > by tight clothes. Averse to coffee.

ABDOMEN: Soreness over liver. Warm drink and salmon produce diarrhea. Itching and burning at anus. Sensation of emptiness at the region of navel, with a desire to draw a deep breath, > bandaging. Ascites, from hepatic disorders. Induration, enlargement and portal congestion.

URINARY: Upward drawing in the urethra. Urine scanty, dark. Increases urine in dropsy.

MALE: Increased sexual desire in old men. Violent erections at night. Oily pungent-smelling sweat on genitals. Edema of scrotum. Varicocele. Enjoyment excessive.

FEMALE: Menses; too early, copious, frequent, too long. Metrorrhagia, with difficult breathing. Copious excoriating leukorrhea. Nymphomania. Nipples sore, cracked. Feels distressed if the flow is slightly delayed.

RESPIRATORY: Oppression in chest, > bending backwards. Hydrothorax. Difficulty in breathing; with or alternating with metrorrhagia.

EXTREMITIES: Felon. Sensation of a splinter under the nail. Nails distorted, crumble, grow rapidly. Dropsy of limbs in old feeble constitution. Feeling of hair on back of fingers. Constant redness of the hands esp. the palms. Ulcer over tibia. Hot sweaty palms. Soreness between toes. Corns sore.

SKIN: *Varicose veins.* Feels as if hot vapor were emitted from all pores. Dry, harsh, itching or cracked skin. Scar, surrounded by pimples, become red around edges. Keloid.

SLEEP: Sensation as if sleeping on side not lain on.

FEVER: Ebullition of heat with pain in bones. *Acrid, eroding sweat, excites itching.* Sweat on hands and feet. Nightly fevers coming on periodically. One sided sweat (L). Sweat on diseased part.

COMPLEMENTARY: Sil.

RELATED: Calc-s; Puls; Sul-ac.

FORMICA RUFA

GENERALITIES: Tincture is prepared from crushed live red ants. It is an arthritic remedy, *for sudden rheumatic or gouty pains.* Tuberculosis. Complaints from over-lifting. Checks the formation of polypi. Atrophy of wounds. Takes cold easily. Carcinoma. It affects spine, liver, kidneys and right side. Checked foot sweat causes chorea.

WORSE: *Cold;* wet. Motion. Before snow-storm.

BETTER: Rubbing. Combing hair. Pressure. Warmth. After midnight.

MIND: Exhilarated, after pain. Forgetful in the evening. Morose; fearful.

HEAD: Brain feels too heavy and large. Headache, > after combing hair. Feels bubbles bursting in forehead.

EYES: Pain in the eyes on waking, > washing.

EARS: Cracking in ear, with headache. Polyp. Parts around ear feel swollen.

NOSE: Coryza and stopped up feeling. Polyp.

THROAT: Pain in neck when hawking or gargling.

STOMACH: Pain shifts from stomach to vertex. Water tastes sweetish.

ABDOMEN: Drawing pain around navel before stool. Light, foaming stools.

URINARY: Quantity of urine increased to double. Urine like saffron.

FEMALE: Ovarian cyst containing water, or blood.

RESPIRATORY: Nervous asthma. Cough mostly at night.

NECK: Pain in neck when chewing, esp. on closing jaws.

EXTREMITIES: Sudden rheumatic pains with restlessness. Weakness of lower extremities. Paraplegia. Muscles feel strained and torn from their attachment. Hands numb. Hard nodes around joints in and out.

SKIN: Red, itching and burning. Hives in flat plaques. Wounds that atrophy.

FEVER: *Profuse sweat without relief.*

RELATED: Rhus-t; Urt.

FRAXINUS

GENERALITIES: It is a uterine tonic for nervous females. It is a useful remedy for all types of uterine displacements and fibroids. Said to be the medical pessary of the first order.

WORSE: Injury. Sprain. Lifting.

MIND: Depression with nervous restlessness and anxiety. Must talk.

HEAD: *Hot spot or dryness on vertex.* Throbbing pain in occiput.

ABDOMEN: Heavy bearing down, extending to the thighs, or falling out sensation; with fibroid.

FEMALE: Uterus enlarged, heavy, prolapsed. Dysmenorrhea. Profuse menses or leukorrhea. Subinvolution. Sensitive ovary (left).

EXTREMITIES: Cramps in feet; after midnight.

FEVER: Cold creeping and hot flushes.

SKIN: Infantile eczema.

DOSE: Ten to fifteen drops of tincture 3 times a day.

GAMBOGIA

GENERALITIES: The action of this medicine is confined to *stomach* and BOWELS. *Burning* in different organs is prominent. Body feels sore all over.

WORSE: Motion in open air. During stool.

BETTER: *After stool.*

MIND: Cheerful and talkative. Irritable.

EYES: Burning in eyes; itching of eyelids, he rubs them. Lids stick together, with sneezing.

NOSE: Violent chronic sneezing in daytime only.

MOUTH: Feeling of coldness at the edge of teeth. Burning, smarting and dryness of tongue and throat.

ABDOMEN: Burning in liver. *Pinching, gurgling in bowels,* then sudden *yellow or green,* THIN STOOLS COMING OUT *in prolonged gushes, with burning at anus and much relief.* Vomiting and purging with fainting.

URINARY: Urine smells like onion.

RELATED: Crot-t.

GELSEMIUM

GENERALITIES: *Gels* centers its action upon the MUSCLES and MOTOR NERVES. In muscles it causes *overpowering* ACHING, TIREDNESS, HEAVINESS, WEAKNESS AND SORENESS, esp. felt in the muscles of the extremities. Affections of motor nerves produce all types of *functional paralysis* - of eyes, throat, larynx, anus, bladder, etc., or TREMORS or twitching of single muscles of face, *chin,* tongue, etc. Circulation becomes sluggish causing *passive arterial or venous congestion,* with *sense of fullness* and heaviness in different organs—heart, liver, etc. Catarrh of MUCOUS MEMBRANES cause watery discharges. General state of paresis, bodily and mental. Complete relaxation and prostration, wants to lie down quietly; half reclined; wants to be held. *Dulness, dizziness, drowsiness; eye or visual effects; tremor; polyuria*—one or two of these symptoms usually accompany most of the diseased conditions in which *Gels.* is indicated. Inco-ordination of muscles, which do not obey the will. Chorea of pregnancy. Convulsions; hysterical. Nervous affections of cigar makers. Body feels light in onanists or hysterical subjects. Influenza. Measles. Pellagra. Post-diphtheritic paralysis. Paralysis agitans. Ill-effects of fright, fear, depressing emotions, anger, bad news, unpleasant surprise. Masturbation, traumatic shock. Pelvic organ symptoms alternate with head symptoms. Weak, tired, delicate, timid, excitable, easily angered persons, children and adolescents. Never well since the flu. Coma. Apoplexy.

WORSE: EMOTIONS. DREAD. *Shock. Ordeal.* Motion. Surprise. *Weather* - HUMID, SPRING, *foggy. Heat* of sun; summer. Periodically. Tobacco. Thunderstorm. Cold damp weather. Dentition. When thinking of his ailment.

BETTER: *Profuse urination; sweating. Shaking. Alcoholic drink.* Mental effort. Bending forward. Continued motion. Afternoon. Reclining, with head held high.

MIND: Confusion; acts as if crazy. Dazed. Apathetic. Desire to be quiet or left alone. Wants to throw himself from a height. DREAD of *falling,* of *ordeal,* death, pain. Indifferent regarding his illness. Answers slowly. Cataleptic immobility, with dilated pupils, closed eyes, but conscious. Child starts, grasps the nurse and screams as if afraid of falling. Discerning power slow. Effects of grief, cannot cry; broods over her loss.

HEAD: VERTIGO, spreads from occiput, as if drunk, with visual symptoms. DULL, HEAVY or band-like headache, around the occiput, to over eyes, < tight cap; > shaking; lying with head high; after profuse urination. Swollen feeling in head. Meningitis - congestive stage, pain at the back of head and dilated pupils. Pressure pain from the vertex to shoulders. Pain in temples extending into ear, wing of nose and chin. Soreness of the scalp. Apoplexy, sub-arachnoid. Blood rushes from the occiput to the forehead. Hot, with cold limbs. Migraine begins at 2 or 3 a.m., > in the afternoon. Cannot hold erect. Fontanelles pulsate strongly.

EYES: Pupils dilated. HEAVY DROOPING EYELIDS. *Diplopia*, when looking sideways, during pregnancy. Blind spells. Sight dim or swimming. Photomania. Affection of vision before migraine. Eyes; red, sore, *aching*, suffused. Detached retina; from injury or myopia. Glaucoma. Orbital neuralgia with contraction and twitching of muscles. Amaurosis from masturbation. Hysterical amblyopia. Eye pain extends to *occiput*. Retinitis. Gauze before. Corrects discomfort in eyes even after accurately adjusted glasses. Vitreous hazy.

EARS: Sudden loss of hearing for a short time. Pain while swallowing. Impaired hearing from cold.

NOSE: Stuffed. *Coryza, with thin acrid watery discharge.* Sensation as of hot water flowing from the nostrils. Summer cold. *Sneezing;* early morning.

FACE: Hot, heavy, *full, dusky red;* besotted or expressionless. Chin quivers. Lower jaw dropped. Lower jaw wags sideways. Paralysis.

MOUTH: Tongue heavy, *numb,* partially paralyzed; *speech thick,* as if drunk, he can hardly speak. Saliva colored yellow as from blood. Tongue numb, trembles while protruding. Thick yellow coating on tongue. Muscles around the mouth seem contracted.

THROAT: Swallowing difficult. Paralytic dysphagia, esp. < from warm food. Swallowing causes pain in the ear. Feeling of a painful lump in throat that cannot be swallowed, in hysterical women. Pain from throat to the ear. Tonsillitis. Post-diphtheritic paralysis. Sore throat during menses. Paralytic dysphagia after cerebral apoplexy.

STOMACH: Usually *thirstless,* but thirst with sweat. Little appetite but can take food or drink. Feeling of emptiness or weakness in the stomach or bowels. Cramps in stomach, < riding or sitting erect. Hiccough, < evening.

ABDOMEN: Passive congestion of liver. Griping in the gall bladder. Periodical colic. Copious yellow stool. Diarrhea; painless; in nervous persons, after sudden emotions as grief, fright, bad news, anticipation of an unusual ordeal. Stool, cream-colored, tea-green. Paralysis of sphincter ani. Prolapse or rectal pain after labor. Involuntary stool.

URINARY: Profuse, clear, watery urine, with chill and trembling, > headache. Incontinence from excitement, from paralysis of sphincter. Alternate dysuria and enuresis. Flow intermittent. Retention. Constant urination; hysterical.

MALE: Involuntary emission without erection. Genitals cold, relaxed. Dragging pain in testes. Profuse warm sweat on scrotum. Sexual power exhausted, slightest caress causes emission.

FEMALE: *Uterus heavy, sore;* feels as if squeezed (antiflexion). Dysmenorrhea, with scanty flow; pain extends to back and hips. Labor pain goes up, backward or down the thighs. Deep yellow leukorrhea, with aching across lower part of the back. Os rigid. False labor pain. Threatened abortion from sudden depressing emotion. Feels a wave from uterus to throat, with choking feeling—impedes labor. Nervous chills-first stage of labor. Coition difficult from contraction of vaginal muscles. Epileptiform convulsions at menstrual period or from suppressed menses. Twitching of muscles of the whole body with drowsiness before puerperal convulsions. Severe afterpains.

RESPIRATORY: Hoarseness, during menses, in hysteria or after depressing emotion. Tiresome, slow breathing. Sensation of a lump felt behind the chest. Spasm of glottis. Long crowing inspiration, sudden and forcible expiration. Dry cough, with sore chest and fluent coryza. Burning in larynx and chest, when coughing.

HEART: Sore. Feeling as if heart would stop beating if she did not move about. Pulse *slow, soft,* weak, *full* and flowing. Weak, slow pulse, of old age. Pain in heart on rising from seat.

NECK & BACK: Neck feels bruised. Unable to hold the head. *Dull pain up and down* spine, > walking; with occipital pain. *Pain under scapula.*

EXTREMITIES: Hard aching in humerus (R). Hands hot, dry, numb, esp. palms. Wants hands dipped in cool water. Cramp in muscles of the forearm. Professional neurosis. Writer's cramp. Heavy lower limbs. Excessive trembling and weakness of limbs. Knees weak < descending; *tottering gait,* cannot direct his legs. Coldness of wrists and hands. Feeling of partial luxation of patella when walking.

SLEEP: DROWSINESS. Starts on falling to sleep. Heavy, stupid sleep. Sleepiness of students. Sleeplessness from mental excitement; thinking or tobacco.

SKIN: Hot, dry; *moist; yellow.*

FEVER: *Chill with aching and languor, mixed with heat or alternating with heat; chill up and down back.* Cold hands and feet. *Heat with drowsiness.* THIRST ABSENT. Fever with trembling. Cold sweat. Bilious; remittent, malarial, typhoid, cerebro-spinal fevers. *Measles.* Nervous, shuddering, chill. Fever preceded by visual disturbances.

COMPLEMENTARY: Arg-n; Sep.

GLONOINUM

GENERALITIES: Nitroglycerine is an explosive substance, therefore its action is quick and violent, with bursting and expansion—a tempestuous remedy. It acts upon the Circulation where it causes VIOLENT PULSATIONS, EBULLITION and *irregular congestion.* BLOOD RUSHES UPWARDS. General pulsation, with numbness. Bursting, expansion or *enlarged* (or even being smaller), feeling in different organs—eyes, head, tongue etc. Pain that comes long after injury. Convulsion, epileptiform, from cerebral congestion or suppressed menses. Burning in small areas or single parts. Climacteric disturbances. Clothing seems tight. Ill-effects of sun heat, bright snow, fire heat, fear or fright. Old scars break out again. Sunstroke. Apoplexy. Troubles due to working under electric or gas light. Eclampsia. Sea-sickness. Walks in shade or with an umbrella.

WORSE: SUN HEAT - ON HEAD. Overheated. HOT WEATHER. MOTION. JARRING. SHAKING. Bending head back. Injury. *Suppressed menses.* Fruit. Weight of hat. Wine. *Gas light. Cutting hair.* Peach.

BETTER: *Open air. Elevating head.* Cold things; cold application.

MIND: Loses sense, sinks down unconscious. Confused, bewildered; loses himself in well-known locality. Frantic with pain, attempts to run away or jump out of window. Shudders and weeps during intermission of pain. Fears she has been poisoned. Shock, sudden attacks of terror, dares not go out into the street. Recognizes nobody, repulses her husband and children. Disinclined to speak.

HEAD: WAVES OF TERRIBLE, BURSTING, POUNDING HEADACHE, with feeling as if standing on head, with expanding and contracting sensation, or as if blood were surging back and forth in the head, from carotids to heart, > vomiting. Pain alternating between temples, < sunshine, damp days. Cracking, snapping, shock, explosion or soreness deep in brain. Head heavy but cannot lay it on a pillow. Headache before, during, after or in place of menses. Numb, sore, hot *vertex*. Veins of temples swollen. Headache > from long sleep. Holds the head tightly, as if skull were too small for the brain.

EYES: Red lower eyeballs or lids. Eyes protrude, look wild. Eyes upturned or rolled outward and upward in convulsion. Sees everything half light and half dark. Lids stick to ball. Blind spells. Eyes sunken. Eyes dry. Black specks, sparks, flashes, before the eyes. Letters appear smaller.

EARS: Throbbing; each heart beat is heard in the ears. Sharp shooting behind ears. Mastoiditis. Deafness; paralysis of auditory nerve.

NOSE: Bleeding on going out in the heat of sun.

FACE: *Bluish*. Flushed, hot. Pain at root of the nose. Chin feels too long. Pain in malar bones, ending in headache. Lower lip feels swollen; or numb. Jaws clenched in sunstroke.

MOUTH: Throbbing pain in teeth; teeth feel enlongated. Tongue heavy, cannot protrude straight; conversation difficult with confused ideas. Saliva increased, thick, in a.m. Froth at mouth.

THROAT: Feels swollen; collar must be opened.

STOMACH: Nausea and vomiting. Horrible faint feeling at the pit of stomach, with throbbing. Rumbling in hypogastrium, esp. < lying on left side. Diarrhea, with sudden stoppage of menses.

URINARY: Profuse, pale, albuminous urine, more frequent at night.

FEMALE: Climacteric flushing. Headache after profuse menses. Sudden cessation of menses with congestion to head. Eclampsia. Throbbing pain begins in breast (L), darts suddenly to head, < motion.

RESPIRATORY: Heavy labored breathing, as from a load on chest. Takes deep breath. Sighing. Numbness in chest, moves upward and down left arm. Oppression of chest alternating with headache.

HEART: *Violent palpitation;* throbbing carotids. Heart seems full, quivers. Pulsations go from the whole body to the fingertips. Purring noise at the region of the heart. Cardiac pain radiates to all parts, to arms, < leaning back or taking wine. Full tense pulse. Venous pulse. Boiling sensation in the region.

NECK & BACK: Neck feels full and stiff, weak and tired, cannot support the head. Hot sensation down back; along spine; burning between the scapulae.

EXTREMITIES: Trembling hands. Knees give way. Thighs and knees weak and knock together, during headache. Unsteady gait. Fingers and toes spread apart during convulsion. Sciatica, > flexing legs on abdomen.

SKIN: Itching all over, < extremities.

SLEEP: Awakes with fear of apoplexy.

FEVER: Heat with hot sweat, sensation as if warm water running upward from nape of neck. Flushes of heat.

COMPLEMENTARY: Bell.

RELATED: Amy-n; Bell.

GNAPHALIUM

GENERALITIES: This remedy is mainly used in affections of the Sciatic nerve, though it has some useful abdominal and female symptoms. Offensive diarrhea with colic, < morning. Weight and heaviness in pelvis. Dysmenorrhea, with scanty menses, very painful the first day. *Intense sciatic pain,* alternating with or followed by numbness, < lying down, motion, stepping, > by flexing the limbs on abdomen, by sitting in a chair. Lumbago with numbness of part and weight, and heaviness in pelvis. Anterior crural neuralgia. Pain in joints as if they lacked oil.

WORSE: Walking. Lying. Cold, damp.

BETTER: Flexing limbs. Sitting in a chair.

RELATED: Coloc.

GOSSYPIUM

GENERALITIES: It was used as a powerful emmenagogue. In homeopathy it corresponds to *many reflex conditions dependent upon disturbed uterine function and pregnancy.* Nausea, with flow of saliva and inclination to vomit, in the morning, before breakfast, with sensitive uterine region. Sensitive stomach with much gas. Vomits on motion or raising up. Hyperemesis. Intermittent pain in ovaries extending towards uterus. *Uterine torpor* sterility. Sensitive womb. Menses late, scanty, watery. Subinvolution. Fibroid. Tumor in breast with swelling of axillary glands. Pain in neck. Menses tardy with sensation that the flow is about to start.

WORSE: Motion.

RELATED: Senec; Ust.

GRAPHITES

GENERALITIES: It is a mineral carbon in which there is a small percentage of iron. It affects the *nutrition* in a peculiar way—one tends to put on unhealthy fat or for those who begin to emaciate. *Circulation* is affected, causing irregular distribution of blood, producing rush of blood esp. to the head; flushing and pallor of the skin and the mucous membranes. Its chief action is on the Skin, esp. *at flexures or folds,* muco-cutaneous junctions, *behind the ears.* It produces Thickening and Induration of skin, glands, tarsi, nails, scars. Thick crusts are formed on the skin. Tendency to callosities. It has a tendency to produce Excoriations, Cracks or Fissures, at muco-cutaneous junction; of eyes, nostrils, mouth, *anus,* nipples, fingertips, *folds of skin.* The patient is usually fat, relaxed, *chilly and costive.* Discharges are thin, foul, scanty, and acrid. *Sourness;* of taste, eructations, stools, urine, blood about teeth, etc. Hemorrhage is watery. *Emaciation* of suffering parts. Sensation of *burning,* numbness and deadness. Pain goes to part not lain on. General sense of uneasiness, tremulousness, which extorts groans. Sudden sinking of strength. Frequently feels faint with partial loss of sense. Aids absorption of cicatricial tissues. Eradicates tendency to erysipelas. Contraction of muscles. Ill-effects of grief, fear, overlifting. Cataleptic condition, consciousness but without power to move or speak. Infiltration. Cramp and burning in different places. Alternate digestive and skin symptoms. *Supersensitive to cold,* which < bone pain, coryza and stomach symptom. Cancerous diathesis; malignance in old cicatrices. Paralysis or sensation of paralysis. Tendency to grow cystic tumor, wens. Dropsy, edema.

WORSE: *Cold;* draft. *Light. During and after menses.* Motion. *Suppression,* of eruption, of secretion. Empty swallowing. Fat. Hot drink. Warmth of bed. Night. Wet feet. Scratching.

BETTER: After walking in open air. Hot drink, esp. milk. Eating. Eructations. Touch.

MIND: *Sad; fearsome; irresolute,* hesitates at trifles. Impulse to groan. Timid. Dread of work. Fidgety, while sitting at work. Feels miserable and unhappy. Weeps; without cause, from music. Forgetful, makes mistake in speaking and writing. Child impudent, teasing, laughing at reprimand. Thinks of nothing but death. Remembers all the events of youth, recent events are forgotten. Fatigue from scientific labor.

HEAD: Vertigo, < looking upwards, reading or sewing. Rush of blood to head, with flushed face and feeling of heat. Brain feels numb. Head feels numb and pithy. Skin of forehead as if drawn into folds. Feeling of cobweb on forehead. Heavy weight or dull pressure at the occiput, as if head is drawn back. Pressive pain or *burning* spot on vertex. Headache, with nausea, during menses. Matted, brittle or falling hair, < vertex and sides. Milk crust. Eczema capitis, scabs sore to touch. Bald spots.

EYES: Shuns daylight. *Photophobia.* Ophthalmia. Eyelids red and swollen. Sore or cracked outer canthi. Ingrown lashes. Sight vanishes during menses. Inflamed or dry, scaly, or pale tarsi. Recurrent keratitis. Eyelids fissured; eczema. Phlyctenae. Hot tears. Eyelids heavy and falling. Letters appear double when writing, seem together when reading. Cystic tumor on eyelids.

EARS: Dryness of inner ear. Thin, white, scaly membrane covering the tympanum. *Moisture and eruptions* behind the ears. Briny otorrhea. Hard body sensations behind ear. Deafness - hears better in a noise. Tinnitus - hissing, detonation like report of a gun. Feels stuffed at full moon, as if air inside or filled with water. Snapping after every eructation.

NOSE: Dryness, with loss of smell. Nosebleed with rush of blood to head, < before menses. Cold at menses. Smell acute, cannot bear the smell of flowers. Stuffed coryza. Scabs and fissures in the nostrils. Sneezing on opening the eyes. Coryza from cold. Painful internally. Chronic catarrh. Discharge offensive, esp. during menses. Excoriated.

FACE: Cobweb sensation on the face. Pale, bloated, haggard, flushed. Acne before the menses. Lips cracked and sore. Moist eczema around the mouth and nose. Barber's itch. Facial paralysis, with distortion of muscles and difficult speech. Formication on lips during menses. Painful nodules on the lower jaw. Falling of hair from chin.

MOUTH: Angles of the mouth ulcerated. Taste sour, like rotten egg. Breath smells like urine. *Dots of thick white fur on tongue.* Burning blisters on tongue. Easy bleeding and swelling of the gums. Sour, foul odor from the mouth. *Blood* from teeth, tastes sour. Salivation at night. Teeth on edge.

THROAT: Nodulated goiter. *Choking* on swallowing from goitre. Falling of a lump in throat, < empty swallowing. Urging to swallow; from constant spasm. Chronic sore throat. Tonsils enlarged. Food would not go down, from spasm.

STOMACH: Aversion to meat, fish, cooked food, salt, sweet. Hot drinks disagree. Excessive hunger or no appetite; worse when hungry. Sour or foul eructations. Burning in stomach, causing hunger, > by eating, hot drinks, esp. milk, lying down. Morning sickness during menses. Vomiting, sour, of food. Periodical gastralgia, with vomiting of food immediately after eating, stomach symptoms < by cold. Cancer of pylorus. Vomiting and purging, icy cold sweat, with headache.

ABDOMEN: *Flatulence.* Cannot bear tight clothes around the waist. *Abdomen distended,* as from incarcerated flatus. Cramp-like pain in abdomen, with deficient secretion of urine, at night. Pain as if intestines were torn. *Stools large, knotty, difficult, stringy,* slimy, or loose, brown, lienteric and very foul. *Intestinal torpor;* constipation for days. Fissure at anus; cutting pain during stool, followed by constriction and aching for several hours; anus bleeds and ulcerates. Stools masses of mucus; slender; pasty. Easy prolapse of rectum. Piles, pain < sitting down, or taking a wide step. Itching of anus and pudenda, before menses. Smarting, sore pain in anus on wiping it. Diarrhea, from slightest indiscretion in eating. Tapeworm.

URINARY: Urine sour smelling, turbid, stream slender. Pain in sacrum or os coccyx while urinating. Stricture of urethra.

MALE: Sexual debility, with increased desire. Averse to coition. Ejaculation too early or failing during coition. Want of sexual enjoyment. Hydrocele. Priapism. Cramp in calves during coition. Impotence from excessive indulgence or masturbation.

FEMALE: Great aversion to coition. Menses *late,* scanty, pale, irregular, painful. Swelling and hardness of ovary (left), < after menses. Induration of ovaries and mammae. Hoarseness, coryza, cough, morning sickness, sweat, swelling of feet or headache, during menses. Leukorrhea pale, thin, profuse, excoriating, in gushes, with weakness in back, < before and after menses. Leukorrhea in place of menses. Cancer of mammae, from cicatrix remaining after mammary abscess. Nipple sore, cracked and blistered. Pain in the uterus when reaching high with arms. Retroversion of uterus; heaviness in hypogastrium with cutting pain down thighs; uterus feels coming out through vagina. Vagina dry, hot or cold. Eczematous eruptions around the vulva.

RESPIRATORY: Constriction of chest, as if too narrow, as if about to suffocate when falling asleep, jumps out of bed, takes hold of something and must eat something, < after midnight. Cramp in the chest. Voice lacks control, > using it. Hoarseness as soon as he starts singing. Voice husky. No control on modulation of voice, > if continues to talk. Asthma, spasmodic, suffocative paroxysms which wake one from sleep, > eating. Dry troublesome cough, with sweat on face. Lacrimation, < taking deep breath.

HEART: Electric-like shock from heart to neck. Strong pulsation in the whole body. Palpitation of heart, with anxiety, with nosebleed. Cold feeling in precordium. Pulse slow during day, fast in the morning.

NECK & BACK: Pain in the nape of neck and shoulders, < looking up and stooping. Sacral pain with crawling. Numbness from sacrum, to legs. Pain in the lumbar region as if vertebrae were broken.

EXTREMITIES: Burning; cramp, jerking. Burning pressure beneath the armpit. Arms and legs go to sleep. Hands or feet either hot or cold. Paralyzed feeling in the limbs. Edema of legs. Nails thick, rough, crippled, crumbling, ingrown. Horny callosities on hands; with cracks. Pain in thumb joint as if sprained, cannot stretch enough. Excoriation of thighs while walking. Cracks and fissures in tips of fingers. Bunions, < fire heat, > pressure. Burning in sole and heel. Feet cold, wet, with *foul excoriating sweat,* < evening. Toes become wet from sweat.

SKIN: Rawness in the folds of the skin. Eruptions cracked, moist and bleed easily, < on head, behind the ears. *Skin*

DRY, *rough, irritable that breaks easily and exudes a gluey moisture,* < in folds, *slow to heal.* MOIST, CRUSTY *eruptions.* Eczema—anal, crural, palmar. Wandering or recurrent *erysipelas. Foul, acrid, footsweat; chafes* the toes. Eruptions < from heat. Old scars ulcerate. Burning in old cicatrices. Old scars with indurated base and margins, with burning.

SLEEP: Excessively tired and sleepy. Sleeplessness till midnight. Sleepy during day. Horrible dreams. Does not feel fresh in the morning.

FEVER: Sweats often on front of the body only. Sweat; offensive, sour, stains yellow, and cold. Inability to sweat. Recurrent periodical fever. Chill in the evening < eating, > open air and drinking water. Wants cover in all stages of fever.

COMPLEMENTARY: Ars; Caust; Ferr; Hep; Lyc; Sulph.

RELATED: Calc-fl; Carb-an; Carb-v; Kali-bi; Puls.

GRATIOLA

GENERALITIES: Though this remedy acts especially on *the gastro-intestinal tract,* it has some mental and sexual symptoms also. *Paralytic pains and feeling of coldness,* esp. in the abdomen, are marked symptoms. Neuralgia due to abuse of coffee. Mental effects from overweening pride. Nervous prostration.

WORSE: Eating. *Drinking too much water,* Summer. Motion. Abuse of coffee. Dinner.

BETTER: Open air.

MIND: Weak will. Ill-humor; tired of life, want of perseverance. Apprehensive of future. Hysteria. Nymphomania. Hypochondriasis.

HEAD: Rush of blood, with vanishing of sight. Vertigo, during or after meal. Forehead wrinkled during headache. Sensation as if brain were contracted and head became smaller.

EYES: All objects seem white, even green trees.

STOMACH: Emptiness after eating. Feels cold water or *loose heavy load* in stomach. Craves nothing but bread.

ABDOMEN: *Profuse, yellowish, green, gushing, watery or frothy, exhausting* diarrhea, with coldness in the abdomen, followed by soreness or burning of anus. Summer diarrhea, from drinking of excess of water.

MALE: Painful rigidity of the penis, after seminal emission, nightly.

FEMALE: Tendency to masturbation; nymphomania. Menses too profuse, premature and too long. Leukorrhea, persistent. Darting pain in mammae (R) when stooping, during menses.

HEART: Palpitation, after stool, with oppression of chest.

NECK BACK: Pain in coccyx, after stool. Neck feels as if seized by hands.

EXTREMITIES: Limb gives way with sciatic pain.

RELATED: Mag-c.

GRINDELIA

GENERALITIES: It produces paresis of the pneumogastric nerve interfering with respiration and profuse secretion in bronchial tubes. *Suffocation on falling to sleep* or on awakening. Asthma and emphysema with dilated heart. Rattling breathing. Bronchorrhea with tenacious whitish expectoration. Cannot breathe when lying down. Cutting, sore pain in the region of spleen extending to hips. Spleen enlarged. Cheyne-Strokes respiration.

WORSE: Falling asleep. Motion. In the dark.

RELATED: Lach.

GUAIACUM

GENERALITIES: It chiefly acts on fibrous tissue of joints, a useful remedy for *arthritic diathesis*. Muscles and tendons are contracted resulting in painful rigidity and swelling of the joints. FREE, FOUL SECRETIONS, expectoration, sweat etc. *Hastens suppuration* of abscess. Tonsillitis with rheumatism. Burning heat; in affected part. Gnawing or sticking pain in chest. *Muscles seem too short* - of eyelids, back, thigh, etc., or FEEL SORE. Contraction between scapulae; palms etc; causing distortion and immobility. Growing pains. Short tendons. Nodes. Unclean odor of the body. Clothes feel damp. Pains often end in stitch, esp. in head. Bones become spongy or suppurate. Progressive emaciation. Feeling that he must yawn, stretch, with uneasy feeling in the whole body. Exostosis.

WORSE: HEAT. *Touch. Motion.* Exertion. Rapid *growth. Mercury.* 6 p.m. to 4 a.m. Puberty. Cold damp weather.

BETTER: Cold (locally). Eating apple. Yawning and stretching.

MIND: *Forgetful,* esp. for names. Strong desire to criticize and despise everything. Thoughtless starting. Indolent, obstinate, fretful.

HEAD: Pain extends to neck, often ending in stitch. Brain feels loose. Headache, > walking, pressure, < sitting, standing.

EYES: Eyeballs seem too big to be covered by the eyelids. Hard pimples around the eyes. Exophthalmos.

FACE: Neuralgia of the left side of the face daily from 6 p.m. to 4 a.m. Face like an old person.

THROAT: *Dry, burning;* painful to touch; acute tonsillitis. Sharp stitches towards the ear on swallowing; cannot swallow without a drink; recurrent tonsillitis, then rheumatism.

STOMACH: Thick white fur on tongue. Aversion to milk, to all food, could not eat anything. Desire for apples, which relieves the gastric symptoms. Burning in stomach. Vomits a mass of watery mucus, then exhaustion. Stomach affections return every summer.

ABDOMEN: Sensation of constriction or stoppage in epigastrium causing cough, dyspnea, etc. Cholera infantum, with face like an old person and emaciation. Flatulent distension.

URINARY: Continuous urging even after urination. Sharp stitches during or after urination.

MALE: Seminal emission without dream. Discharge from urethra.

FEMALE: Ovaritis in rheumatic persons, with irregular menses, dysmenorrhea with irritable bladder. Cold crawling over mammae. Shuddering in the mammae with gooseflesh.

RESPIRATORY: Feels suffocated from stoppage at epigastrium, which causes dry cough, frequently repeated, until expectoration appears. Fetid breath after coughing. Pleuritic stitches, < deep breathing. Recurrent pleurisy. Stitching in apex of (left) lung. Phthisis. Pain in the chest while riding in the open air, > pressure and walking, < sitting and standing.

NECK & BACK: Stiff neck and sore shoulders. One-sided stiffness of back, from neck to sacrum. Constrictive pain between the scapulae.

EXTREMITIES: Tense, short thigh muscles, > sitting. Pricking in buttocks, as if sitting on needles. Pain moves from ankles upward. Arthritis deformans. Burning in affected limb. Hamstrings short.

SLEEP: Yawns and stretches for relief of general ill-feeling. Frequent waking from sleep, sensation as if falling.

FEVER: Sweat profuse on single parts—face, etc. Night-sweat. Fever with chill in the evening. Burning of body. Hot palms. Burning fever with hot face and dry cough.

RELATED: Ferr; Kali-bi; Kreos; Phos-ac; Phyt.

GYMNOCLADUS

GENERALITIES : It causes numbness and bluishness, esp. of the tongue.

WORSE: Cold. Walking.

BETTER: Rest. Leaning against something. Rubbing eyes.

MIND: Forgets everything. Slow grasp; cannot think, comprehend or study.

HEAD: Tight feeling, as if bound.

EYES: Sensation as if being pushed forward; wants to rub them. Pain under brows goes into the nose.

FACE: Crawling as if flies over the face. Erysipelatous swelling.

MOUTH: Teeth sensitive to cold air. BLUISH, WHITE TONGUE.

STOMACH: Hot, sour eructations. Burning spot in stomach.

EXTREMITIES: Violent pain in left radius, as if the bone were crushed.

RELATED: Op.

HAMAMELIS

GENERALITIES: The principal action of this drug is on the VEINS, esp. of rectum, genitals, limbs and throat, producing venous congestion, varicose veins, hemorrhoids and hemorrhage. It is also valuable for painful open wound and burns of the first degree as a local application. It produces *bruised* SORENESS of the affected part; from which blood flows, in blood vessels, in abdomen, etc. Tense bursting feeling, in piles, joints or lower limbs. Congestive fullness. *Veins* painful, sore, cutting, swollen, inflamed. *Painful,* hard, knotty, varicoses. *Hemorrhage,* capillary, dark, fluid, relieves or causes undue weakness. Prickling, stinging pain in veins, muscles, skin. Relieves the pain after operation.

WORSE: *Injury*. Bruise. *Pressure. Air; open,* humid, cold. Jar. Motion. Touch. During day (pain).

MIND: Forgetful. No desire to study or work. Wants due respect to be' shown. Irritable. Hemorrhage with tranquil mind.

HEAD: *Hammering headache*, < left temple. Stupid feeling in head. Pain as if a bolt were passed from temple to temple. Headache after emission.

EYES: Feel forced out, > pressure of finger. Bloodshot eyes. Sore pain in the eyes. Hastens absorption of intraocular hemorrhage. Traumatic effects like iritis, conjunctivitis, etc.

NOSE: Bad odor from nose. Epistaxis, flow passive, non-coagulable, with tightness at the bridge of the nose. Nose-bleeding, in hemiplegia, in old men.

MOUTH: Passive hemorrhage from gums, after tooth extraction, with soreness of the gums. Bloody taste. Tongue feels burnt. Burns of tongue and lips.

THROAT :Sore, with distended veins. Stinging, breaking pain in uvula, while coughing.

STOMACH: Pain and heaviness at the back of stomach. Vomiting of black blood. Averse to water, makes him sick to think of it. Nausea from pork.

ABDOMEN: Piles, bleeding profusely, with soreness. Large quantity of tar-like blood in stool. Bloody dysentery. Varicose veins on abdomen.

URINARY: Hematuria, with increased desire for urination. Dull ache about kidneys.

MALE: Severe neuralgic pain in spermatic cord and testicles, with nausea. Orchitis, < touch. Varicocele. Emission at night without being aware of it. Hematocele.

FEMALE: Menses dark, profuse, with soreness of abdomen. Metrorrhagia, midway between menstrual periods, only in daytime. Ovaritis after a blow, after abortion, with soreness over the whole abdomen. Sore nipples, bleeding. Milk leg. During pregnancy legs become painful, can neither stand nor walk. Leukorrhea, bloody, with soreness of vagina. Vagina sore, tender, vaginismus. Jolting brings on menses.

RESPIRATORY: Hemoptysis, tickling cough, with taste of blood.

NECK & BACK: Sore pain down cervical vertebrae. Breaking backache. Painful scapulae. Dull ache in kidney region.

EXTREMITIES: Tense, bursting feeling in limbs and joints.

SKIN: Phlebitis. Ecchymosis. Varicose ulcer with bloody base. Burns.

COMPLEMENTARY: Ferr; Fluor-ac.

RELATED: Arn; Puls; Vip.

HEKLA LAVA

GENERALITIES: It has marked action on the lower jaw, and has the power to arrest many forms of bone disease—osteo-sarcoma, osteitis, caries, necrosis, exostosis, which are sensitive and painful to touch. Facial neuralgia from carious teeth and after tooth extraction.

HELLEBORUS

GENERALITIES: Commonly it is known as Christmas rose or black hellebore. If the abbreviation "Hell" and the adjective black are any indication, many of its typical symptoms will be understood. It is a remedy for low states of vitality and serious diseases, when everything around the patient looks dark. Patient's face, lips, hands, etc. become dark, nostrils sooty, hence it is a dark and dusky remedy. It affects the MIND and the BRAIN; *senses become blunt and responses are sluggish;* sees, hears, tastes imperfectly. Muscles do not obey the will, hence staggers, drops things, etc. Muscular weakness ending in complete *paralysis.* Convulsion, and twitching of muscles; automatic acts; automatic motion of one arm and leg. Onset of the disease is gradual with progressive weakness. Lies on back, with knees drawn up, or legs spread apart. Dropsical swelling. Epilepsy; with consciousness, followed by deep sleep. Convulsion, with extreme coldness, in sucklings. Noise arrests the paroxysms of convulsion. Ill-effects of checked exanthemata, blows, disappointed love. Feeble and delicate. One side is paralyzed, other keeps up automatic motion. Serous effusion. Parts usually red turn white.

WORSE: *Cold air.* Puberty. Dentition. *Suppression.* Exertion. Evening, 4 to 8 p.m. Touch. Stooping.

BETTER: When thinking of complaints or when mind is diverted.

MIND: Complete unconsciousness. Inattention. *Dull, stupid;* slow of perception or *apathetic. Gloomy;* dismal; *despair;* blank. Envious seeing others happy. Thoughtless staring. Hysterical mania from self-accusation. Involuntary sighing. Irritable, < consolation; does not want to be disturbed. Would not eat or speak. Fixed ideas. Melancholy during puberty. Things look new. Picks at lips and clothes. Believes she is doing wrong, thinks she is going to die on a certain day, just sits and says nothing, does nothing. Idiocy after apoplexy.

HEAD: Stupefying headache, < stooping. Shooting pain causing sudden scream. *Rolls the head constantly,* with moaning (hydrocephalus) or *bores into pillow* for relief (meningitis). Sensation as if water were swashing inside. Headache ends in vomiting. Strikes the head. Forehead wrinkled in folds (brain affection). In concussion of the brain, from blow on the head, after *Arnica* has failed. Electric shock passes through brain before spasm.

EYES: *Half open;* sunken; turned upwards; squinting. *Stupid staring or tired look.* Night blindness. Photophobia, without inflammation.

NOSE: Smell diminished. Nostrils sooty, dilated. Nose pointed, rubs it.

FACE: *Pale;* edematous; red hot, or cold. Neuralgia, unable to chew. Constant chewing motion of the lower jaw which hangs open. Cold sweat.

MOUTH: Grinds the teeth. *Horrible smell from mouth.* Tongue numb, dry, trembling, or covered with yellow ulcers. Ptyalism, with sore corners of the mouth. Aphthous. Bitter taste in the throat, < eating.

STOMACH: Aversion to vegetables, meat, sourkraut. Greedily swallows the cold water, bites the spoon, but unconscious (hydrocephalus). Children nurse greedily. Vomiting of greenish-black substance, with colic. Anorexia, with brain complaints. Thirst absent in most complaints, or thirst with disgust for drink. Intense burning, extending to esophagus, during pregnancy.

ABDOMEN: Gurgling as if bowels were full of water. Distended. Stool loose, watery, or of white *jelly like mucus;* involuntary. Ascites. Lienteria.

URINARY: *Urine,* suppressed, scanty, with dark flakes or sediment, retained, bladder over-distended, during pregnancy. Nephritis. Uremia. Dropsy. Frequent urging to urinate with scanty discharge.

MALE: Hydrocele from suppressed eruptions, on either side.

FEMALE: Suppression of menses, from cold or disappointed love. Uterine dropsy, with piercing pain in limbs. Puerperal convulsion arrested by sudden noise. Pains all over her body forced her menses on.

RESPIRATORY: Sighing respiration. Chest constricted. Gasps for breath with open mouth, propped up in bed (hydrothorax). Cough dry < at night, or suddenly appears, while smoking.

HEART: *Slow, small, soft pulse.*

NECK: Neck rigid (meningitis).

EXTREMITIES: Automatic motion of one arm and leg except when asleep. Thumbs drawn into the palms. Legs drawn up with every attempt to change position. Limbs stretched. Edema of legs.

SLEEP: Sopor, cannot be fully aroused. *Shrieks and starts with soporous sleep.* Muscles twitch during sleep.

SKIN: Pale. Anasarca. Hair and nails fall off. Angioneurotic edema. Gooseflesh.

FEVER: Chill spreads from arms. Chill, with fever, with sweat, with aversion to uncover. Coldness, of sweat.

COMPLEMENTARY: Zinc.

RELATED: Bry; Op; Zinc.

HELODERMA

GENERALITIES: The poison of this lizard which is known as Gila monster causes benumbing paralyses like paralysis agitans and locomotor ataxia. The most peculiar symptom of this poison is the *Intense Icy Coldness,* as if frozen, from within out. Breath, tongue cold; cold feeling in lung and chest; coldness across scapula; burning in spine. Cold creeping ring around the body. In addition patient staggers while walking. Legs lifted high and heels put down hard; sensation as if walking on a sponge or as if with swollen feet. Turns to right when walking.

WORSE: After sleep; at night.

BETTER: Stretching. Warmth.

HELONIAS

GENERALITIES: It is the remedy for FEMALES; who are UNDULY EXHAUSTED by frequent pregnancies, abortion; enervated by indolence and luxury or over domestic work; and who always complain of tired backache and tired feeling. Muscles *heavy, sore,* aching, burning. Constant aching and tenderness over the kidneys. Diabetes insipidus and mellitus. Anemia. *Uterine reflexes.* Dropsy after uterine hemorrhage.

WORSE: *Fatigue.* Stooping. *Pregnancy.* Pressure of clothes. Motion.

BETTER: *If busy.* Diversion. Holding abdomen.

MIND: Extremely gloomy. Melancholy. *Irritable;* cannot endure the least contradiction. Finds fault with everyone. Desires to be left alone. Conversation unpleasant. Always better when doing something, when the mind is engaged.

HEAD: Heat or upward pressure in vertex, as if skull were too full.

MOUTH: Salivation of pregnant women and teething children. Aphthae, during pregnancy. Bitter taste in early a.m.

URINARY: *Dull ache and heat in region of the kidneys,* instead of menses. Urine; profuse, clear; albuminous; saccharine, phosphatic. Nephritis, of pregnancy, with obstinate vomiting. Often an involuntary discharge of urine, after the bladder feels empty.

FEMALE: Menses too frequent, too profuse. Hemorrhage, from atony, dark foul blood. *Uterus heavy, sore, tender, ulcerated* or *prolapsed,* or malpositioned. *Heavy dragging in pelvis.* Menses, suppressed, kidneys congested. Consciousness of womb. Foul, *lumpy* or *curdled leukorrhea.* Dragging in sacral region, with prolapse. Pruritus vulvae. Vulva aphthous, inflamed. Breasts swollen. Nipples painful and tender, < pressure of clothes.

RESPIRATORY: Chest feels as if squeezed.

BACK: Pain and weight in back. Aching between scapulae. Tired and weak. Weakness, weight and dragging down in sacrum, down to buttocks.

EXTREMITIES: Sore pain in outer side of thighs. Sensation as if cool wind streamed up calves. Feet feel numb when sitting.

FEVER: Feels hot when tired.

RELATED: Senec; Sep; Tril-p.

HEPAR SULPHURIS CALCAREUM

GENERALITIES: An impure sulphate of calcium, it affects the NERVES making the patient OVERSENSITIVE *to all impressions—to cold, pain;* touch, noise, odor, draught of air; slightest pain causes fainting. The patient is of *sluggish character* and weak muscles, blondes. CONNECTIVE TISSUE is affected producing TENDENCY TO SUPPURATION; which is very marked. It has a special affinity to RESPIRATORY MUCOUS MEMBRANES producing profuse secretion. *All discharges are profuse, foul, like old cheese, sour—stools,* smell of the body, sweat, etc. SWEATS EASILY and *profusely,* but dares not uncover; sweats without relief. GLANDS inflamed; swell and suppurate. The patient is CHILLY, wears overcoat in hot weather. Sensation *of wind blowing on part.* Takes cold from exposure to damp cold weather. Pains are *sore, Sticking* like *sharp splinters.* Skin is usually affected in folds. EVERY HURT FESTERS. Abscess, threatening, MUCH THICK PUS. Establishes suppuration around and removes foreign body. Yellow, sclerotic expectoration, sweat, etc. Mastoiditis. The side lain on at night becomes gradually very painful; he must turn. Pellagra. Hard, burning nodes. Touchy mentally and physically. Ill- effects of injury, suppressed eruption, mercury. Trembling weakness after tobacco smoking. Pain in bones; caries. Spasm after injury.

WORSE: COLD dry air. WINTER. COLD WIND - DRAFT. PARTS BECOMING COLD. LEAST UNCOVERING. Touch, noise, exertion. *Lying on painful part.* Mercury. Night.

BETTER: HEAT. WARM WRAPS, ESPECIALLY TO HEAD. MOIST HEAT. DAMP WEATHER.

MIND: Dejected and sad. Sudden weak memory. *Touchy* mentally and physically. Quarrelsome, hard to get along with, nothing pleases him, dislikes, persons, places; becomes cross and violent. *Irritable* or DISSATISFIED, with oneself, and others. Ferocious; wants to kill person who offends him; wants to set things affire. Horrid impulses. HASTY in speech, and drinking. The words roll out tumbling over each other. Cross children. Child does not laugh, amuse itself. Sits silent and speechless in a corner.

HEAD: Vertigo, < riding in a carriage or shaking head. Boring headache in right temple and at the root of the nose, < motion, stooping. Hair falls; in spots, after headache. Scalp, sore and sensitive. Sore nodosity on head. Cold sweat on head. Constant pressive pain in half of brain, as from a plug.

EYES: Ulcer on cornea or maculae. Hypopion. Objects appear red and too large. Little pimples surround the inflamed eye. Photophobia. Field of vision one half. Degeneration of retina, from looking at an eclipse.

EARS: Darting pain in the ears. Wax increased. Perforation of the drum. Fetid otorrhea. Mastoiditis. Scurf on and behind the ears.

NOSE: Stops up, or sneezing and running from the nose every time he goes into cold dry wind. Nosebleed, after singing. Sore pain at the root of nose. Stuffed painful nose. Smell like old cheese. Hay fever. Ripened colds and old catarrh.

FACE: Yellow, with blue rings around the eyes. Lower lip cracked in the middle. Bones painful to touch. Shooting in jaw on opening the mouth. Ulcer in the corner of the mouth. Upper jaw projects. Herpes following course of the supra-orbital nerve. Pimples on forehead which disappear in open air. Hard swollen cheek, with a hard growth over it.

MOUTH: Teeth loose. Hollow teeth feel too long. Gums bleed easily. Ulcer of the soft palate that eat away the uvula. Offensive breath. Aphthous pustules on inside of lips and cheeks.

THROAT: Swelling of tonsils and glands of the neck. Quinsy. Sensation as of a fish bone or splinter sticking in the throat, extending to ears on yawning. Sensation of a plug. Hawks mucus. Goitre (R). Pain goes into the head. Stitches extending to ear when swallowing. Chronic tonsillitis, with hardness of hearing.

STOMACH: Longing for acids, *condiments and stimulants;* for vinegar. Stomach weak; burning and heaviness in stomach, after slight meal; stomach easily upset. Constant sensation of acid rising into esophagus. Eating refreshes but causes heaviness. Drinks hastily. Aversion to fatty food. At times desires something but when he gets it, does not like it. Painful on walking, as if it hangs loose.

ABDOMEN: Stitching in the region of liver, < walking, coughing, breathing or touching it. Stools soft but expelled with difficulty. Abdomen; distended, tense. Foul mucus from anus. Bleeding from rectum with soft stool. Diarrhea after drinking cold water. Hepatitis. Hepatic abscess. Stools sour, white. Piles.

URINARY: Urine is passed slowly, with difficulty, drops perpendicularly. Must wait to urinate. Passing of blood or pus after urination. Nephritis, after exanthemata. It seems that some urine always remains in the bladder after urination.

MALE: Chancre like ulcer on prepuce. Flow of prostatic fluid after urination, during stool. Condylomata, foul. Obstinate gonorrhea. Skin of folds between scrotum and thighs become moist and sore. Glands in groins suppurate.

FEMALE: Discharge of blood from the uterus during or after stool. Very foul, hot, membranous, pussy leukorrhea; smells like old cheese. Abscess of labia with great sensitiveness. Itching of nipples and pudenda, < menses. Cancer, with ulceration. Coitus very painful from enlarged and anteverted uterus, with congestion of ovaries.

RESPIRATORY: Larynx sensitive to cold air, painful. Loss of voice and cough when exposed to dry cold wind. Cough from least uncovering. Hoarseness, chronic, of singers. Whistling, choking breathing, must bend head back. Cough *choking,* barking, < cold drinks or in a.m.; hacking as from feather. WEAKNESS AND MUCH RATTLING in chest. PHLEGM LOOSE, *but cannot expectorate,* tightens up in cold air. *Much, thick, yellow expectoration.* Recurrent bronchitis, from every cold. Sensation of hot water dropping in chest. Asthma; after suppression. Cries before cough. Aphonia. Cough, < evening till midnight.

HEART: Palpitation, with stitches.

BACK: Crawling in right scapula.

EXTREMITIES: Encysted tumor at the point of elbow. Whitlow. Nail of great toe painful on slight pressure. Easy dislocation of finger joints. Laming pain in hip joint, < walking. Swelling of knees, ankle and foot. Drawing pain in limbs. Abscess in axilla. Swelling of feet around ankles, with difficult breathing.

SKIN: Sensitive to cool air. Foul moist eruption in folds. Torpid pulsating ulcer, encircled by smaller ones or by pimples or boils. Skin chapped, deep cracks on hands and feet. Very sensitive cold sores. Chronic and recurring urticaria. Angio-neurotic edema. Body exhales a foul odor. Impetigo. Poor granulation.

SLEEP: Sleeplessness; anxious dreams of fire. Unrefreshing. Wakes at night with erection and desire to urinate.

FEVER: Low fever; hectic. Profuse sweat, with least exertion, day and night; sweat sour, sticky, offensive. Night sweat.

COMPLEMENTARY: Iod; Sil.

RELATED: Merc.

HYDRASTIS

GENERALITIES: It acts on MUCOUS MEMBRANES, causing CATARRHAL process, with tendency to *hemorrhage* and ulceration; the catarrh may be anywhere - throat, stomach, uterus, urethra, which is characterized by *thick, yellow, acrid, ropy discharge;* mucus is found in the stool, in the urine; hawks up mucus; hence it can be called a mucus remedy. It produces atonic, cachetic, degenerative conditions, hence suitable for old, *easily* *tired, weak persons* with great debility, and emaciation. Sense of rawness and burning. Cancer and pre-cancerous states. Goitre of puberty and pregnancy. Modifies the course of small-pox when given internally and applied externally. Frequent faint spells with profuse perspiration. Shallow ulcer. Small wounds bleed and suppurate. Clothing feels uncomfortable about groins.

WORSE: *Inhaling air. Cold air.* Dry wind. Open air. Slight bleeding. Washing. Touch. *Old age.* Motion.

BETTER: Pressure.

MIND: Depression; sure of death and desires it. Forgetful.

HEAD: Neuralgia of the scalp and neck. Eczema on forehead along the line of hair, < after washing.

EYES: Ophthalmia, thick mucus discharge. Yellow.

EAR: Otorrhea; thick mucus discharge. Roaring. Deafness from eustachian catarrh.

NOSE: Sore, bleeds; bloody crusts. Ozena. Postnasal dripping. Air feels cold in nose. Blows all the time. Sinusitis after coryza.

FACE: Thin, yellow, sunken. Cancer on lips.

MOUTH: Tongue white, *yellow, dirty,* swollen; large, *flabby,* slimy, with imprint of teeth; feels as if scalded. Stomatitis of nursing mothers, or weakly children. Taste bitter. Aphthae. Bleeding, painful cancerous growth on hard palate.

THROAT: Follicular pharyngitis. Hawks yellow tenacious mucus.

STOMACH: Weak digestion. Gone feeling in stomach with loathing of food, or feels a sharp lump in stomach. Ulcer and Cancer. Painful epigastric tumor, with pulsations. Apt to vomit all foods, retaining only milk, or water. Cannot eat bread or vegetables.

ABDOMEN: Cutting pain from liver to right scapula, < lying on back or right side. Atrophy; cancer, of liver. Jaundice. Lumpy stools, coated or mixed with mucus. Hemorrhoids, even slight bleeding exhausts. *Obstinate constipation* of pregnancy, after purgatives. Raw smarting in the rectum during stools, remaining long afterwards. Pain in the groins as if sprained.

URINARY: Mucus in urine. Gleety discharge, thick, yellow. Putrid odor of urine.

FEMALE: Erosion of cervix. Thick; acrid, yellow; ropy leukorrhea. Pruritus vulvae, with profuse leukorrhea, with sexual excitement. Cancer of breast; nipples; retracted; sore, cracked, in nursing women. Menorrhagia and metrorrhagia; with fibroid. Removes the tendency to habitual adherent placenta. Vagina sore, during coition, bleeding thereafter. Pain in breast (R) on sneezing. Hot watery discharge from uterus.

RESPIRATORY: Bronchitis of old exhausted people. Loose cough, bloody, or thick yellow tenacious sputum, *raises much mucus.* Breathing difficult, < lying on left side.

HEART: Palpitation, from slowly progressing weakness.

NECK & BACK: Neuralgia of neck. Dull, dragging, heavy pain across lumbar region; uses arms to raise himself from a seat.

SKIN: Eruptions like small-pox. Ulcer, cancerous. Atonic ulcer, following removal of tumor.

FEVER: Heat alternating with chill. Tendency to profuse perspiration.

RELATED: Ars; Kali-bi; Puls.

HYDROCOTYLE

GENERALITIES: It is known as Indian pennywort. (Karivana). It produces hypertrophy and induration of connective tissue. Excessive thickening, and marked exfoliation of skin. It is supposed to influence leprosy, elephantiasis, lupus; copper-coloured eruptions in various places. Intolerable itching, esp. of soles, vagina. Cannot stand straight.

HYDROCYANIC ACID

GENERALITIES: Rapidly-acting, most deadly poison; producing convulsion, paralysis, collapse, cramps everywhere. *Effects are sudden*—spasms, collapse, apoplexy. Lacks reaction. Lightning-like jerks from head to feet. Evacuations cease suddenly, sinks down unconscious. Prolonged fainting. Bluishness. Epileptic attacks preceded by nausea and vomiting or waterbrash. Catalepsy. Intense coldness.

WORSE: Full moon. Suppressions. Storm.

MIND: Unconscious. Fear of imaginary troubles; of death, house falling, horses, cars, etc., of crossing the street even when the vehicle is at a considerable distance. Loud involuntary scream before convulsion.

HEAD: *Intense cerebral congestion;* brain feels on fire. Feels as if a cloud were going over his brain.

EYES: Distorted and half open. Eyeballs fixed.

FACE: Pale, or bluish; looks old. Cramp in masseters, jaws clenched in rigid spasm. Lips pale or bluish. Froth at mouth. Frightful contortion of muscles.

MOUTH: Dry. Taste; pussy, metallic, astringent. Tongue cold.

THROAT: *Noisy swallowing;* drink rumbles through throat and stomach. Spasms or paralysis of esophagus.

STOMACH: Great sinking at the pit of stomach. Anorexia. Cholera. Burning from navel to esophagus; chronic dyspepsia.

RESPIRATORY: *Breathing slow,* irregular, gasping. Asphyxia. Dry tickling night cough. Asthma; with choking in the throat. Convulsion, with whooping cough.

HEART: Clutches at the heart as if in distress. Heart failure; compression at heart. Pulse; failing, weak, irregular, unequal, with occasional strong beats. Blood vessels distended, writhing in them. Angina, severe pain.

BACK: Muscles of the dorsal region are contracted.

EXTREMITIES: Hands icy cold.

SKIN: Bluish eruptions.

SLEEP: Yawning, with shivering. Drowsiness. Coma vigil.

FEVER: Icy coldness; < hands.

RELATED: Agar; Cupr; Laur.

HYDROPHOBINUM (See Lyssin)

HYOSCYAMUS

GENERALITIES: Commonly known as Henbane, or Hogbane, it disturbs the MIND, *brain and nervous system* profoundly. Diabolical forces seem to take possession of the brain preventing its functions. It causes a perfect picture of mania, of a quarrelsome and lascivious nature. *Convulsions, trembling, jerks,* twitching, cramps are very marked features. Acute mania or convulsion, alternates with or end in *deep sopor.* Motions of the arms are *clutching* or angular; throws arms about, misses what is reached for; totters while walking. Paralysis after spasm. Epilepsy; vertigo before the attacks. Falls suddenly to the ground with cries. CARPHOLOGY, picks at bed clothes, at fingers. When lying on back, suddenly sits up and lies down again. Child sobs and cries without waking. Eclampsia. *Subsultus,* during fevers. Septic fever. Slides down in bed. Ill- effect of suppressed lochia or milk, fright, disappointed love. Chorea; local, twitching of solitary muscles; squinting, stammering. Suitable for nervous, irritable, excitable persons. Sensation as if walking on and through air.

WORSE: *Emotions; jealousy;* fright; unhappy love. Before and during menses. *Touch.* Cold. Sleep. *Lying.*

BETTER: Sitting up. Motion. Warmth. Stooping.

MIND: *Many bewildering aberrations.* MANIA. *Erotic females,* expose genitals, sing amorous songs. Does foolish things, behaves like one mad. Laughs, sings, *talks, babbles,* quarrels. *Fumbles the genitals. Jealous.* Suspicious. Fears being alone, being pursued, water, being poisoned, being bitten, etc. Laughs at everything, foolishly. Restless, jumps out of bed, *wants to escape.* Utters each word louder. Rage, with desire to strike, bite, fight, insult, scold, and kill. Plaintive cries esp. on the slightest touch even in stupor. Unconsciousness, *can barely be aroused. Muttering* delirium. Thinks one is not at home. Speechless from fright. Confusion. First cannot think, then can scarcely be aroused. Talks with imaginary persons, to dead ones. Imagines things are animals. Fear of being bitten by beasts. Plays with fingers. *Silly,* does comical acts. Looks at hands because they seem too large. Syphilophobia.

HEAD: Waves of pulsation in head. Pulsating headache. Vertigo, before spasm, from smell of flowers, gas, etc. Rolls or shakes the head to and fro; when bending forward, in stupor, after concussion of the brain. Brain feels loose. Feels water swashing in head.

EYES: Aversion to light. Eyes open but does not pay attention. Spasmodic closing of lids. Eyes roll about in orbits. Squint. Constantly stares at surrounding objects. Objects; seem red, large, or with colored border (yellow).

EARS: Deafness, from paralysis of auditory nerve.

NOSE: Nostrils sooty, smoky. Sudden jerks at root of the nose. Loss of smell and taste.

FACE: Pale, flushed, dark red. Muscles twitch. Grimaces, and makes ridiculous gestures. Lower jaw drops. Muscles twitch, when protruding the tongue. Lockjaw.

MOUTH: Sordes on teeth; closes teeth tightly. Foam at mouth. Tongue protruded with difficulty, can hardly draw it in. Speech impaired, lost from fright. Stiff, dark red, cracked tongue, looks like burnt leather. Bites the tongue while talking. Tongue dry, rattles in mouth. Grinds the teeth during convulsion in children. Teeth feel loose when chewing, also too long. Violent pain in teeth, with twitching of muscles of hands, face, etc.

THROAT: Elongation of uvula. Constriction of throat, inability to swallow liquids; solid and warm food >. Fluids come out through the nose, or go down in larynx.

STOMACH: Hiccough; from concussion of brain, of nursing children. Vomiting with convulsion. Cramp in stomach, > after vomiting, < after irritating food. Aversion to water.

ABDOMEN: Colic, as if abdomen would burst. Colic; with vomiting, eructations, hiccough and screaming. Red spots on abdomen. Umbilicus open, urine oozing through. Stools involuntary—bloody, yellow, watery, or even if hard, < mental excitement, during sleep; during fever, while urinating. Gastritis or peritonitis with hiccough. Diarrhea after parturition.

URINARY: Frequent, scanty, painful, nightly urination; or *retention of urine,* after childbirth; paralysis of bladder. Involuntary urination.

MALE: Lascivious; exposes his genitals, plays with genitals, during fever.

FEMALE: Lascivious; uncovers sexual parts. Nymphomania. Hysterical or epileptic spasm, before menses. Convulsive trembling of hands and feet, during menses. Enuresis, during menses. Painless diarrhea in lying-in women. Cold that settles in the womb and brings on labor-like pains. Convulsions during pregnancy. No will to make water in childbed. Milk and lochia suppressed.

RESPIRATORY: Dry, hacking, *spasmodic cough,* from a dry spot in larynx, *at night,* < lying, eating, drinking, talking, singing, > sitting up. Hemoptysis; blood bright red, with spasm. Spasm of chest with shortness of breath, forcing him to bend double. Exhausting cough, with sweat.

NECK: Stiff, contracted to one side.

EXTREMITIES: Trembling of hands and feet. Toes spasmodically contracted while walking or going upstairs. Fists clenched with retraction of thumb (in convulsions).

SLEEP: *Nervous wakefulness.* Falls asleep while answering. Starts out of sleep frightened. Sits up and then goes to sleep again. Profound sleep. Laughs during sleep.

FEVER: Low fever with hot, pale skin. Warm sweat.

RELATED: Bell; Phos; Stram.

HYOSCYAMINE HYDROBROMATE

GENERALITIES: This drug relieves the tremor of disseminated sclerosis and paralysis agitans. Sleeplessness and nervous agitation.

HYPERICUM

GENERALITIES: An excellent remedy for injury to parts rich in sentient nerves, esp. fingers, toes, matrix of nails. LACERATION; when *intolerable, violent, shooting, lancinating* pain shows nerves are severely involved. Injury to the brain and *spinal cord* or after-effects from such injury. Spasm after every injury. *Very painful sore parts,* occiput, coccyx, etc. Pains extend towards the trunk or down the sides with crawling and numbness. Neuritis of *head* or chest, in epigastrium, inter-scapular spine, finger-tips, etc. Shooting up from injured part. Tingling, burning and numbness, with neuritis. Neuralgia of the stump, shudderings. Prevents tetanus, and relieves pain after operation. Joints feel bruised. Convulsion after knocking the body against anything. Jerks in the limbs. Punctured or penetrating wounds, very sensitive to touch. Ill-effect of fright, bite, shock. Wounds are more tender than appearance would indicate. Lies on back, jerking head backwards. Pain in old cicatrices.

WORSE: INJURY. JAR. Concussion of spine, coccyx. *Shock.* Bruises. Exertion. Touch. Change of weather. Fog. Cold damp. *Motion.* After forceps delivery as complication of injury.

BETTER: Lying on face. Bending back. Rubbing.

MIND: Makes mistakes in writing; forgets what she wanted to say. Feels lifted high in air or anxiety lest he should fall from a height. Melancholy.

HEAD: Heaviness or formication in brain. Brain feels loose. Head feels as if touched by icy cold hand. *Head feels larger, drawn to a point.* Throbbing in vertex. Falling of hair, after injury.

FACE: Bloated, hot. Eczema of face; eruptions seem to be under the skin. Intense itching. Toothache, > lying on affected side quietly.

THROAT: Feeling as of a worm moving in. Hot risings in esophagus after a fright or with anxious feeling. Tongue white at the back, tip clean. Craving for wine, with feeling of heat in mouth.

STOMACH: Thirst, with feeling of heat in mouth. Nausea. Belches while drinking water. Desire for pickles, warm drink, wine.

ABDOMEN: Bubbling at navel. Tympanitic distension, > after stool (after laparotomy). Rectum feels dry. Summer diarrhea with eruptions on the skin. Hemorrhoids with pain, bleeding and tenderness (use externally and internally).

FEMALE: Afterpains violent in sacrum and hips with severe headache; pain after forceps delivery.

RESPIRATORY: Spells of short barking cough. Asthma, < foggy weather and > by profuse expectoration.

HEART: Feels as though it will drop down.

NECK & BACK: Pain in the nape of neck. Pressure over sacrum. Consequence of spinal concussion. Coccyx painful, pain radiating up the spine and down the limbs. Painfully sensitive spine. Pain in hips, small of back and coccyx, after labor.

EXTREMITIES: Limbs feel detached. Pressure along ulnar side of the arm. Crawling in hand and feet. Aching in sciatic nerve (left) after prolonged sitting. Hands and feet seem furry, or bones aching. Violent pain and inability to walk or stoop after a fall on coccyx.

SKIN: Painful scars in tissues rich in nerves. Gaping wounds. Skin rough as if full of small knots. Pain in old cicatrices.

SLEEP: Constant drowsiness. Laborious dreams.

FEVER: Shuddering over whole body with desire to urinate.

RELATED: Arn; Led; Rhus-t.

IBERIS

GENERALITIES: This remedy has a marked action on the heart and is useful in cardiac diseases. Cardiac hypertrophy, with thickening of heart walls. Cardiac debility after influenza. Liver region full and painful. Palpitation, *with vertigo and choking in the throat,* < slightest exertion, laughing, coughing. Darting pain through heart. Numbness and tingling in left hand and arm.

WORSE: Lying down; on left side. Motion; exertion. Warm room.

IGNATIA

GENERALITIES: The seeds of Ignatia contain a larger proportion of strychnine than those of Nux vomica, yet there is a great difference between the characteristic features of the two drugs. Though it affects the MIND, EMOTIONAL *element* is profoundly influenced and *co-ordination of functions is interfered with;* causing ERRATIC, *contradictory, paradoxical* mental and physical EFFECTS, which change rapidly, and are opposite to each other. NERVOUS SYSTEM is affected causing SPASMODIC EFFECTS; *often violent with rigidity, twitching and trem-*

ors. It is adapted to the persons of nervous temperament, esp. women of sensitive, easily excited nature, mild disposition, quick to perceive and rapid in execution. SENSE OF LUMP, foreign body or sharp pressure. Jerks run through the whole body. Tendency to start. Globus. Clavus. Hysteria. Chorea after fright, from grief, < after eating, > lying on back. Convulsions of children, during dentition, after punishment, after fear or fright; return at the same hour daily. Spasm, with cry or involuntary laughter. Tonic spasm of single parts, with frothing at the mouth. Spasms alternating with oppressed breathing. Pain in spot, < close attention. Oversensitive to pain. Pains change their locality, come gradually, abate suddenly, or come and go suddenly. Symptoms pass after profuse urination. Plague—preventive and curative. *Nervous shuddering,* with pain. Paralysis after great mental emotion and night-watching, in sick chamber. Suitable for persons who had been starving either from want or from other causes. Ill-effect of grief, fright, worry, disappointed love, jealousy, old spinal injury. Catalepsy with opisthotonos. (Nat-mur should follow in chronic conditions.)

WORSE: EMOTIONS. GRIEF. *Chagrin*. WORRY. FRIGHT. Shock, after losing person or object that was very dear. Air-open, cold. Odor. *Touch. Coffee.* Tobacco. Yawning. Stooping, walking, standing. At the same hour and day.

BETTER: Change of position. *Lying on affected part.* Urination. If alone. Pressure. Deep breathing. *Swallowing. Eating.* Near a warm stove. Sour things.

MIND: ALERT; OVERSENSITIVE AND NERVOUS. *Highly emotional. Moody. Brooding.* GRIEF. *Silent and sad.* SIGHS. *Weeps* or laughs by turns; laughs when she ought to be serious. *Changeable mood. Unhappy love.* Inward weeping; enjoys being *sad.* Angry with himself. Desire to be alone. Everything irks her, intolerant of contradiction, of reprimand. Anguish; shrieks for help. Capricious. Delicately conscientious. Fear of thieves, of trifles, of things coming near him. Introspective. Faints easily; girls who faint every time they go to church; or who fall in love with married men. Sensation as if she had been fasting for a long time. Hurried during menses; no one can do things fast enough for her. Looks about the bed as if to find something. Delights to bring on her fits and produce a scare or a scene. Thinks she had neglected her duty. Sighing and sobbing. Not communicative. Fear of robbers at night.

HEAD: Ache as if a nail were driven out through the sides, ends in yawning and vomiting; alternate with backache. Headache < or > by stooping. Throws head backwards from weight at occiput or during spasms. Vertigo, with sparks before the eyes. Loud talking < headache. Headache; from abuse of snuff, tobacco smoke, coffee, from close attention.

EYES: Asthenopia, with spasm of the lids, and neuralgic pain around the eyes. Flashes of light from violent coughing. Eyelids feel dry. Flickering, zigzags before the eyes.

EARS: Roaring, > by music. One ear red and hot. Deafness, except for human voice.

NOSE: Sensitive to inspired air. Pain over the root of the nose. Sneezing attacks. Cold, with hot knees.

FACE: Twitching of the muscles of face and lips. *Redness and heat of one cheek;* red and pale alternately. Masseters stiff and hard. Emotional trismus. Changes color often when at rest. Facial muscles distort on attempting to speak.

MOUTH: Spasmodic closing of the jaws; bites inside of cheek or tongue when talking or chewing. Corners twitch. Taste sour. Toothache, < after drinking coffee and smoking. Sudden attacks of salivation.

THROAT: Inflamed, hard, swollen tonsils, with small ulcers on them. Follicular tonsillitis. Feeling of a lump when not swallowing *that cannot be swallowed,* > eating solids. Tendency to choke. Globus hystericus. Stitches extend to ear between acts of swallowing. Submaxillary glands painful when moving the neck. Cramps in gullet. Goitre.

STOMACH: Hunger, with nausea. Craves raw or indigestible things, sour things, bread, esp. rye bread. Appetite for various things, but when offered appetite fails. Aversion to warm food, meat, alcohol, tobacco. *Empty sinking or spasmodic ache in stomach,* not > by eating, > by taking deep breath. *Hiccough,* with eructations empty or bitter, after eating, drinking, smoking. Nausea or vomiting, > indigestible things.

ABDOMEN: Colicky, griping pain in one or both sides of the abdomen. Stools painful, difficult although soft. Constrictive sore pain in the rectum, like from blind hemorrhoids, remains for one or two hours after stool. Constipation of neurasthenics. *Pain shoots up in rectum.* Piles, > sitting, < coughing. *Prolapsus of rectum* from moderate straining at stool. Pressure as of a sharp instrument from within outwards. Painless contraction of anus. Hemorrhage and pain, < when stool is loose. Constipation; from taking cold; from riding in a carriage. Urging to stool with erection.

URINARY: Frequent, profuse, watery urine. Urging with inability to pass urine.

MALE: Erection during stool. Sweat on scrotum. Penis contracted, becomes small.

FEMALE: Menses irregular, black, too early, too profuse, or scanty; suppressed from grief. Chronic leukorrhea, with sexual desire. Sexual frigidity.

HEART: Palpitation, during menses. Anxious feeling in the region.

RESPIRATORY: TAKES DEEP BREATH for relief. *Choking*; spasm of glottis. Dry, hacking, spasmodic cough in quick successive shocks shutting off the breath; cough as from dust or sulphur fume. Coughing increases the desire to cough. Cough, everytime he stands still during a walk. Constriction of the chest, feels as if too small. Whispering voice, cannot speak loudly. Sleepy after coughing. Stitches in nipples on deep inspiration.

NECK & BACK: Stiffness of the nape of the neck. Convulsive bending backward of the back.

EXTREMITIES: Jerking in limbs. Warm sweat on the palms. Cramp in calves. Heavy feet. Dislocative pain in joints. Knees are involuntarily drawn upwards when walking. Trembling of hands when writing in anyone's presence. Burning in heels on placing them near one another, when they come in contact they are cold to touch, < at night. Sciatica, < in winter, > in summer. Corns painful as if sore. Knees hot with cold nose. Sensation as if flesh were loose on bones from a blow.

SKIN: Painful, > pressure. Nettlerash over the whole body with violent itching (during fever).

SLEEP: *Violent spasmodic yawning* with running from eyes. Sleep light, every sound wakes. Jerking of limbs on going to sleep. Somnambulism from wounded honor. Same horrid dream over and over again. Child awakes from sleep with piercing cries and trembles all over. Hiccough. Chewing motion of mouth in sleep (children).

FEVER: Chill with red face. Shaking chill with thirst. Sweat, < on eating; sweat often on a small spot on the face. Heat with aversion to uncover, no thirst. Chill during pain. Feeling as if sweat would break out, but does not.

COMPLEMENTARY: Aur; Nat-m; Phos-ac; Sep.

RELATED: Cimic; Nux-v; Sep.

INDIGO

GENERALITIES: It has some reputation in the treatment of epilepsy, when the attacks are preceded by a furious excitable disposition followed by melancholy, timidity and mildness, or there is peculiar undulating sensation in the brain with obscuration of vision, or sensation as if the brain were frozen before the attack. Pain in the limbs, < after every meal. Sciatica - pain from middle of thighs to the knee.

WORSE: Sitting. Rest.

BETTER: Rubbing. Pressure. Walking.

IODOFORMUM

GENERALITIES: A very useful remedy for tuberculous conditions, esp. tubercular meningitis, and for failing of sight due to retro-bulbar neuritis, central scotoma, partial atrophy of the optic disc. Sleep interrupted by sighing and cries. Pupils dilated; contract unequally. Chronic diarrhea, stool greenish, watery, undigested, with irritable temper, due to suspected tuberculosis. Mesenteric glands enlarged. Cannot stand or walk with eyes closed.

WORSE: At night. Warmth. Touch. Motion.

IODUM

GENERALITIES: Iodine has great *absorbent action, which is rapid and intense;* muscles, fat, tissues and glands waste away and general emaciation is the result. GLANDS—THYROID, TESTES, MESENTERIC and mammary first get SWOLLEN, HARD and *heavy,* then begin to dwindle. New growths and hyperplasia come under its action when their growth is rapid. Trembling of limbs or whole body. *Weak and rapidly losing flesh,* even with good appetite. FEELS ALWAYS TOO HOT. Great debility, the slightest effort induces perspiration, cannot talk, becomes out of breath going upstairs. Acute exacerbation of chronic inflammation. Arthritis deformans with swollen joints after acute attack of rheumatism. *Secretions are hot,* acrid or watery, persistent or salty. ACUTE CATARRH OF THE MUCOUS MEMBRANES, ESP. LARYNX and lungs, pneumonia with rapid extension. Vasoconstriction, causing edema, ecchymosis, hemorrhage. Vascular degeneration. Atrophy or induration of testes, ovaries, uterus. Wasting diseases of scrofulous patients. Adenoids. Goitre. Pancreatic diseases. Arthritic affections. Tuberculosis. Affections of connective tissue, with torpidity and little pus. General pulsations or local throbbing in large arterial tracks. Burning. Infiltration. Internal tickling. Ill-effect of nervous shock, disappointed love. Plastic exudation. Facial paralysis or epilepsy, from suppression of goitre. Emaciation, with glandular enlargement. Feels well only while eating, in any diseased condition. Sluggish reaction, hence chronicity of many affections. Suitable for over-grown boys with weak chest and aged persons.

WORSE: HEAT OF: *room;* air wraps. Exertion; ascending, talking. Fasting. Night. Rest. Touch. Pressure.

BETTER: COLD AIR; cold *bathing.* Walking about in open air. Eating. Sitting up.

MIND: Anxiety about the present (no reference to the future) when quiet. Dejected, with tendency to weep, or *intolerably* CROSS AND RESTLESS. Excited. Sudden impulse to run and do violence, but motion < and exhausts; > if busy. Thinks he is well. Fear of people, of physician;

shuns everyone. Suicidal tendency. Fretful; forgets what is to be spoken or done, does not know what. Does not understand why he has done some particular things. Tendency to do some strange things without any cause, to kill somebody, to kill himself. Heart palpitates when thinking of real or imaginary wrongs.

HEAD: Reverberations in head. Throbbing, rush of blood and feeling of a tight band. Vertigo; chronic, congestive. Headache of old people, < in warm air, from fatigue, walking fast, riding in car. Sensation as if brain were being stirred around with a spoon.

EYES: Protruded. Convulsive movement and quivering of the eyes; of lower eyelids. Profuse lacrimation. Acute dacryocystitis. Staring with wide open eyes; eyelids seem to be retracted.

EARS: Chronic deafness with adhesion in the middle ear. Eustachian catarrh.

NOSE: Pain at the root of the nose and frontal sinuses. Coryza, < open air. Nose red and swollen; sudden much sneezing, with dripping of hot water. Acute nasal engorgement associated with high blood pressure. Alae feels as if spread wide apart. Descending colds.

FACE: Withered, *brownish,* sallow or dusky; miserable look. Coldness of face in fleshy children. Facial paralysis, after reduction of goitre.

MOUTH: Profuse fetid, soapy saliva. Metallic taste. Foul ulcers; aphthae. Offensive odor from the mouth. Tongue; hypertrophied, painful, nodular or fissured.

THROAT: Constriction, impending deglutition. Burning and scrapping in throat. *Goitre; hard,* with sensation of constriction. Uvula swollen. Submaxillary glands swollen.

STOMACH: *Ravenous hunger yet emaciates, or variable appetite,* with thirst. Gets anxious or worried if he does not eat. Drinking cold milk > constipation. Pulsation in the pit of the stomach. Bitter taste to solid food, not drinks. Hiccough. Empty eructations.

ABDOMEN: Liver and spleen enlarged and sore. Stool frothy, wheyey, fatty, cheesy, or lienteric; pancreatic affections. Trembling in abdomen. Chronic morning diarrhea of emaciated, scrofulous children. Jaundice—eyes, skin, nails yellow. Swelling of mesenteric glands.

URINARY: Urination frequent and copious; urine; dark, yellow-green, milky, with variegated cuticle on its surface; sediment like red pepper. Incontinence in old people with prostatic enlargement. Milky white fluid runs from urethra after stool.

MALE: Testicles swollen and indurated. Twisting in spermatic cord. Atrophy of testes; with loss of sexual power. Sarcocele. Hydrocele.

FEMALE: Great weakness during menses. Menses brown; renewed after every stool. Mammae dwindle away and become flabby. Wedge-like pain from ovary to uterus. Nodosities in the skin of mammae with black points. *Leukorrhea acrid,* eroding thighs and linen, < during menses. Mammae heavy, as if would fall. Sterility from atrophy of ovaries and mammae.

RESPIRATORY: *Painful, choking hoarseness;* child grasps the throat while coughing. Laryngitis. Diphtheria. *Dry, tickling, croupy cough. Short breath,* esp. on going upstairs. Edema of glottis. Expectoration of cast of larynx; or of blood streaked mucus. Voice rough. Tickling all over chest. Bronchi raw. Violent pulmonary congestion. Pneumonia, hepatization spreading rapidly with high temperature and absence of pain. Pleuritic effusion. Asthma, breathes heavily when quiet. Itching low down in lungs behind sternum.

HEART: Feels squeezed as if by an iron band followed by great weakness and faintness. Palpitation, < least exertion. Feeling of vibration or purring over heart. Tachycardia. Myocarditis. Pulsation in large arterial trunks.

NECK & BACK: Swelling of the neck when speaking; grows thick.

EXTREMITIES: Chronic arthritic affections; stiff and enlarged joints. Synovitis. Cold hands and feet. Acrid sweat on back of feet. Edema of the feet. Back of hands brown, as if swollen; painful when turning hand, not when closing fingers. Painful corns.

SKIN: Hot, dry, dirty; *brown spots* on skin. Nodosities on skin. Anasarca of cardiac origin. Itching pimples and itching in old cicatrices. Scars break open.

SLEEP: Restlessness in blood, prevents sleep.

FEVER: *Hyperpyrexia,* or external coldness with anxiety or stupor. Hectic fever. Flushes of heat all over the body; heat waves to head. Sweats easily. Early morning sweat >.

COMPLEMENTARY: Lyc; Sil.

RELATED: Ars; Fluor-ac; Phos; Spong.

IPECACUANHA

GENERALITIES: It acts chiefly on the *pneumo-gastric* nerve producing gastrointestinal disturbances, and RESPIRATORY AFFECTIONS, with CONTINUOUS NAUSEA. *Discharges are foamy and profuse.* BRIGHT RED, GUSHING HEMORRHAGE, with nausea. Nausea and shortness *of breath* usually accompany most of the complaints. Convulsions, infantile, body rigid, stretched out, followed by spasmodic jerking of arms towards each other. Awkward, stumbles against everything. Tetanic spasms from swallowing tobacco. Convulsions; in whooping cough, from suppressed exanthema, from indigestible food. It is indicated in fat children and adults who are feeble and catch cold in warm moist weather. Ill-effects of vexation, reserved displeasure, injury, suppressed eruption, quinine, morphia, indigestible food, loss of blood. Over-sensitive to heat and cold. Opisthotonos and emprosthotonos.

WORSE: WARMTH, *damp room. Overeating.* Ice, pork, veal, mixed or *rich food;* candy, fruits, raisins, salad, lemon peel, berries. Periodically. Heat and cold. Vomiting. Motion. Lying.

BETTER: Open air. Rest. Pressure. Closing eyes. Cold drink.

MIND: Holds everything in contempt, and desires others also should do the same. Cries, screams, howls, and is hard to please (children). Full of desires but knows not for what. Sad. Faints suddenly; in summer or in hot room.

HEAD: Aches as if bruised or crushed, which goes down into the root of the tongue. Migraine, with nausea and vomiting. Pain in occiput, < vomiting, during chill. Cold sweat on forehead.

EYES: Inflamed, red; conjunctivitis. Profuse gushing lacrimation, with nausea. Shooting pain through the eyeball. Nausea from looking at moving objects.

EARS: Cold (right), during fever. Cannot endure the least noise.

NOSE: Bleed, blood bright red. Coryza with stoppage of nose and nausea. *Sneezing.*

FACE: Pale; blue about the eyes or lips; white linea

nasalis. Periodical orbital neuralgia, with lacrimation, photophobia and smarting eyelids.

MOUTH: Child thrusts its fist into the mouth and screams. *Clean or red pointed tongue.* Saliva increased. Toothache, with a jerk radiating to temples; > while eating. Tongue, clean, yellow, or white, pale. Taste; bitter, sweetish, bloody.

STOMACH: Desire for dainties, sweets. *Feels miserable or sinking or relaxed as if hanging down. Horrid nausea, not > by vomiting.* Vomits; blood, bile, food, mucus, < stooping. Aversion to food. *Thirstless.* Vomiting of infants at the breast.

ABDOMEN: Griping, drawing or *cutting pain about the navel,* < motion, > by repose; pain extending towards the uterus. Stool brown, grass or yellow green, frothy, molasses-like or *bloody,* slimy. Dysentery, with head hot and cold legs. Lumps of mucus in stools.

URINARY: Unsuccessful *urging to urinate.* Hematuria, with nausea and cutting in abdomen and urethra, with oppression in chest and short breath. Shooting from kidney down the thighs to the knees.

FEMALE: Uterine hemorrhages, profuse, bright, steady flow or gushing, with nausea and gasping with each gush of blood. Cutting pain in uterus from left to right. Stitches from navel to uterus. Menses; too early and too profuse. Vomiting during pregnancy. Prolapse of uterus, < during menses. Hemorrhage of placenta previa. Steady flow of bright red blood, which does not coagulate. Great weakness with scanty menses.

RESPIRATORY: Painless hoarseness at the end of a cold. Constant constriction in chest and larynx, < least motion. Spasm of vocal cord. *Gasps for breath. Asthma. Cough incessant and violent,* with every breath. *Paroxysm of suffocative cough,* with retching; child *stiffens* *out,* becomes red or blue in face and finally is nauseated, gags and vomits, > stepping into open air, warmth and repose. Whooping cough with bleeding from the nose and from the mouth. LOOSE coarse RATTLE IN CHEST WITHOUT EXPECTORATION. Bronchopneumonia. Hemoptysis, < slightest exertion. Asthma accompanied with skin disease. Suffocative attacks from foreign substance in windpipe.

NECK & BACK: Tetanic spasm of back which bends it backward or forward. Shooting from kidney region into thighs. Cramps between scapulae during motion.

EXTREMITIES: Coldness of one hand, other is hot. Femur feels dislocated on sitting down. Bruised pain in all the bones.

SLEEP: Shocks in limbs on falling to sleep. Eyes half open during sleep, with moaning and groaning. Loss of sleep causes nausea and fatigue.

SKIN: Itching, with nausea, scratches until he vomits.

FEVER: Short chill with long heat. Chill alternating with heat. Heat without thirst. Suppressed or mixed intermittent fevers, *nausea in all stages.* Catarrhal or gastric fever. Hands and feet drip cold sweat. Infantile remittent fever.

COMPLEMENTARY: Ars; Cupr.

RELATED: Ant-t; Lob.

IRIS VERSICOLOR

GENERALITIES: Iris acts powerfully on GASTRO-INTESTINAL MUCOUS MEMBRANES, on salivary glands, LIVER and PANCREAS, producing *profuse secretion* which *is sour, acrid and burning. Oily nose, greasy taste and fatty* *stool* are other characteristics. Promotes the flow of bile. Symptoms set in suddenly, accompanied by rapid elimination. Cholera morbus and sick headache.

WORSE: Periodically. *Weekly,* 2-3 a.m. Spring and Autumn. After midnight. *Mental exhaustion. Hot weather.*

BETTER: Gentle motion.

MIND: Low-spirited. Fear of approaching illness. Dullness of mental faculties.

HEAD: Aches begin with blurring of vision. Sick headaches, with diarrhea. Shooting in temples with contractive feeling of the scalp. Tired headache with mental exhaustion (studying, sewing), < coughing, cold air; > gentle motion.

EYES: Sunken. Violent supraorbital pains. *Periodic visual disturbance,* blindness, hemiopia etc. with headache.

EARS: Aural vertigo with intense noises in ears.

NOSE: Oily. Constant sneezing.

FACE: Neuralgia, < after breakfast, involving the whole face, with copious urine, and urging for stool.

MOUTH: Feels greasy, burnt or scalded. Tongue burns or feels cold. *Greasy or sweetish taste. Profuse ropy saliva,* drops when talking.

THROAT: Heat and smarting in throat. Burning from fauces to stomach, > inhaling cool air or drinking cold water. Goitre.

STOMACH: Sour, bitter eructations. *Burning of whole alimentary canal,* not > by cold drinks. Continuous *nausea.* Bitter, sweetish water; acrid, *watery, Sour Vomiting With Burning.* Deficient appetite. Periodical vomiting spells—every month, six weeks, last for two or three days.

ABDOMEN: Liver sore. Colicky pain before each spell of vomiting and purging. STOOLS BILIOUS, ACRID, WATERY; BURN LIKE FIRE. *Painless cholera morbus.* Urging to stool with headache, facial neuralgia, and pain in teeth. *Stools fatty.* Anus feels sore or as if sharp points sticking in it.

URINARY: Profuse, clear urine, with headache. Burning along the length of urethra after urination. Diabetes.

FEMALE: Protracted nausea and vomiting during pregnancy; profuse flow of saliva.

EXTREMITIES: The hips feel wrenched out. Shooting, laming pain along limbs; sciatica.

SKIN: Herpes zoster, with gastric derangement, right side. Psoriasis, irregular patches with shining scales. Sweat smells of vinegar.

RELATED: Ars; Merc; Phos.

JABORANDI

GENERALITIES: Pilocarpus is a powerful glandular stimulant. It produces hypersecretion from upper respiratory tract and salivary glands, and *abnormal sweat.* In addition it produces very important eye affections. *Tendency to take cold and to sweat.* Hot flushes, salivation, nausea and profuse perspiration. Limits the duration of mumps. *Colliquative states.* Exophthalmic goitre.

WORSE: Start of menses. Cold. Exhaustion.

MIND: Very nervous and tremulous. Has fixed idea that she will murder all her family members with a hatchet.

HEAD: Aches, with vertigo and nausea on using the eyes.

EYES: Visual disturbances. Eyes easily tire from slightest use. Retinal images retained long after using eyes.

White spots before the eyes. Lids twitch. Smarting pain in the eyes. Near-sighted. Pupils contracted. Exophthalmos. Squint, convergent, after operation. Vitreous opacity.

EARS: Nervous deafness, > in noise. Tinnitus. Serous exudation into tympanic cavity. Mumps, esp. when metastasizes to the testes.

MOUTH: *Salivation;* saliva viscid - like white of an egg. Tension in salivary glands.

THROAT: Exophthalmic goitre, with increased heart's action; pulsation in arteries, tremors and nervousness.

STOMACH: Nausea on using eyes or looking at moving objects. Stubborn vomiting of pregnancy. Diarrhea, with flushed face and profuse perspiration.

MALE: Orchitis—metastasis of mumps.

FEMALE: Menses, start with coldness, throbbing in head and pelvis, and backache.

HEART: Violent ebullitions to heart and chest. Nervous cardiac affections.

RESPIRATORY: Much inclination to cough, with difficult breathing. Edema of lungs. Frothy or profuse, thin, serous expectoration.

SKIN: Red. *Sweat,* with palpitation, general pulsation and tremor. Nervous sweat. Unilateral sweat.

RELATED: Agar; Ant-t; Ip.

JALAPA

GENERALITIES: It is a powerful purgative, hence it affects intestines and stomach. *Child is good all day, but screams and tosses about all night,* or child may be troublesome and restless day and night, with any complaint. Colic. *Stools watery,* muddy or sour, bloody. Infantile diarrhoea, with general coldness, blueness of face.

WORSE: Night. Eructation.

RELATED: Coloc.

JATROPHA

GENERALITIES: It is also an active purgative, hence it affects *stomach and intestines.* Vomiting easy, albuminous. Hiccough followed by copious vomiting. *Loud gurgle like water from a bunghole in abdomen, then profuse gushing stool.* Unquenchable thirst. Rice-water stool. Violent cramps that draw the muscles of calf flat. Icy coldness of the whole body, esp. lower limbs.

WORSE: Covering. Morning. Summer.

RELATED: Crot-t.

JUSTICIA

GENERALITIES: Very useful remedy for acute catarrhal conditions of the respiratory tract. Fits of sneezing with lacrimation and *loss of smell and taste.* Coryza fluent, acrid, with violent sneezing, coughing or asthmatic attack. Cough with tightness of chest, as if it would burst; cough *with bronchial rattle, obstruction of breath* and sneezing. Stiffening out, trembling and convulsion, with cough or fever. Whooping cough. Tough expectoration. Puffy hands and feet in a.m. Chilliness. Sensitiveness.

WORSE: Close room. Dust. Noise. Eating.

RELATED: Ip; Dros; Puls.

KALI ARSENICUM

GENERALITIES: It is a valuable remedy for inveterate skin diseases and when patient's condition tend towards malignancy. All the sufferings are < at night. Sudden noise or touch throws the whole body into a tremor. Tongue burns, numb; neuralgia of tongue. Palpitation, with nephritis. *Burning in throat.* Aching in stomach. Passes much gas, then diarrhea. Cauliflower-like excrescences of os uteri, with flying pain, foul smelling discharges, and pressure below the pelvis. Intolerable itching, < undressing, walking, warmth. Chronic eczema. Psoriasis. Numerous small nodules under the skin. Black leg ulcer running bloody, foul water, with cutting, burning, itching and dyspnea. Chilly and sensitive to cold. Cannot get too warm even in summer.

WORSE: *Touch. Noise.* Cold feet. 1-3 a.m.

BETTER: Rainy days.

KALI BICHROMICUM

GENERALITIES: Potassium bichromate specially affects the MUCOUS MEMBRANES *of the air passages, Nose, pharynx,* stomach and duodenum producing ADHESIVE, STICKY, STRINGY, *tough, lumpy or thick discharges.* Diseased conditions progress *slowly* but *deeply,* causing great weakness bordering on paralysis, but little fever. Plastic or fibrous exudations spread downwards. It is adapted to fat, fair, fleshy, light-complexioned persons, subject to *catarrh* or with syphilitic or scrofulous history. *Pains occur in small spots or migrate quickly from place to place,* and finally attack the stomach. Rheumatic and gastric symptoms alternate. Diagonal pain. Ascending symptoms—gastric pain, chill, heat, etc. Formation of crusts on mucous membranes and skin. Ulcers; with dark dots; deep, perforating, round, punched out, with over-hanging edges or thick crusts. Septal or peptic ulcers. Sensation of heaviness in different parts. Feels a hair on tongue, in nostril, etc. Yellowness of discharges, eyes, vision, tongue, etc. Sharp stitching pain. Itching internally in vagina, ear, lung, etc. *Cracking of joints.* Indolent or sluggish reaction, in many conditions—ulcers; inflammation, etc. Affections of root of the nose, tongue, penis, etc. Stubborn suppuration. Plugs of pus; stringy. Ill-effects of indulgence in beer and malt liquor. Neuralgia, daily at the same hour. Sickly, chilly and cachectic. Biting like bugs. Membranes look furred. Pains appear and disappear suddenly. Epilepsy; ropy saliva from mouth during convulsion. Weakness and weariness; after pains.

WORSE: COLD, *damp.* Open air. Spring. *Undressing. Morning,* after sleep, 2-3 a.m. Protruding tongue. *Hot weather.* Alcohol, beer. Suppressed catarrh. Stooping. Sitting.

BETTER: Heat. Motion. Pressure.

MIND: Indifferent. Indolent - aversion to mental and bodily labor. Anthropophobia, avoids human society.

HEAD: Vertigo with nausea when rising from a seat. Blindness, followed by violent headache; *over eye brows* or outward along the brows, < cold, > pressing at the root of the nose, by warm soup. Aching and fullness in glabella. Periodical headache. Migraine, in small spots and from suppressed catarrh. Bones of head feel sore; sharp stitches in bones. Sensation of a solid block in forehead.

EYES: Ulcer on cornea, no pain or photophobia. Conjunctiva yellow, puffy, covered with yellow-brown spots. Discharges ropy and yellow. *Blindness,* before headache. Vision seems crossed, > looking with one eye. Eyelids; swollen; winking during convulsions, with itching; granular. Dense opacity of cornea. Photophobia only by daylight. Eyelids twitch on opening.

EARS: Sharp stitches in ears (left). Thick yellow fetid discharge. Violent tickling in ears. Tympanum perforated.

NOSE: Pain at bridge or root. *Pressure or stuffed* at root of the nose. Snuffles, esp. of fat chubby children. Discharges; thick, ropy, greenish, yellow, *acrid.* Tough elastic plugs, leave a raw surface. Expired air feels hot. Fetid smell from retention of discharge in nose. Tickling as from a hair in left nostril. Coryza with obstruction of nose. Violent sneezing, < in the morning. Chronic inflammation of frontal sinuses with stopped up sensation. Septum ulcerated. Abscess. Ozena. *Nasal diphtheria.* Sensation as if two loose bones were rubbing together on blowing the nose. Loss of smell. Nose feels heavy, dry. Nasal polyp.

FACE: Pale, yellowish. Blotchy. Red, florid. Mumps on the right side. Sweat on upper lip.

MOUTH: Toothache, radiating, with swelling of the glands. *Tongue* glistens, cracked, smooth or heavy; dry, red, lemon-yellow, furred in dysentery. *Tongue pains when protruded,* at the root. *Sticky mouth.* Sweet, metallic taste. Tongue; thickly coated, broad, flat, indented. Aphthous ulcers deeply corroding. Feels a hair on back part of the tongue, not > by eating or drinking. Mouth dry, > by drinking cold water.

THROAT: *Hawks up thick mucus,* must wipe it away. Uvula edematous, relaxed, bladder-like. Fissured pharynx. Dry, burning. Something sticks in, with pain into neck and shoulders. Throat pains when putting the tongue out. Aphthae. Diphtheria. Tonsils swollen with deafness, in children.

STOMACH: Craving; for beer, for acid drink. Dislike for meat, water. Vomiting more than he drinks, of bright yellow water. Regurgitates liquids. Round ulcer of the stomach. Gastric symptoms > by eating. Sore spot in stomach or food lies like a load. Nausea with heat in the body, > eating and open air. Nausea with burning in anus and erections.

ABDOMEN: Feeling of constriction from liver to shoulder (right). Stitches in spleen extending to lumbar region. Chronic intestinal ulceration with vomiting and emaciation. Stools gelatinous, jelly-like, *or gush of brown frothy water,* then burning and tenesmus, < after rising in the morning. Periodical dysentery - every year, in summer. Diarrhea or dysentery after rheumatism. Sensation of a plug in anus and as if something eating into bowels.

URINARY: Heavy kidneys. Feels one drop of urine had remained behind after urination, which cannot be expelled. Nephritis with scanty albuminous urine. Bloody urine with pain in back. Hematochyluria.

MALE: Constrictive pain at the root of penis at night after waking. Chancre ulcerating deeply. Gleet, with stringy or jelly-like profuse discharge clogging the urethra. Sexual desire absent in fleshy persons. Stitches in prostate when walking, must stand still.

FEMALE: Menses; with suppression of urine or red urine. Leukorrhea acrid, yellow, ropy with pain across sacrum and heaviness in the hypogastrium. Prolapsus uteri < hot weather. Milk; stringy, watery. Itching, burning of vulva with sexual excitement. Vomiting of pregnancy.

RESPIRATORY: Voice hoarse, < evening. Laryngitis. Tickling in larynx with cough, < eating, with eructation, > heat; then vertigo. *Rawness,* under sternum; *pains through to back* and shoulders on coughing. Expectoration yellow, stringy, profuse, with deep cough. Sensation of a bar across the chest. Asthma, < coition. Cough, > by expectoration. Dry, metallic, hacking cough.

HEART: Dilated, with kidney lesions; insufficiency of aortic valve. Feeling of coldness about heart. Heart weak. Pulsation felt in all the arteries.

NECK & BACK: Stiffness of neck, < bending head forward. Cutting through loins; cannot walk. Pain in coccyx < walking, sitting and touching it, extending up and down. Coccyx pains before urination, > after. Feels as if something cracked across sacrum, < stooping.

EXTREMITIES: Paralytic weakness of hands. Sciatica, > motion and flexing the leg, < standing, sitting or lying in bed. Pain along border of the foot. Wandering pain along the bones. Rheumatic pain, < eating. Tendo-achilles swollen and tender. Shin bones, painful; periosteitis from blow.

SKIN: Pustules, with black apices. Skin hot, dry, and red, > cool air. Brown spots. Blisters on soles. Depressed, round scar after healing of eruption or ulcer.

SLEEP: Unrefreshing, feels debilitated in extremities.

FEVER: Hot flushes; then *sticky sweat,* then chill. Cold sweat on hands and feet. Chill with sweat.

COMPLEMENTARY: Ars; Phos; *Psor.*

RELATED: Kali-c; Merc; Phyt; Puls.

KALI BROMATUM

GENERALITIES: Potassium bromide affects the MIND AND NERVES producing failure of mental power, general numbness, and *anesthesia* of mucous membranes, esp. of eyes, throat and skin. Its power over sexual sphere is very great; patient is sensual, with lascivious fancies;

satyriasis and nymphomania. Epilepsy is associated, with sexual excess or abuse in men, and in women fits occur during menses; fits usually occur during new moon and are followed by headache. Onset of disease is slow, *without any pain.* Paralysis. Weakens the heart and lowers temperature. Ill-effects of worry, loss of business, reputation, and embarrassment, sexual excess, illness or death of a near friend. Chorea from fright. Paralysis agitans.

WORSE: *Mental exertion.* Emotions — anger, fright, worry, grief. Periodically; night, 2 a.m. Summer; new moon. *Sexual excess.* Puberty. Unsatisfied sexual desire.

BETTER: When busy mentally and physically.

MIND: *Depressive delusion*—thinks he is pursued, will be poisoned, will commit some great crime, will murder her children or husband. Nervous. Brain fag from grief and anxiety. Suspicious, looks on all sides, fears people yet cannot remain alone in the dark. Fidgety, *busy hands,* fumbles. Moves arms about wildly. *Complete loss of memory,* forgets how to talk, has to be told the word before he can speak it. Amnesic aphasia. Melancholy, much concerned about health, complains without cause. Remorse; *wrings hands;* bursts into tears. Slow, hesitates, omits or mixes up words in talking and writing. Profound indifference and disgust for life. Imagines he cannot pass a certain point. Frequent shedding of tears. Night-terror in children, awake screaming, unconscious, recognize no one, followed by squinting. Senile softening of the brain. Suicidal mania with trembling.

HEAD: Numb feeling in head, < occiput. Vertigo, as if ground gave way and staggering gait, < stooping. Symptoms of apoplexy. Violent headache or numbness felt in occiput; from concussion of brain.

EYES: Sunken. Eyeballs move in every direction. Squinting after night-terror of children.

EARS: Hardness of hearing. Sounds echo in ears. Roaring at night synchronous with pulse.

NOSE: Smell impaired. Coryza descends to larynx.

FACE: Flushed, yellow, cachectic. Expressionless. Acne on face.

MOUTH: Difficult speech, stammering. Breath fetid. Numb. Tongue protrudes with a jerk; Chorea.

THROAT: Numb. Dysphagia of liquids (children), can swallow only solids.

STOMACH: Vomiting—with intense thirst; after each meal; hysterical; after exciting emotion. Persistent hiccough.

ABDOMEN: Spasm with retraction of walls. Sensation as if bowels were falling out. Cutting colic. Internal coldness. Green watery stools, with rapid collapse. Cholera infantum, with twitching and jerking of muscles, and retraction of abdomen. Rectal polyp. Persistent diarrhea, much blood expelled.

URINARY: Diabetes mellitus. Dribbing of urine at the beginning of stool. Urethra numb. Enuresis.

MALE: Excessive sexual desire with constant erection at night. Desire lessened, even impotence. Impotence with melancholy, epilepsy, nervous prostration.

FEMALE: Nymphomania; during puerperal state. Sterility from excessive sexual indulgence. Ovarian neuralgia from ungratified sexual desire. Cystic tumors of ovary. Flooding in young women, with sexual desire. Menorrhagia, from strong sexual desire. Fibroid. Subinvolution. Sexual feeling lost, aversion to coition.

RESPIRATORY: Croupy cough. Reflex cough during pregnancy. Breath hot; hurried. Asthma, with dry cough, tosses arms about wildly.

EXTREMITIES: Hands and fingers in constant motion. Twitching of fingers. Trembling of hands during voluntary motion. Unsteady gait. Cannot stand erect, legs weak.

SKIN: Acne. Moist eczema of legs. Psoriasis. Skin cold; numb. Scar remaining after eruptions.

SLEEP: Drowsiness; often broken by start. Sleeplessness, due to worry, grief and sexual excess. Night-terror. Somnambulism in children.

FEVER: Painful flushing of the face, during climacteric.

RELATED: Calc; Con; Op; Stram.

KALI CARBONICUM

GENERALITIES: Weakness caused by all potassium salts is more pronounced in this typical salt of potassium group. WEAKNESS *of the muscles of heart,* of the back, of limbs; *weakness of intellect.* Fibrous tissues and ligaments of joints, uterus, and lumbar back are particularly affected producing relaxation; *joints give way, back feels broken;* the patient is compelled to lie down or lean on something. *Sweat, backache and weakness* are the three characteristic symptoms of Kali-carb. It is adapted to *fleshy, aged, soft, thin- blooded and cold persons* sensitive to atmospheric changes, to every draft of air, always shivering, with *dropsical* and paralytic tendency. The cold air feels hot. Those who have vague symptoms or *with old* their symptoms. SHARP STITCHING, *stabbing* or catching pains are felt in various parts of the body--joints, *chest,* muscles, head, when lying on affected side, or with any other affection. *Throbbing pain, numbness or coldness of single parts*—abdomen, fingers. Parts lain on are painful or go to sleep.

Discharges are profuse and acrid. *Convulsions* seem to pass off with eructations. Sudden unconsciousness. Twitching of the muscles; rigidity and atony of the muscles. Whole body feels as if it were hollow. Fatty degeneration. Tubercular diathesis. Hypothyroidism. Sensation as if bed were sinking under her. Never well since pneumonia. Burning like fire. Tendency to start, with loud cry; when touched even lightly, esp. in the soles, which generates a thrill throughout the body. Pain goes to the part uncovered, not lain on. Ill-effects of suppression of eruptions in childhood, closing of ulcer or fistulous opening, catching cold and overstrain. Debilitating states after miscarriage and labor. Disposition to phlebitis.

WORSE: *Cold*—AIR; draft; cold water; after overheating; after exertion. *Winter.* 2-3 a.m. Before menses. *Lying on painful* or left side. Loss of fluids. After parturition, abortion. Stooping. By a sudden or unguarded motion. Change of weather. After coition. Touch. Motion.

BETTER: Warmth. Sitting with elbows on knees. By day. Open air. Motion.

MIND: Peevish. Easily startled. Starts when touched, esp. on feet, on dropping to sleep. *Anxiety, with fear when alone.* Anxiety felt in stomach. At a loss to know how to say what she wishes. Very irritable. Weeps much. Hypersensitive to pain, noise, touch. Never quiet or contented. Fear; of future, ghosts, death. Anxious about his own disease. Quarrels with one's bread and butter, with ones family. Feels as if bed were sinking under him.

HEAD: Ache goes into eyes, < motion of carriage, sneezing, coughing, stooping, yawning, > when raising the head and pressing the forehead. Constant sensation as if something loose in head, turning, twisting towards the forehead. Wakes from headache. Hair; dry; falls out from eyebrows, temples and beard. Painful tumors on scalp.

EYES: Weak; after coition, after measles, after abortion. Vision spotted—bright sparks, blue or green spots, drops before the eyes. Inner angles of the eyelids *swollen,* or swelling like a bag between upper eyelids and the brows. Painful sensation of light penetrating the brain on shutting the eyes. Eyelids cold.

EARS: Stitches in ears from within outwards. Cracking in ears. Right ear hot, left pale and cold. Noises in ear; with headache.

NOSE: Descending coryza. Swollen, hard, red. Obstruction, > walking in open air. Foetid yellow-green or crusty discharge. Nose-bleed on washing the face in the morning. Nostrils ulcerated. Nose red, covered with pimples. Chronic cold. Breathes through mouth.

FACE: Bloated. Pale, sickly, sallow, with sunken eyes. Freckles. Swelling of lower jaw and sub-maxillary glands. Cramps in jaws.

MOUTH: Toothache; alternating with stitching pain in left breast, only while eating. Mouth slimy. Tongue, gray-white. Gums separate from teeth. Itching in gums. Pus oozes out, pyorrhea. Aphthae; much salivation. Burning, soreness or painful pimples on the tip of tongue.

THROAT: Hawks up tough mucus in a.m. Swallowing DIFFICULT, food slowly descends, remains half way in esophagus, with gagging and vomiting; stricture of esophagus. Small particles of food go easily in windpipe. Sticking pain as from fish bone.

STOMACH: Salty, sour regurgitation. Vomiting of sour mucus. Desire for sweets, for acids. Stomach *distended and sensitive.* Fullness even after little drink or food. Milk and warm food disagree. Feeling as if *stomach were full of water.* Feeling of lump deep in epigastrium which is sensitive to touch. *Throbbing* at back of stomach. Gastric pains go to back, chest, limbs etc. Wants to eat frequently but least food oppresses her. Nocturnal vomiting of food. Nausea, > lying. Sour eructations. Feels sleepy and weary while eating, cannot finish her meal. When hungry, feels anxious, nauseated, nervous, tingling, palpitation, etc.

ABDOMEN: *Distended, hard, tympanitic* and cold. Throbbing at navel. Feeling as if cold fluid passed through intestines during menses. Flatulence. Stitches in liver or sore liver. Pain from left hypochondrium through abdomen; must turn on right side before he can rise. Cutting pain as if intestines were torn to pieces. *Stools difficult; large, hard lumps,* then burning or torn feeling. Piles; inflamed, bleeding, descend when urinating or coughing, > riding on horseback. Stitching like fine needle during pregnancy, or red hot poker in rectum, > cool bathing. Easy prolapse of rectum. Chronic diarrhea of dyspeptics during day only. Constipation, after or during menses. Sensation of a lump rolling and rising from the abdomen (right) to throat and back again, on coughing. Anal fistula. Dropsy. Jaundice. Constipation alternating with diarrhea.

URINARY: Burning in left kidney. Nocturnal enuresis of adults, < coughing, sneezing. *Urine foamy,* with thick red sediment. Stitching pain in kidneys going from buttocks to thighs. Pressure on bladder long before urination; the more it is pressed the less the urine flows. Urination slow with burning in urethra. Nephritis, from exposure to cold or injury.

MALE: Complaints after coition. Copious painful pollution; with subsequent painful erection. Prostration after coition; often with shuddering. Sleeplessness and uneasiness for 2 or 3 days after coition. Aversion to coition. Strange uneasy feeling in genitals. Chronic gonorrhea; painful scanty discharge, burning during and after urination.

FEMALE: Delayed first menses; with chest symptoms and ascites. Amenorrhea. Menses; too late; acrid, profuse. Violent colicky pain before menses which are irritating and of pungent odor. Fine stitches in mammae. *Leukorrhea, with labor-like pain causing itching and burning in pudendum;* > washing. Labour pains inefficient; felt in back, down the hips and thighs. Complaints after parturition and abortion. Haemorrhage, after curetting, and all sorts of other treatment. Eclampsia, > eructations. Puerperal fever with cutting pain in hypogastrium, with black and scanty urine. Uterine tumor, cyst. Menorrhagia, > taking bath. Soreness of genitals during coition and during menses. Menses early, with profuse discharge; late, with scanty and pale discharge. Severe uterine spasms without appearance of menses, with feeling of heat and restlessness.

RESPIRATORY: Catarrhal aphonia with violent sneezing. Breathing difficult, *asthmatic,* < least motion or walking, alternating with diarrhea, with vertigo. Incessant hard retching or *choking,* futile cough, then vomiting. Whooping cough. Lungs seems to stick to the ribs. *Stabbing chest pains.* Hydrothorax. Whole chest very sensitive, during coughing. Cough with relaxed uvula. Coldness of chest. Expectoration difficult, or small round balls come flying from the mouth without effort; salty, thick, bloody, yellowish, greenish, offensive and profuse expectoration which tastes sour or pungent.

HEART: Seems to hang by a thread. Palpitation, then weakness, in valvular disease; pulsation when becomes hungry. Burning in heart region. Heart pain extends to left scapula. *Pulse small, soft, variable; intermittent* or *dicrotic.* Arrhythmia. Cardiac degeneration. Violent palpitation, shakes the whole body; throbbing extending to tips of fingers and toes.

NECK & BACK: Everything affects the small of the back or pain starts there. Neck feels large. *Backache, with given up feeling,* must lie down; feels as if broken. Small of the back feels weak. Lumbago; with sudden sharp pains extending up and down, back and down the thighs. Backache after delivery or abortion. Spine painful while eating. Burning in the right side of spine.

EXTREMITIES: Weakness in arms. Arms feel numb, cold. Numb pinching in left arm. Burning like fire in fingers. *Legs give out;* feel heavy. Tips of toes and fingers painful. Edema of left foot. *Soles very sensitive.* Pain from hip to knee. Knees painful < going down stairs or upstairs. Jerks the limbs, esp. when the feet are touched. Sciatica, tearing pain in the thighs, with jerking of muscles.

SKIN: Sensitive, dry. Burning as from mustard plaster. General itching or hives, during menses. Itching of warts. Tension, pressure, rending in scars.

SLEEP: Falls asleep while eating. Talks in sleep. Awakes at about 2 a.m. to 4 a.m. with nearly all complaints. Wakes at 1 or 2 a.m., cannot sleep again. Yawns with headache, etc.

FEVER: Chilly; with hot hands; and sleepiness; in open air. Internal burning. Sweat scanty, foul on feet. Sweats with slightest exertion; sweat on painful part, on affected part.

COMPLEMENTARY: Ars-i; Carb-v; Nit-ac; Nux-v; Phos.

RELATED: Ars; Calc-hyp; Fl-ac; Lyc; Phos; Sep; Sulph.

KALI CHLORICUM

GENERALITIES: This remedy disorganizes the blood and affects the mouth, kidneys and rectum. Profound prostration; *coldness* in different parts and organs, even in blood. *Easy hemorrhage*—nosebleed, bloody stools, etc. scurvy. These are most marked symptoms. Discharges are *fetid.* Gray, white, plastic exudates. Lardaceous and fatty degeneration of liver, spleen, kidneys and other solid organs. Toxemia of pregnancy.

WORSE: Cold. Mercury. Jar. Coughing. Sneezing.

BETTER: Nosebleed (mental symptoms).

NOSE: Bleeding at night only from right nostril.

FACE: Swollen; she can hardly see in the morning. Neuralgic pains, < talking, eating, or slight touch, followed by numbness.

MOUTH: Fetor. Acute ulceration and follicular *stomatitis;* aphthous and gangrenous. Noma (ulcerative stomatitis). Tongue swollen, cold. Scurvy. Salivation.

STOMACH: Coldness felt. Sudden vomiting, incessant, of all food, of offensive dark green mucus. Throat cold.

ABDOMEN: Griping colic, with shifting of flatulence and diarrhea, followed by continuous rectal pain. Dysentery, much blood passing with profuse, greenish mucus. Cries with violent cutting pain in the rectum in dysentery and diarrhea.

URINARY: Nephritis. Urine albuminous, scanty, suppressed. Hematuria.

RESPIRATORY: Constriction of chest, as from sulphur fumes.

HEART: Coldness in precordial region. Right pulse full, left small. Coldness in blood.

EXTREMITIES: Ankles swell in the evening. Arms, feet cold.

SKIN: Cold. Pimples between lip and chin.

KALI CYANATUM

GENERALITIES: This most poisonous drug should be remembered in agonizing neuralgia, esp. orbital and supramaxillary region with screaming and loss of consciousness. Cancer of the tongue, with indurated edges. Sudden sinking sensation. Power of speech lost but intelligence intact. Sciatica, gait unsteady.

WORSE: 4 a.m. to 4 p.m.

BETTER: Motion in open air.

KALI IODATUM

GENERALITIES: Potassium iodide was used as an anti-syphilitic remedy. It acts prominently on fibrous and connective tissues, producing infiltration, edema. *Glands are swollen* or atrophied. Exostosis, swelling of the bones, rickets, purpura and hemorrhagic diathesis come under its influence. Diversity of lesions, diversity of aggravations, with many tedious symptoms without any one feature being in prominence calls for this remedy. Gouty, rheumatic, syphilitic diathesis. *Stubborn chronicity.* Feels used up. Crushing or sharp stitching pain. Discharges are COPIOUS, *watery, acrid, salty;* thick, green or foul. *Diffused soreness* after pain of affected parts. Pain long after injury. *Weakness,* emaciation. Arteriosclerosis. *Craves motion in open air.* Cachexia. Contraction of muscles and tendons, chronic arthritis, with spurious ankylosis. Actinomycosis. Coldness; of painful parts; in bones. Fungoid disease. Dropsy, from pressure, from swollen glands.

WORSE: *Heat.* Pressure. Touch. *Night.* Damp. Mercury. Changing weather. Jarring. Cold food, esp. milk. Sunset to sunrise.

BETTER: *Motion. Cool air.* Open air.

MIND: Irritable, irascible, esp. towards his children, his family. Harsh-tempered and cruel. Trivial details of life seem insupportable. Cannot think. Despondent. Bad temper. Abusive. Nervous, must walk. Talkative, disposed to jest.

HEAD: Vertigo in the dark; < railway travelling. Violent headache, as if screwed through sides of head, < warmth and pressure. Hard painful lumps on cranium, with headache. Pain in scalp on scratching, as if ulcerated. Big head and small jaws - rickets. Brain feels enlarged. Hair changes color and falls off. Bilateral headache. Scalp fissured, and sore. Tender spots on head.

EYES: *Puffy,* burning, watery; conjunctiva red. Syphilitic iritis. Constant oscillation of the eyeballs. Winking is painful. Chemosis. Edema around eyes. Lower lids twitch.

EARS: Tinnitus. Boring pain in the ears. Deafness.

NOSE: Red, swollen. Coryza descending with profuse *acrid,* hot, watery discharge, < cool air; coryza with salivation and dyspnea. *Tightness at the root of the nose.* Ozena with perforated septum. Cool, greenish, irritating discharge from nose. Burning, throbbing in nose and sinuses. Violent sneezing. Takes cold on every damp day.

FACE: Neuralgia. Tight pain at zygoma. Glutinous mucus on lips in a.m.

MOUTH: Toothache nagging, as if a worm were digging in it. Taste bitter; on waking; salty. Salivation. Bloody saliva, with sweetish or disgusting taste in mouth. Severe pain at the root of tongue at night. Ulcers in mouth, looking as if coated with milk.

THROAT: Sore throat of speakers. Goitre sensitive to contact. Dry. Tonsils enlarged.

STOMACH: Cold food and drinks, esp. cold milk < . Much thirst. Sensation as if waterbrash is occurring. Throbbing; painful burning. Aversion to all food; to broth.

ABDOMEN: Flatulence, with air hunger. Squeaking or clucking noise. Diarrhea with pain in lumbar region as if broken, or as if menses would appear. Early morning diarrhea of phthisis. Stools frequent. Fissured anus; of infants.

URINARY: Frequent urination of copious, clear, urine, < before menses, at night.

MALE: Atrophy of testicles. Chronic gonorrhea; discharge thick green. Excoriation by least friction.

FEMALE: Uterus feels as if squeezed, during menses. Leukorrhea; corrosive, like meat washing. Atrophy of mammae. Menses late and profuse.

RESPIRATORY: Larynx feels raw. *Air hunger,* with flatulence in a.m., awakes strangling. Whistling asthmatic breathing. *Air passage raw.* Dry bronchitis. Frothy, greenish, soapsuds-like expectoration. Pleuritic effusion. Pneumonia. Chest pains go backwards. Pain from sternum to back.

HEART: Palpitation and darting pain, < when walking. Aneurism.

NECK & BACK: Small of the back feels as if in a vise. Bruised pain in lumbar region, < sitting bent. Pain in coccyx as from a fall.

EXTREMITIES: Pain in hips forcing limping. Sciatica, pain < lying on the affected side, sitting, standing; wakes him at night; > walking and flexing legs. Rheumatism of the knee, with effusion. Tip of thumb ulcerates and turns yellow.

SKIN: Acne. Giant urticaria. Small boils, leaving scars. Rough nodules all over.

SLEEP: Weeps loudly during sleep, but unconscious of it.

FEVER: Chilly in bones; in painful parts. Heat in evening. Chilly when uncovers. Alternate heat and chill. Heat with shudders. Hot and dry, then drenching sweat. Profuse night-sweat which >.

RELATED: Iod; Sulph; Syph.

KALI MURIATICUM

GENERALITIES: Potassium chloride is Dr. Schuessler's tissue remedies. It causes *catarrhal condition,* producing MILKY WHITE, viscid, *sticky, thick,* slimy or lumpy discharges. *Tough* plastic or *fibrinous* exudates. *Hard* deposits. *Glandular swelling. Sore, cutting or sticking, shifting pains.* Crawling. Numbness. Ill-effect of vaccination. Sprain. Burn. Blows, cut. Embolism. Crosswise symptoms. Slow reaction. Stubborn infiltration.

WORSE: *Open air. Cold* drink. Draft. Heat, of bed. Lying. Night. Dampness. Motion. Sprain. *Fat; rich food.* During menses.

BETTER: Cold drink. Rubbing. Letting hair down.

MIND: Discontented, discouraged. Fears evil. Sits in silence. Imagines he must starve. Habitual loss of appetite or refuses food. *Irritable and angry;* at trifles.

HEAD: Stunning shock in head or a leaden load holds down the occiput, > letting hair down and warmth. Brain feels loose. Copious white dandruff. *Sweating of head.* Crusta lactea.

EYES: Pustules on cornea. Cataract. Trachoma. Corneal opacity. Scintillation on coughing. Exudation in retina.

EARS: *Deafness;* from *catarrhal condition and occlusion of eustachian tube.* Crackling noise on blowing nose or swallowing. Snapping, itching or plug sensation in ears. Glands about the ears are swollen. Soreness of eustachian tube.

NOSE: Stuffy cold in head. Discharge white, thick. Hawking of mucus from posterior nares.

FACE: Bluish; sunken. Cheeks swollen and painful. Paralysis, following pain in face. Muscles of face twitch and tremble, < eating, speaking or coughing. Mumps without fever.

MOUTH: Eruptions around the mouth. Aphthae. Thrush. White ulcers in the mouth. Scorbutic gums. Tongue mapped; gray or white at base. Taste; salty, bitter, with coldness of tongue. Sensation as if a tumor were growing on the tongue.

THROAT: Grayish-white, ulcerated. Chronic sore throat. *Tonsils swollen,* inflamed, swallowing excessively painful, can hardly breathe. *Hawks out thick white mucus, cheesy.*

STOMACH: Fatty or rich food causes indigestion, he loathes it. Nausea, with shiver. Stomach heavy at night. Vomits food. Hunger disappears after drinking water.

ABDOMEN: *Fullness after eating. Pale,* hard or flocculent stools. *Anus sore,* < walking or after stool. Itching or crawling in anus after stool. Piles, bleeding; blood dark and thick.

URINARY: Dribbling urine. Cystitis. Discharge of white thick mucus.

FEMALE: Menses dark, clotted, black like tar, excessive. Leukorrhea, milky white, thick, bland. Soft, tender nodes in mammae. Painful mammae before or at menses.

RESPIRATORY: *Difficult or oppressed breathing.* Bronchitis. Expectoration sticky, milky, or flies from the mouth. Rawness in chest. Flushes of heat in chest.

HEART: Coldness at heart.

NECK & BACK: Heaviness under right shoulder. Buzzing under right scapula. Backache, > lying. Lightning pain from small of back to feet. Must get out of bed and sit up.

EXTREMITIES: *Cold hands* and feet. Hands get stiff while writing or knitting. Cramps in limbs—in legs. Twitching thighs. Tension in leg alternating with tension in arm. Cold foot-sweat. Cutting in bones. Exudation and swelling around the joints. Cracking of tendons, back of hand.

SKIN: Branny. Bursitis. Eruptions connected with stomach or menstrual disorder.

SLEEP: Anxious dreams.

COMPLEMENTARY: Calc-s.

RELATED: Bry; Ferr-p; Puls.

KALI NITRICUM

GENERALITIES: Potassium nitrate affects *respiratory organs,* kidneys, heart and blood vessels. Secretion into cavities is increased. Sudden dropsical swelling of the whole body. It is often indicated in suppurative nephritis, asthma and cardiac asthma. Pains are *dull, stitching,* throbbing. Wooden, *numbness.* Relapsing phthisis. Very weak. *Hemorrhagic tendency.*

WORSE: *Walking.* Cold. Damp. Taking cold. Eating veal. Lying with head low. Breathing.

BETTER: Gentle motion. Drinking water in sips.

MIND: Mental weariness from lack of occupation of interest. Discouragement and fear of death.

HEAD: Fainting fits, with vertigo in morning, < on standing, > sitting down. Pain in occiput, > letting hair down. Head pain > by motion of carriage. Sensation as if hair were being pulled during pain.

EYES: External angle of right eye twitches, < chewing.

EARS: Chronic deafness from paralysis of auditory nerve. Vertigo and tinnitus.

NOSE: Swollen feeling, more in right nostril. Point red and itching. Polyp.

MOUTH: Tongue, red with burning pimples.

STOMACH: Nausea, as if about to vomit, < at night. Epigastric or substernal pain goes towards axilla.

ABDOMEN: Diarrhea from eating veal. Thin, watery, dark, bloody stools.

URINARY: *Frequent and profuse emission of clear urine.* Diabetes insipidus. Dull kidney pain.

FEMALE: Profuse menses, black like ink.

RESPIRATORY: Rapid gasping breathing, sits upright. *Violent dyspnea,* with burning in chest, dull stitches and nausea; *can only drink in sips* though thirsty. Congestion of right lung. Asthma. Free sour expectoration gives relief.

HEART: Palpitation, < lying.

BACK: Pain extends into the chest.

EXTREMITIES: Hands and fingers feel swollen.

FEVER: *External coldness*—chin, skin. Internal burning.

RELATED: Cam; Glon.

KALI PHOSPHORICUM

GENERALITIES: Dr. Schuessler's great remedy for conditions arising from *want of nerve power.* The patient is NERVOUS; SENSITIVE, WEAK, AND EASILY FAGGED by *pain,* worry, mental fatigue, etc. *Neurasthenia.* Paralysis; infantile, during dentition. Paralytic weakness, or pain with sensation of paralysis. It is also useful in states of adynamia and decay; gangrenous conditions, suspected malignant tumor. PUTRID, carrion-like odor of secretions; foul odor of the body. Secretions are golden yellow. Stitching pains. After operation, when in the healing process, the skin is drawn tight over the wound, esp. cancer. Ill-effect of mechanical injuries, grief, vexation. Sexual excitement from indulgence or suppression. *Irregular menses,* pulse, etc. Little pain. Emaciation; wasting diseases. Septic state and septic fever. Carbuncle. Hemorrhage. Progressive muscular atrophy. Seasickness without nausea.

WORSE: Slight causes—excitement, *worry, mental* or physical fatigue. Touch. Pain. Cold. Dry air. Puberty. Eating. Coition.

BETTER: Sleep. Eating. Gentle motion. Leaning against something.

MIND: Shy—nervous dread; starts easily. Slightest labor seems a heavy task. Indisposed to meet people, or to talk with them. Depressed, gloomy. Angry. Perverted affection, averse to her own; cruel to husband, to baby.

Irritable; children cry and scream, fly into passion, can hardly articulate. Apprehensive, about future, his health. Fear of crowd, death, etc. Forgetful. Night terror. Religious melancholy.

HEAD: Vertigo when facing sun, < looking up, on standing, from sitting up. Headache; of students, < before and during menses, > by gentle motion. Brain fag. Cerebral anemia. Hunger with headache.

EYES: Burn, sting; swim in tears. Yellow-gray, milky secretion. *Eyelids droop (left).* Retinitis. Weakness of eye. Loss of perceptive power. Squint, after brain disease. Black spots before eyes.

EARS: Humming and buzzing in the ears. Hearing sensitive, cannot endure noise. Deafness, from atrophic condition of nerve.

NOSE: *Itching in posterior nares.* Violent *sneezing* with symptoms of fresh cold; sneezing at 2 a.m. Hay fever, as a prophylactic.

FACE: *Sad, care-worn look.* Brown stripe at the edge of hair. Neuralgia, > cold application.

MOUTH: Palate feels greasy. Tongue yellow, like liquid mustard. Aphthae. Breath fetid. Mouth excessively dry, feels as if tongue would cleave to the roof of the mouth. Gums; spongy, receding, bleeding, with toothache. Speech, slow, becoming inarticulate. Creeping paralysis of the tongue. Nervous chattering of teeth. Noma (ulcerative stomatitis).

STOMACH: Craves ice-water, vinegar, sweets. *Hungry soon after eating.* Nausea, > eructation, < coughing. Nervous gone sensation at the pit of stomach, > eating. Aversion to food, esp. bread and to meat. No appetite except for sweets.

ABDOMEN: Diarrhea, stools of foul, putrid odor, hot; golden yellow stools, painless, from fright, followed by weakness. Cutting pain in abdomen. Dysentery - stool consists of pure blood. Rice-water stools in cholera. Paretic condition of rectum and colon after removal of piles. Entero-colitis. Feels cold, > covering.

URINARY: Urine saffron yellow or milky. Nocturnal enuresis, obstinate in nervous, excitable children, in old people. Bleeding from urethra. Urine stops and starts.

MALE: Sexual excitement, but prostration, and weak vision after coition, or after nightly emissions.

FEMALE: *Menses; irregular,* too late, too scanty. Horribly foul leukorrhea. Periodical discharge of copious orange coloured fluid from vagina and rectum. Feeble and ineffectual labor pain. Sexual desire intense for 4 or 5 days after the menses. Delayed menses, with depression.

RESPIRATORY: Aphonia, from paralysis of vocal cord. Nervous asthma, < least food. Short-breath < going upstairs. Cough, with yellow sputum.

HEART: Pulse irregular. Palpitation, < slightest motion or ascending stairs.

NECK & BACK: Paralytic lameness of back, must lean on a chair. Axillary sweat smells of onion. Spinal irritation. Creeping sensation and intense pain along spine, relieves the headache.

EXTREMITIES: Prickling in hands and feet. Numb finger tips. Foot feels frost bitten. Pain in soles. Paralytic weakness of limbs. Feet fidgety.

SKIN: Blue spots on skin. Skin inactive. Cold. Jaundiced.

SLEEP: Night-terror; of children. Drowsy. *Yawning.* Somnambulism. Sleeplessness, from worry, business trouble, etc. Amorous dreams; restlessness and heat during sleep.

FEVER: Subnormal temperature.

RELATED: Caust; Pic-ac; Zinc.

KALI SULPHURICUM

GENERALITIES: This Dr. Schuessler's tissue remedy affects respiratory mucous membranes, and skin where it causes *desquamation.* DISCHARGES ARE PROFUSE AND DEEP YELLOW, *Thin or sticky.* Processes are torpid in nature. *Suppuration. Stitching,* tearing, festering pain, *that shifts about.* Lack of reaction. Cancer, epithelial. Ill-effect of chill when overheated. *Injury.* Growth of nails interrupted.

WORSE: *Warmth*—of room, air. Noise. Consolation. Evening.

BETTER: *Cool air.* Walking. Fasting.

MIND: *Hurried.* Irritable. Desire to lie down, but lying <, so one must walk for relief. Frightened at trifles. Desires and then rejects things.

HEAD: Yellow dandruff, moist, sticky. Scald head. Bald spots (after gonorrhea).

EYES: Ophthalmia neonatorum. Purulent yellow mucus in eye diseases.

EARS: Eustachian deafness. Watery, sticky, thin yellow discharge, offensive; with polyp.

NOSE: Engorgement of nasal and laryngeal mucous membranes, with mouth breathing, snoring, etc., after removal of adenoids.

FACE: Aches in heated room. Epithelioma.

MOUTH: *Yellow, slimy tongue.* Loss of taste and smell.

STOMACH: Feels a heavy load on stomach. Dread of hot drinks. Craves sweets.

ABDOMEN: Feels cold, during colic. Hard tympanitic, in whooping cough. Empty feeling in hypogastrium, > passing flatus.

URINARY: Oxaluria. Pyelitis.

MALE: Gonorrhea; gleet; slimy yellowish green discharge.

FEMALE: Menses with a feeling of weight in abdomen. Leukorrhea, yellowish, watery.

RESPIRATORY: *Coarse rattle in chest.* Croupy hoarseness. Bronchitis. Asthma, with easily expelled yellow, slimy expectoration.

EXTREMITIES: Shifting, wandering pains. Rheumatism, < heat. Arthritic nodes.

SKIN: Yellow - jaundice. Abundant *desquamation.* Ulcers, ooze thin YELLOW WATER. Psoriasis. Nettle-rash. Dry skin. Eczema; intertrigo.

FEVER: *Profuse easy sweat.* Intermittent fever; rise of temperature at night.

RELATED: Puls; Tub.

KALMIA LATIFOLIA

GENERALITIES: Kalmia affects the NERVES, HEART, *circulation. Pains are neuralgic, with tingling, numbness. Trembling or paralytic weakness. Pains shift rapidly,* shooting *outward along the nerves,* with much nausea and slow pulse. *Aching, bruised, stiff feeling.* Dull, tearing, crushing pain, *moving downwards;* pain alternating with cardiac symptoms, or between upper and lower limbs. Rheumatism, syphilitic. Neuralgia, after the disappearance of herpetic eruptions. Motion brings on complaints. Albuminuria. Great weakness with neuralgia.

WORSE: MOTION. Lying on left side. Bending forward. Looking down. Heat, of sun. Becoming cold. With the sun. Sunrise to sunset. Stooping. During leukorrhea.

BETTER: *Eating*. Cloudy weather. Continued motion. Recumbent posture.

MIND: Memory and mental faculties are perfect in a recumbent posture.

HEAD: Vertigo; with headache, blindness, pain in the limbs and weariness, < stooping, looking down. Cracking in head frightens him, it sends in a sound in ears like blowing of a horn. Head symptoms < and > with the sun. Shooting from nape to vertex and face. Maddening supra-orbital pain (R).

EYES: Stiff drawing sensation when moving the eyes. Vision becomes black on looking downwards. Iritis. Scleritis. Eyelids stiff. Retinitis. Albuminuria, esp. during pregnancy.

EARS: Sound like blowing of a horn.

NOSE: Coryza; with increased sense of smell.

FACE: Flushing with vertigo. Neuralgia, < right side, from exposure to cold, > food. Stitching and tearing in jaw bones. Lips stiff, dry, swollen.

MOUTH: Stitches in tongue. Tingling in salivary gland. Bitter taste, with nausea, > eating. Tired feeling in chewing muscles.

STOMACH: Pain in pit of stomach, < bending forward, > sitting erect. Feeling as if something were being pressed under the epigastrium. Wine > vomiting.

URINARY: Albuminuria, with pain in lower limbs. Frequent urination of large quantity of yellow urine, > headache.

FEMALE: Suppressed menses, with severe neuralgic pain throughout the whole body. Leukorrhea one week after menses; symptoms < during leukorrhea.

HEART: Fluttering of heart with anxiety. Pains sharp, *burning,* shooting, stabbing, radiating to left scapula and arm, *take away the breath, with slow pulse.* Palpitation, < bending forward; palpitation felt in throat, after going to bed. Trembling all over visible, < lying on left side, > lying on back. Hypertrophy; valvular insufficiency. Aortic obstruction. Tobacco heart. *Pulse slow, weak,* tremulous.

NECK & BACK: Pain from neck down arm; brachialgia. Pain down back, as if it would break. Lumbar pain of nervous origin, with heat and burning.

EXTREMITIES: Deltoid rheumatism - right. Pains affect large part of the limb. Weakness, numbness, pricking and sense of cold in limbs. Tingling and numbness of the left arm (heart pain). Pain along ulnar nerve goes into little or fourth finger. Joints red, hot, swollen.

SKIN: Stiff; dry.

SLEEP: Sleepless; turns often; wakes very early in the morning.

FEVER: Protracted and continued fever, with tympanites.

COMPLEMENTARY: Benz-ac; Spig.

RELATED: Acon; Dig; Rhus-t; Spig.

KREOSOTUM

GENERALITIES: This medicine is a mixture of phenols obtained from distillation of wood tar. It affects the mucous membranes of the DIGESTIVE TRACT, THE *female genitals and* disorganizes the BLOOD. Excoriations. *Burning like fire. Profuse,* ACRID, HOT, FOUL DISCHARGES, *eructations,* sputum, etc., *redden the part.* Lumpy discharges, menses, etc. *Hemorrhage passive,* brown, dark—from small wounds. Tumefaction. Fullness. Heaviness.

Scurvy. Cancerous affections. Gangrene. Great debility, with miserable feeling. It is suitable for lean persons, old women (post-climacteric diseases), over grown poorly developed children—marasmus. *Blackness* of teeth, leukorrhea, lochia, etc. Rapid emaciation. Complaints are accompanied by yawning. Children would not sleep unless caressed and fondled. *Pulsations* all over the body. Severe old neuralgia. Congenital syphilis.

WORSE: DENTITION. Pregnancy. *Rest.* Cold. *Eating. Lying.* Summer. Bad smell. During menses. From 6 p.m. to 6 a.m. Coitus. Touch. Sprain.

BETTER: Warmth. Hot food. Motion. Pressure. After sleep.

MIND: Dissatisfied with everything; wants things then throws them away and wants something else. Screams at night (children). Music causes weeping and palpitation. Fear at the thought of coition in women. *Cross, wilful and obstinate.* Stupid. Longs for death. Child moans constantly or dozes with half open eyes or is cross and sleepless during dentition.

HEAD: Dull pain as from a board pressing against the forehead. Buzzing in head. Scalp sensitive, < combing hair. Falling of hair.

EYES: Hot, acrid, smarting tears. Lids red and swollen. Suffering of eyes alternating with suffering of limbs. Constant quivering of eyelids.

EARS: Difficulty of hearing during and before menses.

NOSE: Offensive smell and discharge. Chronic catarrh of old people.

FACE: Yellow pallor with red blotches during chill or heat. Sick, suffering expression; old-looking children. Burning pains, < talking or exertion, > lying on affected side.

Lips red, bleeding. Moistens lips frequently without being thirsty.

MOUTH: *Very rapid decay of teeth,* with putrid odor from mouth. Black spots on teeth. *Puffy, bluish, spongy, bleeding gums.* Intolerable toothache during pregnancy. Very painful dentition. Aphthae or salivation during pregnancy. Taste bitter low down in throat. Foul breath. Pegged teeth.

THROAT: Burning; choking sensation. Bitter taste when swallowing food, after drinking water.

STOMACH: Eructations hot; frothy. Nausea. Vomiting of food several hours after eating; vomiting of sweetish water in the morning. Vomiting in pregnancy; of undigested food. Vomiting in uterine ulcer and cancer of the stomach. Icy coldness in stomach. Hematemesis. Craves smoked meat. Cold food, fasting <, dare not remain fasting. Disgust of food during convalescence. Painful hard spot at stomach.

ABDOMEN: Distended. Diarrhea—bloody, dark, brown, lienteric, offensive stools. Green stools during dentition. Child struggles and screams during stool, as if it would go into a fit. Sore pain, < deep breathing. Constriction of rectum, with uterine cancer.

URINARY: Sensation of a lump pressing down on bladder. *Urination* hurried; *involuntary when lying,* on coughing. Can urinate only when lying. Dreams of urinating. Enuresis in the first part of the night. Urine offensive. Frequent urination, with copious urine during day. Diabetes. Drinks much but passes little at a time.

MALE: Burning in genitals during coition from coming in contact with acrid vaginal discharge, penis swells next day. Prepuce bluish black, with hemorrhage and gangrene.

FEMALE: Menses profuse; lumpy intermittent, < lying, > sitting or walking. *Leukorrhea; gushing,* like bloody water, offensive, corrosive, causing itching, staining the linen yellow, with accompanying complaints, white, having odor of green corn. Violent pain during coition, burning in parts followed by discharge of dark blood next day. Violent itching of vulva and vagina, < during urination. Lochia lumpy, offensive, intermits. Cancer, erosion of cervix. Dwindling of mammae with small hard painful lumps in them. Menses < lifting, overexertion. Stitches in vagina, make her start.

RESPIRATORY: Hoarseness with pain in larynx, > sneezing. Cough with little expectoration or copious purulent expectoration after every cough; cough after influenza. Winter cough of old people, with heavy pressure on sternum. Deep pain in chest. Burning as from hot coal in chest. Gangrene of lungs. Periodical hemoptysis. Neglected phthisis.

HEART: Stitches in heart region. Pulsation in all arteries when at rest.

BACK: Dragging pain in back extending to genitals and down the thighs. Feels as if everything would come out (in women); pain with urging to stool and urination, pain with leukorrhea. Burning in sacrum; scapulae feel bruised.

EXTREMITIES: Pain in the hip joint (left), with sensation as if leg were too long when standing. Pain in left thumb as if sprained.

SKIN: Violently itching, moist or scurfy eczema on eyelids, face, joints, back of hands. Small wounds bleed freely. Ulcers break out and heal, bleed after coition. Urticaria, after menses.

SLEEP: Disturbed, caused by restlessness of the whole body or with sensation of fatigue and pain in all limbs.

Tosses about whole night without any apparent cause. Dreams of urinating.

FEVER: Cold sweat.

COMPLEMENTARY: Sulph.

RELATED: Ars; Arum-t; Carb-ac; Graph; Nit-ac; Psor.

LAC CANINUM

GENERALITIES: Milk of bitch acts upon THROAT, NERVES and *female genital organs.* It causes oversensitiveness of NERVES producing restlessness, nervousness, prostration and abnormal sensations; cannot bear one part of her body to touch the other, must keep even her fingers apart. SYMPTOMS ALTERNATE SIDES. Symptoms of throat, ovaries, skin, etc. *go from right to left,* then back again or *reverse;* throat, ovaries, skin troubles etc. *Glistening parts*—inflamed, ulcer, etc. It dries up milk in woman who cannot nurse the baby. Diphtheria and diphtheritic paralysis. Ozena. Erratic pains or disposition of symptoms. Results of fall.

WORSE: TOUCH. *Jar. During menses. Cold air, wind* draft. Morning of one day and evening of the next. After sleep.

BETTER: Open air. Cold drink.

MIND: *Full of imagination*—horrid; of snakes, vermin. Very forgetful, makes mistakes in writing and speaking. Every symptom seems a settled disease which is incurable. Fear of disease, of falling downstairs. Child cross and irritable, screams all the time, esp. at night. *Despondent.* Attacks of rage. Hysteria at the height of sexual orgasm. *Feels as if walking on air* or not touching the bed when lying down. Thinks himself of little consequence. Absent-minded. Imagines that he wears someone else's nose, thinks that whatever she says is a lie. Fits of weeping. One's own body seems disgusting.

HEAD: Aches change side. Blurred vision. Nausea and vomiting at the height of attack of headache which is < by noise, talking; > by quiet. Sensation as if brain were alternately contracted and relaxed.

EYES: Sees faces before her eyes, < in the dark. Sees vermins, creeping things. Eyelids heavy.

EARS: Noises in ears. Reverberation of voice, as if speaking in a large empty room. Sound seems very far off. Deafness from hereditary syphilis.

NOSE: Coryza - one nostril stuffed up, other free and discharging. Profuse nocturnal nasal discharge, purulent, staining pillow greenish-yellow. Fluids escape through nose while drinking. Cracks in alae nasi. Smell of flower seems to send chill over her.

FACE: Pale, careworn, anxious. Jaws crack while eating.

MOUTH: Tongue coated white, with bright red edges. Putrid taste, < sweets. Talking difficult, talks through the nose (nervous throat affection). Drooling in diphtheria (saliva drops down.) Tongue stiff. Crack in corners of the mouth. Stutters when talking fast, has to speak slowly. Salivation.

THROAT: Sore; has *glistening patches of china whiteness* or red glistening in tonsillitis and diphtheria. Symptoms change repeatedly from side to side, > by cold drink or warm drink, but < empty swallowing. Sore throat beginning and ending with menses. Swallowing difficult, < solids. Pain extend to ears.

STOMACH: Craves; milk and drinks much of it, highly seasoned dishes. Aversion to liquids, esp. water; to anything sweet. Sinking at epigastrium with nausea. Salty food only tastes natural. Nausea >, eructations. Everything except fish makes her worse.

URINARY: Urine scanty, infrequent; urination once only in twentyfour hours, then copiously, but with some difficulty and slight irritation. Nocturnal enuresis (specific). Bladder feels full after urination.

FEMALE: Menses; gushing, hot as fire; too early; bright red; profuse, green or of ammoniacal odor. Breast swollen, painful, < least jar, has to hold breast firmly when going up and down; before menses, > on appearance of menses. Constant pain in nipples. Flatus from vagina. DRIES UP MILK. Galactorrhea. Milk scanty. Leukorrhea; profuse, during day, none at night, < standing and walking. Sexual organs extremely excited, < by putting hand on breast; pressure on vulva while sitting, or from slight friction caused by walking.

RESPIRATORY: Hoarseness during menses. Cough from constant tickling in the throat. Clavicles sore to touch.

HEART: Pain when going up and down the stairs.

NECK & BACK: Stiffness of neck. Spine aches from base of brain to coccyx; very sensitive to touch or pressure. Cold creeping down back.

EXTREMITIES: Sciatica. Legs cold up to knees. Constant pain of right hip. Rheumatic pains shifting from one side to other. Heels sore. Cramps in feet.

SLEEP: Dreams of snakes. Lies with one leg flexed and other stretched. Dreams of urinating. Wakes at night with a sensation as if bed were in motion.

RELATED: Lach; Lyss; Puls.

LAC DEFLORATUM

GENERALITIES: Skimmed milk is useful in diseases with faulty NUTRITION and anemic condition of *blood.* Feels completely *exhausted* whether she does anything or not; great fatigue when walking. Sensation as if cold air was blowing on her, even while covered up; as if sheets were damp. Sufferings from loss of sleep. Dropsy; from organic heart disease; and from chronic liver complaints. Persons or children who become sick on taking milk. Obesity.

WORSE: Cold; *least draft.* Wet. Hands put in cold water. *Milk.* Loss of sleep. Weekly. Shut places.

BETTER: Rest. Pressure of bandage. Conversation.

MIND: Despondent; > conversation; does not care to live; has no fear of death, is sure he is going to die. Horror of shut places.

HEAD: Vertigo; < lying on left side, moving head from pillow, turning while lying; must sit up. Blindness, then throbbing frontal headache, with much pale urination, < noise, light, motion, during menses, > by bandaging, conversation. Migraine, ceases at sunset. Distress in head after injury. Faintness on extending arms overhead. Skull feels lifted up. Persistent headaches, for years. Head becomes sore on coughing.

EYES: Photophobia, even candlelight unbearable. Feels as if eyes were full of little stones, during headache.

FACE: Pale, sickly look. Painless swelling of the face.

STOMACH: *Aversion to milk.* Nausea and vomiting, deathly sickness. Vomiting incessant with no relation to eating, first of undigested food, sour, then of bitter water. Vomiting of pregnancy. Children suffer from coryza after drinking milk.

ABDOMEN: Constipation, with ineffectual urging. Stools *large, hard, with great straining, lacerating anus.* Persistent constipation, > only by purgatives or enema, with violent attacks of sick headache.

URINARY: Boring, sore pain in kidneys. Frequent and profuse urination, with headache or other pains. Urination involuntary, while walking in cold air, while riding, or when hurrying to catch a train. Lack of sensation when the bladder is full.

FEMALE: Menses delayed; in girls who drink much milk; suppressed by putting hands in cold water. Scanty flow of milk; restores the milk.

EXTREMITIES: Tips of fingers, icy cold, rest of the hand warm.

SKIN: Very sensitive to cold. Symmetrical patches, itching and burning after scratching. Skin thickened at the edges of feet.

SLEEP: Restlessness from loss of sleep.

FEVER: *Always feels chilly.*

RELATED: Nat-m.

LACHESIS

GENERALITIES: Native American name of this snake is *surukuku* (bushmaster). Poison of this snake was first proved by Dr. Hering. Like other snake poisons it decomposes BLOOD; affects the *Heart and Circulation.* NERVES become very sensitive, esp. CUTANEOUS and VASO-MOTOR. Excessive sensitiveness of the surface with intolerance of touch, or constriction; intense nervous irritability, restless, tossing, moving. Symptoms appear on LEFT SIDE, then *go to right* - THROAT, OVARIES. GREAT FEMALE REMEDY. *Intensively rapid onset of the disease with great prostration. Malignant* or septic states; diphtheria; gangrene, diabetic, traumatic, senile; carbuncle, erysipelas come under its influence. HEMORRHAGE thin, containing dark particles like charred straw; vicarious—nosebleed, bloody urine, etc. Small wounds bleed much. *Blueness of the affected part;* of hand. Discharges acrid, OFFENSIVE. ASCENDING SENSATION; *in throat; chills.* FLUSHES OF HEAT; rushes of blood. Sensation of a LUMP in throat, abdomen, liver, rectum, etc.; rolling about in bladder. EXCESSIVE PAINFULNESS—*of throat;* ulcers; spots on body. Sensation of *constriction* in throat, in head like a skullcap; of anus. *Drawing;* vertex to jaws, in rectum, etc. Great physical and mental weakness. Trembling of the whole body, of hands, tongue, etc. Hard throbbing, or *hammering* pain. Neuralgic pain changes locality, with palpitation. Epilepsy comes on during sleep; from jealousy; onanism; loss of fluids. Left-sided paralysis after apoplexy or cerebral exhaustion. Fainting, with pain in heart, nausea, pale face, vertigo. Chorea from piercing ears. Awkward gait; left side weak. Dropsy from liver and spleen diseases; after scarlatina. Cellulitis with burning and blue color of the skin. Purpura. Bubonic plague. Cancer. Diphtheritic paralysis and other affections. Carriers of diphtheria. Ill-effects of injury, punctured wounds. Grief, fright. Vexation; anger. Jealousy; disappointed love. Masturbation; sprain (blueness of part). Never well since climaxis. Symptoms develop in sleep and the patient wakes up at any time day and night. Hysteria. Catalepsy. Sensation of thread drawing the part or spreading *over.*

WORSE: SLEEP, AFTER SLEEP. MORNING. HEAT OF SUMMER, SPRING, *room,* SUN. SWALLOWING EMPTY, LIQUIDS. SLIGHT TOUCH OR PRESSURE. PRESSURE OF CLOTHES *around neck, waist.* RETARDED DISCHARGES. Start and close of menses. CLIMAXIS. ALCOHOL. Cloudy weather. Standing or stooping. Motion. Closing eyes. HOT DRINKS.

BETTER: OPEN AIR. FREE DISCHARGES. Eructation. *Hard* pressure. COLD DRINKS. Bathing affected part. Sitting bent. Eating, esp. Fruits. Warm applications.

MIND: Nervous; excitable. LOQUACITY, *rambling,* frequently jumping from one subject to another, then sadness, or repeats the same thing. *Compelling delusions,* Thinks herself under superhuman control, thinks she is dead and preparations are being made for her funeral; thinks herself pursued, hated and despised. Persistent erotic ideas, without ability. *Insane jealousy. Suspicious.* Sad in the morning; no desire to mix with the world. Malice. Mischievous. Mania from over-study. Delirium; tremens from over-watching; fatigue; loss of fluid; over-study. Feels full of poison. Fears; going to sleep, lying down; or that heart will stop. Restless, uneasy; does not want to attend to business, wants to be off somewhere all the time. Derangement of time sense. Aversion of women to marry. Religious insanity. Talks, sings, whistles; makes odd motions. Mocks. Crawls on the floor; spits often, hides, laughs or is angry; during spasms. Weak memory. Mistakes are made in writing and speaking. Mind symptoms < after sleep. Predicts the future correctly. Proud and lazy. Hateful.

HEAD: Vertigo; < turning to right, closing eyes, looking at one and same object; from walking in open air. Headache: heavy, bursting, down to nose, side (right) feels cut off. Migraine, pain extending to neck and shoulders. Weight, pressure on the vertex, or burning of the vertex. Sun headache, with glimmering of vision. Falling of hair, esp. during pregnancy. Perforating tumor of the skull. Numbness, crawling (left). Does not want hair touched.

EYES: Feel small or as if drawn together by cord tied in a knot at the root of the nose. Blindness with lung or heart affections. Eyes water, from pain. Fistula lacrimalis, with eruptions on face. Intra-ocular hemorrhage. Feels as if eyes were forced out on pressing the throat. Dim sight. Unsteady look, eyes roll vacantly.

EARS: Hardness of hearing with want of wax. Ear wax too hard, pale, dry. Ear pain with sore throat. Pulsations. Ear wax like chewed paper. Stricture of eustachian tube.

NOSE: *Stopped coryza.* Discharge with every cough. Nosebleed, with amenorrhea, on blowing the nose. Blood and pus from nose. Paroxysms of sneezing in hay asthma. Red pimples on nose (rum-blossom) of drunkards. Cannot bear anything before nose.

FACE: Purple, mottled; dusky during heat. Netted veinlets on face. Neuralgia (left side); heat rises to the face. Lower jaw drops (coma). Septic mumps. Flushes of heat. Enormous swelling of lips.

MOUTH: Gums; bluish, swollen, easily bleeding. Tongue swollen, trembles when protruding; catches on teeth, rolls about, red, dry, cracked at tip. Bad odor from mouth. Aphthae and denuded patches, with burning and rawness. Much thick, pasty saliva. Thick blundering speech; cannot open mouth wide. Peppery, sour taste. Cannot bear anything infront of mouth. Toothache extends to ears. Chattering of teeth. Teeth feel long. Sudden forcible protrusion and retraction of tongue.

THROAT: Feeling of a lump in throat; ascending and is swallowed back again—a hot lump or soft body or crumb of bread. *Throat pain* extends to ear. *Choking.* SWALLOWING PAINFUL, the wrong way, returns through nose, < empty swallowing, less from liquids and > by solids. Excessive tenderness of throat to external pressure, *must loosen collar.* Diphtheria, laryngeal. Tonsillitis, Quinsy. Hawks out foul pellets from throat in chronic sore throat, or thick mucus which cannot be forced up or down. Throat pit feels swollen or sensation of a sore spot back of pit. Constriction, > eating. Cannot swallow sweet or acrid things.

STOMACH: Cravings; for alcohol, oysters, for coffee which agrees. Hungry, cannot wait for food, or loss of hunger alternately. Thirsty, but fears to drink. Gnawing pressure in stomach, > eating, but returning in few hours (cancer); *soreness or cramp in epigastrium.* Vomits during menses, with headache. Eructations; before epilepsy, at menses. Nausea comes on after going to bed, after drinking ice-water.

ABDOMEN: Sore festering, throb, deep in liver; cannot bear anything around waist. Inflammation and abscesses. Septic gall-bladder. Cutting pain in right side of abdomen causing fainting. Swelling in cecal region, must lie on back, with knees drawn up. Appendicitis. Pain from loin down thighs. Constipation of pregnancy. Anus feels tight. Pain, up the rectum every time he coughs or sneezes. Hemorrhage from bowels containing charred particles. Piles, protrude, painful < coughing or sneezing. Constant urging in rectum, not for stool. Offensive stools. Beating in the anus as with hammer, with menses. Sensation as of a ball rolling when turning over. Diarrhea from fruits and acids.

URINARY: Ball-rolling sensation in the bladder when turning over. Bloody urine. Urine frequent, foamy, dark. Small tumor in urethra causing retention. No urine, no stool.

MALE: Strong sexual desire, without physical power. During coition the emission is tardy or does not occur at all. Lascivious ideas without erection of penis. Prepuce thickened. Semen with pungent odor. Ill-effects of masturbation. Cheerful after night emission.

FEMALE: Left ovary swollen, indurated, painful, must lift covers. *Menses black, scanty,* lumpy, acrid, vicarious from nose. Uterine and ovarian pains > by flow of blood. Feels as if the os is open. Mammae; inflamed, bluish. Nipples swollen, erect, painful to touch. Milk; thin, blue.

Leukorrhea copious, smarting, staining and stiffening the linen greenish. Climacteric troubles—palpitation, flushes of heat, hemorrhage, etc. Nymphomania. Less the flow more the pain. Ovarian tumors. Dysmenorrhea on the first day. Desire to go in open air and run about before menses.

RESPIRATORY: *Suffocation* and strangulation on lying down, *on dropping to sleep,* must spring from bed and rush for open air window. Feels he must take deep breath. Air-hunger. Tickling, choking cough, < touching neck or auditory canal, > retching out a little expectoration. Cough during sleep without being conscious of it. Feels as if a skin hanging in or a valve in larynx, as if a plug were moving up and down with cough. Larynx painful to touch. Last stage of pneumonia. Abscess of the lungs. Expectoration; frothy, purulent, difficult, bloody, with excessive perspiration. Loss of voice from paralysis of vocal cords, or edema. Cough as if some fluid has gone through wrong way; cough mostly during day.

HEART: Palpitation, with fainting spells. Restlessness, trembling, anxiety about the heart. Heart, *weak,* sensation as if it turns over or is too big, or as if hanging by a thread. Pulse weak, intermittent, slow, irregular. Cyanosis neonatorum. Carditis; metastatic. Senile arteriosclerosis.

NECK & BACK: Neck sensitive to least pressure. Neck stiff, moves jaws with difficulty. Neuralgia of coccyx, < rising from sitting, feels as if sitting on something sharp. Sensation of thread stretched from back to arm, legs, eyes.

EXTREMITIES: Swollen glands in axilla. Left arm, fingertips numb. Trembling of hands (in drunkards). Garlic odor of sweat in axilla. Felon, bluish swelling. Tingling, pricking in left hand. Cracks in skin at the corners of nails. Knees cold, or as if hot air is going through. Foot sweat foul or cold. Sciatica, must lie still, < by least motion. Tendons contracted. Toes feel broken. Pain in the shin bones in affections of throat. Cramps in calves, from fear. Phlegmasia alba dolens.

SKIN: *Mottled* or livid; dark marks; ulcer; eating; on legs with bluish, purple areolae. Fungoid ulcer. *Varicose* ulcer, carbuncle, boil, with bluish areolae. Bedsore with black edges. Cellulitis. Erysipelas of old age. Purpura with intense prostration. Cicatrices redden, hurt, break open and bleed. Capillaries dilated. Small wounds bleed much.

SLEEP: Sleeps into aggravation. Sleeplessness, from cerebral irritation; of drunkards. Frightful dreams; of snakes. Children toss about moaning in sleep. Sleepiness yet cannot sleep.

FEVER: Chill, < drinking; with sweat. HEAT on *vertex;* heat IN FLUSHES, *on waking; on falling to sleep.* Sweat—about neck, during sleep, in axilla, bloody, staining, blackish, yellow, garlicky. Feet icy cold.

COMPLEMENTARY: Lyc; Phos; Zinc-i.

RELATED: Caust; Sep; Zinc.

LACHNANTHES

GENERALITIES: A remedy for torticollis and rheumatic symptoms about neck. Bubbling and boiling about the heart, rising to head. Stiffness of neck, drawn over to one side, in sore throat. Pain in nape as if dislocated, when turning the neck, or bending the head back. Bridge of nose feels pinched. Feeling of icy coldness in mid-scapular region.

LACTICUM ACIDUM

GENERALITIES: This acid is found in buttermilk and is a valuable remedy for morning sickness, diabetes, rheumatic affections, breast troubles. It is suitable to anemic, pale women. Nausea—on waking, > by eating; in diabetes or pregnancy. Thirst. Voracious hunger. Fullness or lump like puff ball in throat. Pains in the breast with enlargement of axillary glands. Pain extending to head. Rheumatic pains in joints, knees, < by motion. Flying pain in the limbs. Trembling of whole body while walking. Frequent passing of large quantities of saccharine urine. Hot, acrid eructations, < smoking. Salivation - waterbrash. Sweaty feet.

LACTUCA VIROSA

GENERALITIES: This remedy seems to be a true galactogogue, increases the milk in breast. Urine smells of violets. Sensation of a drop continuously passing along the urethra when seated.

LAPIS ALBUS

GENERALITIES: It is silico-fluoride of calcium, a remedy for new growths and glandular affections. Pains are burning, stinging, shooting. Uterine carcinoma, fibroid tumor, with intense burning pain and profuse hemorrhage. Severe menstrual pain causing swooning. Enlargement of the glands esp. cervical, which are elastic and pliable rather than stony hard. Sarcoma. Lipoma. Glandular swellings where no glands are usually found.

LAPPA

GENERALITIES: This remedy chiefly affects the *skin,* liver, joints and uterus. *Heavy, sore, aching* as if lying uncomfortably. Numbness—lumbar region, of aching calves. Constriction.

WORSE: Cold; wet. Shaking. Lying on right side. Violent exertion.

BETTER: Cloudy weather.

HEAD: Vertigo, with nausea and vomiting. Weight on vertex.

EYES: Redness about eyes. Styes, crops of.

NOSE: Red across nose.

FACE: Inveterate acne, < touch.

STOMACH: SOURNESS; sour taste to meat; all food turns sour; vomits it. Diarrhea alternating with rheumatic symptoms.

URINARY: Profuse and frequent urination; urine milky. Phosphaturia.

FEMALE: Bruised, sore, heavy feeling in uterus, with great relaxation of vaginal tissue. Uterine displacement, < standing, walking, a misstep, sudden jar.

CHEST: Trembling in chest.

EXTREMITIES: Front of thigh weak. Old sores about joints.

SKIN: Eruptions; sticky on head, face, etc. Moist, foul eczema; of infants. Many small painful boils. AXILLARY SWEAT COLD, *runs down chest,* foul.

COMPLEMENTARY: Mag-c.

LATHYRUS SATIVUS

GENERALITIES: Affects the anterior and lateral columns of the cord, causing many paralytic affections of lower extremities. Athetosis; infantile paralysis. Useful in wasting and exhaustive diseases when there is much weakness and heaviness, and slow recovery of nerve power. Reflexes increased.

WORSE: Cold damp weather.

MIND: Depressed.

HEAD: Vertigo when standing with eyes closed.

MOUTH: Burning of the tip of tongue. Tongue feels as if scalded. Tongue and lips numb.

URINARY: Urination involuntary, hurried.

EXTREMITIES: Tremulous tottering gait. Excessive rigidity of legs; spastic gait. Knees knock together when walking. Knee jerks exaggerated. Cannot extend or cross legs when sitting. Heels do not touch the ground when walking. Sits bent forward, straightens up with difficulty. Gluteal muscles and muscles of lower limbs are emaciated. Stiffness and lameness of the ankles and knees. Feet are dragged or put down suddenly and forcibly while walking. Sensation of a damp cloth around the waist. Legs are cold during day, become hot and burn at night, > uncovering. While lying down legs can move from side to side but cannot be lifted.

SLEEP: Continuous yawning with sleepiness.

LATRODECTUS MACTANS

GENERALITIES: This spider poison affects the HEART producing a typical picture of *angina pectoris.* Blood become thin, watery. Tetanic effects lasting for several days. *Restless; with cardiac pains,* and *prostrated.*

WORSE: Least motion, even of hands. Exertion.

MIND: Anxiety. Screams fearfully with pain exclaiming that she would lose her breath and die.

STOMACH: Nausea then abdominal pains. Vomiting of black vomit. Transfixation of pain or sinking at epigastrium.

RESPIRATORY: *Gasping breath; fear of losing breath and dying.* Apnea.

HEART: *Violent* CARDIAC PAINS; sharp, extending to shoulders or *both arms,* to fingers, *with numbness.* Precordial anxiety. *Restless; with cardiac pain,* and prostration. Quick, feeble, thready pulse.

EXTREMITIES: Pain in left arm, feels paralysed. Hard aching pain in axilla. Paraesthesia of lower limbs.

SKIN: Cold as marble.

SLEEP: Dreams of flying.

RELATED: Tarent.

LAUROCERASUS

GENERALITIES: The small quantity of Hydrocyanic acid which this medicine contains produces symptoms accompanied by SUDDEN DEBILITY and *lack of reaction,* esp. in chest and heart affections. It affects the MIND and BRAIN causing *bluntness of special senses.* CYANOSIS. COLDNESS NOT > by warmth. Weak sphincters. Long-lasting fainting. Sensation of falling down—in brain, in abdomen in heart, etc. Epilepsy: clonic spasm of all limbs, with paralytic weakness. Twitching. Chorea: emotional, with constant jerks, cannot keep still; speech indistinct after every excitement, gasping for breath.

Gasping - before, during and after spasms. Nervous collapse. Apoplexy. Internal burning. Hemorrhage; of thin, bright blood, mixed with gelatinous clots. Effects of fright. Blue baby, asphyxia neonatorum. Antidotes the effects of Digitalis given in crude doses. Well chosen remedies do not act.

WORSE: *Sitting up.* Exertion. Cold. Fright. Stooping.

BETTER: *Lying with head low.* Eating. Sleep. Open air.

MIND: Loss of consciousness, with loss of speech and motion. Fear and anxiety about imaginary evils. SUDDEN LOSS OF MEMORY from fright, pain, etc. Dulness of special senses. Gets angry when not understood.

HEAD: Vertigo with sleepiness. Head pain, < 11 a.m. to 1 p.m. Nightly tearing in vertex. Sensation as if a cold wind were blowing on head, as if brain were falling. Brain feels contracted and painful.

EYES: Protrude, staring, open. Objects look larger.

FACE: *Blue,* with gasping. Feels as if flies and spiders are crawling over the skin. Lock-jaw. Twitching of the muscles of face.

MOUTH: Foam at the mouth; in convulsions. Speechlessness from pain in stomach. Tongue stiff, cold, burnt or numb.

THROAT: Spasmodic contraction of throat and esophagus. DRINKS ROLL AUDIBLY *through esophagus and intestines.*

STOMACH: Persistent hiccough. Bitter eructations. Vomiting of food during cough. Disgust for food during pregnancy. Violent pain in stomach with loss of speech. Pain during urination. Nausea near a hot stove.

ABDOMEN: A sensation of a lump falling down in abdomen from above the navel to small of back, < talking or overexertion. *Gurgling flatulence.* Pain in the liver as though abscess were forming. Liver; indurated, atrophied; nutmeg. Paralysis of sphincter ani; involuntary stools. Cancer of rectum; with bleeding of bright red blood.

FEMALE: Pain in uterus with cancer, with oozing of bright blood, with gelatinous clots, > sleep. Faints with coldness during menses. Burning and stinging in and below mammae.

URINARY: Urine; retained, suppressed, involuntary; with palpitation and suffocation, and fainting.

RESPIRATORY: Larynx and trachea raw. *Suffocation, gasps for breath, on sitting up.* Shallow breathing. Dyspnea, with sensation that he is unable to raise the chest walls; > lying down. *Cough—tickling,* spasmodic, nightly; of phthisis; short, dry of cardiac origin; < lying down. Bloody, or scattered with bloody dots. Gelatinous expectoration. Asphyxia neonatorum. Burning in chest on inspiration. Low voice.

HEART: *Holds hands over the heart,* as if there were some trouble there, < by any exercise. Palpitation. Mitral regurgitation. Pain in the region of heart. Pulse weak, variable, slow, or irregular.

EXTREMITIES: Clubbing of fingers. Toe and finger nails become knotty. Veins of hands distended. Cold clammy feet up to the knees in chorea, heart disease. Feet numb on crossing the legs.

SKIN: Cool; livid.

SLEEP: Fearful anxiety and restlessness; cannot fall to sleep. Coma vigil.

RELATED: Am-c; Gels; Hyd-ac; Prun.

LECITHIN

GENERALITIES: Prepared from the yolk of egg and animal brain it is a phosphorus containing complex organic body. It improves the nutrition, esp. of blood, hence very useful in anemia, convalescence, neurasthenia and insomnia. Excellent galactogogue, renders milk more nourishing. Tired, weak, short of breath; loss of flesh; symptoms of general breakdown. Sexually weak. Ovarian insufficiency.

LEDUM PALUSTRE

GENERALITIES: This remedy affects the fibrous tissue, of JOINTS, esp. small, *ankles, tendons,* heels and SKIN; hence it can be called a rheumatic remedy, where rheumatism *begins in the feet and travels upwards.* Affected parts become *purple, puffy, and then emaciate. The patient is always chilly, affected parts are cold, yet averse to external warmth. There is a general lack of* vital heat. Painful, cold, edematous, joints. Shifting, tearing pains. Weakness and numbness of the affected parts. Torpidity of integuments, esp. after suppression of discharges from the eyes, ears and nose. *Hemorrhage* of bright frothy blood. Dropsy. Petechiae. Tetanus with twitchings of muscles near the wound. Ill effects of alcohol, hair-cutting; suppressed discharges, punctured wounds, recent or chronic injury, bites, stings, bruises. Drunkards. Rush of blood. Abscess and septic conditions, > by cold. If Ledum is given immediately after punctured wounds, it prevents tetanus. *Hypericum* when tetanus develops. It is adapted to full-blooded, plethoric, robust or pale, delicate patients.

WORSE: Warmth; of covers, stove, air. Injury. Motion (joints). Night. Egg. Wine. Spitting.

BETTER: *Cold bathing,* air. Reposing.

MIND: Angry, out of humor. Dissatisfied, hates his fellow beings, avoids their company.

HEAD: Raging, pulsating headache, < least cover. Affected after getting wet. Misstep causes concussion of the brain. Itching as from lice. Blood-boils on forehead.

EYES: *Blood shot or bruised.* Tears acrid, make the lower lids and cheeks sore. Hemorrhage into the anterior chamber after iridectomy. Ptosis of eye (R) from injury.

EARS: Hardness of hearing; feels as if the ears were stuffed up by with cotton, < cutting hair, wetting the head.

NOSE: Persistent nosebleed; soreness of the nose with violent burning.

FACE: Mottled. Red pimples on forehead and cheeks, stinging when touched. Submental glands swollen. Crusty eruptions around the nose and mouth.

MOUTH: Bitter taste in the mouth; mouldly when coughing. Sudden flow of watery saliva, during colic.

STOMACH: Nausea on spitting.

RECTUM: Anal fissure. Blind smarting piles.

URINARY: Much uric acid and sand in urine. Urine often stops during the flow. Copious clear, colorless urine, deficient in salts.

MALE: Pollution of sanguinous or serous semen.

FEMALE: Bleeding fibroids. Great coldness during menses, yet desires cold air.

RESPIRATORY: Cough; tormenting; from tickling in larynx, with epistaxis; then sobbing respiration, < in receding eruptions. Double inspiration. Hemoptysis, alternating with rheumatism, or coxalgia. Yellow, purulent sputum. Chest hurts when touched.

NECK & BACK: Back stiff; *cramps in back, < rising from sitting.* Lumbago.

EXTREMITIES: Cramp over hip-joint. Swollen, blotchy, ecchymotic legs and feet. Heels sore. Soles painful, can hardly step on them. Trembling of hands when moving them or grasping anything. *Easy spraining of ankles.* Feet (dorsum) itch by night and are stiff in a.m. Balls of great toes swollen. Feet held to earth as by a magnet when attempting to move. Pain in shoulder on raising arm.

SKIN: *Wounds—punctured,* twitches in; from nails, stings, etc. Foul pus. Eruptions on only covered part. Edematous swelling. Red spots and rash.

FEVER: *Coldness* of parts, < limbs; coldness with the pain, during fever, as if in cold water. Foul sweat; Profuse night sweat.

RELATED: Arn; Bry; Rhus-t; Sec.

LEPTANDRA

GENERALITIES: It affects the right side and *liver,* causing hemorrhage. *Burning in hepatic region.* Bilious states Weakness, hardly able to stand or walk. Jaundice.

WORSE: Cold drink. Motion. Periodically. Wet weather.

BETTER: *Lying on abdomen,* on side.

MIND: Hopeless; despondent and drowsy; with hepatic affections.

HEAD: Dull frontal headache, with aching in navel.

EYES: Smarting and aching.

MOUTH: Tongue yellow, or black down center.

STOMACH: Craving for cold drinks which < burning and aching in stomach. Bilious vomiting. Sinking at the pit of stomach. Meat and vegetables disagree.

ABDOMEN: *Sore or dull; burning ache over liver or near gall-bladder, extending over bowels to navel or towards left scapula* or along spine, which feels chilly. Liver swollen transversely. Acute liver conditions. *Gall-stones.* Constant dull aching in umbilical region. Stools muddy, watery, < morning, *tarry or black;* FOUL. *Stringy,* waxy or spurting, in the morning; with pain at navel. Dysentery, after diarrhea. Prolapsing piles, with *hemorrhage.* Jaundice, with clay colored stools. Feeling as if something was passing out of the rectum.

URINARY: Red or orange-colored urine, with dull aching in lumbar region.

FEMALE: Menses suppressed or retarded, with liver affections. Leukorrhea; warm, watery; runs down the limbs; from ulceration of the os.

HEART: Soreness. Pulse slow and full.

EXTREMITIES: Pain in sciatic nerve (left), < on sitting. *Nails very thin,* soft and splitting.

FEVER: Chilly along the spine and down the arm.

COMPLEMENTARY: Phos.

RELATED: Bapt; Card-m; Chion.

LILIUM TIGRINUM

GENERALITIES: It manifests its chief action upon the VENOUS CIRCULATION *of the heart* and FEMALE ORGANS—*ovaries and uterus,* and is useful in many reflex conditions dependent on some pathological condition of these organs. It also affects *rectum and bladder* and left side. Often indicated in unmarried women. FULL, HEAVY OR FORCED OUT feeling in uterus, ovaries, heart, etc. *Utero-ovarian sagging.* Wandering, flying, shooting pains or opening and shutting pains; radiating from ovary to heart, to left breast, down the legs, etc. *Backward* pains about eyes, to occiput, from nipples through chest, from heart to left scapula. Pain in small spots. *Pulsation,* ebullition, gurgling and burning. *Nervous tremors,* in hypogastrium, spine, knees, etc. Venous congestion. Discharges acrid. Nervous, hysterical. Faints in warm room or after standing for a long time. Women exhausted by sexual excess. Symptoms from sexual excitement. Rheumatism. Mental and uterine or/and cardiac symptoms alternate.

WORSE: WARMTH of room. Motion. *Miscarriage.* Walking. Standing. Consolation. Pressure of bed clothes. Jarring.

BETTER: *Cool, fresh air. When busy.* Lying on left side. Sunset. Pressure. Support. Crossing legs. Rubbing.

MIND: *Hurried. Nervous. Snappish. Depressed. Erotic.* Fruitless activity. Despondent. Disposed to curse, strike. *Dread* of insanity, being incurable. Desires finery. Wild, crazy feeling. Inclination to weep, weeps much; is very timid and indifferent to anything done for her. Dissatisfied with her own things, envious of others. Dementia from business worries and sexual excess; tears the hair. Feels hurried, walks fast, does not know why. Wants to talk, yet dreads saying anything, lest she should say something wrong. Has to keep very busy to repress sexual desire. Consolation <. Sits alone and broods over imaginary troubles. Sexual excitement alternating with apprehension of religious ideas. Prefers society.

HEAD: Wild feeling in head, as though she would be crazy. Headache, burning; dependent on uterine disorders, < before and after menses; > at sunset. Headache over left eye to vertex, with vertigo and visual effects.

EYES: Feel sprained; bite and burn, < reading. Wild look. Myopic astigmatism, has to turn the head sideways to see clearly. Pain in eyes extend to back of head. Weak ciliary muscles.

EARS: Rushing sounds in ear after going to bed.

NOSE: Sneezing, > pain in head and eyes.

MOUTH: Tongue; coated yellowish, white in patches. Sweet taste at back of mouth; foul tastes > eating.

THROAT: Hawking of mucus, with constant nausea.

STOMACH: Craving for meat, or for sour or sweet dainties. Aversion to coffee, bread. Hunger, as if from spine. Thirsty, before severe symptoms. A hard body felt rolling around during day only. Vomiting from displacement of uterus.

ABDOMEN: Skin of abdomen feels stretched and stiff. Sore, distended; cannot bear weight of cover after menses. Weak, tremulous feeling extending to anus. *Heavy dragging-down* of whole abdominal contents extending even to organs of chest, must support the abdomen; with dysuria. Pressure on rectum with constant desire for stools, > urination, < standing. Sharp pains, > gentle rubbing, with warm hand. Early morning diarrhea, after rising, urgent, cannot wait a moment; stools small, frequent, with tenesmus. Dysentery, < change of life in plethoric women. Sharp pains, >

doubling up. Tenesmus of the rectum and bladder. Piles; after delivery.

URINARY: Constant pressure on bladder, with constant desire to pass urine; with sensation of a ball in rectum. Urine milky, scanty, hot. If desire is not attended to, feeling of congestion in chest.

FEMALE: *Heavy dragging or outward pressing in pelvis,* with dysuria, as if all organs would escape through vagina, must hold it. Menses early, scanty, dark, clotted, offensive. Flow only when moving about. Ovarian (left) pain travels down thighs or up below the left breast. Leukorrhea thin, brown, acrid; stains brown, < after menses. Neuralgic pain in uterus, cannot bear pressure of clothes. Prolapse or anteversion of uterus. Subinvolution. Sexual desire increased; obscene; to repress must keep herself busy. Feels a rivet or ball under (left) mamma; sensation a hard body pressing upon rectum and ovaries, > walking.

RESPIRATORY: Oppressive load on chest; air hunger; takes long deep breath. Sensation of a lump in centre of chest moving up and down on empty swallowing. Suffocates in a warm or crowded room, theater or church.

HEART: *Feels clutched, full to bursting; cold,* weak; as if hanging by a thread. Angina pectoris, with pain in right arm, < stooping, lying on right side, > rubbing and pressure. *Palpitation.* Pulse irregular, very rapid. Pulsations all over the body.

NECK & BACK: Neck aches, when tired. Broken feeling between scapulae. Sensation of pulling upward from tip of coccyx.

EXTREMITIES: Pain from hip to hip. Cannot walk on uneven ground. Legs ache, cannot keep them still. Feeling of a cool wind blowing on legs. Burning in palms and soles. Trembling of knees. Pricking in fingers. Paralytic stiffness of fingers. Staggering gait; cannot walk straight. Joints feel dry.

SKIN: Tingling, formication, burning in various parts.

SLEEP: Unable to sleep on account of wild feeling in head.

FEVER: Chilly, > in cool open air.

RELATED: Aloe; Plat; Puls; Spig.

LITHIUM CARBONICUM

GENERALITIES: This remedy affects notably head, eyes, *heart, small joints* and urinary organs. Rheumatism connected with heart or eye lesion. Whole body feels SORE *and heavy*. Bruised spot from fall and blow. Violent lancinating pain, as from red hot needles. Pressing from within out in head, abdominal ring, perineum, chest. Pain as from a dull point. Uric acid diathesis. Paralytic stiffness of the whole body. Prostration. *Acidity.* Increase of bulk and weight. Gout.

WORSE: Night. After suppressed menses.

BETTER: *Eating.* Urinating. Motion.

MIND: Disposed to weep about his lonesome condition. Difficulty in remembering names.

HEAD: Ache, > eating but returns again and remains until food is taken again . Vertigo with ringing in the ears. Headache from sudden suppression of menses. Head feels too large.

EYES: Feel dry and painful, < reading. Vertical hemiopia, right half of object is invisible, < during menses. Sunlight blinds him.

NOSE: Swollen and *red,* esp. right side. Coryza, dripping from nose in open air.

EAR: Pain behind ear (L), extending to neck.

FACE: Both cheeks are covered with dry bran-like scales.

THROAT: Lumps of mucus drop into throat. Soreness extending to ear.

STOMACH: Gnawing in stomach, with pain in left temple, > eating. Acidity. Cannot endure slightest pressure of clothes from fullness in pit of stomach.

ABDOMEN: Pain in abdominal ring (left) like a pressing from within outward. Diarrhea after fruits or chocolates.

URINARY: Pain in the region of bladder extending to spermatic cord after urination. Urine scanty, with much thirst, with red-brown sediment. Urine less inspite of taking normal drinks.

MALE: Erection after copious urination.

FEMALE: Pain in mammary glands which extends to arms and fingers.

RESPIRATORY: Air feels cold on inspiring, even in lungs. Constriction of chest.

HEART: *Pain sore,* with eye symptoms, going to head, with pain in bladder, < bending forward, before menses, > urinating. Trembling and fluttering of the heart, < vexation.

EXTREMITIES: Soreness of fingers, > grasping. Ankle joint pains while walking. Pain in the joints is relieved by very hot water.

SKIN: Barber's itch. Dry, harsh skin. Eczema.

RELATED: Lyc; Nat-p; Sul-ac.

LOBELIA INFLATA

GENERALITIES: It stimulates *vaso-motor nerves,* causing *increased secretions,* RELAXATION, and *weakness,* with sweat, with deathly sickness all over, with oppressed *rattling respiration.* Sits with elbows on knees. Prickling all over. Cannot bear the odor of tobacco although addicted to it. Nausea and vomiting with nearly all respiratory troubles, and gastric affections.

WORSE: Cold bathing. Suppression. After sleep. Tobacco. Tea. Foreign body. Slightest motion.

BETTER: Rapid walking. Eating a little.

MIND: Despondent. Sobbing like a child.

HEAD: Dull heavy pain. Vertigo with fear of death.

EARS: Deafness due to suppressed discharge (otorrhea) or eczema.

FACE: Bathed in cold sweat. Neuralgia of face (L), with retarded menses.

MOUTH: *Profuse flow of saliva,* with retching, hiccough, dyspnea, with good appetite.

THROAT: *Feeling of a lump in throat;* impeding deglutition.

STOMACH: Feeling of a lump. *Deathly nausea,* with vertigo, > by a little drink or food, < night and early morning. *Nausea and vomiting,* with profuse sweat, on face (cold), with respiratory symptoms. *Faintness and weakness in epigastrium.* Acid, burning taste.

URINARY: Deep red urine; with red sediment. Urine suppressed or infrequent.

FEMALE: *Morning sickness,* suddenly disappears, > by a little food and drink. Labor pain with shortness of breath. Pain in sacrum and sense of weight in her genitals.

RESPIRATORY: *Dyspnea,* nervous, with labor pain; as if from a wedge in larynx, with general prickling, > rapid walking. Asthma. Spasmodic cough, with sneezing, belching, or gastric pain. *Rattle in chest but does not expectorate. Constriction or oppressive fullness in chest.* Senile emphysema.

HEART: Feels as if it would stop. Pulse weak or soft, flowing.

BACK: Pain in sacrum; cannot bear slightest touch; sits leaning forward.

SKIN: Plaques of edema, with ecchymoses. Prickling and itching, with nausea.

RELATED: Ant-t; Ip; Tab.

LOLIUM TEMULENTUM

GENERALITIES: This remedy is useful in paralytic conditions. Tremor and convulsion; paralysis agitans. Prostration and restlessness.

WORSE: Wet; wet season.

MIND: Anxious and depressed.

HEAD: Vertigo, must close eyes. Head heavy.

MOUTH: Tongue tremulous. Speech difficult, cannot pronounce the whole word.

STOMACH: Nausea, vomiting. Severe purging.

EXTREMITIES: Gait unsteady. Trembling of all limbs, cannot write, or hold a glass of water. Spasm of arms and legs. Violent pain in calves, as if bound by a cord.

FEVER: Cold rigor all over, esp. in limbs.

RELATED: Lathy; Sec.

LYCOPERSICUM

GENERALITIES: Tomato has marked action on deltoid and pectoral muscles; pain is > by lifting arm upward and outward. Pains remain after influenza.

HEAD: Headache begins in the occiput, spreads all over the head and settles with great violence in temples, < tobacco smoke.

RELATED: Sang.

LYCOPODIUM

GENERALITIES: It is called vegetable sulphur. It affects the NUTRITION DUE TO WEAKNESS OF DIGESTION. Acts upon URINARY ORGANS. Most of the symptoms develop on the RIGHT SIDE and *go to the left:* THROAT, *chest,* ovary. Ailments develop gradually weakening the functional power; the function of liver is seriously disturbed. Deep-seated progressive chronic diseases. *Repeating symptoms or alternating symptoms*—chill after chill, flushing then paling; flexion then extension; automatic acts. *Relapsing conditions.* Prostration of mind and body. It is adapted to old personS, or who become old early, where the skin shows yellowish spots, or to precocious weakly children. *Lyc.* patients are *intellectually* keen but of weak muscular power, lack vital heat; circulation poor, it seems to stand still, with cold, numb extremities, or numbness may appear in spots. Sudden symptoms, pains come and go suddenly; or cause anger, jerking, etc. The patient is *thin,* withered and FULL OF GAS. ACIDITY; *sour* taste, eructations, etc. Descending symptoms, colds, emaciation etc. *Calculi;* gall-stone, gravel. Dropsy; ascites in liver diseases. *Coldness,* partial: head, throat, etc. *Dryness;* of palms, soles, vagina, skin, etc. *Rawness,* in folds, anus, nipple etc. Formication of affected limbs. Paralysis. Carcinoma. Inflammation of bones, mostly at ends; softening and caries of bones. Spasms with screaming, foaming at the mouth, throwing the arms about. *Oversensitive to pain,* patient is besides himself. Sense of internal paralysis. Lithic acid diathesis. Ill-effects of fear, fright, chagrin, anger, anxiety, fevers, overlifting, masturbation, riding in a carriage, tobacco chewing, wine. One side of the body hypertrophied at change of life in women. Atrophy of infants. Hemorrhage, dark blood. Erectile tumor. Boils recurring periodically. Emaciation and debility from loss of fluid.

WORSE: PRESSURE OF CLOTHES. WARMTH. *Awakening.* Wind. *Eating,* even a little fills to satiety; oysters. *Indigestion.* 4 to 8 p.m. Wet weather, stormy weather. Pressure. Before, or suppressed, menses. Milk. Vegetables—cabbage, beans; bread, pastry.

BETTER: WARM DRINKS, food. Cold application. *Motion. Eructations. Urinating.* After midnight.

MIND: *Confusion over daily affairs. Mentally active but grows weaker.* Melancholy; afraid, to be alone, of men, of his own shadow. *Sensitive,* weeps when thanked; or when meeting a friend. *Fearsome;* dread of men; presence of new persons, of everything, even ringing of door bell. Loss of self-confidence, from anticipation; averse to undertaking new things yet when he undertakes it he goes through with ease and comfort. AWAKES ANGRY, sad and anxious. Vehement; headstrong. *Domineering, exacting,* reserved, or despairing. Spells or writes wrong words or syllables. Cannot bear to see anything new. Cannot read what he writes. Hurried when eating. Incipient paralysis of brain. Weeps all day. Sad, on hearing distant music, or cheerful and merry. Hateful. Cranky. Miserly. Brainfag, after influenza. Anxious thoughts as if about to die. Indecision. Timidity. Resignation. Misanthrophic, flees even from his children. *Amative.* Distrustful; fault finding; suspicious.

HEAD: Shakes head without any cause, or involuntarily, slow first then rapid. Vertigo when looking at anything turning. Head cold. Pain in temples as if screwed together, < menses. Pain begins on one side goes to other where it is worse. Headache, < if not eating regularly, lying down, stooping, > uncovering. Pulsating pain in occiput, at night, < when hot. Hair falls, becomes gray early. Premature baldness, after abdominal affections, parturition. *Deep furrows on forehead* in abdominal, pulmonary and brain affections, and in misers. Dandruff. Hydrocephalus. Meningitis, tubercular. Catarrhal headache, < when discharge from nose is slacked up. Throbbing after every spell of cough; pain when pressing at stool.

EYES: Half open. Hemiopia. Day-blindness. Sparks before the eyes, in the dark. Styes on lids towards the inner canthi. Polypus on external canthi. Cataract, with suppressed menses. Feel cold, or hot; seem too large.

EARS: Humming and roaring, with hardness of hearing; every noise causes peculiar echo in ear. Thick, yellow, offensive discharge, with deafness. Eczema about and behind the ears. Feels as if hot blood rushed into ears.

NOSE: Nose stopped up; snuffles; breathes through mouth; child starts from sleep rubbing the nose. *Fan-like motion of alae nasi;* in brain, lung and abdominal troubles. Feeling of dryness posteriorly. Ozena, acrid. Chronic coryza; blows nose often. Nasal troubles from childhood. Acute smell.

FACE: *Yellowish,* pale, gray, with blue circles around the eyes. Face withered, shrivelled and emaciated. Flushes of heat. Twitchings. *Mouth hangs open.* Sore lips. Twists face and mouth. Silly expression.

MOUTH: Toothache, with swelling of cheek, > warm application. Tongue dry, black, cracked, stiff, heavy, *swollen,* moves to and fro or is darted out rapidly; trembling. Painful ulcer on tip or below tongue. Speech indistinct; stammers the last word. Saliva dries on palate and lips. Dryness without thirst. Lower jaw drops in fever. Teeth yellow. Mouth waters. Gums bleed when touching or cleaning teeth. Taste; too acute; sour; bitter; mouldy; small tumors in mouth in various places.

THROAT: Feeling of a hard body in esophagus. A ball rises and sticks in throat. *Sore throat,* < cold drink. Swelling and suppuration of tonsils. Chronic enlargement of the tonsils. Diphtheria - deposits spread from right to left. Food and drinks come through nose on swallowing. Throat cold. Feeling of contraction provoking constant swallowing.

STOMACH: Digestion weak. Loss of appetite. *Hunger, but quick satiety.* EATING EVER SO LITTLE CREATES FULLNESS. Hiccough. *Incomplete burning eructations,* rise only to pharynx which then burns for hours. Farinaceous and flatulent food, cabbage, beans, oysters disagree. Sensation as if fasting after meals, but without hunger. Desire for sweet things. Aversion to soup, to bread. Canine hunger, the more he eats, the more he craves. Wakes at night feeling hungry. Vomits food and bile, coagulated blood, dark greenish masses, after eating and drinking. Cancer; perforating ulcer. Churning sensation. Gnawing in stomach, > drinking hot water. Desire for sweets, delicacies, pastries, etc. Food tastes sour. Likes to take drink and foods hot. Coldness in stomach. Bad effects of onions.

ABDOMEN: *Epigastric anxiety, pressure.* Feels a band about waist. *Flatulence much, Noisy,* pressing out, *of lower bowels.* Sensitive, congested liver. Chronic hepatitis; atrophic; nutmeg liver. Sensation of something moving up and down, or a hard body rolling, when turning to the right side. Ascites from liver diseases. Soreness, < hypogastrium, alternating sides. Brown spots. Colic in babies, < evening. Constipation, of children, ineffectual urging from contraction of sphincters, feeling as if much remained unpassed after stool. Stool, contains sand; small, difficult; first part is hard, is difficult to expel, last part is soft or thin and gushing; followed by faintness and weakness. Hemorrhoids aching, painful to touch, > hot bathing. Alternate diarrhea and constipation. Rawness of anus. Constipation when away from home or travelling. Chilliness in the rectum before stool. Constipation or diarrhea during pregnancy. Gastro enteritis from fright. Diarrhea from cold drinks. Continued burning in rectum.

URINARY: Frequent urging to urinate, > riding in car. Renal colic in ureter (right) goes to bladder. Urine, scanty; *cries before urinating,* esp. children who wake up from pain, with screaming, and toss the limbs about; *red sand in urine;* slow in coming, must strain; suppressed, retained. Urine, milky, turbid. Polyuria, during the night. Hematuria. Involuntary urination, esp. in fever or from fright during coition. Urine bloody, with paraplegia or sometimes with constipation. Urine burning hot.

MALE: *Sexual exhaustion;* impotence; erection feeble; falls asleep during coition. Yellow tumor on corona glandis. Exhausting pollutions. Enlarged prostate. Premature seminal emission.

FEMALE: Menses in clots and serum; discharge of blood from genitals during stool. Vagina burns < during and after coition. *Leukorrhea acrid; periodical;* milky; < before full moon. Physometra. Cutting from right to left ovary; ovarian tumor; dropsy. Dropsy of uterus. Hard burning nodosities in mammae with stitching, aching pain and soreness. Rawness of nipples which are sore, fissured, bleed easily. Fetus seems to be turning somersaults. Dysmenorrhea violent, with fainting. Menses suppressed, for months. Delayed menses with undeveloped mammae at puberty. Milk in breast without being pregnant. Child vomits blood after sucking bleeding nipples.

RESPIRATORY: Craves air but is chilled by it. Short, rattling breathing, < lying on back. Cough: dry, tickling, teasing; in puny boys with emaciation; day and night; deep hollow; as from sulphur fumes, < on descending; with emaciation; < on empty swallowing, stretching the throat; deep breathing. Salty greenish-yellow, lumpy or foul expectoration. Unresolved pneumonia. Brown yellow spots on chest. Abscess of the lungs, tuberculosis. Difficult respiration due to hydrothorax or hydropericardium, with flapping of nose. Feeling of tightness in chest with burning.

HEART: Aneurism. Aortic disease. Palpitation: with flapping of alae nasi at night, < lying on right side; with cold face and feet. Pulse fast, < after eating, evening. Sensation as if the circulation stood still. Hypertrophy.

NECK & BACK: One side of the neck stiff and swollen. Burning as from hot coals between the scapulae. Pain in the back and right side from congestion of liver. Pain in the small of the back, < sitting erect, > urination. Stiff back. Emaciation about the neck. Bubbling sensation. Lumbago, < slightest motion (after *Bry).*

EXTREMITIES: Axillary abscess (right). Hands and feet numb; cramps in hands and feet. Fingers twitch during sleep. Sticky sweat on fingers. Pain jerks legs upward. Cramps in calves, when walking, at night. One foot hot, other cold, or cold sweaty feet. Constant troublesome heat of hands. Sciatica right side; cannot lie on painful side, pressure, > hot application and walking. Cramp in toes, at night. Pain in heels as if treading on pebbles. Heels numb. Palms dry. Varicose veins on legs. Edema of feet, rises until ascites forms. Pain in bones at night. Curvature and caries of bones. Emaciation of one hand or one leg. Hands and feet become heavy, relaxed, tremble, > by motion. Painful corns on soles. Toes and fingers contracted. Toes bend when walking. Profuse fetid foot sweat.

SKIN: Dry; rawness in folds. Abscess beneath the skin. Urticaria, chronic, < warmth. Erectile tumor, < before menses. Blood-boils. Boils which do not mature but remain blue. Sites of old boils and pustules indurate and form nodules that remain long. Vesicular swellings. Eczema associated with urinary, gastric, hepatic disorder. Psoriasis. Ulcers, fistulous. Scabs do not separate. Viscid and offensive sweat.

SLEEP: Drowsy during day; on waking, the child starts; becomes cross, kicks, scolds, or holds his mother. Awakes terrified. Anxious dreams of fatal accidents. Child sleeps all day and cries all night. Laughs or weeps n sleep.

FEVER: Coldness, icy; partial-of head, abdomen, stomach, throat, etc., < coughing. Body becomes cold during cough, feels as if lying on ice. Chill; followed by another chill, then vomits, after first sleep. Foul, viscid sweat—axillary, of feet; odor of onions. Fever: continuous, remittent, intermittent.

COMPLEMENTARY: Calc; Iod; Kali-c; Lach; *Puls;* Sulph.

RELATED: Carb-v; Sil.

LYCOPUS VIRGINICUS

GENERALITIES: A HEART REMEDY; lowers the blood pressure, reduces the heart rate and increases the length of systole. Heart ailments with many side-symptoms, or associated with RAPID TUMULTUOUS HEART BEATS. Hemorrhage due to valvular heart disease; or passive, from nose, piles, lungs, etc. Shifting pains—from heart to eyes, head to heart, heart to wrist, etc. Toxic goitre. Ill effects of suppressed hemorrhoidal flow.

WORSE: *Excitement. Exertion. Heat. After sleep.* Lying on right side. Abuse of heart remedies. Suppressions. Thinking of it.

MIND: Nervous, hurried and *tremulous.* Slow comprehension.

EYES: *Protruding* (exophthalmic goitre), with tumultuous action of the heart. Supra-orbital pain (right) with aching in testicles (left).

FACE: Brownish-yellow; expressionless; bloated.

STOMACH: Eructations taste of tea. Diarrhea in jaundice from weakness of heart.

URINARY: Drinks large quantity of water and passes large quantity of urine, with irritability of the heart. Bladder feels distended when empty.

MALE: Neuralgic pain in testicles with supra-orbital pain.

RESPIRATORY: Choking when lying down. Cough with hemoptysis and feeble, weak heart. *Heart cough.* Deep, violent cough in the evening, and night without waking. Sweetish expectoration.

HEART: Action *tumultuous, violent, excessively rapid,* stormy. Labored heart at night. Palpitation and cardiac distress, < when thinking of it. *Oppression at heart.*

Pains sore, aching, constricted. Pulse large, full, soft, slow, weak irregular, intermittent; does not synchronize with heart.

BACK: Hot, ache beneath scapula (right).

FEVER: Coldness.

RELATED: Cact; Coll; Crat.

LYSSIN

GENERALITIES: This nosode is prepared from the saliva of rabid dog. It affects the nervous system, throat and sexual organs. *Senses become over acute.* Convulsion, spasm brought on by dazzling light or sight of running water. Aching in bones. Complaints from abnormal sexual desire. Ill effects of dogbite. Bluish discoloration of wound. Trembling or quivering sensation throughout the body.

WORSE: *Noise of or sight of running water.* Heat of sun. Glistening objects. Wind, draft. Thinking of fluids. Stooping. Bad news. Emotion. Riding in a carriage.

BETTER: Bending backward. Gentle rubbing. Steam or hot bath.

MIND: Fear of becoming mad. Anger. Rapid speech. Impatient. *Violent temper,* impelled to do reckless things such as throwing a child through the window. Roams about. Strange notions and apprehension, during pregnancy. Rude, abusive, bites and strikes. Feels he cannot physically endure his fear much longer.

HEAD: Ache from bite of dog, whether rabid or not, < by noise of running water, bright light. Throws the head back when sneezing. Dry hair becomes oily.

MOUTH: Saliva tough, ropy, viscid, frothy; *spitting constantly.* Speech impeded from spasm of throat.

THROAT: Sore; constant desire to swallow which is difficult; gagging when swallowing water from spasm of gullet.

URINARY: Desire to urinate or for stool on seeing running water, or cannot urinate unless he hears water run.

MALE: Abnormal sexual desire. Painful erection of penis and frequent seminal emission. Semen is discharged too late or not at all during coition.

FEMALE: Consciousness of uterus. Vagina sensitive, rendering coition painful. Uterine displacement. Leukorrhea profuse, running down the legs. Strange notions, desires or cravings, during pregnancy.

RESPIRATORY: Barking cough.

HEART: Stitch on hearing church-bell. Pain as if needles were running into it.

NECK: Pain in neck, > bending head backward.

SLEEP: Yawns frequently without sleepiness, esp. when listening to others.

RELATED: Lac-c; Lach.

MAGNESIA CARBONICA

GENERALITIES: This remedy produces a catarrhal condition of *stomach* and bowels, with marked *acidity. Sour*—smell of the body (esp. children), vomiting, regurgitation, *stool,* etc. It affects the nerves (facial and dental), causing sharp, shooting pains *along them; must walk about.* Numbness, and a feeling of distension in various parts. Affections of malar bones. Whole body feels tired and painful, esp. legs and feet. It is suitable for ailing, worn out, *nervous, flatulent and flabby* persons, esp. women, children, nurslings. Sensitive to slight impression. *Emaciation.* Marasmus, children will not thrive in spite of feeding and medicines. Cannot bear hands covered, yet chilled by uncovering. Spasms. Epileptic attack, while walking or standing; he frequently falls down suddenly, with consciousness. Ill effects of shock, blow, mental distress, vexation, fit of passion, pregnancy, excess of care and worry, dentition, injudicious feeding; milk. Dryness of mucous membranes, skin. Children disposed to boils. Glands enlarged.

WORSE: *Cold;* wind, drafts. *Change of weather.* Night. Starchy food, milk. Rest. Slight causes, touch, etc. Uncovering. Every second day, every three weeks.

BETTER: *Motion. Walking about;* in open air. Warm air.

MIND: Trembling; anguish and fear as if some accident would happen, > when going to bed. Least touch causes starting. Sad and taciturn. Dazed feeling, packs and unpacks her clothes, without consciousness of having done so.

HEAD: Vertigo, < when kneeling. Pain in the head, as if the hair were pulled, < mental exertion, stooping. Itching of scalp, < in damp weather. Brain heavy. Sinking of occipital bone in marasmic children.

EYES: Black moles before the eyes. Eye-balls feel enlarged and sensitive to pressure. Opacity of cornea. Cataract, lenticular.

EARS: *Deafness, comes suddenly* and varies. Feeling of distension in middle ear. Ears numb. Deafness on taking cold, cutting wisdom tooth.

NOSE: Coryza and nasal stoppage before menses. Dry coryza; breathes through mouth. Chronic affection of nose.

FACE: Tearing, digging, boring pain on one side, must move about. Pain and swelling of the malar bones, < cold wind. Tumor of the malar bones. Waxy pallor. Slovenly expression. Tension as of white of an egg dried on face.

MOUTH: Tearing, digging, burning toothache, < during pregnancy, motion of carriage, cold, and when quiet. Ailments from cutting wisdom teeth. Teeth feel too long. Mouth dry at night. Taste bitter, sour. Frequent sudden stammering speech.

THROAT: Sore throat, < before menses. Hawks up cheesy masses from throat. Sticking pain in throat, < talking and swallowing .

STOMACH: Craving for meat, fruits, acids, vegetables. Nibbling appetite. Sour eructations. Heartburn. Vomits undigested milk or bitter water. Violent thirst. Aversion to green food. Cabbage, potato disagree. Milk is refused, causes pain in stomach.

ABDOMEN: *Cutting;* griping; pressing colic, followed by thin green stools, which <. STOOLS *frothy,* GREENISH, LIKE WATER, LIKE A SCUM OF FROG POND. *Milk* passes undigested in nursing children. Sour stool. Constipation after mental shock or nervous strain. Stool lienteric, with gelatinous fatty masses; grass green, or dry, hard, crumbling; white clay, putty-like. Colic followed by leukorrhea. Cutting about navel, > passing flatus.

URINARY: Involuntary urination while walking or rising from a seat.

MALE: Discharge of prostatic fluid when passing flatus.

FEMALE: Menses, like thick dark molasses, *tarry,* viscid; too late, or scanty; flow only in sleep, *at night* and on rising or when lying down, ceases when walking, or by pressure on abdomen and on stooping. Leaves a fast stain. Leukorrhea white, acrid, preceded by colic, regularly after the menses. Falls down in a dead faint at each menstruation period.

RESPIRATORY: Craves open air. Cough paroxysmal, with difficult, thin, salty, bloody expectoration. Chest sore, constricted. Cough from tickling in the larynx, at night.

EXTREMITIES: Heavy, weary feet. Right shoulder painful, cannot raise it. Cannot bear hands covered, yet chilled by uncovering. Cannot put left foot on ground when walking. Swelling in poplitea.

SLEEP: Unrefreshing, more tired in the morning than on retiring. Awakes at 2 or 3 a.m. and cannot fall asleep again. Sleepiness during the day, sleepless at night.

SKIN: Sore, dry, sensitive to cold. Nodosities under the skin. Hair and nails unhealthy.

FEVER: Chilly, takes cold, before menses. Fever at night. Sour, greasy, indelible sweat.

RELATED: Rheum.

MAGNESIA MURIATICA

GENERALITIES: The action of this remedy centers around the LIVER, NERVES, *uterus and rectum,* so it is adapted to *nervous* women suffering from utero-hepatic complaints or cardiac symptoms, or for those who have suffered for a long time from indigestion and biliousness; for men with disordered liver and sexual disorders; for puny rickety children during dentition. Spasmodic, *hysterical complaints.* Globus. It is an after-dinner remedy, complaints such as fainting fit, dyspnea, nausea, trembling, etc., occur after dinner, > by eructations. Pains are boring, spasmodic, contractive, *crampy,* darting. *Burning.* Chronicity. Ill effects of sea- bathing, esp. weakness. Shocks through the body electric-like, when wide awake. Perversions of taste and smell. General soreness, and sensitiveness to noise.

WORSE: *Lying on right side. Noise. Night. Eating. Salty foods. Milk. Touch.* Sea-bathing. Mental exertion.

BETTER: Hard Pressure. Lying bent. *Hanging down affected part. Gentle motion. Cool open air.*

MIND: Uneasiness; nervous excitability with tendency to weep. Feels as if some one was riding after her and she must keep riding faster and faster. Disinclined to talk.

HEAD: Bursting headache; < motion, open air; > hard pressure, wrapping warmly. Much sweating of head. As of boiling water on the side lain on. As if hair were pulled.

EYES: Lacrimation and burning of the eyes when looking at anything in broad daylight. Yellow sclera. Tinea ciliaris.

EARS: Sensitive to noise. Pulsations in ears.

NOSE: Red, swollen. Acrid, crusty ozena. Loss of smell and taste, following or with coryza. Nocturnal obstruction of nose, must breathe through the mouth.

FACE: Pale, yellow. Pimples on the face and forehead itching, < night, warm room and before menses. Blisters on lips.

MOUTH: Toothache, < if food touches the tooth. Tongue feels burnt, mouth feels scalded. Continued rising of white froth into the mouth. *Loss of taste. Broad yellow scalloped tongue.*

THROAT: Sensation of a ball rising into the throat, > by eructation.

STOMACH: Craves sweets, dainties. Hunger but knows not for what. Regurgitation while walking. Milk, salty food, <. Eructations like rotten egg, like onion. Hiccough during and after dinner, causing vomiting.

ABDOMEN: *Sore, enlarged liver,* with bloating of abdomen, < lying on right side, drags if lies on left side. Cramp in the gall-bladder, > by eating. Flatulence. STOOLS DRY, *knotty,* of little balls, like sheep dung, gray, crumbling at anus. Absence of desire for stool. Jaundice. Tapeworms. Colic, hysterical, followed by leukorrhea. Pain from liver to spine or epigastrium.

URINARY: Urine can only be passed by bearing down with the abdominal muscles. Urethra numb; in the dark one cannot tell whether urine is passing or not. Stricture after dilatation. Urine passes in drops, some always seems to remain.

MALE: Pain in testes and cords, < after coition, or after unrequited sexual excitement. Burning in back after coition.

FEMALE: Menses: *profuse, dark, lumpy,* like pitch; with cramps, backache and pain in the thighs; more copious when sitting than walking. Dysmenorrhea, > by pressure on the back, or lying on a hard pillow. *Gushes of leukorrhea, follow* colic in abdomen, uterine spasms, after every stool, in hysteria. Metrorrhagia of old maids, blood clotted.

RESPIRATORY: Spasmodic dry cough, < for e part of the night. Bloody sputum or congestion and soreness of chest, after sea-bathing. Oppressed breathing, globus hystericus.

HEART: Palpitation and cardiac pain while sitting, > by moving about or lying on left side. Functional cardiac affections, with liver enlargement.

NECK & BACK: Throbbing below left scapula. Bruised sensation or burning in hips; or in back after coition (male). Cramp in back, < walking.

EXTREMITIES: Cramp in thighs, < sitting. Thighs and calves tense; must move limbs. Finger tips numb. Ankles cold or nervous, < night. Cutting in heels. Feet sweaty.

SKIN: Formication all over the body. Abscess, yellow thin foul pus. Jaundice. Sweat on head and feet.

SLEEP: Anxiety and restlessness of the body as soon as she closes the eyes, from heat of the body or from shock. Sleep unfreshing, tired in morning.

FEVER: Chill even near a stove, > open air.

RELATED: Nat-m; Puls; Sep.

MAGNESIA PHOSPHORICA

GENERALITIES: Dr. Schuessler's remedy for *cramps, convulsions, neuralgic* pains and spasmodic effects, showing its influence on NERVES and *muscles*. Suitable for tall, slender, dark and neurotic persons, or tired, languid, exhausted subjects. *Nervous, tense, and subject to sudden violent paroxysms of neuralgic pain,* sharp, *shooting like lightning, suddenly changing places,* radiating, boring, constricting, extorting cries, causing restlessness and prostration. *Twitchings.* Tic. Spasmodic effects—hiccough, yawning, chorea. writer's cramps, piano or violin player's cramp. Much pain. Ill effects of standing in cold water, cold bathing, working in cold clay, catheterization, dentition, study. Complaints of teething children. Chorea, > during sleep, < at stool and by emotions. Palsy, paralysis agitans.

WORSE: COLD AIR, draft, water. Lying on right side. *Touch. Periodicity.* NIGHT. Milk. *Exhaustion.*

BETTER: *Warmth. Hot bath. Pressure. Doubling up. ubbing.*

MIND: *Always talking of her pain.* Indisposition to study and mental work. Drowsiness on every attempt to study. Talks to himself constantly, or sits in moody silence, or carries things from one place to another and back.

HEAD: Aches after mental labor, > by warmth. Sensation as if contents were liquid, as if parts of brain were changing places, as if a cap on head, as if an electric shock in the head extending to all parts of the body.

EYES: Supra-orbital pains > warmth. Twitching of eyelids. Eyes hot, aching, tired. Nystagmus, strabismus, ptosis. Photophobia.

EARS: Severe neuralgic pain, < going into cold air, washing face and neck with cold water; worse behind right ear.

FACE: Neuralgia, < when body gets cold, from washing or standing in cold water, on opening mouth to eat or drink.

MOUTH: Cracks in angles of lips. Toothache, > heat and hot liquids. Tongue clean, with colic. Painful contraction of jaw joint with backward jerking. Taste of banana. Food does not taste right. Spasmodic stammering.

THROAT: Stiff, sore; parts seem puffy (right), with chilliness and aching all over. Nervous angina.

STOMACH: Hiccough day and night. Burning pain, vomiting and hiccough > by hot drink; cancer of stomach. Thirst for very cold drinks.

ABDOMEN: Enteralgia, flatulent colic, > bending double, rubbing, warmth, pressure; with eructations which may or may not relieve. Bloated, full sensation in abdomen, must loosen the clothes, walk about, and constantly pass flatus. Cutting into thighs. Abdomen, contracted. Diarrhea ceases and spasm or brain troubles set in.

URINARY: Noctural enuresis from nervous irritation. Vesical neuralgia after use of catheter.

FEMALE: Menstrual colic, > by flow. Membranous dysmenorrhea. Menses too early, dark, stringy, tarry, flowing at night, leaving a fast stain. Ovarian neuralgia. Vaginismus.

RESPIRATION: Spasmodic. Whooping cough, > cool air. Spasmodic nervous asthma.

HEART: Angina pectoris. Pulse irritable. Nervous palpitation.

NECK & BACK: Stiffness of neck and back. Cramps. One vertebra seems absent.

EXTREMITIES: Skin of fingers tight. Pain in lower limbs, alternating sides. Paralysis agitans. Trembling of hands. Writer's, instrument cramp. Cramp from prolonged exertion, prolonged use of tools. Crampy contraction of fingers. Sciatica with tender feet.

SKIN: Barber's itch. Herpetic eruptions with white scales.

SLEEP: Sleepy when attempting to study. Spasmodic yawning as if it would dislocate the jaw, with tears.

FEVER: Chill runs up and down the back, with shivering followed by suffocation.

RELATED: Coloc; Dios.

MAGNESIA SULPHURICA

GENERALITIES: Skin, urinary and female symptoms are marked. Diarrhea with diuresis. Greenish urine with red sediment. Profuse, dark intermittent menses. Thick leukorrhea as profuse as menses. Lumpy feeling between shoulders. Back feels broken. Left arm and foot numb. Crawling in fingertips. Small pimples all over the body which itch violently. Warts large, soft.

WORSE: Morning, on awakening.

BETTER: Rubbing. Walking.

RELATED: Nat-s.

MAGNETIS POLUS AUSTRALIS

GENERALITIES: South pole of magnet is useful for ingrowing toe nails, with sore pain on the inner side of the nail of big toe, < walking or slight touch.

MALANDRINUM

GENERALITIES: This nosode is prepared from the virus of grease - a horse disease. It is very effectual protection against small pox and for ill effects of vaccination. Clears the remnants of cancerous deposits.

MANCINELLA

GENERALITIES: This remedy produces marked *skin*, throat and mental symptoms, esp. depressed states at puberty and climaxis with exalted sexuality. Acridity. Burning, smarting, in various parts. Favors rapid healing of wounds.

WORSE: *Cold drink, cold* feet. Anger. Dampness. Eating. Touch. Puberty, climaxis.

MIND: Sudden vanishing of thoughts, forgets what she wishes to do next, her errand. *Fear of insanity,* of evil spirits. Depressed with sexual erethism. Bashful. Melancholic. Homesick.

HEAD: Feels empty, with vertigo, while walking about. Hair falls after acute sickness. Pain in vertex, < lying.

EYES: *Lids heavy* and sore. Eyes smart or *burn on closing* them. Dull ache behind the eyes. Intense inflammation; with loss of vision (for some days). Photophobia.

NOSE: Illusion of smell—of gunpowder, dung, etc.

FACE: *Swollen*, spotted. Herpes on lips.

MOUTH: *Profuse foul yellow saliva*. Burning and pricking in the mouth, not > by cold water.

THROAT: *Cutting pain, < cold drink. Choking sensation* rises in the throat when speaking, preventing drinking though thirsty. Diphtheria. Tonsils swollen.

STOMACH: Craves cold water. Swollen epigastrium. Vomiting of food, followed by severe colic and profuse diarrhea. Aversion to meat, bread, wine. Feels flame rising from stomach. Repeated green vomit.

ABDOMEN: Bowels sore and burn. Colic, < cold drink.

RESPIRATORY: Cough, < cold drink. Aching behind the sternum.

HEART: Pulse weak, very large and soft. Needle-like stitches at heart.

EXTREMITIES: *Biting vesicles on soles;* desquamation and dryness of soles. Pain in thumb. Acrid, sticky foot sweat.

SKIN: Vesicles. Large blisters as from scald. Brown crusts and scabs. Pemphigus. Dermatitis; with extensive vesiculation, oozing sticky serum and forming crusts.

RELATED: Arum-t; Canth; Rhus-t.

MANGANUM

GENERALITIES: *Manganese* is closely associated with iron and like iron it causes anemia with destruction of red blood corpuscles. Moreover, it has special affinity for INNER EAR, *larynx, trachea, periosteum* of *shinbone, joints, ankles* and *lower limbs*. Motor paralysis, ascending. Paralysis agitans, paraplegia, come under its influence. *Bones are very sensitive. Pain, deep soreness* of the whole body, every part of the body feels sore when touched—*ears, joints,* skin. Pain extends to ear from other parts. *Everything affects the ear. Diagonal pains.* Yellow-green lumpy or bloody discharges. Chronic arthritis; with infiltrated glistening joints. Weak joints. *Festination,* walks backward. Growing pains and weak ankles. Progressive muscular atrophy. Cellulitis, subacute stage. Suppuration of skin around joints. Asthmatic persons, who cannot lie on a feather pillow. Fatty degeneration. Wants to lie down in bed which > all the troubles. Typhoid fever, badly treated, with prolonged convalescence. Valuable for boys and girls whose voices are changing. Necrosis and caries of bones. Malignant ulcer with blue border, following slight injury.

WORSE: Change of weather. *Touch. Cold. Damp. Night. Speaking. Feather bed.* Laughing. Motion. Bending backward.

BETTER: *Lying down.* Open air. *Sad music.* Eating. Swallowing. Change of weather.

MIND: Constant moaning or groaning. Weak and nervous. Anxiety and fear. Involuntary laughing and weeping. Anxiety and fear when moving in the room > lying down. Anxiety, as if something bad is going to happen. Sad, weeping, silent. All mental conditions are > lying down. Does not enjoy joyous music, but immediately affected by the sad.

HEAD: Feels heavy, seems larger. Pains from above downward, < straining at stool, jarring, stepping.

EYES: Field of vision contracted. Aching in the eyes, from sewing, reading fine print.

EARS: *Everything affects the ears;* pain extends to ear from other parts. Ears feel stopped. Deafness in damp weather. Tinnitus. Swelling of the parotid glands, in fever. Blowing the nose > deafness. Stitching in the ears, from talking, laughing, swallowing. Cracking, < blowing nose and swallowing.

NOSE: Blowing is painful. Crampy pain at the root of the nose. Dry coryza, with complete obstruction. Obstruction of nose and fluent coryza alternately.

FACE: Pale, sickly; stolid mask-like. Twitching, jerking pain from lower jaw to temples, < laughing.

MOUTH: Nodes on palate and tongue. Toothache, < by anything cold or sucking; goes up in the ears. Flow of saliva, while speaking, with colic, paralysis, etc. Taste oily.

THROAT: Hemming and hawking all the time annoying everybody.

ABDOMEN: Chronic enlargement of the liver. Jaundice. Feels as if intestines were loose and shaking when walking about. Pain and constriction at the navel. Passes much flatus with stools. Bowels are irregular, he has constipation or diarrhea. Cramp in the anus while sitting, > lying down. Cutting in umbilical region, < on taking deep breath.

URINARY: Darting in urethra on passing flatus.

FEMALE: First menses delayed. Menses early, scanty, pale in anemic patients. *Climacteric flushings.* Discharge of blood between periods.

RESPIRATORY: Chronic hoarseness, voice rough, < a.m., > by expectoration of greenish or yellow lump of mucus, or smoking. Cough, > lying down, < reading, laughing; with aphonia. Every cold rouses up as bronchitis. Aphonia from laryngeal tuberculosis. Larynx dry and sore.

EXTREMITIES: Weak, uncertain legs. Cannot walk backwards without falling. Walks stooping. Slapping gait. Walks on metatarso-phalangeal joint; walks backward. Tendency to fall forward. Inflammation of bones and joints, with nightly digging pains; pain in shin bones. Inflamed ankles. Children are unable to walk on account of affection of ankles. Paralysis, with inclination to run forward if he tries to walk. Knees pain and itch. Hands, when closed and stretched, feel swollen.

SKIN: Rough, cracked (flexures), bluish. Suppuration of skin around joints. Red elevated spots. Chronic eczema, with amenorrhoea, < menses or menopause. Dry hard ulcers. Pruritus of diabetes. Chronic eruptions, inveterate, like psoriasis.

SLEEP: Many vivid dreams which are well remembered. Much yawning.

FEVER: Sudden flushes of heat, in face, chest and over the back.

RELATED: Chin; Psor.

MARUM VERUM (TEUCRIUM)

GENERALITIES: NASAL AND RECTAL symptoms are very marked. *Excitable* and *oversensitive*, from abuse of medicines and when they fail to act. Delicate old persons and children. Internal tremor, < excitement. Desire to stretch. Threadworms. Polypi—nasal, vaginal, in ear, etc. Fibrous tumor.

WORSE: Weather changing; damp cold. In bed. Touch. Stooping. Sitting. Side lain on. Rubbing gently.

BETTER: Open air. Sweat.

MIND: Desire to sing. Mental excitement and loquacity. Very indolent, does not want to do mental or physical labor.

HEAD: Frontal pain, < stooping.

EYES: Smarting in canthi. Eyelids red and puffy. Tarsal tumor.

EARS: Hissing sound when passing hand over ear, when talking or forcibly inspiring through the nose. Itching. Polypus.

NOSE: *Crawling, must pick it,* with lacrimation and sneezing. Stoppage of nose, < side lain on, on reading aloud. Chronic catarrh; atrophic; discharge of large, lumpy, irregular clinkers. Loss of smell. Mucous polypi. Solid lumps from posterior nares.

MOUTH: Itching in palate.

THROAT: Mouldy taste in throat when hawking or coughing. Follicular pharyngitis.

STOMACH: Constant hiccough; jerking, in emaciated children after nursing, with stitch from stomach to back. Vomiting of large quantities of dark green masses.

ABDOMEN: *Itching anus; prevents sleep.* Threadworms.

RESPIRATORY: Dry cough, < coughing.

EXTREMITIES: Ingrowing toe nails, with ulceration, > moving. Burning in the tips of fingers. Staggering walk, places one foot over the other.

SLEEP: Sleepless after excitement, from itching anus or skin, which lasts all night.

COMPLEMENTARY: Calc.

RELATED: Cina; Sil.

MEDORRHINUM

GENERALITIES: Prepared from gonorrheal virus, this nosode is a powerful deep-acting medicine indicated for chronic ailments due to suppressed gonorrhea. It affects the *mind, nerves, mucous membranes;* is useful in chronic pelvic disorders of women; for dwarfish and stunted, *sour*-smelling children. *Profuse acrid discharges, causing itching.* Fishy odor of the secretions. Offensive odor of the body, esp. children and women. Poor reaction due to *sycotic taint. Many different kinds of pain—stiffness, aching, soreness; edema of limbs;* dropsy of serous sacs. Emaciation. Trembling all over (subjective); intense nervousness and profound exhaustion. *Numbness*; formication internal. *Arthritic,* rheumatic pains. Diseases of the spinal cord, even organic lesions ending in paralysis. Enlargement of the lymphatic glands all over the body, with heat and soreness. Loss of power in the joints; joints feel loose. *Burning.* Small, very sore aphthae; blisters. States of collapse, wants to be fanned all the time. Tumor, Cancer, scirrhus, etc., with history of sycosis. Body smells bad to her, cannot wash.

WORSE: *Damp*; cold. *Daytime*; sunrise to sunset; 3-4 a.m. After urinating. Touch, even slight. Closed room. Before storm.

BETTER: Lying on Abdomen. Bending backward; stretching out. *Fresh air;* being fanned. *Hard rubbing.* Seaside. Dampness. Sunset. Damp weather.

MIND: Weak memory. Cannot concentrate. Forgets names, word, her errand. Cannot finish sentences. Loss of thread of conversation. Wild feeling. *Things seem strange.* Cannot speak without weeping; tells it over and over again. *Hurried*, and anxious; irritable. Time passes slowly. Fear in the dark, as of someone is behind her, whispering to her. *Sensitive, nervous,* impulsive, abrupt, rude, mean, cruel. Apprehensive, anticipates events. *Feels far off,* as though things done today occurred a week ago. Many ideas but uncertain of execution. *Sad,* dismal outlook, > weeping. Persistent ideas; alternating or erratic states. Cross through day, merry at night. Dread of saying wrong thing. Everything startles her. Noncommital. Suicidal thoughts. Fears going insane. Feels life *unreal*, everything seems unreal. Desperate. *Sad.* Tearful. Fearful.

HEAD: Vertigo, < in vertex, and on stooping. Head-pain, with a sense of tightness, < jarring of ears; pulls her hair. Burning in occiput; occipital pain goes to behind eyes. *Hair tousled.* Burning deep in brain. Head heavy and drawn backwards. Itching; dandruff.

EYES: Feels as if she stared at everything at one go, as if sticks in the eyelids. Ptosis. Eyelashes fall out, objects look double or small. Swelling under eyes. Sees imaginary objects. Upper lid hard as if it had cartilage in it.

EARS: Partial or total deafness. Ringhole sore and gathered. Pulsation in ears. Quick darting pains. Hears voices.

NOSE: Coryza, with loss of smell and taste. Snuffles in children, not relieved by other remedies. Epistaxis. Post nasal discharge, thick yellow. Exhalation *hot.* Hay fever. Nose dirty (children). Tip of nose cold. Intense itching of the tip. Coryza, > sea-bathing. Nasal catarrh running down throat.

FACE: Grayish, greasy, greenish; *yellow at the edges of hair. Red spiderlets* on face. Acne on face, < after menses. Small boils break out during menses. Lips thickened from mouth-breathing.

MOUTH: Small, very sore aphthae. Blisters on inner surface of the lips and cheeks. Water tastes like perfume. Teeth serrated, soft, crumbling, yellow. Tongue coated brown and thick.

STOMACH: Craving; for liquor which she used to dislike, salt, sweets, oranges, ice, sour things, green fruits, refreshing things. *Vomiting of pregnancy,* pernicious. Morning nausea. Excessive thirst, dreams of drinking water. Ravenous appetite, hunger after eating.

ABDOMEN: Heavy lower abdomen. Grinding colic, > bracing feet, lying on abdomen. Can pass stool only by leaning very far back, then shivering. Burning in epigastrium. Flatulence with numbness. Dark fetid oozing from anus, of fish brine odor. Anus *fiery red, moist, violently itching.* Cholera infantum, with opisthotonos. Agonizing pain in solar plexus, applies his right hand to stomach and left lumbar region.

URINARY: Noctural enuresis. Scalding ammoniacal urine. Pain in kidney region > by profuse urination, with craving for ice. Bubbling in kidney region. Slow flow.

MALE: Heaviness of prostate, painful and enlarged, with frequent and painful urination. Impotency. Prostration after seminal emission. Heaviness in perineum. Persistent gleety yellow discharge.

FEMALE: Intense menstrual colic, > pressing feet against support. Menses profuse, dark, clotted, foul; stain which difficult to wash out; with frequent urination. Mammae; cold, sore. Sore, oozing or icy nipples during menses. Blistering leukorrhea, thin, of fishy odor. Os uteri sensitive, ulcerated. Breast sore at non-menstrual periods. Itching vagina, > rubbing and by bathing with tepid water. Drawing in ovaries, > pressure. Sycotic sterility. Breast cold, icy, the rest of the body warm.

RESPIRATORY: Air hunger. *Cough, > lying on stomach,* < from sweet things. Dyspnea, cannot exhale. Asthma, sycotic, infantile. Lungs feel stuffed with cotton. Feels a cavity in chest. Coldness in chest.

HEART: Sensation of cavity where heart ought to be.

BACK: Spine sore and tender. Burning heat in spine. Cutting, burning, crawling above left scapula. Pain from left to right shoulder. Lumbago from lifting.

EXTREMITIES: Arms hairy. Bites nails. Burning of hands and feet. Legs heavy, ache all night, cannot keep them still. Cramps in legs, > stretching them. *Heels, balls and soles tender and itching,* cannot walk on them, has to walk on knees. Fingertips crack and burn. Ankles easily turn when walking. Edema of limbs. Nails depressed, as if bent. Edema of feet followed and > by diarrhea.

SKIN: Itching, sore. Sycotic red nodes. Deep red spots. Condylomata. Yellow. Continuous itching, < thinking of it. Skin cold but feels the blood hot. Copper-colored spots, remaining after eruption.

SLEEP: A short sleep seems a long one which > . *Sleeps in knee-chest position.* Dreams of drinking something.

FEVER: Burning heat with sweat; wants to uncover but is chilled thereby. Sweat easy, towards morning. Hay fever. Limbs become cold.

RELATED: Bar-c; Nat-m; Psor; Thuj.

MELILOTUS

GENERALITIES: This medicine produces *congestion,* esp. to the HEAD, and profuse bright red hemorrhage which gives relief. Infantile spasms. Epilepsy from blow to head. Pain with debility. Feeling of rawness.

WORSE: *Climacteric.* Walking. Weather *changing,* stormy, rainy.

BETTER: Bleeding. Profuse urination. Vinegar (application).

MIND: Wants to run away and hide. Fear of danger, of being arrested, of talking loudly—she whispers. Treacherous memory. Thinks everyone is looking at her. Wants to kill himself, or threatens to kill those who approach. Religious melancholy. Weeping.

HEAD: Rush of blood to head. VIOLENT THROBBING. Congestive, nervous, periodical headaches, threatens his reason, > nosebleed, menstrual flow, application of vinegar. Fulness all over the head. Headache alternates with backache.

EYES: Hot, heavy, wants to close them tightly for relief, as if they were too large.

NOSE: Dry, must breathe through the mouth. Profuse and frequent epistaxis, with general >.

FACE: *Intensely red;* and flushed with throbbing carotids and headache. Red before hemorrhage from nose, lungs, uterus.

URINARY: Frequent profuse urination (which relieves headache).

FEMALE: Recurring sharp darting pain in vagina and vulva at close of menses.

RESPIRATORY: Feels as if smothering, < rapid walking, as if clothes were too tight across chest.

SKIN: Dry.

RELATED: Bell; Calc; Glon.

MENYANTHES

GENERALITIES: It produces *icy coldness of prominent, single, or affected parts*—nose, ears, fingers, knees, abdomen, etc. Tensive and compressive pains. Spasmodic jerking and visible twitchings, with neuralgia. Jumpy, fidgety women with urinary troubles.

WORSE: Walking, even lightly. Ascending. Rest. Light. Noise. Jar.

BETTER: *Hard pressure.* Twilight. Lying on hand. Stooping.

HEAD: *Bursting headache,* pain ascends from nape, > stooping, sitting bent. *Heavy pressure on vertex,* > hard pressure with hand. Feels weight in nape. Head cold, as if cold wind blowing on it.

EYES: Misty vision.

EARS: Tinnitus, when chewing.

NOSE: Cold. Nauseous smell before nose, like that of rotten egg.

FACE: Visible twitching of the facial muscles, < rest.

STOMACH: Coldness extending to esophagus. Desire for meat. Aversion to bread and butter.

ABDOMEN: Coldness, < pressing with it hard.

URINARY: Frequent desire to urinate with scanty urine.

HEART: Anxiety, as if some evil were going to happen. Slightest exertion causes irregular action.

BACK: Boring at scapula (left). Bruised pain in sacrum, < stooping, walking.

EXTREMITIES: Cramp in posterior thigh, < sitting. Cramp from ankle to calf (right). Icy coldness of hands and feet. Legs jerk and twitch, < lying down.

SKIN: Feels tight.

SLEEP: Vivid dreams, with agitated sleep.

FEVER: Shivering with yawning. Quartan malaria.

RELATED: Verat.

MEPHITIS

GENERALITIES: This medicine is prepared from the liquid contained in the anal glands of skunk. It produces *spasmodic effects* and is a very great remedy for whooping cough. Should be given in the lower dilutions. Nervous exhaustion. Debility after severe illness. Wants to bathe in ice-cold water. Trembling and choking, with exophthalmos. Fine vibrations cause great uneasiness.

WORSE: Lying. Night. After menses.

BETTER: *Cold bath* or weather, *icy water*.

MIND: Excitable, full of fancies. Talkative. Disinclination to work, with inclination to stretch.

HEAD: Violent vertigo, < sitting, stooping, turning in bed. Feels a finger pressing on occiput. Headache from motion of carriage.

EYES: Hot, red, and painful. Inability to read fine print.

FACE: Bloated.

MOUTH: Foul breath.

THROAT: Food goes the wrong way. *Chokes easily,* when drinking and talking.

STOMACH: Vomits food hours after eating. Desire for salted food.

RESPIRATORY: Dyspnea; cannot exhale. Asthma, < ice water. Spasmodic or whooping cough; few paroxysms during the day-time but many at night. Cough violent, suffocative, spasmodic, nervous, < talking or drinking. Foul expectoration. Asthma of consumptives or drunkards.

SLEEP: Short, seems to refresh. Awakes at night with rush of blood to legs.

RELATED: Cor-r; Mosch.

MERCURIUS

GENERALITIES: The first potency is prepared (originally by Hahnemann) from soluble black oxide of mercury or from pure metallic mercury. There is no difference between the symptoms of these two preparations, but it seems that when Merc sol fails when indicated, Merc vivus acts. *Merc.* affects more or less every organ and tissue of the body. Blood decomposes producing profound anemia. LYMPHATIC GLANDS are enlarged, glandular activity, esp. of SALIVARY AND MUCOUS GLANDS, increases. SECRETIONS ARE FREE, *thin, slimy, acrid; burning, foul, thick greenish-yellow. Ulceration* of the mucous membranes, esp. of mouth and the throat. Manifestations of hereditary syphilis; bullae; abscess, marasmus. Snuffle, destructive inflammations of bones, *cellular tissues,* joints comes under its range. Patient suffers from great variety of symptoms; he is uncertain in his mental and physical behaviour, *tremulous,* weak and *sweaty. Swellings* edematous; continued exudations. Redness. Livid congestions. Pains stick to one point. *Suppuration;* pus bloody, thin, greenish. *Offensiveness* of secretions, breath, body. *Yellowness of* eyes, teeth, nasal discharges; biliousness; jaundice. Parts are much swollen, with raw, sore feeling. Sensitive to heat and cold—human barometer. Everything seems too short. *Weak, exhausted and ready to sink down,* < after stool. Rheumatism. Emaciation. Salty lips, taste, expectoration, etc. Oily perspiration. Syphilis, sycosis, scrofula. Convulsions. Cataleptic rigidity of the body. Paralysis agitans; paraplegia. Contraction of joints. Ill-effects of fright, suppressed gonorrhea and footsweat. Feels body made of sweets. Burning, stinging pains. Trembling; disorderly motion of paralyzed parts. Stricture after inflammation. Indurations. Exostoses, painful. Softening of the bones.

WORSE: NIGHT air. SWEATING. LYING ON RIGHT SIDE. WHEN HEATED *in bed* or from fire. DRAFT to head. *Weather - changing, cloudy, damp cold. Taking cold.* Heat and cold. Wet feet. Fire light. Before stool. During and after urination. Touching anything cold.

BETTER: Moderate temperature. Coition. Rest.

MIND: *Hurried,* in speech. Stammering, nervous, with tremors. Violent, hurried impulses—homicidal, suicidal. Restless and sweaty. Changes the place constantly. Fear with desire to escape. Uncontrollable desire to travel far away. Indifference to everything, does not even care to eat. Inclination to catch passing strangers by the nose. Filthy in mind and body; does foolish, mischievous, disgusting actions. Slow in answering questions. Weary of life. Suicidal thoughts during menses, > weeping. Thinks he is losing his reason. Memory weak; forgets everything. Loss of willpower. Senses impending evil. Precocious. Groaning and moaning. Suspicious. Time passes slowly.

HEAD: Vertigo, < lying on back; feels as if on a swing. Band feeling about the head. Headache, with ear and toothache. Exostosis with feeling of soreness. Scalp tense, oily sweat on head. Meningitis. Hydrocephalus. Child turns head from side to side and moans. External head painful to touch. Cephalohematoma. Falling of hair from sides and temples.

EYES: Lids; red, thick, swollen; tarsii scurfy and swollen. Scanty or profuse burning acrid discharge. Eyes drawn together. Black spots, flames, sparks before the eyes. Photophobia, < heat and glare of fire; of foundrymen. Arcus senilis. Iritis; with hypopion. Keratitis. Lacrimation profuse, burning, acrid. Conjunctivitis from taking cold. Lids spasmodically closed. Periodical loss of sight. Optic nerve and eye affection in those who work in foundries. Foggy vision.

EARS: *Pains extend to ear from teeth,* throat, etc. Otorrhea thick yellow discharge, fetid and bloody. Deafness on becoming heated; > on swallowing and blowing nose. Boil in external canal. Sensation of cold water running from the ear, of coldness in ears, during pregnancy.

NOSE: Much sneezing. Sneezing in sunshine. Nostrils raw, ulcerated. *Colds travel upward* or attacks eyes. Coryza acrid, purulent, too thick to run. Heavy nose. Red, raw, dirty nose of children. Nosebleed, when coughing, during sleep, blood hangs in dark coagulated strings. Frequent sneezing, without coryza. Sinusitis.

FACE: Pale, yellow, dirty looking; puffy under eyes. *Cheeks swollen,* red, hot. Aching in jaws. Mumps. Lips salty, dry, cracked in angles (right), burn when touched. Masseter muscles contracted. Facial paralysis from cold.

MOUTH: Offensive, putrid odor from mouth. Painful ragged, swollen, *bleeding gums.* Gumboil. Teeth hollow, black; pain, < heat and cold, night; feel tender and elongated. Aphthae. SALIVA INCREASED, *flows during sleep; yellow, bloody,* bad-tasting, offensive. Tongue broad, flabby, yellow, INDENTED; needle pricks at tip. Furrow across upper portion of the tongue, with pricking.

Sweetish, Metallic Taste. Speech difficult from trembling of tongue. Loss of speech, replies by signs and grimaces. Stammering. Ranula, with salivation and sore gums. Itching palate. Ulcers behind the tongue. Tonsils enlarged. Feels something rising in the throat, with desire to swallow it down. Taste sweetish, bread tastes sweet. Stomatitis from chewing gum.

THROAT: Sore, raw, smarting, burning. Sensation of hot vapor ascending; an apple core, choke pear, or something hanging. Ulcers on tonsils, on pharynx. Quinsy, with difficult swallowing, after pus has formed. Stitches into ears on swallowing. Hawks large lumps from throat. Constant inclination to swallow. Drinks return through nose.

STOMACH: Intense thirst for cold drink and beer. Weak digestion, with continuous hunger. Feels replete and constricted. Aversion to meat, coffee, butter and oily things. Sweet things and milk disagree, though he craves them. Rancid eructations. Frequent hiccough. Heartburn.

ABDOMEN: Liver *enlarged, sore,* indurated. *Jaundice.* Bowels feel weak, holds them. Intestines feel bruised when lying on right side, or as if they fall to side on which one is lying. Inguinal glands swollen or suppurating. Stools painful, scanty, bloody, *greenish slimy;* ashen white, acrid; then tenesmus or chill; never-get-done feeling. Rectal tenesmus with tenesmus of bladder. Appendicitis, > lying on back. Prolapsus ani after stool. Swelling of inguinal glands on taking cold. Dysentery. External abdomen cold to touch.

URINARY: Frequent urging to urinate day and night, with copious or scanty urine. Urine causes itching. Urinates more than drinks. Albuminuria, urine black, bloody. Burning after urination. Stream of urine very small. Dysuria. Hematuria, painless.

MALE: Glans and prepuce inflamed and swollen; phimosis. Testicles swollen, hard, with shiny red scrotum. Pulls and scratches at the genitals from a kind of itching which makes him do so. Bloody emissions. Gonorrhea. Red meatus. Vesicles, ulcers, soft chancres. Herpes preputialis. Swelling of lymphatic vessels along penis.

FEMALE: Collapse and fainting at start of menses. Menses; profuse with abdominal pains. Genitals feel raw. Leukorrhea thick, white, when urinating, > coition. Itching, < urination, > washing with cold water. Prolapse of uterus with vagina, > coition. Mammae painful and full of milk at menses. Sterility, with too profuse menses. Easy coitus and certain conception. Stinging pain in ovary. Pain below (right) mammae through to scapula. Tendency to abortion from sheer weakness. Abscesses appear anywhere on body during menses and disappears after menses. Leukorrhea in small girls causing prostration. Mammae swollen, become hard, with ulcerative pain during menses. Cancer of mammae and uterus. Itching of vulva. Milk spoiled. Milk in breast of boys; and in girls instead of menses.

RESPIRATORY: Hoarse, rough voice. Cough in double bouts, dry at night, yellow-green sputum by day. Respiration difficult, < lying on left side, but cough < lying on right side. Stitches from lower right chest to back, < sneezing or coughing. Sensation of bubbles or hot steam in chest. Epistaxis during whooping cough. Cough < by smoking. Jaundice; in pneumonia. Shortness of breath on going upstairs or walking quickly. Asthma, > tobacco smoke and cold air.

HEART: Palpitation on slight exertion. Awakes with cardiac tremor. Pulse irregular, quick, strong and intermittent, or soft and trembling.

NECK & BACK: *Neck stiff;* cervical glands enlarged. Burning pain in back, < emission. Tearing pain in coccyx, < pressing on abdomen. Pain goes forward from right scapula.

EXTREMITIES: Weakness and trembling of the limbs, esp. of hands. Fingers numb. Cold sweat on feet in a.m., in bed. Phlegmasia alba dolens. Dropsical swelling of feet and legs. Icy cold hands after emission. Bone-pains deep or near the surface, < at night; must get up and walk about. Cold heels. Sensation as if knees were larger.

SKIN: General tendency to free perspiration but patient is not relieved thereby, skin always moist. Skin yellow, tender, excoriated, like raw meat. Moist crusty eruptions. *Ulcers;* irregular, spreading, shallow, bleeding, with cutting and proud flesh. Pimples around the main eruption. Boils and abscesses form at the time of menses. Jaundice with itching on abdomen. Itching at night in bed. Moist eczema. Insensible.

SLEEP: Sleepless at night from ebullition of blood (to chest and head), from nervous excitability, from pain or other troubles.

FEVER: Easily chilled or *overheated.* Alternate chill and heat. Creeping chills. Chilly with abscesses. Catarrhal, gastric, bilious fever. Measles. Fever after suppression. EASY PROFUSE SWEAT *without relief,* during sleep, with pains; oily, foul, sour or with strong sweetish penetrating odor; on head, chest; stains indelibly yellow.

COMPLEMENTARY: Bell; Sil.

RELATED: Kali-i.

MERCURIUS CORROSIVUS

GENERALITIES: *Merc cor* is a powerful disinfectant and has much greater rapidity of action, causing *violent effects*. It causes tenesmus of RECTUM along with tenesmus of bladder. Inflammation with swelling and feeling of constriction. *Burning, internal*, in throat, stomach, *rectum, neck of bladder*, kidneys, etc. *Constriction* of throat, rectum, bladder, etc. Discharges acrid—tears, nasal discharge, etc. Cracks on palms, soles, corners of mouth. Phagedena. Syphilis. Albuminuria in early pregnancy (Phos later and at full term). Gonorrhea. Lies on back with knees drawn up.

WORSE: AFTER URINATION AND STOOL. *Swallowing. Night. Cold. Autumn*. Hot days, cool nights. Acids.

BETTER: Rest.

MIND: Anxious and restless; *rocks hard*. Stares at persons who talk to him, and does not understand them. Difficult thinking. Disturbed speech. Stupid.

HEAD: Pain in temples, < looking sideways. Vertigo with deafness when stooping.

EYES: Excessive photophobia and acrid lacrimation. Burning. Soreness of the eyes. Iritis. Keratitis. Retinitis—albuminuric, hemorrhagic. Ophthalmia neonatorum. Lids edematous, red, excoriated. Objects appear smaller, or double vision.

EARS: Violent pulsation in ears. Fetid pus.

NOSE: Fluent acrid coryza. Ozena with perforation of septum. Gluey nasal discharge. Swollen red nose.

FACE: *Pale about mouth*. Cracks in angles of the mouth. Edematous swelling of the face. Lips black, dark red, swollen. Upper lip swollen and turned up. Jaws stiff.

MOUTH: Tongue patchy, swollen and inflamed. Could not be protruded. Salivation, with salty taste. Pyorrhea, Gums purple, swollen, with toothache; spongy. Aphthae, ulcers. Burning, scalding sensation in mouth. Teeth loose, nightly toothache. *Taste; astringent,* salty, bitter. Necrosis of lower jaw.

THROAT: Uvula red, swollen, elongated. Sore, red, painful swelling, < heat; sharp pain goes into ears, < pressure. Burning pain and great swelling, < slightest pressure. All glands about the throat swollen. Tonsils swollen, covered with ulcers. SWALLOWING DIFFICULT; spasmodic constriction, on attempting to swallow a drop of liquid.

STOMACH: Insatiable thirst, for cold drink. Distension and soreness of the pit of stomach; cramp in epigastrium, < least touch. Vomits mucus and blood. Gastritis. Regurgitation, astringent. Great desire for cold food.

ABDOMEN: Bloated, painful to least touch. Cutting colic, below navel. Painful flatulence. Appendicitis. *Continuous urging to stool and urine.* A NEVER-GET-DONE FEELING. STOOLS BLOODY, SHREDDY, SLIMY; HOT WITH TORMENTING TENESMUS. Passes pure blood or bloody water. Dysentery. Spasm of rectum during coition. Sweat before and after stool.

URINARY: Intense burning in urethra. Urine HOT, BURNING, PASSED DROP BY DROP, *scanty,* suppressed, bloody, frequent; dribbling, < sitting. Urethra bleeds after urinating. *Tenesmus of bladder* with tenesmus of rectum. Nephritis. Albuminuria, of pregnancy. Cystitis. Gonorrhea. Paraphimosis. Bleeding kidneys. Sweats after urination.

MALE: Penis and testes enormously swollen. Chordee, < sleep. Hard chancre. Gonorrhea, discharge thick greenish.

FEMALE: Leukorrhea, pale yellow, with sweetish nauseous smell. Glandular swellings about the nipples. Nipples crack and bleed; pain, < when nursing. Menses too early and too profuse.

RESPIRATORY: Breathes as if through a metallic tube. Constriction of the chest, Breathes through pectoral muscles. Cutting pain in larynx. Frequent stitches shoot through thorax.

HEART: Palpitation during sleep.

BACK: Pott's disease, lies on back with knees drawn up.

EXTREMITIES: Deltoid feels relaxed. Sensation as if legs had gone to sleep. Cramp in calves, in dysentery. Paralysis of limbs; trembling. Feet icy cold. Exostoses on shin, sternum, ribs.

SKIN: Cold. Ulcers—perforating; spreading; serpiginous. Nails grey-colored.

SLEEP: Violent hiccough during sleep.

FEVER: Chilly after stools. *Sweats from every motion*; partial, < forehead and lower parts; foul; at night. Heat when stooping and coldness when rising.

RELATED: Ars; Canth.

MERCURIUS CYANATUS

GENERALITIES: A valuable remedy for toxemia of acute infectious diseases, esp. diphtheria, when there is *early, rapid and extreme* prostration, with *cyanosis, coldness* and *tremor*. Affects most prominently MOUTH, THROAT and LARYNX. Rapid local destruction. *Putridity.* Hemorrhage of dark fluid blood. Twitching and jerking of muscles. Efficient prophylactic in diphtheria.

WORSE: Swallowing. Speaking. Eating.

MIND: Great excitement; fits of passion. Fury. Talkativeness.

HEAD: Atrocious headache, < night.

EYES: Sunken; fixed.

NOSE: Profuse epistaxis several times a day.

MOUTH: Covered with ulcerations, with gray membrane. Free salivation. Fetor of breath.

THROAT: *Cutting pain*, on swallowing. Much thick grayish membrane in the throat. Looks raw in spots esp. in public speakers. Tonsils enlarged. Necrotic destruction of soft parts of palate and fauces. Septic diphtheria.

STOMACH: Early and complete anorexia. Incessant hiccough. Thought of food causes retching. Milk >

ABDOMEN: Frequent diarrhea preceded by severe colic. Stools; offensive, green, slimy, bloody, black.

URINARY: Urine albuminous, amber-yellow, scanty, suppressed.

RESPIRATORY: Cutting pain in larynx. Hoarseness, talking painful. Croupy cough, causes suffocation.

HEART: *Weak.*

EXTREMITIES: Varicose veins with great tenderness of leg (left). Cold limbs.

SKIN: Moist and cold. *Sweatiness.*

RELATED: Lach.

MERCURIUS DULCIS

GENERALITIES: Calomel produces catarrhal inflammation of the *ear* and is useful in *eustachian catarrh* and deafness. Inflammation with plastic exudates; peritonitis; meningitis; pleurisy. Has a reabsorbent action. Pale mucous membranes. *Biliousness*, remittent bilious fevers. Pallor; *flabby bloatedness*. Pale scrofulous children who have swelling of cervical and other glands. Dropsy due to combined renal and cardiac diseases, esp. with jaundice. Biliary stasis.

WORSE: Acids.

BETTER: Cold drink.

HEAD: Painful scalp.

EYES: Rapid winking. Closure of lacrimal duct. Eyes; red, dry, gummy.

EARS: Closure of eustachian tubes. Membrana tympani retracted, thickened. Deafness; from every cold; of old age. Sudden fluttering.

NOSE: Blows lumps of mucus from nose.

FACE: Pallid.

MOUTH: Tongue; indented; indurated; black. Constant flow of dark putrid saliva. Foetor oris.

THROAT: *Tonsils inflamed* (right), > cold drink. Dysphagia. Granular pharyngitis.

STOMACH: Cyclic vomiting of infants.

ABDOMEN: Bloated, hot, painful. Acrid, *grass-green* diarrhea of infants. Anus sore and burning. Hypertrophic cirrhosis of liver (use 1x).

MALE: Acute inflammation of prostate, after suppressed gonorrhea.

RESPIRATORY: Slimy, pussy sputum. Pleurisy.

SKIN: Flabby and ill-nourished. Copper-colored eruptions.

FEVER: Remittent bilious fever. Sweatiness.

RELATED: Kali-m.

MERCURIUS IODATUS FLAVUM

(Mercurius protoiodatus)

GENERALITIES: This remedy has a strong affinity for *glands,* of the THROAT, lymphatic and mammary glands. Right side is usually affected and like Lyc. symptoms go from right to left. Syphilis Mammary tumor. Deep bone pains, esp. at night.

WORSE: *Odor.* Raising up. Warm drink. Lying on left side. Cold and damp weather. Touch.

BETTER: Open air.

MIND: Lively, merry, talkative.

HEAD: *Faint or dizzy on rising from a chair,* or when reading. Dull frontal headache, with pain at the root of nose, > when mind and body are actively engaged. Head pain follows heart pain.

EYES: Keratitis; cornea looks scratched or chipped out by fingernail. Photophobia. Dark circles around the eyes. Swelling below right eye.

EARS: Sudden sharp pain in ears, < touch.

NOSE: Mucus descends through posterior nares into the throat, causing hawking.

MOUTH: Desire to clench the teeth; jaw is stiff and tired from grinding pain in teeth, during sleep. Teeth feel on edge, < heat, cold and sweets. Teeth feel too long, cannot eat. Pyorrhea. *Tongue moist, filmy coated,* or THICK YELLOW AT BASE; tip and edges red. Toothache after filling.

THROAT: *Sore* (right then left). Constant inclination to swallow. Tonsils swollen, > cold drink. Lacunar tonsillitis. Goitre with suffocation. Cervical glands swollen. Adenitis.

STOMACH: Weak, empty feeling in stomach. Nausea at the sight or smell of food. Thirst for sour drink.

ABDOMEN: Pain in abdomen with pain in heart. Faint sick feeling in hypogastrium before stools. Black discharge with or without stool.

URINARY: Urine copious, dark red, scanty.

MALE: Hard chancre, painless, with enlarged inguinal glands, not disposed to suppuration. Dreams of urination followed by seminal emission of which he knows nothing.

FEMALE: Yellow leukorrhea, of very young girls. Mammary tumors, with knots in axilla, blueness of the part, warm perspiration and gastric disturbance.

HEART: Pain preceded by head pain. Palpitation with dyspnea, < lying on back. Feeling as if heart had jumped out of its place.

EXTREMITIES: Knees numb. Laming pain in right arm, < writing. Pain right forearm, with pain in left hip.

SKIN: Flat warts.

RELATED: Lyc., Merc.

MERCURIUS IODATUS RUBER

(Mercurius bin iodatus)

GENERALITIES: Like *Merc-i-fl.* this salt also affects the *lymphatic glands,* THROAT, but on the left side. It acts on cellular tissue also, has wandering rheumatic pain with weariness. Early case of cold, esp. in children. Cuts short attack of asthma when given in 2x or 3x or prevents it developing during the night if given at bedtime. *Much hard glandular swelling.* Chronic suppurating buboes. Swellings.

WORSE: Empty swallowing, or swallowing food. After sleep. Weather changes. Washing floor. Getting wet. Touch and pressure. After dinner.

MIND: Ill humour. Disposed to cry.

HEAD: Painfully heavy occiput. Frontal region feels as if bound by a cord.

EYES: Granular eyelids. Trachoma.

EARS: Closure of eustachian tube, opens with a pop. Deafness, > after becoming warm on walking.

NOSE: Coryza with right side of nose hot and swollen.

FACE: *Aching, sore malar bones.* Slimy, sticky lips on waking. Eczema on chin.

MOUTH: Tongue wrinkled, stiff at base, pains when moving.

THROAT: *Dark red fauces.* Throat Sore (left to right). *Tonsils and glands greatly swollen.* Disposition to hawk with sensation of a lump in throat. Stiffness of muscles of throat and neck. Hawks much mucus from posterior nares. Uvula elongated. Diphtheria; submaxillary glands painfully enlarged.

STOMACH: Desires food more salted.

URINARY: Urethra indurated.

MALE: Hard chancres. Stubborn suppurating buboes. Sarcocele of left testicle.

FEMALE: Profuse acrid green leukorrhea. Fibroids stony hard.

RESPIRATORY: Asthma. Hoarseness on getting little wet. Catching pain under right breast, oppressing breathing. Cough from elongated uvula, with sore throat.

NECK: Stiff. Cervical adenitis.

EXTREMITIES: Wandering rheumatic pains, esp. muscular. Middle humerus feels as if about to break. Pain from calf to sacrum.

SKIN: Small fissures and cracks. Moist cracks on palms.

FEVER: Intense shivering followed by feverishness. Night sweat, hot.

RELATED: Lach.

MEZEREUM

GENERALITIES: It affects SKIN, *bones*, nerves and mucous membranes of the mouth and stomach. It produces *violent* burning, darting, like fire, in the muscles. *Irritation, burning itching* or burning smarting on the skin; burning, boring pains in bones, esp. long bones and neuralgia of the teeth and face, and after shingles. *Sudden pains of various kinds* followed by chilliness, numbness and soreness. Lacrimation with pain. *Affected parts become cold,* or emaciate. *One-sided symptoms;* whole or partial. Ill effects of suppressed eczema capitis; vaccination and mercury. Gouty-rheumatic, syphilitic dyscrasia. Excessive sensitiveness to air, even of a fan. Sensation of a cool breeze blowing on the part. Internal *burning* with external violent itching, in small areas, or in single parts. Caries, exostosis of bones. Periostitis. Bones seem enlarged. Acrid secretions, pus, leukorrhea, etc. Ulcers. Twitching of eyelids, right side of face, etc. Convulsion, > by tight grasping. Cystic osteoma. Abscess of fibrous parts or tendons. Body feels light.

WORSE: NIGHT. *Suppression. Warmth of bed,* of fire, etc. *Cold, air,* draft; damp. Motion. Touch. Mercury. Vaccination.

BETTER: Wrapping up. Heat of stove (prosopalgia). Eating. Open air.

MIND: Indiffeence to everything and everybody, looks through a window for hours without being conscious of the objects around. Apprehensive at the pit of the stomach when expecting some very unpleasant intelligence or pain or shock. Forgetful. Religious and financial melancholy. Aversion to talk, it seems to him to be hard work to utter a word. Reproaches or quarrels with others.

HEAD: Pains extend to eyes, malar bones, neck, etc. with lacrimation, > stooping, < talking, anger. Numbness of one side of scalp or top of head. Milk-crust. Skull painful. White scabs. Hair falls in handful; dandruff, white, dry.

EYES: Pain outward along the brows. Dryness of the eyes; they feel too large. Ciliary neuralgia after operation upon the eyes, removal of eyeball. Inclination to wink, jerking of eyelids. Feeling of coldness, with pain in the eyeballs.

EARS: Feel too open, as if tympanum was exposed to cool air which blew into the ear. Deafness after suppression of head eruptions. Desire to bore fingers in it. Thickening of tympanum.

NOSE: Visible twitching at the root of nose. Frequent sneezing, with pain in chest. Post nasal adenoid.

FACE: Neuralgic pains come and go quickly, and leave part numb, < eating, > near hot stove. Euptions around the mouth, with coryza. Cracks in corners of mouth. Twitching of muscles (right).

MOUTH: Burning in tongue, extending to stomach. Breath smells like rotten cheeze. Root of the tooth decays. Toothache radiates into temples, > with mouth open, and from drawing in air. Teeth feel dull and elongated. Dry, dark red mouth. Middle of the tongue fissured.

Watering of the mouth. Tongue coated along one side only. Ranula, < talking and chewing, ejects a watery fluid.

THROAT: Dark red, burning, sore, < winter. Nausea felt in throat, > eating.

STOMACH: Constant longing for food. Taste bitter, sour; beer tastes bitter, which is vomited. Craving for ham, fat, coffee, wine. Gastric pain burning corroding, > milk, and eating. Gastric ulcer. Vomiting of chocolate-colored substance, with nausea. Waterbrash. Chronic gastritis. Induration of stomach.

ABDOMEN: Constipation after confinement. Prolapse of rectum and constriction of anus about the prolapse, which makes it difficult to replace. Diarrhea; stools contain glistening particles. Stools hard, large, as if they would split the anus. Contraction of diaphragm. Swelling of glands with large abdomen in children.

URINARY: Hematuria, hot, preceded by cramp in bladder. Few drops of blood are passed after urination. Red pellicle on urine.

MALE: Painless swelling of the penis and scrotum. Testicles enlarged. Gonorrhea, with hematuria. Itching glans penis.

FEMALE: Stubborn, albuminous, serous, corroding leukorrhea. Obstinate ulceration of vagina and cervix. Menses scanty, frequent, profuse, long-lasting; with faceache.

RESPIRATORY: Dry tickling cough, causes vomiting, < hot things. Chest feels too tight on stooping. Snoring in children.

BACK: Coccyx painful, after a fall.

EXTREMITIES: Aching, itching in poplitae. Pain and burning in tibia and long bones. One hand hot. Limbs feel cold, and as if shortened. Paralysis of flexors of fingers, cannot hold anything.

SKIN: *Intolerable itching,* < by warm bath; changes place on scratching, coldness after. Pruritus senilis. Eruptions, ooze acrid, gluey moisture, form *thick crusts, with pus beneath;* or chalky white. Deep, hard, painful *ulcers,* < touch and warmth.

FEVER: Chill of single parts as if dashed with cold water.

COMPLEMENTARY: Merc.

RELATED: Ars; Guai; Kali-i; *Merc.*

MILLEFOLIUM

GENERALITIES: This remedy affects the CAPILLARIES of LUNGS, *nose*, and uterus. It causes *bruised soreness, congestion* and is very valuable remedy for *profuse, painless, bright red, fluid hemorrhages*—nose-bleed, hemoptysis, oozing of blood from the edges of closed wounds, from over exertion, etc. Profuse mucus discharges. Spasms or convulsion, esp. after suppression of hemorrhages - menses, lochia, milk, etc. Ill effects of operation for stones, biliary, renal, etc.; fall from a height; sprain. Varicose veins in pregnancy. Piercing thrusts of pain.

WORSE: Injury. Violent exertion. Stooping. Coffee.

BETTER: Bleeding. Discharges. Wine.

MIND: Seems to have forgotten something; does not know what he is doing or wants to do. Moaning children. Sad. Aversion to work.

HEAD: Piercing thrusts of pain, beats the head against the wall. Headache, < stooping.

EYES: Inward piercing, pressing goes to the root of the nose. Vision nebulous, with contortion of facial muscles.

EARS: Sense of cool air passing through the ears.

NOSE: Bleeding, with congestion to head and chest.

STOMACH: Hematemesis. Cramps in stomach, with sensation of a liquid flowing in intestines to anus.

ABDOMEN: Wind colic. Hemorrhage from bowels after much exertion. Bloody dysentery.

URINARY: Urine bloody. Stone in bladder with retention of urine. Pus-like discharge after lithotomy.

MALE: The seminal discharge fails during coition. Wounds and injuries of penis.

FEMALES: Uterine hemorrhage, bright red, fluid. Painful varices during pregnancy. Useful for the prolonged bleeding of hard labor. Curative in post-partum hemorrhage. Sterility from profuse menses.

RESPIRATORY: Oppression of chest, with bloody expectoration or palpitation. Cough with bloody sputum in suppressed menses or hemorrhoids.

HEART: Palpitation, with bloody sputum.

FEVER: Continuous high fever.

RELATED: Arn; Led.

MOSCHUS

GENERALITIES: Musk is a well known perfume, which produces fainting in some by mere smelling of it, hence easy fainting in any diseased condition is its chief indication. It is suitable for persons of sensitive nature, *hysterical women* and men. *Spasmodic, nervous effects* with a feeling of coldness. FAINTS easily-while eating, during menses, from heart disease, etc. *Twitching, choking*, globus hystericus, ending in unconsciousness. Feels a cool wind blowing on part. *Tension* in muscles, skin, mind. Nervous shuddering, laughter, hiccough, etc. Buzzing, squeezing, plug-like sensation. *Poor reaction*; diseases do not follow the normal course. Complains without knowing what ails him. Epilepsy, with shuddering as from a rigor or chilliness. Catalepsy. Imaginary diseases. Girls who are selfish, obstinate, self-willed, and much pampered; resort to all kinds of cunning to have their whims gratified. *Coldness*, general or of single parts. Parts lain on feel dislocated or sprained.

WORSE: Cold. *Excitement. Suppression of* menses, etc. Side lain on. During or after a meal. Pressure. Motion.

BETTER: Open air. Rubbing. Smell of musk.

MIND: Hurried, tremulous and *awkward*; bursting activity, with weakness, so everything falls from the hands. Violent anger, talks excitedly, raves, scolds, till mouth becomes dry, lips blue, eyes staring and she falls unconscious. Fears *noise*, dying, to lie down lest one should die. *Imaginary sufferings*. Uncontrollable laughter. Sexual hypochondriasis. One feels being rapidly turned around. Talks to himself and gesticulates. Sudden loss of memory.

HEAD: Vertigo, with fainting, as if falling from a height, $<$ stooping, $>$ rising. Headache, with coldness, fainting, involuntary stool, and polyuria. Shivering in scalp.

EYES: Turned upward, fixed and glistening.

EARS: Sounds as from reports of cannon. Rushing, fleeting sound. Nervous deafness.

NOSE: Bleed, with spasmodic jerking of muscles.

FACE: One cheek red but cold, other pale and hot. Lips blue. Chewing motion of the lower jaw.

STOMACH: Desire for black coffee, beer and brandy. Everything tastes flat. Violent eructations. Spasmodic nervous hiccough. Aversion to food. Faints while eating. Nausea on seeing of at thought of food.

ABDOMEN: Tension in abdomen as if clothes were too tight. Incarceration of flatus. Stools of sweetish odor. Stools are passed involuntarily in sleep.

URINARY: Copious watery urine. Diabetes. Urine normal during day, but dark red, offensive at night.

MALE: Sexual desire increased, with insupportable tickling in the parts and tensive pain in penis. Impotence from diabetes. Nausea and vomiting after coition. Emission without erection. Erection with desire to urinate.

FEMALE: Sexual desire increased, with intolerable titilations in parts (in old women). Dysmenorrhea, with fainting.

RESPIRATORY: *Sudden nervous suffocation,* wants to take deep breath, < becoming cold, > belching. Chest oppressed; hysterical spasm of the chest. Cough ceases; mucus cannot be expectorated. Cough with pain under left breast. Asthma.

HEART: *Anxious palpitation,* with fear of death, says he shall die. Hysterical. Trembling around the heart.

NECK & BACK: Tension in back, before menses.

EXTREMITIES: One hand hot and pale, the other cold and red. Limbs tense, feel too short. Coldness in tibia. Painful; restless.

SLEEP: Sleepy by day, sleepless at night, awakes frequently.

FEVER: *Sensitive to cold air* which makes him shudder. *Skin cold.* Burning heat with restlessness. Sweat smelling like musk.

RELATED: Carb-v; Castor; Ign; Nux-m; Valer.

MUREX

GENERALITIES: Like Sepia the juice of purple fish affects the FEMALE SEXUAL ORGANS prominently. It is adapted to sensitive, nervous, lively, affectionate women, who are very tired, weak and run down, must lie down which <. Pains are diagonal, ovary to opposite breast. Climacteric sufferings.

WORSE: *Touch.* In sun. Sitting. Lying down. After sleep.

BETTER: Before menses. Eating. Pressure and support. Putting head back.

MIND: Great depression of spirits, a sort of deep hypochondriacal state. Anxious, apprehensive, > leukorrhea. Memory weak, cannot find correct words to express himself.

HEAD: Squeezing at the back of head, > putting hand on it or by throwing head backward.

NOSE: Distressing coldness of the nose all day.

STOMACH: Violent hunger even after eating. *Sinking, all-gone sensation.*

ABDOMEN: Painful weariness of loins. Weight in hypogastrium.

URINARY: Frequent urging to urinate. Urine smells like valerian. Slight discharge of blood while urinating.

FEMALE: Pain, stitching in genitals; moves up through abdomen into the breasts. *Painfully sore uterus;* consciousness of womb. Feeling as if something was pressing on a sore spot in the pelvis, > sitting. *Violent nervous sexual desire, nymphomania,* from least contact with the parts. Bearing down pain, *must keep legs tightly crossed.* Copious menses with large clots. Leukorrhea thick, yellow, bloody; alternating with mental symptoms. Pain in mammae during menses. Walking difficult, all joints are weak during pregnancy. Prolapse, enlargement of the uterus. Discharge of blood through the vagina or bloody leukorrhea during stools. Feels as if bones of pelvis are getting loose.

BACK: Lumbar pain impels walking which <.

SKIN: Dry, as if about to crack. Hives.

RELATED: Lil-t; Plat; Sep.

MURIATIC ACID

GENERALITIES: Hydrochloric acid has an elective affinity for blood, producing septic conditions similar to that found in low fevers with high temperature and *great prostration*. MUSCLES are affected, esp. of HEART, bladder, anus, tongue, etc., causing paresis. MUCOUS MEMBRANES *of the* MOUTH and *digestive tract* are dry, bleeding, cracked and *deeply ulcerated. Soreness* of the body causing RESTLESSNESS, frequently changes the position *but soon grows weak and very debilitated;* wants to lie down; slides down in bed; eyes fall shut, lower jaw drops. *Bluish*; tongue, piles, ulcers. *Burning*. Tearing pains. Violent hemorrhage. Scorbutic states. Pulsation in single parts. Parts are dry, *deeply ulcerated*, bleeding or cracked. Bloody mucous membranes. *Muscular exhaustion*. Dropsical swelling.

WORSE: *Touch. Wet weather*. Walking. Cold drink, bathing. Sitting. Human voice. Sun.

BETTER: Motion. Warmth. Lying on left side.

MIND: Introvert. *Sad and taciturn*. Suffers in silence. Irritable. *Muttering. Persistent loud moaning*.

HEAD: Vertigo, < moving eyes slightly, lying on right side or on back. Occipital pain, *leaden heaviness*, < looking intently at any object. Brain feels bruised; with headache,.sound of voice is intolerable. Periodical pain over left eye, with numbness down right arm and aphasia. Hair feels as if standing on end.

EYES: Vertical hemiopia. Eyes close on sitting; from exhaustion.

EARS: Deafness. Distant voice (talking) causes headache. Cutting from mastoid to nape. Tingling, creeping, cold pain running upto vertex.

NOSE: Bleed; much sneezing.

FACE: *Dark or glowing red face*, with cold hands and no thirst. *Lips sore, cracked and scabby*. Lower jaw fallen. Freckles due to exposure to sun.

MOUTH: *Dry*. Tongue; bluish, heavy, stiff, hinders talking; shrunken or burnt-looking. Aphthae. Teeth troubles, < acids and sweets. Sordes on teeth. Gums swollen, bleeding, ulcerating. Hard lumps in the tongue. Lips, burn, heavy, bloated. Everything tastes sweet. Beer tastes like honey. Cancer of tongue.

THROAT: *Dry*, with burning in chest. Attempt to swallow produces spasm and choking. Involuntary swallowing.

STOMACH: *Aversion to meat*. Achlorhydria. Stomach will neither tolerate nor digest food.

ABDOMEN: Fulness and distension in abdomen from small quantity of food. Empty sensation in the stomach, also in the abdomen after stool, and in a.m. *Involuntary stools* or prolapse of rectum *on urinating* or *passing flatus. Very sore piles,* > heat, < during pregnancy, protruding like a bunch of grapes. Anus sore during menses. Liver enlarged, sore. Ascites from cirrhosis of liver.

URINARY: Atony of bladder, must wait a long time before urine will pass, or has to press so hard that anus protrudes. Cannot urinate without also passing stool. Urine; red, violet, milky, copíous, night and day; escapes from passing wind.

FEMALE: Leukorrhea, with backache. Pricking in vagina. Genitals very sensitive, cannot bear least touch.

HEART: Large, full and soft pulse. Pulse drops every 3rd beat. Pulse feeble, rapid and small. Palpitation felt in face.

EXTREMITIES: Red swollen, burning fingers and toes. Weak thighs. Staggers when walking, from weakness of thighs and knees. Eczema of dorsum of hands. Cramps in the ball of thumb (right) when writing, goes off when moving it. Pain in tendo-achilles. Forearms heavy.

SKIN: Ulcers throb on walking. Scarlet fever, livid with petechiae.

FEVERS: Cold in bed, in early morning. *Intense burning heat, with aversion to covers.* Adynamic fever—typhoid, septic, etc.

RELATED: Bapt; Bry.

MYGALE LASIODORA

GENERALITIES: The chief clinical use of this spider poison is in chorea, esp. of upper parts. Twitchings and contraction of facial muscles and head, which is jerked to the right side. Mouth and eyes open in rapid succession. Words are jerked out in the effort to talk. Nausea, with palpitation and dim vision. Violent erections, chordee. Usteady gait, limbs drag while walking. Convulsive uncontrollable movements of arms and legs. Constant motion of whole body. Intense red streaks along lymphatics.

WORSE: Eating. Sitting. Morning.

BETTER: During sleep.

RELATED: Agar; Tarent.

MYRICA CERIFERA

GENERALITIES : It has a marked action on the *liver* and heart. Mucous discharges are offensive, tenacious and difficult to detach. *Combined liver and heart affections.*

WORSE: Warmth of bed. After sleep. Morning. Motion.

BETTER: Open air. Eating, breakfast.

MIND: Despondent, dejected. Irritable.

HEAD: Dull heavy aching in forehead and temples on waking in the morning.

EYES: Yellow sclera. *Very red eyelids.*

FACE: Yellow, jaundiced.

MOUTH: Dry; water relieves only partially. Tongue coated thick yellowish, dark. Tenacious, thick nauseous mucus in mouth and throat. Taste bitter. Offensive breath.

STOMACH: Imagines he cannot eat; the taste is so foul. Loss of appetite; loathing of food. Desire for sour things. Sinking in epigastrium, < eating, > fast walking.

ABDOMEN: Dull pain in the liver, with pain under either scapulae. *Liver affections with heart complaints*, with urticaria, with jaundice. Jaundice of infants, from cancer of the liver, with bronze-yellow skin. Fulness and burning in gall-bladder. Adhesive mucus in stools. Flatus is passed continuously while walking. Urging to stool but passes only great amount of flatus. Stools foul, pasty, of grey color.

URINARY: Beer-colored urine, with yellowish froth.

FEMALE: Leukorrhea acrid, fetid, thick, yellow, long lasting.

HEART: Pulse slow, feeble, irregular.

BACK: Pain under scapulae with liver complaints.

SKIN: Itching of jaundice.

SLEEP: Drowsiness. Ugly dreams.

COMPLEMENTARY: Dig; Kali-bi.

RELATED: Chel.

NAJA

GENERALITIES: The action of cobra poison settles around the HEART—hypertrophy and valvular diseases. Affects medulla and cerebellum, *respiration, throat, ovary.* Left-sided symptoms. *Nervous, excited and tremulous, with heart affection,* often reflex. Feeling of intoxication; loss of power over limbs, over sphincters; unable to speak. Swooning fits. Sensation of wasting away. Parts seem drawn together. *Constriction* in chest, throat, etc. Burning as from hot iron. Many pains. Screwed up sensation. Collapse. Sepsis. Ill effects of grief. Insensible right side. Affections of heart with paucity of symptoms.

WORSE: *Lying on left side.* After sleep. After menses. *Cold* air, draft. Pressure of clothes. Alcohol. Touch.

BETTER: Walking or *riding in open carriage.* Sneezing. Smoking.

MIND: Broods constantly over imaginary troubles and makes himself wretched. Suicidal, brooding insanity. Depressed, with distress about sexual organs, > in the evening. Aversion to talking. Dreads to be left alone. Fear of rain. Notion as if everything were done wrong and could not be rectified.

HEAD: Pain in the left temple and in left orbital region, extending to occiput with nausea and vomiting, > smoking. Entire head feels hollow. Sensation of a blow on occiput. Vertex sensitive to cold. Headaches after cessation of menses. Pain in forehead and temples, with heart symptoms.

EYES: Staring. Ptosis of both lids. Hot pains at back of eyeballs.

EARS: Noises in ears, with nauseous taste in mouth. Black discharge, smelling like herring brine.

NOSE: Flow of water from nose, then intense sneezing which > the breathing. Hay asthma.

MOUTH: Wide open; flow of saliva. Tongue cold. Loss of speech.

THROAT: Feels a lump in throat. Suffocative *choking,* grasps the throat. Stricture of esophagus, swallowing difficult or impossible.

STOMACH: Craving for stimulants which <. Eructations tasting like barley water; or hot, foul.

FEMALE: *Pain from left ovary to heart,* < one week before menses. Obscure pain in left groin, post-operative.

RESPIRATORY: Puffing breathing. Cardiac asthma; or cough. Dry or empty feeling in left lung. Ribs feel broken. Oppressive weight on chest; as if a hot iron had been run in. Asthma preceded by coryza, < lying; > sitting up.

HEART: *Weakness.* Violent pain, shooting to left scapula, *shoulder* or neck, holds hand over it, < after riding in carriage. Visible palpitation; hypertrophy. Endocarditis, septic. Damaged heart after infectious diseases. Pulse slow (up to 45), irregular, weak, tremulous; changes force. Chronic nervous palpitation, < after preaching. Choking. Tension low.

EXTREMITIES: Cramps in shoulders, nape or thigh bones. Numb left arm. Violent racking in marrow of thighs. Puffy or sweating hands and feet, with cough. Acute pain under the left thumb nail running up the arm. Loss of power.

SKIN: Itching cicatrices.

SLEEP: Deep comatose, with stertorous breathing.

FEVER: Sweat on lumbar back and ankles.

RELATED: Cimic; Lach; Laur; Spig.

NAPHTHALINUM

GENERALITIES: A product from coal tar, has a special affinity for eyes. It produces detachment of retina, deposits an exudation in the retina. Opacity of cornea; cataract; amblyopia.

NATRUM ARSENICUM

GENERALITIES: *Nat-ars.* is a valuable remedy for miner's asthma; from coal dust. Racking cough with profuse greenish expectoration. Oppression of chest and about the heart. Lungs feel as if smoke had been inhaled. Feels tired all over; sensation as if the thyroid gland were compressed by a thumb and finger.

NATRUM CARBONICUM

GENERALITIES: Sodium carbonate affects the *digestion and nerves.* The patient is *oversensitive* to open air, music, noise, dietetic errors. *Great debility* from any exertion, from summer heat. *Puffiness.* Relaxation; easy dislocation. *Pains cause tremor, cold sweat,* anxiety, etc. Twitching in the muscles and limbs. Contraction of muscles, tendons. Emaciation. Anemia. Ill effects of sunstroke (chronic); overstudy, strain. Children who cannot tolerate milk but thrive better on cereals. Children when asleep jump, cry, grasp the mother; startled, nervous children. Swelling and induration of glands.

WORSE: HEAT — *of sun,* weather (body). 5 a.m. Music. *Mental* or bodily *exertion*. Onanism. Milk. Dietetic error. *Draft*. Thunder-storm. Alternate days. Full moon. Vegetable diet; strachy food. Cold drink when overheated.

BETTER: Eating. Rubbing. Motion. Pressure. Wiping with hand. Boring into nose or ears with finger. Sweating.

MIND: Cross and *irritable*. Aversion to society, even that of their own family, her husband. *Gloomy*. Lively, talkative. Anxious and fearful, < thunderstorm, electric changes in the atmosphere. Playing on piano causes anxiety and trembling. Sensitive to presence of certain persons. Difficult, slow comprehension. Music causes tendency to suicide, sadness, religious insanity. Occupied with sad thoughts. Indiffierent.

HEAD: Vertigo from wine, mental exertion; from exposure to sun. Headache in hot weather, slightest mental exertion, working under gaslight. Head pains out through eyes; head bent backwards. Feels too large. Falling of hair.

EYES: Dazzling flashes or stars before vision, on awakening. Dim eyes, has to wipe them constantly. Cannot read small print.

EARS: Deafness; with recurring earache, with amenorrhea. Feels as if a bubble bursting in, as if something moved in ear on swallowing.

NOSE: Swollen or peeling. Red nose with white pimples on it. Catarrh. Foul, thick, yellow or green discharge. Coryza, < least draft, alternate days. Stoppage at night. Violent sneezing. *Post-nasal discharge*.

FACE: Pale, withered, bloated. Freckles, yellow spots, pimples. Lips swollen.

MOUTH: Dry. Bitter taste in the mouth, food tastes bitter. Vesicles and smooth ulcers in mouth with burning; mouth open. Toothache, < sweetmeats and fruits. Taste perverted; too sensitive. Affections of the under-surface of the tongue. Tongue heavy, unwieldy, patient has difficulty in talking.

THROAT: Hawks much mucus from the throat. Must drink to swallow solids, from roughness, dryness of esophagus and throat. Throat painful when yawning, and swallowing.

STOMACH: *Digestion weak,* < by slightest errors in diet. *Acidity.* Aversion to milk, which causes diarrhea. Acid dyspepsia with belching and rheumatism, > by soda biscuits. Greedy, always nibbling. Gastric pains, > eating. Hungry at 5 a.m. Always belching. Ill effects of drinking cold water when overheated. Waterbrash. Heartburn after fat.

ABDOMEN: Flatus changes places, abdomen pouts here and there. Epigastrium painful to touch and when talking. Diarrhea from starch, milk. Stools; like orange pulp; in women at change of life. Sudden call to stool without result or stools escape with haste and noise. Stools; black, hard, smooth, crumble. Colic with retraction of navel and hardness of skin.

URINE: Urine of bright or dark yellow color. Urine smells like horse's urine, from vegetable or milk diet. Burning in urethra during and after urination.

MALE: Increased sexual desire with priapism and painful pollutions. Incomplete coition. Glans penis easily becomes sore. Nightly emissions. Sweats after coition. Discharge of prostatic fluid at stool and when urinating; prostate affections.

FEMALE: Induration of cervix. Sterility from non-retention of semen. Leukorrheal discharge offensive, irritating, thick, yellow, ropy; preceded by colic. Menses late, scanty, like meat washing. Motion as of fetus in uterus. Promotes conception.

RESPIRATORY: Cough dry, tickling < when entering a warm room, at 9-11 a.m. Loose, hollow, cough with salty purulent greenish sputum. Cough, with coldness of left side of breast.

HEART: Palpitation; from noise, rattling of paper etc., on going upstairs, when attention is directed to something, when lying on left side.

NECK & BACK: Cracking in cervical vertebrae when moving the neck. Boring at tip of left scapula. Cold between scapulae. Goitre hard, with pressing pain. Tingling in back.

EXTREMITIES: Heaviness of legs and feet, with tension in them, when sitting or walking. *Ankles weak.* Unsteady walk. Dislocation and spraining of ankles. Little obstruction on pavement causes him to fall, or falls without apparent cause. Burning wrists and ankles. Locomotor ataxia, fulgurating pain, > eating. Soles tender, as if from needles, burn while walking. Jerking of hands on going to sleep. Cramp from ankles to toes. Contraction of fingers. Poplitea painful on motion. Folds of fingers and toes sore.

SKIN: Dry, rough, milky, watery. Blisters on small joints, tips of toes or fingers. Pustular eruptions. *Sweats easily.* Formication.

SLEEP: Drowsy during day, after meals. Wakes too early in the morning. Amorous dreams. Sleeps with mouth open.

FEVER: *Easy sweat.*

COMPLEMENTARY: Sep.

RELATED: Lyc; Nat-m.

NATRUM MURIATICUM

GENERALITIES: Common salt profoundly affects the *nutrition.* Its excessive intake produces symptoms of salt retention, such as dropsy and edema, but it also affects the *blood* causing anemia and leukocytosis. MIND, HEART, liver and spleen come under its influence. The patient is *thin, thirsty, poorly nourished* on account of *digestive* disturbances, and his MENTAL BEHAVIOR and physical symptoms are *hopeless* or awkward in nature. Emaciation, descending, of *neck* or abdomen. MUCOUS MEMBRANES and skin may be DRY or may produce thick, *white or clear, watery, acrid discharges.* Dryness of mouth, *throat*, rectum, vagina, etc. *Numbness* of one side, of parts lain on, with paralysis; fingers, *parts seem too short.* Easy exhaustion. Contraction of muscles, tendons. Neuralgic pains with tears. *Trembling.* Prostration. Hysterical debility. Emaciation even while living well. Great weakness and weariness. Tendency to take cold. *Coldness.* Children talk late; are cross, irritable, cry from slightest cause. Cachexia, malarial. Oversensitive to all sorts of influences. Goitre, hyperthyroidism. Addison's disease. Diabetes. Twitching in muscles. Frequent starts in upper part of the body. Chorea, jumping, after fright. Ill effects of disappointment, fright, grief, fit of passion, loss of fluids, masturbation, injury to head; silver salts; salt. Young girls become lovelorn and fall in love with married men. Paralysis from emotion, sexual excess. Likes to be covered but it does not >. Trembling of the whole body from smoking tobacco.

WORSE: *Exact periodicity.* 9 to 11 a.m.; *with the sun.* Alternate days. After menses. HEAT *of sun*, summer; dampness. *Exertion* - of eyes, mental, talking, reading, writing. Violent emotion. *Sympathy. Puberty.* Quinine.

Bread, fat, acid food. Coition. Seashore. Chronic sprain. Noise; music. Touch. Pressure. Full moon.

BETTER: *Open air*. Cool bathing. *Sweating*. Rest.. Going without regular meals. Tight clothing. Deep breathing. Before breakfast. Rubbing. Lying on right side. Talking long.

MIND: Hateful to persons who had offended him. Detests consolation or fuss. *Sad* during menses; sad without cause. *Reserved*. Easily angered, < if consoled. Company distresses. Hypochondriac. Weeps bitterly, or wants to be alone to cry. Weeps involuntarily, without cause or cannot weep. Cheerful. Laughs, sings, dances, alternating with sadness. Boisterous grief. Dwells on past unpleasant memories. Anxiety. Apprehension. *Fear or dreams of robbers*. Awkward in talking; hasty; drops things from nervous weakness. Absent-minded. Scattered thoughts. Revengeful. Thinks he is pitied for his misfortunes and weeps. Immoderate laughter with tears. Abrupt. An idea clings, prevents sleep, inspires revenge. Alternating mental conditions. Extremely forgetful. Aversion to men (females).

HEAD: Vertigo; as if falling, < standing near a window, on closing eyes, > lying with head high. HEADACHE bursting, on coughing, maddening, *hammering*; heavy *over eyes*, on vertex, with partial numbness or disturbed vision, < on *awakening*, from sunrise to sunset, menses, motion; even of eyes, frowning, reading, > sleep, pressure on eyes, lying with head high, sitting still. Nodding motions of the head. Headache of school children. Migraine. Falling hair. Injured part tender to touch. Loss of hair in children or lactating mothers.

EYES: Painful, on looking down. Letters run together while reading. Stricture of lacrimal duct, escape of mucus when pressing on the sac. *Lacrimation* with redness; burning, acrid; from affected side; from sneezing; coughing; laughing etc. Eyes feel drawn together. Itch and burn, must wipe them. Ptosis on lying down. Vision blurred, wavering. Hemiopia, then headache. Eyelids close with headache, spasmodically. Cannot read by artificial light. Sparks, black spots, fiery zigzag before eyes. Incipient cataract. Protruding eyes due to goitre. Retinal images are retained too long. Eyes give out in reading and writing.

EARS: Noises, buzzing, humming, ringing. Painful cracking in the ear when masticating. Itching behind ears.

NOSE: Violent fluent coryza, lasts one to three days, then stoppage of nose high up making breathing difficult. Sneezing early in the morning. Alternate fluent and dry coryza; cold commences with sneezing, gushing of fluid. Little ulcers in nose. One side numb. Loss of smell and taste. Nosebleed; on stooping, or when coughing, at night.

FACE: Pale, muddy, or shiny as if greased. HERPES about the lips or at the edge of hair; pearly. Crack in the middle of the lower lip. Lips tingle, feel numb. Throbbing in lower jaw, < biting; heat and cold. Upper lip swollen. Prosopalgia. Falling of whiskers and beard.

MOUTH: TONGUE MAPPED, *beaded* or *striped along edges*. Aphthae. Loss of taste and smell, Numbness and stiffness of one side of tongue. Tingling of the tongue. Tongue heavy, difficult speech. Children learn to talk slowly. Fistula dentalis. Epulis or small tumor on the gums. Sensation of hair on the tongue. Tongue feels dry. Vesicles and ulcers in mouth and on tongue, smart and burn when touched by food. Teeth sensitive to air or touch; pain < on chewing. Toothache with tears or salivation.

THROAT: Hawks much mucus, bitter, salty. Uvula hangs to one side. A dry, sore spot in the throat, tickles and causes cough, etc. Food goes down the wrong way; post-diphtheritic paralysis. Only fluids can be swallowed. Solids reach a certain point and then are violently ejected. Throat glistens. Exophthalmic goitre. Sore throat; with sensation as if she has to swallow over a lump, as if a plug in throat. Tobacco smoker's throat.

STOMACH: Desire For Salt, bitter things, sour things, farinaceous food, oysters, fish, milk. *Thirsty, drinks large quantity of water.* Great hunger yet emaciates; with depressed mind. *Averse to bread,* meat, coffee, tobacco. Hunger without relish. Hiccough. Burning eructations, after eating. Sweet risings from stomach during menses. Anxiety in stomach rises into head. Waterbrash. Sweats while eating; on face. White slimy mucus is vomited with relief. Heartburn with palpitation. Feels better on an empty stomach.

ABDOMEN: Epigastric pulsation. Epigastrium swollen and painful. Sudden distension. Tense abdomen, < in groins. Pain in abdominal ring on coughing. Rigidity of the left side. Colic with nausea, > flatus. *Stools dry, hard, crumbling;* tear the anus or cause burning. Stools coated with glassy mucus. Constipation on alternate days from inactivity of rectum; painless watery diarrhea, chronic; morning, on moving about; from abuse of opium. Constriction of rectum. Herpes about anus. Abdominal viscera loose, as if dragging, when walking. Red spots on epigastrium. Herpes ani.

URINARY: Involuntary urination; on coughing, laughing, sneezing, walking, sitting. Polyuria with thirst for large quantities of water. Has to wait long for urine to pass in presence of others. Urine clear with red sediment. Must wait before the urine will start. Pain just after urination.

MALE: Backache and weak legs with depression after coition. Pollution shortly after coition. Sexual desire, with physical weakness. Suppressed gonorrhea. Weakness, even paralysis, after sexual excess. Loss of hair from pubes.

FEMALE: Aversion to coition which is painful from dryness of vagina. Burning-smarting in vagina during coition. Delayed first menses. Dysmenorrhea with convulsions. Sterility with too early, too profuse menses. Debilitating leukorrhea, white, thick, instead of menses. Prolapse of uterus with aching in lumbar region or with cutting in urethra, < in the morning, > lying on back. Hot during menses. Mammary glands emaciate. White leukorrhea turns green gradually. Stitches beneath nipples.

RESPIRATORY: Cough from tickling in the pit of stomach, with asthma or palpitation, < winter. Respiratory catarrh after suppressed sweats. Sticking in liver while coughing. Dyspnea on ascending. Whooping cough; with lacrimation. Breath; hot, offensive. Exertion of arms > breathing.

HEART: *Palpitation* shaking body or alternating with beating in head. Fluttering of the heart, with weak, faint feeling, < lying down. Palpitation; anxious, < exertion, emotion, lying on left side. Pulse full and slow or weak and rapid, intermittent every third beat, < lying down. Coldness, soreness at the heart.

NECK & BACK: Painful stiffness of neck. Bruised backache, early in a.m., < coughing, coition, > lying on back, on something hard; or pressure. Can stoop readily, but hurts to straighten. Buttocks emaciated in infants.

EXTREMITIES: Trembling of the hands when writing. Cracked fingertips. Hangnails. Palms hot and sweaty. Hamstrings seem short, painful, drawing in. Numbness and tingling in fingers and lower extremities. Catch in knee. Housemaid's knee. Cracking in joints on motion. Ankles weak and turn easily. Legs cold. Convulsive jerking of the limbs on falling asleep. Scurfs, scales in axilla. Bending the joints of fingers difficult. Children do not learn to walk. Soreness of toes or between toes.

SKIN: Oily, dry, harsh, unhealthy or yellow. Chaps or *herpetic eruptions,* < flexures, or about knuckles. Dry eruptions on margins of hair. Warts of palms and hands. Hives, whitish, < exertion. Corns. Scars painful, Redness of old scar.

SLEEP: Sobs during sleep. *Awakes feeling weak.* Dreams of robbers. Somnambulism, rises and sits about room. Starts and talks in sleep.

FEVER: Coldness of many parts—hands, feet, heart. Morning chill with thirst. Chilly but < in sun. Sweat scanty, at edge of hair, on nose, on face while eating.

COMPLEMENTARY: Ign; Sep.

RELATED: Puls.

NATRUM PHOSPHORICUM

GENERALITIES: This remedy is useful for conditions arising from excess of lactic acid as a result of too much sugar. It affects duodenum, bile ducts, mesenteric glands and genitals. SOURNESS— *eructations*, vomiting, stomach, stools, leukorrhea, expectoration, sweats, etc. Ailments with *excess of acidity. Infants who have been fed to excess with milk and sugar. Deep yellow*, creamy *discharges. Debility*. Pricking sensation. Tightness of muscles and tendons. Jaundice (1x trit.). Oxaluria. Worms. Swelling of lymphatic glands. Ill effects of mental exertion or sexual vice or both. Marasmus of bottle-fed babies. Trembling and palpitation from thunderstorm. Cracking in joints. Nervousness; tired feeling. Leukocytosis.

WORSE: *Sugar.* Milk. Mental exertion. Thunderstorm. Gaslight. Coitus. Bitter foods. Fat food.

BETTER: Cold.

MIND: Mental weakness. Fear at night that something will happen. Imagines that pieces of furniture are persons; he hears footsteps in the next room. Nervous; forgetful. Sad from music. Indifferent to everything, to his family. Sits quite still for a long time. Easily frightened.

HEAD: Feels dull in the morning. Cutting pain in temples (right) while studying. Pressure and heat on top of head as if it would open.

EYES: Golden yellow creamy matter from the eyes. White of the eyes dirty yellow. Eyes weak, < gaslight. Squinting with worms. One pupil dilated.

EARS: One ear red, hot, itching, scratches until it bleeds, with gastric affections and acidity. Sensation as if water falling in from a height.

NOSE: *Itching.* Offensive odor before nose. Yellow thick offensive mucus. *Child picks nose.* Prickling with lacrimation.

FACE: Itching about mouth. *Pale* or red on alternate sides. Florid.

MOUTH: Blisters on tip of tongue. YELLOW CREAMY COATING AT THE BASE OF TONGUE on tonsils, or roof of mouth. Thin moist coating on the tongue. Sensation of hair on tongue. Grinding of teeth in children. Pricking, numbness of whole mouth.

THROAT: As if a lump were preventing speech. Swallowing difficult. Yellow coating on tonsils.

STOMACH: Sour eructations. Vomiting of sour cheesy masses. Desire for strong-tasting things, eggs, fried fish, beer which >. Aversion to bread and butter.

ABDOMEN: While at stool sensation as if a marble dropped down descending colon. Noisy flatulence. Fulness in abdomen, < standing or eating a little. Gastro-duodenal catarrh. Jaundice. Urging to stool and urination after coitus (men). Stools hacked. Greenish diarrhea. Itching at anus. Afraid to pass flatus lest stool should escape. Sclerosis of liver and hepatic form of diabetes, esp. when there is a succession of boils. Round or threadworms.

URINARY: Urging to urinate and burning and itching at meatus after coition. Must wait for urine to start.

MALE: Semen thin, watery, smells like stale urine. Emissions followed by weak back and trembling of knees. Itching of scrotum, prepuce.

FEMALE: Sterility with acid secretions from vagina. Leukorrhea sour, creamy, honey-colored, or acid and watery. Morning sickness, with sour vomiting. During menses feet icy cold during day, burn at night in bed.

RESPIRATORY: Respiration difficult. Cough, < sitting. Chest feels empty after eating. Pain in chest, < deep breathing and pressure.

HEART: Trembling about heart, < going upstairs, after menses. Feeling as if a bubble from heart forced the way through arteries. Heart pain is > when big toe pains. Heart pains alternating with rheumatic pains. Anxious palpitation after thunderstorm.

NECK & BACK: Weakness after coition. Heavy dragging in the back. Swelling of glands of neck extending to chest. Goitre with feeling of pressure.

EXTREMITIES: Aching in wrists and finger joints. Trembling of limbs after coition. Rheumatism. Feet icy cold during day, burn at night. Synovial crepitation. Cramps in hands while writing. Legs give way while walking.

SKIN: Itching in various parts, esp. ankles; eczematous eruptions. Hives. Skin smooth, red, shining.

SLEEP: Sleepy in the forenoon, but sleepless before midnight. Dreams anxious, amorous, of dead people. Very drowsy, falls asleep while sitting.

FEVER: Feet icy cold in daytime, burn at night.

RELATED: Cina; Kali-s; Kreos.

NATRUM SALICYLICUM

GENERALITIES: Produces marked effect upon the internal ear, with vertigo, deafness, noises in the ears with loss of bone conduction. Hence it is useful in Meniere's disease. Vertigo when objects seem to move to the right, < on rising from lying. Temperature subnormal with slow pulse. Prostration after influenza.

NATRUM SULPHURICUM

GENERALITIES: Sodium sulphate or Glauber's salt is a remedy for hydrogenoid constitution where complaints are such as due to living in damp houses, basements, cellars; patient cannot eat even plants growing near water, nor fish. It specially affects OCCIPUT, LIVER and pancreas. Sudden violent effect in ailing patients. *Piercing pain* at short ribs (left), in hip (left), < rising or sitting down. *Yellow watery secretions*, stools, skin, vesicles, etc. Thick yellow green pus. *Fulness*. Sour, bilious and lithemic. Sycosis. Pains < on thinking of them. Epilepsy, or petit mal after head injuries. Suppressed gonorrhea. Dropsy. Fistulous abscess. Mental trouble arising from a fall or other injuries to head. Trembling.

WORSE: DAMP weather; *night air*. Cellar. *Lying on left side. Injury to head*. Lifting. Touch. Pressure. Wind.

Light. Music. Subdued light. *Late evening*. Vegetables, fruits. Cold food and drink. Lying long in one position.

BETTER: Open air; warm dry air. Change of position. Breakfast. Lying on back.

MIND: Sensitive and suspicious. Sadness, < music or subdued light, sitting near a stained glass window. Fear of crowd, of evil. Suicidal impulse, has to use self-control to prevent shooting himself. Melancholy. Cheerful after stool. Mental troubles arising from injury to head or fall. Intermittent attacks of mania. Does not want to speak, and feels that nobody should talk to him.

HEAD: Crushing or gnawing in occiput. Headaches, < by noise, stooping, during menses, light, eating, > in dark room, vomiting. Salivation with headache. Vertigo, > head sweat. Meningitis, spinal. Scalp sensitive, hair combing painful. Vertex hot. Brain feel loose when stooping. Head jerks to right side.

EYES: Granular lids. *Photophobia* on waking in morning. Heavy lids. Conjunctiva yellow. Crawling. Eyes feels hot.

EARS: Piercing stitches in ears, < damp weather.

NOSE: Runs water at night. Nosebleed before and during menses, stops and returns often. Sneezing with fluent coryza. Thick yellow discharge.

FACE: Yellow, pale, sickly. Itching of face.

MOUTH: Slimy, thick, tenacious white mucus. Bitter taste. *Dirty brown, or greenish yellow, thick, pasty tongue, esp. at base*. Tip of tongue feels burnt. Toothache, > by holding cold water in mouth. Gums burn like fire. Salivation during headache. Blisters on palate. Burning in mouth as from pepper.

THROAT: Thick yellow mucus drops from posterior nares. Swallowing impeded. Burning in pharynx during menses.

STOMACH: Desire for ice and cold water. Thirst at the start of fever only. Aversion to meat and bread. Slow digestion. Concomitants to nausea. Green *bilious* vomit. Acid dyspepsia with heartburn and flatulence. Starchy food, milk and potatoes disagree.

ABDOMEN: Liver region sore, tender, < deep breathing, stepping, jar; heavy, < *lying on left side.* Hepatitis; duodenal catarrh. Feeling of a lump below liver. Clawing in gall bladder. Colic, > rubbing or kneading abdomen, lying on sides. Cramps at umbilicus. FLATULENCE; incarcerated, painful, pushes here and there in right abdomen. *Rumbling, gurgling in bowels, then sudden noisy spluttering stool,* after rising in a.m., or drives from bed. Foamy or yellow diarrhoea; mixed with green slime. Stool involuntary when passing flatus, etc. Loose morning stools. Great size of the fecal mass. Jaundice, after anger.

URINARY: Frequent urination. Diabetes, brick dust or white sandy sediment, polyuria.

MALE: Gonorrhea, chronic; discharge thick, greenish; little pain. Condylomata. Itching of glans penis, scrotum.

FEMALE: Herpetic vulvitis. Leukorrhea yellowish green, following gonorrhea, with hoarseness. Nipples retracted.

RESPIRATORY: Dyspnea. Asthma, sycotic; in children; as a constitutional remedy, < early morning. Loose but violent cough, > sitting, must hold the chest or sides. Piercing through lower left chest. Every fresh cold or any unusual exertion brings on an attack of asthma. Breathing short while walking; constant desire to take deep, long breath. Asthma, with early morning diarrhea. Expectoration greenish, copious.

BACK: Piercing pain between scapulae. Sharp cutting pain in back spreading upwards like a fan. Violent pain in back of neck and base of brain. Lumbar region pains on attempts to retain the urine.

EXTREMITIES: *Inflammation around root of nails.* Hangnail. Pain in hip joint, < rising or sitting down, compelling the patient to move constantly because of its severity. Sciatica on rising from sitting or turning in bed, no relief in any position. Throbbing, piercing in heels. Vesicles on soles. Burning below knees. Edema of feet. Trembling of hands on waking and also when writing.

SKIN: Itching while undressing. Watery yellow blisters, wart-like red lumps all over the body.

SLEEP: Dreams of fighting, of running water. Awakes; from pain, from flatulence.

FEVER: Chilly, cannot get warm even in bed. Heat with aversion to uncover. Foul axillary sweat.

COMPLEMENTARY: Ars; Thuj.

RELATED: Coloc; Glon; Med; Puls.

NICCOLUM

GENERALITIES: Nickel is a remedy for periodical nervous headache, with asthenopia, weak digestion, constipation, of debilitated literary persons. Must sit up and hold the head with hands or has to put the arms on thighs when coughing, < night. Violent hiccough; with thirst. Child must be held up during the cough otherwise it would be seized by spasm.

WORSE: Periodically; every two weeks, yearly.

NITRICUM ACIDUM

GENERALITIES: This acid has a marked affinity for the MARGINS OF THE OUTLETS, esp. of the throat, anus and mouth; in addition it affects GLANDS — *liver*, prostate and salivary. It causes HEMORRHAGES—easy, bright, or bloody water. Patients are greatly debilitated, trembling, shivery, sensitive, and sore. Pains STICKING LIKE SPLINTER or *ulcerative gnawing*. Slight pain affects him violently. Discharges are ACRID, thin, dirty or brown, cause redness or destroy hair. OFFENSIVENESS—ozena, foot or night sweats. Mucous membranes are dark, smooth. Orifices are red, swollen and cracked. *Sensation of a band about* or weight hanging to the part. Sore, *stiff* during pain. Hard, gritty exudates. Cracking joints. Pains come and go quickly. Suitable for yellow, *brunettes* of spare habit, or persons suffering from chronic diseases, having a tendency to catch cold, or diarrhea. Cachexia. Bleeding after curettage. Malignancy. Phagedena. Fistula. Syphilis. Sycosis. Cancer. Stubborn suppuration. *Bones painfully sore*. Convulsions, epileptiform, at night and on going to bed. During the day, frequent vertigo, > riding in carriage. Ill effects of loss of sleep from nursing the sick. Pain as if flesh is torn from the bones. Caries and exostoses of bones. Sensitive to medicines given in high potency. Sensation of a mouse running up and down left side.

WORSE: Slight causes—TOUCH, JARRING, *noise*, rattling. *Motion*. Milk. Fat food. After eating. COLD *air*. *Dampness*. *Night*. Evening. Changing weather. Heat of bed. Mental exertion or shock. *Mercury*. Loss of sleep.

BETTER: *Gliding motion*. Riding in a carriage. Mild weather. Steady pressure.

MIND: Irritable, hateful, vindictive. So angry, he trembles. Profane, cursing using vulgar language. Quarrelsome delirium; talks to spirits in other tongue. Confusion. Thoughts vanish, after exertion of mind. Sadness. Despondency. Taciturn. Refuses consolation on one's misfortune. Anxiety about his disease, fear of cholera; of death. Constantly thinks about past troubles. No disposition to work, to perform any serious business. Hopeless despair. Weeps from discontent of himself. Easily frightened.

HEAD: *Crushing* head pain; < pressure of hat, street noise. Sensation of a band around head. Skull sore. Puffy swelling on scalp. Falling of hair, from vertex.

EYES: Sensation of warm water flowing over eyes, > cold water, or water running from the eyes. Conjunctiva pouts in spots. Diplopia. Eyelashes; stiff, all point towards nose (right). Paralysis of upper lids. Fistula lacrimalis.

EARS: Deafness, > noise, in train, riding in a carriage, deafness from enlarged and indurated tonsils; after measles. Cracking in ears when chewing. One's speech echoes in ears. Caries of mastoid. Cystic tumor on lobes of ears.

NOSE: Bleeding, dark, clotted, with chest affections, < weeping. Dripping from nose in diphtheria. Sneezing frequent without coryza, during sleep. Coryza with shortness of breath. Red, scurfy tip. Cutting pain in the nose; caries of bone. Fetid yellow discharge. Ozena. Green casts from nose every morning.

FACE: *Yellow*; sickly. Peeling of lips. Angles of lips raw, cracked or scabby. Cracking in jaws when chewing.

MOUTH: Loose teeth. Gums swollen, sore, flabby, bleeding at inner side. Moist, fissured or mapped tongue. Tongue, clean, red with center furrow. Sore palate. Ulcers in soft palate, with sharp splinter-like pain. Salivation, bloody, with green coating on tongue. Fetor oris. Ranula.

Bites the tongue and cheek. Teeth yellow; caries of teeth. Teeth feel soft and spongy.

THROAT: Sticking pain as from splinters, goes into ears, < swallowing. Tonsils red, swollen, uneven, with small ulcers thereon. Cannot swallow even a teaspoonful, difficult swallowing. Hawks out mucus from posterior nares.

STOMACH: Longing for fats, salt, indigestible things, chalk, earth, etc. Hunger, with sweetish taste. Milk disagrees. Nausea; with occasional vomiting, > riding in a carriage. Dislikes meat, things sweetened with sugar, bread. Nausea with eructations, cannot take food.

ABDOMEN: Stools tear the anus, even though soft. Prolonged pain after stool; walks in agony. Rectum feels torn; fissures in rectum. Painful, easily bleeding piles. Colic, > tightening clothes. Anus; itching, eczematous or oozes moisture. Ulceration after dysentery which have been badly treated. Feels a dry, hot cloth on abdomen. Inguinal hernia; of children. Burning in rectum after urination. Hemorrhage from rectum; after removal of piles.

URINARY: Urine *strong as horse's,* or offensive; cold when it passes; alternately profuse and scanty. Urine contains oxalic acid, uric acid and phosphates. Hematuria with shuddering along the spine. Sensation of a *hot wire* in urethra. Cramps from kidney to bladder. Infective nephritis. Stream thin, as due to stricture. Red scurfy spots on prepuce or on corona glandis. Painless retention or incontinence of urine. Contracted kidney.

MALE: Itching, burning foreskin. Chancre; phagedenic. Edematous prepuce. Phimosis. Stricture from gonorrhea or syphilis.

FEMALE: Voluptuous itching of vagina after coition. Bloody water from vagina, or hemorrhage from overexertion. Menses irregular, early, profuse, like muddy water. Metrorrhagia after parturition, after curetting. leukorrhea brown, flesh-coloured, watery or stringy; stains yellow or leaves spot with black border. Hard nodes in or atrophy of mammae. Pain in the back, buttocks, and thigh during menses.

RESPIRATORY: *Cough shattering;* from a dry spot in larynx; with stitching pain in lumbar region, < cold, winter. Short breath on going upstairs. Cough in sleep without waking. Expectoration muco-purulent, yellow, bitter, offensive, smeary, accompanied with sweat. Empyema. Hemoptysis. Cavernous phthisis. Short breath from uterine displacement. Congestion in the chest with palpitation and fear. Cutting in larynx. Panting breathing when reading or stooping.

HEART: Palpitation and anguish on going upstairs. Pulse intermits at fourth beat; irregular. Nervous palpitation caused by slightest mental excitement.

BACK: Stitching pain in lumbar back when coughing. Stitches in and between scapulae; neck stiff. Pain in back at night, > lying on abdomen.

EXTREMITIES: Finger-joints swollen. *Warts* on back of hands. Herpes between fingers. Fetid foot-sweat causing soreness of toes. White spots on nails. Tibia painfully sore. Pain in patella, impeding walking. Chilblain of toes. Sweating of palms and hands, cold. Blue nails. Weak ankles; cracking when walking. Ingrowing of the nails with ulceration and feeling of splinter, < touch. Nails distorted, discolored, yellow, curved.

SKIN: Dry, *eroded*, cracked in every angle. Coppery spots on shin bones. Skin itches on undressing. Crusts form and fall. *Ulcers* rapid, raw, ragged, with proud-flesh or plugs of pus. Stubborn suppuration. Burrowing pus. Warts large, jagged, bleed on touch or washing. Condylomata. Old scars become painful in cold weather.

SLEEP: Shocks on going to sleep. Pains come during sleep. Anxious, unrefreshing sleep, with frightful dreams.

FEVER: Icy *coldness* of soles. Chill continuous. *Sweats easily*, then takes cold. Exhausting (urinous) profuse sweat in morning—in axillae, on feet, and hands (in spinal injury). Night-sweat on part lain on.

COMPLEMENTARY: Calc; Thuj.

RELATED: Ars; Kali-c; *Kreos;* Merc.

NITRO-MURIATIC ACID

GENERALITIES: This remedy is prepared by mixing 18 parts of nitric acid with 82 parts of hydrochloric acid. It is almost a specific for oxaluria.

NUX MOSCHATA

GENERALITIES: Nutmeg is a popular domestic medicine for putting off the menstrual period, or for bringing it on, and also for diarrhea. It profoundly disturbs the SENSORIUM, *mind and* NERVES, causing exaltation of senses and nervous sensibility. *Digestion* is disturbed. FEMALE ORGANS are affected. When any complaint causes DROWSINESS, or is accompanied by drowsiness; and if in addition there is *chilliness* or *coldness* and THIRSTLESSNESS; *Nux Mos.* should be considered and given. *Dryness* as a sensation, or actual, is another characteristic symptom, of mouth, tongue, eyes, etc., but NO THIRST. *Heaviness* of eyes, tongue, etc. Marked tendency to *fainting fit*, with heart failure, < at stool, menses with slight pain, from sight of blood, while standing (when dressing). *Hemorrhage dark. Fleeting pains.* It is useful in scrawny, delicate, hysterical women who have small breasts and who *laugh or cry* by *turn.* Feeling of a hard lump in stomach, liver, throat. Hysteria. Mania. Automatism. Parts lain on feel sore. Feels as if drunk, staggers on trying to walk. Catalepsy. Spasm of children, with diarrhea. Epilepsy with consciousness. Little pain. Puffiness. Clairvoyance. Paralysis with spasms, and trembling of tongue, eyelids, esophagus. Mental depression from grief. Ill effects of fright, mental exertion, suppressed eruption. Humming, buzzing, funny feeling in body. Marasmus of little children. Hard parts feel soft.

WORSE: *Cold bath, damp, wind*, drafts. Fog. Cold feet. *Pregnancy.* Change of season. EMOTION, excitement. Exertion. MENSTRUATION. Jar. Bruise. Slight causes. Mental exertion or *shock.* Summer, hot weather. Motion. Lying on painful side. Overheating. Milk. Shaking head.

BETTER: Moist heat. Warm room. Dry weather.

MIND: *Dreamy.* Clairvoyant state. Changeable, laughing and crying. Bewildered; objects seem changed or grow larger. Thoughts suddenly vanish while talking, reading or writing. Uses wrong words (during headache). Slow ideation. Talks loudly to herself. Sense of duality—thinks she has two heads; seems to be two persons. Fickle and wavering in his undertakings. Entire loss of memory of his past life. Sense of impending dissolution. Mania with odd speeches and ridiculous gestures. Mockery. Laughing. Jesting. Surrounding seems changed, does not known well-know streets. Listless; indifferent. Answers irrelevantly. Short time seems very long. Sense of levitation. Does her household duties automatically, does not recollect what she has done.

HEAD: Aches; bursting in temples, > hard pressure. Vertigo as if drunk, staggering when walking in open air. Head feels full and expanding. Cerebral congestion. Brain feels loose; striking the sides on motion. Painless pulsating in head, in small spot. Convulsive movements of the head, could not talk or swallow. Raising head from pillow causes deathly sickness. Head drops forward while sitting.

EYES: Objects; look larger, or too small, very distant, oblique, too close together; vanish, red. Blindness, then fainting. Eyes seem dry, which impedes the movement of the eyelids. Pterygium over cornea.

EARS: Oversensitive hearing; for distant sounds increased.

NOSE: Oversensitive to smell. Nosebleed of dark blood. Dry; stopped up, must breathe through mouth.

FACE: Pale. Retracted lips. Foolish, childish expression, diabolic grin. Jaws feels paralyzed, cannot close them. Lips swollen, stick together.

MOUTH: Teeth seem pulled. Mouth *dry,* disappearing when entering the house, *without thirst*, < sleep. Tongue adheres to the roof of the mouth. Thick cottony saliva. Tongue numb, paralyzed, speech difficult. Chalky taste. Toothache of pregnant women, > warmth, < touch or sucking. Teeth seem loose. Saliva lessened, feels like cotton in mouth.

THROAT: *Dry.* Difficult swallowing; from paralysis of muscles.

STOMACH: Craving for highly seasoned food which only is digested. Loathing when eating or thinking of food. Digestion weak; all food turns to gas. Nausea and vomiting from irritation of uterine pessary. Flatulent dyspepsia. Eating a little too much causes headache. Hiccough.

ABDOMEN: Excessively bloated. *Flatulent colic.* Sensation of a board across the hypogastrium. Navel sore, even ulcerated, festering. *Stool; soft, but unable to expel it;* putrid; bright yellow and lienteric, < at night. Faintness during or after stool. Summer diarrhea from cold drink, boiled milk. Inactive rectum.

URINARY: Dysuria, from beer or wine, in hysteria, with dysmenorrhea, after eating, from uterine complaints. Urine smells like violet.

FEMALE: *Menses irregular, in time and quantity; thick, dark.* Leukorrhea muddy, bloody; replaces menses. Mammae too small. Nipples retracted. Flatus from vagina. Pain of uterus from pessary. Menses suppressed. Deficient labor pains. Continuous and obstinate flooding.

RESPIRATORY. *Hoarse voice, when walking against wind, hysterical.* Cough, < when getting warm in bed. Dyspnea, with feeling of weight in chest; asthma hysterical, difficult inhalation. Loss of breath when standing in water.

HEART: Trembling, fluttering, as from fright, fear or sadness. Palpitation, > walking about, drinking warm water. Sensation as if beating in vacuum, as if something grasped the heart. Pulse intermits at long intervals; exciting fear of death. Pulse weak, irregular.

NECK & BACK: Neck so weak, head drops forward on chest. Pain in back, now in sacrum, now in lumbar region. Pain along spine. Backache and neuralgia of sacrum and coccyx < riding in a carriage. Feels a piece of wood stretched across sacrum, < before menses.

EXTREMITIES: Fatigue on slight exertion. Limbs seem floating in the air. Rheumatism; drawing, wandering pains, < cold damp air, cold wet clothes, > warmth. Dry palms. Hysterical paralysis. Soles always moist. Feels as if treading on hard peas when walking. Feet cold with appearance of menses.

SKIN: Dry, cold. Blue spots.

SLEEP: *Sleepy attacks*, sudden, with vertigo. Great sleepiness with all complaints. Dreams; of falling from high place, of being pursued.

FEVER: Alternate chill and heat. Chill with stupor. Sweat; red or bloody or absent.

COMPLEMENTARY: Calc; Lyc.

RELATED: Cann-i; Croc; Gels; Mosch; Op; Rhus-t.

NUX VOMICA

GENERALITIES: *Nux-v.* is an everyday remedy. It corresponds to many diseased conditions to which a modern man is prone. It is useful for those persons who lead a *sedentary life,* doing much mental work, or remain under stress and strain of prolonged office work, business cares and worries. Such persons in order to forget their worries are apt to indulge in wine, women, rich stimulant food and sedative drugs; and suffer in consequence. The typical *Nux* patient is rather thin, spare, quick, active, nervous and irritable. It affects the nerves, causing hyper-sensitiveness, and overimpressionability— mentally and physically. Produces DIGESTIVE DISTURBANCES, partial congestion and hypochondriacal states. Dyspeptic persons who always select their food for experimenting that is little digested. He is subject to spasm, convulsions, and fainting. The patient seems to be always out of tune. THE ACTION IS VIOLENT, often irregularly fitful or inefficient. *Twists and jerks.* Spasms, tetanic, with consciousness, < by slightest touch, but > by grasping tightly, or when elbow was stretched. Tense contracted feeling. Lightning-like pains. Neuralgia, prodromal. Sensation of a rough body internally. Sensation of heaviness and lightness alternately. *Bruised soreness* OF ABDOMEN, brain, etc. Internal scrapy sensation or RAWNESS, in throat, larynx. *Takes cold. Fainting,* after stool, vomiting. labor pain, etc. Biliousness. *Hemorrhage.* Debauches; much drugged patients. *Trembling.* Epilepsy during stool. Paralysis from apoplexy in high livers; partial, with vertigo and nausea; with sticking pains. Reflexes increased. Firm-fibered brunettes. Reverse peristalsis. Ill effects of masturbation, sexual excess. Varicose veins, without tortuosity, black hard cords, from much standing, or from sedentary habit.

WORSE: EARLY MORNING. COLD—OPEN AIR (dry), *draft*, seat, wind. UNCOVERING. HIGH LIVING. Coffee, condiment, *liquor, drugs, purgatives*, over eating. *Sedentary habits. Debauchery. Mental exertion,* fatigue, vexation. Disturbed sleep. SLIGHT CAUSES—*anger, noise, odor, touch,* PRESSURE of clothes at waist. Yawning. Tobacco. Music. Disappointment of ambition. Wounded honor. Mental shock.

BETTER: FREE DISCHARGES. Naps. *Wrapping head.* Resting. Hot drinks. *Milk.* Fat. *Moist air. Lying on sides.*

MIND: *Active.* ANGRY AND IMPATIENT; *cannot stand pain,* so mad, he cries. *Zealous; fiery* temperament. *Nervous and excitable.* Aversion to work. Fears poverty. Sullen. Spiteful. Nagging. *Violent.* Ugly, suicidal, homicidal impulses. Fear of knives, lest she should kill herself or others. Fault finding. Reproaches others. Frightfully apprehensive about getting married (girls). Time passes too slowly. Talks about one's condition. Even the least ailment affects her greatly. Hypochondriasis. Melancholia. Delirium tremens. Cannot bear noise, light, odor, touch, music, conversation or reading. Angry when consoled. Head-strong, self-willed.

HEAD: Vertigo: brain and objects turn in circle, with momentary loss of consciousness, with black spell, on empty stomach. Bruised sensation of the brain. Dizzy and faint in a crowd or where many lights are burning. Headache in the sunshine. Sensitive scalp. Swollen forehead. Head seems larger than body. Takes cold, > wrapping head warmly. Migraine. Frontal headache with desire to lean it on something.

EYES: Bloodshot. Lacrimation on affected side. Atrophy of the optic nerve. Photophobia. Paresis of ocular muscles. Lower eyeballs yellow. Loss of vision due to alcohol and tobacco. Exudation of blood from eyes. Spring conjunctivitis.

EARS: Itching in ear through eustachian tubes. External meatus dry and sensitive. Pain, stitching, when swallowing. Loud sounds are painful.

NOSE: Oversensitive to strong odors, even fainting. Nose stopped, but runs water, on one side. Snuffles of the newborn. Nosebleed during sleep from suppressed flow of piles, from coughing. *Sneezing* violent, *abortive,* from intense crawling in nostril (left). *Coryza,* fluent by day, and in open air, dry at night. Smell before nose like old cheese, burning sulphur. Smell acute. Nose looks sharp and pointed.

FACE: *Red, turgid* or yellowish < about nose and mouth. Left angle of the mouth drops. Infra-orbital neuralgia, with swelling of cheek, intermittent, > when lying in bed. Jaws snap shut, stiff. Acne from eating cheese. Pimples from excessive use of liquors. Child passes its hand constantly over face (brain disease).

MOUTH: Teeth chatter. Toothache, > warm drink. Fetor oris; sour. Small aphthous ulcers in the mouth. TASTE BITTER, sour, bad in a.m., low down in throat. Itching palate, eustachian tube. Gums swollen, white, and bleeding. Needles at edges of tongue, < after eating, washing face in cold water.

THROAT: *Rough, raw, as if scraped.* Putrid taste on coughing. Small ulcers in the throat; pain < during empty swallowing. Stitches extend into ears.

STOMACH: Craves piquant food—beer, fat food, chalk, stimulants. HICCOUGH from overeating, cold or hot drink. Violent retching, < hawking. *Eructations* sour. Heart-burn. *Waterbrash. Nausea, > if he can vomit.* VIOLENT VOMITING, bilious, sour, wants to vomit but cannot. *Food lies like a heavy knot in stomach.* Gastralgia; pain goes into back and chest, > vomiting and hot drinks, < from food. Indigestion. Hunger, yet aversion to food. Eructations difficult, sour, bitter. Severe pain in stomach from injury, < least food.

ABDOMEN: Sensation of a band about waist, *clothes oppress it.* Bruised *soreness of abdominal wall.* Liver sore, enlarged; sticking pain. Gailstone colic. *Jaundice* from anger. Bowels gripe here and there. SORE BOWELS, < COUGHING AND STEPPING. Hernia; infantile; from constipation or crying; umbilical hernia. Flatulent colic. UNEASY, FITFUL AND FRUITLESS URGING FOR BOWELS TO ACT, > STOOL. Constipation. Inactive peristalsis. Strains hard at stool; feeling as if part remained unexpelled; passes small quantity at each attempt. Rectum: spasms flatus retained, constant uneasiness. Piles itching, blind, bleeding, > cool bathing. Dysenteric stools > pain for a time. Diarrhea with jaundice, after debauch during fever. Colic in nursing infants from stimulating food taken by the mother. Colic from suppressed hemorrhoidal flow. First part of stool soft, last hard. Prolapse of rectum from diarrhea. Dragging in anus when not at stool. Sense of goneness in the groins.

URINARY: Renal colic (right), extends to genitals and legs, with dribbling urine; > lying on back. Painful ineffectual urging to urinate. Spasmodic strangury. Hematuria from suppressed hemorrhoidal flow or menses. Spasmodic urethral stricture. Paralysis of bladder, urine dribbles, in old men with enlarged prostate or gonorrhea. Involuntary urination when laughing, coughing, sneezing.

MALE: Desire easily excited. Penis becomes relaxed during embrace. Bad effects of onanism, sexual excess. Premature ejaculation. Cannot be in female company without having emission. Increase of smegma.

FEMALE: Desire too strong, with burning in vulva. *Menses profuse, early and prolonged;* intermittent; of dark, lumpy blood; irregular; with fainting spells. Dysmenorrhea; cramps extend to the whole body, with constant urging to stool. Leukorrhea fetid; stains yellow. Inefficient labor pains; faints at every labor pain. Profuse bleeding after abortion. Prolapse of uterus from straining or lifting. All old symptoms are < after menses. Lochia scanty, offensive. Nipples sore; white spot in centre. Tensive pain when nursing. Painless gathering of milk in breast from not nursing the child.

RESPIRATORY: *Cough violent,* throwing the patient down, paroxysmal, whooping, with splitting headache, has to hold his head. Shallow respiration. Oppressed breathing. Asthma from disordered stomach, with fulness of stomach. Hoarseness, with painful roughness in larynx and chest. Cough with sensation as if something torn loose in the chest. Intercostal neuralgia, < lying on painful side. Asthma with feeling as if clothing were too tight, > belching. Desire to eat during cough.

HEART: Palpitation on lying down. Heart feels tired. Angina pectoris, patient lies on knee with body bent backward.

NECK & BACK: Cervico-brachial neuralgia; painfully stiff neck; pain down shoulder (right), < touch. Wry neck from cold or nervous shock. Lumbar ache, as if breaking, *must sit up in order to turn in bed.* Crawling along spine. Acute lumbago. Sacral region feels lame after parturition.

EXTREMITIES: Arms go to sleep; numb, stiff feeling. Tense cramp in calves and soles, must stretch feet, or stand still while walking. Feet feel clubby and raw. Shooting from toes to thighs, < after stool. Drags his feet while walking, (chorea), legs tremble, unsteady gait. Knee joints feels dry, cracking during motion. Paralysis of lower limbs from overexertion or from being soaked. Automatic motions of hand (r) towards mouth (apoplexy). Legs stiff.

SKIN: Goose skin. Skin red and blotchy. Urticaria with gastric derangement. Bluish spots.

SLEEP: *Yawning.* Sleepy in the evening or sleepless from rush of ideas. *Awakes too early, cannot go to sleep again,* finally sleeps, until aroused. Nightmare. Dreams; anxious being pursued by animals, dogs and cats; amorous. Weeping and talking during sleep.

FEVER: Chill with thirst, and heat without thirst. EASILY CHILLED, CANNOT UNCOVER, < *motion and* drinking even during the heat. Body burning hot, esp. face, but unable to move or uncover without feeling chilly. Excessive rigor with blue fingernails. Sweat sour; one sided; warm on uppermost side, on lying down.

COMPLEMENTARY: Kali-c; *Phos*; Sulph.

RELATED: Ign; Lyc.

OCIMUM CANUM

GENERALITIES: This remedy is useful in diseases of kidneys, uterus, bladder and urethra. Symptoms of renal colic, esp. of right side, are pronounced. *Sore pain* *in ureters.* Renal colic with hematuria and violent vomiting, with wringing of hands, moaning and crying all the time. Red sand in urine, which may be of saffron color and of musk-like odor. Swollen inguinal and mammary glands. Nipples painful to least contact. Vaginal prolapse. Urine scanty; which <.

OENANTHE CROCATA

GENERALITIES: It is a valuable convulsive remedy; useful in epileptiform, puerperal and uremic convulsions. *Epilepsy;* with priapism, < during menses or instead of menses; during pregnancy. Falls backward and utters a loud cry before falling. Status epilepticus. Sensation of a bug creeping under the skin about the waist; < touch of clothes. Insanity; hallucination. Face swollen; convulsive twitching of facial muscles; foaming at mouth, lock-jaw. Tendency to cry over little things. Rosy red blotches on face, chest, arms, abdomen. Burning heat, < head and throat. Profuse offensive sweat. Obstinate vomiting for days not relieved by any thing.

WORSE: *Injury*. Sexual and menstrual disturbances. Water.

RELATED: Bell; Cic.

OLEANDER

GENERALITIES: It has a marked action on *nervous system*, heart, skin and *digestive tract. Paralytic condition,* with cramp-like contraction of upper extremities. Paresis after infantile paralysis. General cramps. *Numbness. Weakness,* with trembling, in nursing women. Sense of vibration. Emptiness in stomach and chest after eating, > brandy. Hemiplegia. Paralytic rigidity.

Sopor. Unable to speak or speaks with difficulty. Discharges involuntary.

WORSE: Rubbing. Undressing. After suckling. Friction of clothes.

BETTER: Looking sideways. Brandy.

MIND: Sadness, with lack of confidence and power. Morose, peevish. Distraction. Slow comprehension.

HEAD: Vertigo; < looking fixedly at an object or looking down, turning to either side in bed; with diplopia. Headache, > by looking crossways, sideways or squinting. Vertigo for a long time before paralysis. Biting, itching of scalp. Moist milk-crusts, < occiput. Corrosive itching on forehead and at edges of hair, < heat.

EYES: Feels as if drawn back into head. Can see objects only when looking at them sideways. Diplopia. Lacrimation when reading.

FACE: Pale. Sunken. Numb upper lip. Lower jaw trembles when yawning.

MOUTH: Toothache only while masticating. Tongue numb. Loss of speech.

THROAT: Sensation as if cool wind blowing in throat (left).

STOMACH: Empty feeling even after eating, > brandy; from nursing. Canine hunger with hurried eating. Throbbing in pit. Desires cold water. Aversion to cheese. Extreme debility of digestive power.

ABDOMEN: Passes food undigested in the morning, which he ate the day before. Stools thin, lienteric, involuntary; escape with flatus; in children.

URINARY: Involuntary urination.

FEMALE: Tremor after nursing; so weak she can scarcely walk across the room.

HEART: Palpitation, with weakness and empty feeling in chest, > brandy. Pain on stooping.

EXTREMITIES: Crampy contraction of upper limbs in paralysis. *Numbness* of limbs. Weakness of lower limbs. Painless paralysis. Veins on hands swollen. Hands tremble, while writing. Trembling knees when standing. Feet constantly cold. Fingers rigid and thumb turns on palm. Limbs stiff and cold.

SKIN: Sensitive, *chafes* and oozes or bleeds. Eruptions with itching, biting as if lice. Skin numb.

SLEEP: Sopor, yawning with trembling of lower jaw.

FEVER: *Heat from mental exertion.*

RELATED: Anac; Chin.

OLEUM ANIMALE

GENERALITIES: This volatile oil was prepared by Dippel first by distillation of stags' horn. It affects the NERVES, esp. pneumogastric nerve; digestive organs. Symptoms appear here and there or in single parts. Affected parts feel *sore.* Tremulous weakness of hands, knees, feet, etc. Pain in spots. Stitches; burning pains as from red hot needles. *Pulled upward* and *from behind forward pains* in malar bones, testicles, mammae, etc. Icy *coldness* from tips of teeth to throat, stomach, etc. Shuffling gait. *Urinous;* eructations, leukorrhea, etc. Flesh feels torn from bones. Ill effects of suppressions, esp. of foot sweat. Neurasthenia.

WORSE: Cold. *Eating.* Suppression. Menses. Hot drink. Noise. 2 to 9 p.m.

BETTER: Rubbing. Pressure. Stretching. Open air. Changing position. Eructation.

MIND: Indolent, inclined to sit. Nervous irritability. Sad, introverted, absorbed in self, speaks in whispers. Vanishing thoughts. Faintness; of gastric origin.

HEAD: Pain in spots. Migraine with polyuria. Vertigo of gastric origin, > bending head backwards.

EYES: Glistening bodies before eyes. Lacrimation on eating. A skin seems to overhang the eyes. Twitching of lids.

FACE: Malar bones feel pulled up. Twitching lips. White of an egg felt dried on lips. Swelling beneath right lower jaw.

MOUTH: Toothache, > pressing teeth together. Sensation of coldness coming out from tips of teeth. Mouth feels greasy. Snow-white cottony saliva. Tongue sore as if scalded. Bites cheek while eating.

THROAT: Sore, dry, constricted; empty swallowing difficult though food and drink pass easily. Sensation as if cold air penetrates the throat. Hawks out gluey brown lumps. Acrid vapor or raw streak in throat, < cough.

STOMACH: *Water-brash,* > chewing tobacco. Pulsation or feeling of water in stomach. Sensation of coldness (lump of ice), burning, constriction, > eructation. Urinous eructations.

ABDOMEN: Flatulence and rumbling.

URINARY: *Profuse, pale urine, of fish-brine odor,* < hysteria, migraine. Frequent scanty urine, then headache. Greenish urine. Small stream of urine.

MALE: Seminal losses; on straining at stool. *Testes swollen alternately; feel pulled* forcibly upward and seized. Neuralgia of spermatic cord. Pressure in perineum. Prostate hypertrophy.

FEMALE: Menses early, scanty; black flow. Sore mammae before menses; outward stitches in nipples in scirrhus.

Stitches in breast from behind forward. Urinous leukorrhea.

RESPIRATORY: Asthma from suppressed foot-sweat. Stitches at clavicle.

HEART: Anxious palpitation. Pulse slow.

BACK: Aching scapula (right), > pressure. Sprained feeling in sacrum. Unsteady gait. Cracking in cervical vertebrae on raising the head.

SKIN: Excoriation in bends of joints.

FEVER: Alternate chill and heat. Cold foul foot-sweat, fishy on heels.

RELATED: Sulph; Tell.

OLEUM JECORIS

GENERALITIES: Cod liver oil is a nutrient and affects the chest, liver, pancreas and tendons. Phthisis and scrofulous diathesis. Soreness. Burning in spots. Faulty nutrition. *Atrophic infants;* children who cannot digest milk. Emaciation; hot hands and head. Lassitude. Discharges yellow. Always taking cold.

WORSE: Milk. *Cold damp* air or place. Motion.

FACE: Growth of short thick hair on chin and upper lip in women.

MOUTH: Tongue yellow. Fetid breath.

ABDOMEN: Soreness and heaviness in the region of liver, < exercise.

FEMALE: Establishes menses. leukorrhea yellow, with weak back.

RESPIRATORY: Hoarseness. Dry, tickling, hacking cough, > as fever comes on. Early phthisis. *Soreness or stitches* *in chest.* Hemoptysis. Yellow sputum. Cough with palpitation.

BACK: Chill, or fluttering from sacrum up back to occiput.

EXTREMITIES: Chronic rheumatism with rigid muscles and tendons. Palms hot toward evening.

SKIN: Yellow. Milk-crust. Ringworm (local application). Cold abscess.

FEVER: Hectic. Night-sweat.

RELATED: Phos.

ONOSMODIUM

GENERALITIES: This remedy acts upon *nerves* and *muscles.* It causes loss of power of concentration and coordination, and disturbance in the sense of proportion. *Aching, soreness and stiffness of* muscles, after the pain. Prostration, weariness and *tiredness*; acts as if born tired. Seems to tread on cotton. Staggering. Neuralgic pains. Neurasthenia, sexual, from loss of sexual desire in both sexes.

WORSE: *Sprain.* EYE STRAIN. *Sexual excess.* Darkness. Tight clothing. Warm. Humid air. Jarring.

BETTER: Rest. Sleep. Eating. Cold drink. Undressing.

MIND: *Irresolute.* Confused. Forgetful. Slow thinking. Aphasia. Fear of falling on going up or downstairs.

HEAD: Migraine. Headache from eyestrain and sexual weakness, < dark. Vertigo, with headache, < lying on left side, raising the hands above the head. *Occipital headache* as if screwed, < eyestrain and lying down. Pain up and down from occiput (left) to shoulder, < exertion. Dull, heavy up-pressing in occiput.

EYES: *Aching, heavy, tired and stiff.* Eye troubles combined with ovarian symptoms. *Misjudges distance.* Vision blurred. Color-blindness for red and green.

THROAT: Dry and stiff; all symptoms are > by cold drinks and eating.

ABDOMEN: Distended feeling, > loosening clothes. Stools yellow, mushy; hurying him out of bed in morning. Craving for icewater and cold drink.

URINARY: Urination frequent, scanty. Aromatic urine.

MALE: *Loss of sexual desire.* Psychical impotence. Speedy emission, deficient erection. Sexual excitement. Constant severe erection.

FEMALE: Sexual desire completely destroyed. Pain alternates between ovaries. Uterine pain, > undressing and lying on back. *Soreness of ovaries with that of rectum.* Feels as if menses would appear. *Leukorrhea; excoriating,* yellowish, offensive, profuse, running down the legs. Mammae swollen, aching. Nipples itch.

RESPIRATORY. Hacking cough, with sticky white sputum, > drinking cold water.

BACK: Tired feeling in lower part of the back.

EXTREMITIES: *Tired* and numb feeling in legs and poplitiae.

RELATED: Cimic; Hyper; Lil-t; Rhus-t.

OPIUM

GENERALITIES: Opium contains about eighteen alkaloids, of which apomorphine, morphine and codeine are well known. It affects the NERVES, MIND AND SENSES, producing *insensibility of nerves*, PAINLESSNESS, *depression; drowsy, stupor; torpidity and general sluggishness* *of function and lack of vital reaction*—a kind of negative state. *Excretions* except of skin, are checked. Voluntary motions are lessened. Loss of power; of concentration, self-control, and judgment. *Paralysis*, painless, of brain, tongue, *bowels,* etc. Tremors, twitchings, jerking during sleep. Convulsion, < heat of room or hot bath. *Bed seems hot,* hunts for a cold place. Hot sweat, *hand. Stupid sleep* accompanies all complaints—during spasm, violent chill, etc. Epilepsy in sleep, from approach of strangers (children), from fright, < glare of light, anger, insult. Throws limbs or stretches arms at right angle to the body; stupor between spasms. Want of susceptibility to medicines even though indicated. Faints every fifteen minutes. Sensation of bodily well-being, great happiness. Painless ulcer. Suppuration. Dropsical swelling of the whole body. *Internal dryness.* Ill effects of fear, fright, anger, shame, sudden joy; charcoal fumes, sun. Complaints appear with sweat. Complete idiocy from masturbation.

WORSE: EMOTIONS, FEAR, *fright*, shame, joy. Odors. ALCOHOL. *Sleep*. SUPPRESSED DISCHARGES. *Receding eruptions.* If heated. Sunstroke.

BETTER: Cold. Uncovering. Constant walking.

MIND: Complete loss of consciousness. Apoplectic states. PLACID. Wants nothing, says nothing ails him. Exaltation of mind, vivid imaginations. *Gaiety.* Talkative. Rash. Bold; increased courage. *Dreamy.* Sluggish. Dull. Stupid. No will-power. Tendency to lie. Fear after fright remains. Delirium tremens, with terror. Wants to go home, thinking that he is not at home. Carphology. Indifferent to pain and pleasure. Sees frightful visions, mice, scorpions, etc. Deceptive; vision, taste, touch; perversion of all senses. Imagines part of his body very large. Nervous, irritable; tendency to start.

HEAD: Vertigo after fright; of old people with lightness of head; from injury to head. Heavy occiput. Paralysis of brain. Head hot, with hot sweat.

EYES: Glassy; staring, immovable. Pupils contracted, dilated, insensible to light. Half-closed. Upturned. Ptosis. Visual hallucination. Red, bulging. Embolism of central artery of retina.

EARS: Acuteness of hearing. Clocks striking at a great distance keep her awake.

NOSE: Loss of smell.

FACE: Dark, turgid, *sweaty* or hot red or pale and red alternately. Besotted look. Corners of the mouth twitch. Trembling, twitching of the muscles of face. *Old look* after cholera infantum, of a suckling child three or four weeks old. Hanging down of lower jaw. Lock-jaw. Lips swollen, protruding.

MOUTH: Tongue paralyzed; protrudes to right side; black, dry. Difficult speech. Bloody froth.

THROAT: Dry. Inability to swallow; on swallowing food either goes the wrong way or returns through the nose.

STOMACH: Hungry; but no desire to eat. Vomiting, in peritonitis; of fecal matter, of urine. Very thirsty. Retching from emotions.

ABDOMEN: Hard, tympanitic. Feeling of a weight in abdomen. Bowels feel completely obstructed. *Paralytic atony of bowels*, after laparotomy. Lead colic. Incarcerated umbilical or inguinal hernia. Obstinate constipation. *Stools of hard black balls.* Bloody mucus oozes from open anus. Retention of stool from ileus. Stools involuntary, after fright. Violent pain in rectum as if pressed asunder. Difficult emission of flatus. Intestinal spasms, child cries day and night.

URINARY: *Paralytic atony of bladder*, after laparotomy. Retention of urine—in children from nursing an angry nurse, from spasms of neck of bladder, from fright. Urine slow to start, feeble stream. Involuntary from fright. Renal colic, pain radiates to bladder and testicles.

MALE: Spasmodic stricture from drinking poorly fermented liquor, and in drunkards.

FEMALE: Dysmenorrhoea, forcing her to bend double, with urging to stool. Amenorrhea from fright. Softness of uterus. Lively or violent fetal motion. Puerperal convulsions. Threatened abortion, and suppression of lochia from fright. Convulsions come from stoppage of labor pains. Prolapsus from fright. Hiccough during pregnancy.

RESPIRATORY: Rattling, *unequal breathing*. Sighing, snoring, continuous stertor. Cough; tickling, with dyspnea and blue face, or profuse sweat on whole body, > drinking water. Heat in chest. Breathing stops on going to sleep and it does not start unless the patient is moved. Hemoptysis. Aphonia from fright. Yawning after cough.

HEART: Burning about the heart. Weak. *Full slow pulse*. Palpitation after alarming events, fright, grief, sorrow, etc.

BACK: Opisthotonos. Pulsating arteries and swollen veins on neck.

EXTREMITIES: Trembling of the limbs after fright. Painless paralysis. Twitching and spasmodic movement of limbs. Veins of hands distended. Feels as if lower limbs were severed and belong to someone else. Numbness; weakness. Shuffling and trembling gait. One or other arm moves convulsively to and fro.

SKIN: Crawling here and there. *General itching*. Rough and dirty. Dry. Painless, indolent ulcer. Whole body looks red. Blue spots.

SLEEP: *Somnolence.* Heavy stupid sleep of the aged. Tired and sleepless drunkards. Sleeplessness from acuteness of hearing. Coma vigil. Sleepy but cannot go to sleep. Dreams of cats, dogs, black forms.

FEVER: General low temperature with inclination to stupor. *Hot, sweaty and drowsy*, with cold limbs. Hot sweat over whole body except lower limbs. Sweats; without relief.

COMPLEMENTARY: Alum; Bar-c; Phos; Plb.

RELATED: Arn; Nux-m.

ORIGANUM

GENERALITIES: Sweet marjoram strongly affects the female sexual organs. Increased desire for coitus. Eratomania, with inclination to commit suicide. Great sexual excitement driving her to masturbation. Lascivious ideas, impulses, dreams. Swelling and itching of nipples and pain in breast. Thoughts of marriage, which dispel sadness. Desire for active exercise impelling her to run.

RELATED: Canth; Hyos; Plat.

OSMIUM

GENERALITIES: This metal is found associated with platinum. It affects the *respiratory tract*, esp. *Trachea*. Though secretions are foul, urine smells like violet, eructations are like radish and axillary sweat like garlic. Crawling on back and shoulders. Pains go up and down. Causes adhesion of the nail fold.

WORSE: Coughing. Talking.

MIND: Weeping mood, screaming with cough.

EYES: Greenish or rainbow colors around the light. Glaucoma, with iridescent vision.

NOSE: Coryza, fluent, with a feeling of stoppage. Snuffling.

STOMACH: Feels full of broken stones or lumps. Eructations smelling like radish.

URINARY: Urine; albuminous; smelling like violet.

MALE: Steady aching in glans penis. Pain in testes and spermatic cord.

RESPIRATORY: Spasmodic cough; sounds as if coughing in an empty tube; with torn loose feeling and tenacious sputum. Talking causes pain in larynx. Sensitive air passages.

BACK: Crawling on back and shoulders.

EXTREMITIES: Axillary sweat smells like garlic. Twitching of fingers with spasmodic cough. Fold of skin remains attached to growing nail.

SKIN: Eczema. Itching pimples.

RELATED: Ars; Iod; Phos.

OXALICUM ACIDUM

GENERALITIES: Though oxalates are found in certain sour vegetables which are eaten the acid itself is a very violent poison not only producing *gastro-enteritis* but affecting also the *nerves* and *spinal cord*, causing motor paralysis. The patient becomes weak, cold, livid and numb all over, < lower limbs. *Excruciating pains*, like lightning, in streaks, *in spots*, burning, etc. Symptoms < by motion and thinking of them. Thinking will bring on the conditions when they are not actually present. Rheumatism of the left side. Neurasthenia. Neuralgia.

Paralysis; of left side, from spinal meningitis. Periodical affections.

WORSE: *Thinking of it. Cold. Touch. Shaving.* Mental exertion. Motion. Strawberries, sour fruits, grapes.

BETTER: After stool.

MIND: Nervous and sleepless. Very much exhilarated; quicker thought and action. All conditions made worse by thinking about oneself.

HEAD: Vertigo; swimming sensation on lying down, while looking out of window. Band-like sensation about the head; sensation of a screw behind each ear, > after stool. Numb pricking in occiput. Sore tender spot on scalp.

EYES: Small, and especially linear objects appear larger and more distant than they are. Sight vanishes with epistaxis. Hyperesthesia of retina.

FACE: Pale, cold, livid. Feeling of heat.

MOUTH: *Sour taste*, eructations, with difficult swallowing.

STOMACH: Emptiness with gnawing compelling one to eat. Burning pain goes upwards, < slightest touch, sugar. Cannot eat strawberries. Sugar, coffee and wine disagree.

ABDOMEN: Colic about the navel, or involuntary muddy brown stools, > lying. Flatus passes with difficulty. Stitching pain in the liver, > deep breathing. Fainting and vomiting during stool. Diarrhea from coffee. Chronic inflammation of bowels.

URINARY: Thinking of urinating causes necessity to urinate. Pain in glans penis, when urinating. Oxaluria.

MALE: Neuralgic pain in spermatic cord, < from slightest motion. Testes throb or feel crushed.

RESPIRATORY: Low voice. Hoarseness with cardiac derangement. Aphonia from paralysis of vocal cord.

Dyspnea, nightly. Short, jerking inspiration, and sudden forced expiration. Pain from lower chest (left) to epigastrium. Chest fixed. Left lung painful. Voice altered.

HEART: Sharp darting in heart and left lung, extending to epigastrium, depriving of breath; sits erect with arms folded across chest. Palpitation, < lying. Angina pectoris. Heart symptoms alternate with aphonia. Beats of heart intermit when thinking of it. Fluttering heart.

BACK: Numb pricking in back. *Back feels too weak to hold the body.* Cold creeps up spine.

EXTREMITIES: *Weak trembling hand and feet.* Drawing, lancinating pain shooting down extremities. Lower limb, blue, cold, insensible, immobile. Numbness extends from shoulders to fingertips. Hands cold as if dead. Wrist (R) constantly painful, as if sprained; wants to stretch it, cannot hold anything. Pain in fleshy part of thumb (R).

SKIN: Sensitive, sore, smarting, < shaving. Perspires easily. Mottled in circular patches.

RELATED: Ars; Pic-ac.

OXYTROPIS

GENERALITIES: Commonly known as Loco or crazy weed, it has a marked action on nervous system producing uncertain, staggering or backward gait. Great mental depression. Urging to urinate when thinking of it. Trembling and sense of emptiness.

WORSE: Thinking of it. Every other day.

BETTER: After sleep.

PAEONIA

GENERALITIES: Anal and skin symptoms are marked. Skin is very *sensitive*; ulceration, from pressure of tight boots, bedsore, etc. Shooting or splinter-like pains. Varicose veins. Rolls on floor from pain.

WORSE: *Touch* or pressure. Night. Motion. STOOL.

MIND: Much affected by bad news.

RECTUM: *Excruciating pain at anus*, continues long after stool; must rise and walk about at night. Fissures or fistula in anus. Hemorrhoids - large, ulcerated. Painful ulcer oozing, offensive moisture on perineum. Anus covered with crusts.

SLEEP: Terrifying nightmares.

SKIN: Sensitive. Ulcer from pressure, bedsore. Bunion.

RELATED: Rat.

PALLADIUM

GENERALITIES: This metal is closely associated with platinum and gold. It affects the *ovaries,* esp. the right, uterus and mind. *Pains fleeting,* transient. Weakness, aversion to exercise. Bruised soreness. Ailments from bad news.

WORSE: *Emotion, lively*; chagrin. *Social functions*. Standing. Exertion.

BETTER: Touch. Pressure. Diversion. Rubbing. After sleep, stool.

MIND: Love of approbation, seeks the good opinion of others and attaches great importance to them. Easy prey to slights, real or imaginary; wounded pride and fancied neglect, sometimes finding vent in violent expressions. Depressing news < all symptoms. Time passes too slowly. Keeps up brightly in company, much exhausted afterwards.

HEAD: Feels as if swung backward and forward. Headache across the top of head from ear to ear, > fixing attention on it.

FACE: Blue, sallow.

THROAT: Feels as if crumbs of bread had lodged in, as if something hanging near hyoid bone. Glairy mucus from throat.

ABDOMEN: Shooting pain from navel goes into breasts or pelvis, > after stool. Hollowness in groins. Feels as if intestines were bitten off. Coughing, sneezing, < pain in abdomen. Stools white; constipated.

URINARY: Cutting pain in bladder, > stool. Bladder feels full but little urine is passed.

FEMALE: Uterine prolapse or retroversion. Sub-acute pelvic peritonitis. Bearing-down pain, > rubbing. Cutting in uterus, > after stool. Menstrual discharge while nursing. Glairy, yellow leukorrhea before and after menses. Pelvis leaden heavy, < standing. Ovarian pain, > pressure. Abdomen feels sore after menses and apprehension that something horrible will happen.

BACK: Tired feeling in small of back.

EXTREMITIES: Fleeting neuralgic pains in various parts of the body. Drafting pains from toes to hips.

SKIN: Itching all over the body after undressing.

RELATED: Asaf; Plat.

PAREIRA BRAVA

GENERALITIES: Genito-urinary organs and left side is affected by this remedy. Constant urging to urinate; violent pain in the glans penis and down the thighs during efforts of urination; *must get on knees and hands pressing* head firmly to the floor to urinate. Cartilaginous induration of mucous membranes of the urethra and bladder. Renal colic; enlarged prostate; with retention of urine and catarrh of the bladder. Dysuria. Urine contains thick, stringy, white mucus or *red sand.* Edema of the lower limbs.

RELATED: Berb; Med.

PARIS QUADRIFOLIA

GENERALITIES: If affects head, spine, eyes and one side. Sensation of *heaviness*; numbness; *parts feel too big* or drawn together. Disorder of sense of touch, objects felt rough. Coldness of right side of the body while left side was hot. Whole body painful, esp. when touched. Mucus secretions are green and tenacious. Sensitiveness to offensive odors. Broken feeling of joints. Ill effects of injury, suppressions.

WORSE: Thinking. Eyestrain. Touch.

BETTER: Pressure. Eructation.

MIND: *Garrulous loquacity.* Silly conduct. Loquacious mania. Inclination to treat others with rudeness and contempt.

HEAD: Vertigo on reading aloud. Headache, < by thinking. Head feels large, expanded. Occipital headache with a feeling of weight. Headaches as from pulling a string from eyes to occiput. Scalp sensitive, cannot comb hair. Left side numb. Chronic headache.

EYES: *Balls seem pulled back or feel too large*, and heavy.

EARS: Pain as if ears were pressed out, or forced apart by a wedge, < swallowing.

NOSE: Imaginary foul smells. Bread, fish, milk smell putrid.

FACE: Seems drawn into root of nose. Neuralgia; hot stitches in malar bones.

MOUTH: Dry on awakening. Tongue dry, feels too large.

THROAT: Hawks up *tough green mucus.* Sensation of a ball in the throat. Burning when eating and drinking.

STOMACH: Heavy as from a stone, > by eructation. Weak digestion. Red curved streak above navel.

RESPIRATORY: *Periodical* painless *hoarseness.*

NECK: Weight and weariness in nape of neck. Stitches in coccyx on sitting. Violent pain on both sides of neck extending down to fingers, < mental exertion.

EXTREMITIES: Fingers feel numb. Everything feels rough. Joints feel broken, swollen or dislocated at every motion.

SKIN: Painfully sensitive.

FEVER: Unilateral coldness or heat. Heat descending from the neck to back.

RELATED: Bell; Nux-v.

PASSIFLORA INCARNATA

GENERALITIES: Has a quieting effect on the nervous system, hence an efficient antispasmodic remedy. Convulsions of children during teething. Breaks off morphine habit. Insomnia of infants and the aged, and mentally worried and over-worked persons. Tetanus.

Hysteria. Puerperal convulsions. Asthma (10 to 30 drops). General atonic condition (30 to 60 drops repeated several times).

PETROLEUM

GENERALITIES: Rock oil chiefly acts on the *skin, esp. of folds*, scalp, face, and genitals. Produces catarrhal condition suited to long-lasting deep-seated wasting diseases; complaints following mental states fright, vexation, etc. Lingering gastric and intestinal troubles. Tremulous weakness. Feels sick internally. *Internal itching.* Dread of open air; with shivering when exposed to it *Dryness* in ear, nose, etc. Discharges are thick, purulent and yellowish green. Hemorrhage; blood light red, < lifting or riding. Burning. Twitching. Catalepsy. Dropsy. One of the first remedies for car, train or sea sickness. Ill effects of sprain, suppressed eruption. Wooden feeling. Emaciation, esp. of chest. Coldness in spots; in abdomen, in heart, after scratching. Bruised soreness, < in joints. Glands enlarged. Cracks. Unhealthy granulations after severe burns. FEAR, *long lasting.*

WORSE: MOTION; OF CAR, CARRIAGE, BOAT. *Weather—cold, winter*, changing; thunderstorm. *Eating. Vexation.* Cabbage. Coition. Touch, even of clothes.

BETTER: Warm air. Dry weather. Lying with head high.

MIND: Excited, irritable, after coition; inclination to be angry and to scold. Irresolute. Sense of duality, thinks he is double or someone else lying alongside or one limb is double. Death seems near and must hurry to settle the affairs. Worries but does not know why. Loses his way in the street; loss of memory. Fearful.

HEAD: VERTIGO, like that produced by swinging motion, *felt in occiput. Occiput; aching, heavy.* Headache, < shaking, coughing, must hold temples for relief. Falling of the hair. Moist eruptions on scalp, < occiput and ears. Head feels numb as if made of wood. Cold air as if blowing on head.

EYES: Inflamed tarsi. Loss of eyelashes. Fistula lacrimalis (of recent origin). Canthi fissured.

EARS: Deafness; with noises in ears in old people. Noise from several people talking is unbearable. Dryness in ears. Discharge of pus and blood from the ears. Moist spots behind the ears. Itching deep in the ears, in eustachian tube. Painful externally.

NOSE: Dry. Nostrils ulcerated, cracked, burning. Ozena, purulent discharge. Tip of nose itches.

FACE: Dry, as if covered with albumin. Pale or yellow, hot after eating. Easy dislocation of jaw.

MOUTH: Dry. Offensive smell, like garlic. Ulcers on the inner cheek, painful when closing the teeth. Soreness while chewing. Tongue white in centre, dark streak along edges.

THROAT: Foul mucus in throat. Hawks out in the morning. Dry.

STOMACH: Hunger, causing nausea, awaking at night, after stool. Pungent acrid eructations. Thirst for beer. Desire for dainties. Aversion to meat, fat, cooked or hot foods. Vomits bitter green substance. *Nausea; train and seasickness*; nausea during pregnancy, must stoop.

ABDOMEN: Inflated; internal coldness. *Diarrhea* or dysentery *by day only*, < cabbage, then miserable empty feeling. Itching of anus, after stools. Pinching colic, > bending double. Navel ulcerated in infants. Piles and fissure of anus with great itching. Herpes on perineum.

URINARY: Involuntary urine on rising. *Stricture from chronic* urethritis. Enuresis, at night. Sudden urging, if not attended to immediately causes severe pain. Cystitis, urethritis. Dribbling of urine after urination.

MALE: Itching and burning herpes on the scrotum, between scrotum and thighs, on the perineum. Genitals sweaty (both sexes).

FEMALE: Aversion to coition. Menstrual flow causes itching. Soreness and moisture on genitals with violent itching. Leukorrhea—albuminous, profuse, with lascivious dreams. Itching and mealy covering on the nipples. Dry obstinate eruptions. Prolapsus uteri from constant diarrhea.

RESPIRATORY: Cough, coming from deep down chest, waking the patient up at night (in young girls and boys). Cough at night only or < then, shatters the head, > pressing. Oppression of chest from cold air.

HEART: Cold feeling about heart. Fainting, with ebullitions, heat and palpitation.

NECK & BACK: Neck stiff, cracks when moved. Pain in spine and all over the body with sciatica. Coccyx painful on sitting. Pain in sacrum, < standing erect. Sharp pains shooting up dorsal spine into occiput.

EXTREMITIES: Cracking in joints. Joints stiff. Limbs go to sleep. Ragged, chapped hands and fingers, bleeding, in housemaids. Psoriasis of the palms. Stitches, blisters in heels.

SKIN: DIRTY, HARD, ROUGH, THICKENED, like parchment; *it gets raw, festers or won't heal,* < in folds. *Deep cracks* in angles, nipples, fingertips. Brown spots. Eruptions having thick, hard, moist or yellow green crusts; on occiput; on genitals, < cold. Eczema. Herpes. Vesicles. *Itching* orifices, with burning. Cold spots. All eruptions itch violently, must scratch until they bleed, part becomes cold after scratching. Chilblains that itch, burn and become purple.

SLEEP: Restless, with frightful dreams.

FEVER: Chilly with dry mouth. Palms and soles hot. Sweat in spots; foul on feet or axillae. Flushes of heat all over in frequent attacks during day.

COMPLEMENTARY: Sep.

RELATED: Graph; Sep.

PETROSELINUM

GENERALITIES: This remedy has influence on the genitourinary sphere. Sudden, irresistible urging to urinate, with drawing, tingling, crawling, itching from perineum throughout the whole urethra. Gonorrhea, milky or yellow discharge. Dysuria, with prostatic enlargement. Urinary difficulties of babies. Very painful urination causing him to shiver, dances around the room in agony.

PHELLANDRIUM

GENERALITIES: Produces *catarrhal condition* of the respiratory tract. Phthisis. Acts on *mammae* and nerves. Feeling of tiredness while walking. Feels as if all the blood-vessels were in vibratory motion.

WORSE: Cold, open air. Using eyes.

BETTER: While nursing.

MIND: Peevish arrogance.

HEAD: *Clang, like striking on metal, in brain,* waking him. Weight on vertex; aching and burning in temples and above the eyes.

EYES: Ciliary neuralgia, < attempting to use the eyes. Intolerance of light. Only half open, and looks as if one has been crying for a week.

FACE: Livid red in the evening.

STOMACH: Eructations smelling of bed-bugs. Everything tastes sweet. Desires sour things; milk or beer. Aversion to water.

FEMALE: Pain in nipples on nursing, goes into abdomen. Intolerable pain in milk ducts between nursing.

RESPIRATORY: *Expectoration horribly offensive* (like bed-bugs), loose, profuse, smeary, causing dyspnea. Cough compels him to sit up. Sticking pain from left border of right breast to between shoulders. Pains going backwards through chest.

SLEEP: So sleepy would fall asleep while standing at work.

RELATED: Asaf.

PHOSPHORICUM ACIDUM

GENERALITIES: *Phos-ac affects the* MIND, esp. its EMOTIONAL SIDE; in addition it influences sensory nerves, sexual system and *bones*. WEAKNESS and DEBILITY common to all acids is very marked in this acid, *with free secretion*—profuse urination, loss of fluids, sweating, etc., except with diarrhea. Mental debility appears first, then physical. *Slowness* of mind, and special senses. Pains go to part lain on. Sensitive to light, sound and odor, which takes away her breath. Sense of pressure, weight in forehead, sternum, vertex, eyes, navel, breasts, etc. Formication at root of hair, *along the spine* in limbs. Useful for those young people who grow rapidly and who are overtaxed mentally and physically. When the system is ravaged from acute diseases, venereal excesses, grief, loss of vital fluids, it calls for this acid. Bruised soreness, like growing pains. Hemorrhage, blood dark. Bone diseases—osteitis, periosteitis, caries. Rachitis. Diabetes. Neurosis of stump after amputation, > from deep breathing. Relieves the pain of cancer. Coldness of parts. Ill effects of bad news, disappointed love, grief, chagrin, injuries, shock. Pining, with emaciation. Neurasthenia. Formation of abscesses after fever. Gnawing pain in bones. Loose joints. External parts become black. Senile gangrene.

WORSE: LOSS OF FLUIDS. *Sexual excess. Fatigue. Convalescence* after fever. EMOTION, *grief,* chagrin. Mental shock. In home-sickness. Unhappy love. *Drafts; cold.* Music. Talking. Sitting. Standing. Overlifting. Operation. Fright (chronic).

BETTER: *Warmth.* Short sleep. Passing stool.

MIND: *Quiet,* unwilling to speak, or hasty speech. *Indifferent to everything.* APATHETIC from unequal struggling with adverse circumstances, mental and physical; obtuse, or torpid, with tendency to diarrhea or sweatiness. *Slow grasp.* Cannot collect his ideas; hunts for words. Poor memory. Settled despair. Aversion to talking. Answers reluctantly or slowly, briefly, incorrectly. Hysteria at change of life. Home-sickness with inclination to weep. Mild delirium, easily aroused. Brainfag. Hopelessness. Dread of future; broods over one's condition.

HEAD: Crushing weight on vertex; pain as if temples were crushed; < shaking or noise. Vertigo as if floating in the air, while lying in bed, with ringing in the ears and glassy eyes, < standing, walking. Hair thins out, turns gray early. Falling of hair. Schoolgirl's headache from overuse of eyes. Headache after coition.

EYES: Lusterless; glassy; staring; *sunken*; *blue rings around.* Pain as if eyeballs are pressed together and into head.

Eyeballs feel large. Yellow spots on conjunctiva. Loss of vision from masturbation. Sees rainbows. Photophobia.

EARS: Intolerance of noise, esp. music, which causes stitches, even while singing himself. Nervous deafness after typhoid-like fevers. Every sound re-echoes loudly in the ear. Shrill sound in ears on blowing nose. Illusions of hearing, hears bell peeling. Earache on blowing nose.

NOSE: Bleeding. Itching, bores fingers into nose. Nose swollen, with red patches or pimples on tip of nose.

FACE: Pale, sickly. Tense as if white of an egg had dried on it. One side cold. Acne from onanism. Hair of beard fall out.

MOUTH: Bleeding, swollen gums, retract from teeth. Teeth become yellow and feel dull. Slimy tongue. Red streak in middle of tongue. Bites sides of tongue involuntarily, in sleep. Mouth dry. Lips dry, cracked. Painful nodosities on the gums. Taste of rotten eggs.

THROAT: Hawks up tough mucus. Dryness of palate.

STOMACH: Craving for refreshing and juicy things, for cold milk. Acidity. Sour food and drink disagree. Pressure as from a weight. Loss of appetite.

ABDOMEN: Aching in umbilical region. Distension and fermentation. Loud rumbling. Cold. PROFUSE, PAINLESS, DIRTY WHITE, WATERY or LIENTERIC STOOLS BUT LITTLE DEBILITY. Stools involuntary, escape with flatus, when moved in children. Stools odourless. Liver; seems to be too heavy, painful, during menses. Flatus offensive, garlicky.

URINARY: Urine frequent, profuse, watery, MILKY. Diabetes. Phosphaturia. Burning in kidney region. Enuresis in first sleep. Whey-like urine shortly before menses.

MALE: Weak, relaxed genitals, suddenly during coitus, preventing emission. Weakness and pollution after coition. Nightly emission with lascivious dreams. Testes tender and swollen. Prostatorrhea when passing a soft stool. Herpes preputialis. Eczema of scrotum. Sycotic excrescences.

FEMALE: Uterus bloated, as if filled with wind. Menses too early and too profuse, with pain in the liver. Itching yellow leukorrhea after menses. Health deteriorated from nursing. Sharp pressure in left mamma. Infants vomit milk constantly. Dysuria during pregnancy.

RESPIRATORY: Weak feeling in chest, < by talking, coughing or sitting, > walking. Takes cold, > draft on chest. Spasmodic tickling cough. Pressure or twisting behind the sternum rendering breathing difficult. Expectoration salty.

HEART: Palpitation; in children and young persons who grow too fast; after grief; after self-abuse. Pulse irregular, intermittent.

NECK & BACK: Paralytic *weakness along spine.* Formication along spine. Spondylitis of cervical vertebrae. Lumbar region heavy, increases pain in legs. Burning along the spine. Fine stitches in coccyx and sternum. Boils on buttock.

EXTREMITIES: Heavy forearms. Wens on hands between metacarpal bones. Formication in limbs. Pain at night as if bones were scraped. Stumbles easily and makes mis-step. Burning below waist. Cramp-like pressure in arms, hands and fingers. Numbness along radial nerve.

SKIN: Clammy, wrinkled. Pimples, acne, blood boils. Tendency to abscess after fever. Painless ulcer with stinking pus. Formication in various parts.

SLEEP: SLEEPY BY DAY, hot and wakeful at night. Sleep deep but when aroused fully conscious, during fever. Short sleep > weakness.

FEVER: Cold parts—one side of face, abdomen, etc. Heat with sweat. *Profuse sweat,* < at night, as a sequel. *Sluggish painless fevers.*

COMPLEMENTARY: Chin.

RELATED: Gels.

PHOSPHORUS

GENERALITIES: Phos causes inflammation and degeneration of the MUCOUS MEMBRANES OF STOMACH AND BOWELS; inflames the spinal cord and NERVES; causing paralysis; disorganises the *blood* causing fatty degeneration of the BLOOD VESSELS and every tissue and organ of the body. Thus it produces a picture of *destructive metabolism*. It is suited to those young people who are grow rapidly and are inclined to stoop. Chorea of children who grow too fast. *Tall, slender* persons of sanguine temperament; *nervous weak delicate* persons who like to be magnetized. Insidious onset. Gradually *increasing debility,* ending in severe or rapid disease. HEMORRHAGE recurrent, vicarious; small wounds bleed much. Blood streaked discharges. Purpura hemorrhagica. Recurrent cold, croup, etc. Great susceptibility to external impressions, light, sound, odor, touch, electrical changes, etc. Suddenness of symptoms; prostration; fainting weak spell, sweat, shooting pain. Uncertain, involuntary acts. Emptiness in chest, stomach, etc. TIGHTNESS in chest, of cough, etc. Pain or soreness in *spots.* Paralysis; pseudo-hypertrophic muscles; of insane; internal paralyses—throat, rectum. Internal itching, tickling, throbbing here and there. Numbness. Burning. Jerking localized; subsultus. Joints; stiff, with little pain. Sprains; easily dislocated; weak spells in joints, < exertion. Symptoms due to heart and lung affections. Caries of the bones, spine, upper jaw. Hard swelling here and there. Osteomyelitis. Exostoses. Bone fragility. Polypi, easily bleeding. Jaundice, as a concomitant, hematogenous. Hemophilia. Polycythemia. Erectile tumors. Pyemia. Acidosis. Phthisical habit. Emaciation. Spasms on the paralyzed side. Epilepsy with consciousness. Petit mal. Totters while walking. *Human barometer.* Flabby muscles. Ill effects of anger, fear, grief, worry; exposure to drenching rains, washing clothes; tobacco; having hair cut; iodine, excessive use of salt. Healed wounds break out again and bleed. Lipoma. Cancer.

WORSE: LYING ON painful side, LEFT SIDE, BACK. SLIGHT CAUSES; EMOTION; talking; touch; odors; light. COLD; open air. Putting HANDS in cold water. WARM INGESTA. Puberty. Salt *sexual excess.* Loss of fluids. *Sudden change in* weather—windy, cold; thunderstorm, lightning. *Morning and evening. Mental fatigue.* Twilight. Shaving.

BETTER: *Eating. Sleep.* Cold food and water, washing face with cold water. Rubbing (magnetic). Sitting. Dark.

MIND: *Amative*, will uncover his body and expose his genitals. Excitable, easily angered and vehement from which he afterwards suffers. Anxious. Fear—being alone, at twilight, of ghosts, about future, of thunderstorm, senses something creeping out of every corner. Quickly prostrated by unpleasant impressions. Timid and irresolute. Melancholy; disinclined to work, study, converse. Weary of life. Sheds tears, or attacks of involuntary laughter. Destroys everything; spits at nurse, kisses who comes near her. Apathy, indifference even towards her own children. Insanity with exaggerated idea of one's own importance; grandeur. *Any lively impression is followed by heat* as if immersed in hot water. Clairvoyant. Weeps before menses. Wants sympathy. Laughs at serious things. Anxious restlessness, patient cannot sit or stand still for a moment, esp. in dark or twilight.

HEAD: VERTIGO accompanies many symptoms—of aged; floating; on waking; whirling, > stool. Head heavy; *aches over one eye;* with hunger, < children, lying on right side, > cold washing of face. Brain-fag with coldness of occiput. Burning temples. Vertex; throbs, hot, after grief. Softening of brain, with formication, numbness of limbs, feet drag. Congestion to head. Dandruff copious. Itching of scalp. Falling of hair in large bunches, in spots. Occiput cold; shocks; epilepsy. Feels as if pulled by hair.

EYES: Lacrimation in wind. Photophobia. *Flashes*, haloes, *red*, green, black, > shading by hands. Narrow field of vision. Balls feel large, stiff. Colored vision then migraine. Glaucoma. Degenerative changes in retinal cells. Retinitis albuminurica. Partial loss of vision from abuse of tobacco, sexual excess, lightning. Optic atrophy. Choroiditis. Long curved lashes. Yellow. Cataract. Eyes hollow with blue rings around them. Vitreous opacities. Letters appear red when reading. Sensation as if everything were covered with mist, dust or veil, or something pulled over tightly over eyes. Eyes turned outward.

EARS: Difficult hearing of human voice. Echoes and reverberations of sounds, esp. music. Polypi in the ear. Otitis media. Mastoiditis. Dulness of hearing after typhoid. Feels as if foreign bodies were lodged. Something seems constantly in front of ears.

NOSE: *Nervous fan-like motions of alae nasi.* Coryza alternately fluent and dry, on alternate sides. Epistaxis—instead of menses; of youths, then pneumonia; with cough, during stool. Nose swollen. Caries. Ulcers in the nose. Nasal polypus, bleeding easily. Chronic catarrh, blows blood from the nose. *Sneezing*, < odors, smoke, etc.; with dyspnea, causes pain in the throat. *Descending nose cold.* Oversensitive to smell. Sneezing and coryza on putting hands in water. Swollen, red, shiny. Bad smell.

FACE: *Pale about nose and mouth;* sickly; changing color. Necrosis of the lower jaw. Burning heat and redness of cheek. Lips blue, dry, cracked, sooty, scabby. Skin as if too tight.

MOUTH: Teeth numb. Toothache from washing clothes, from having hands in cold or warm water. *Gums* bleeding; *sore behind central incisors.* Tongue dry, smooth, red. Persistent bleeding after tooth extraction. Itching of palate. Abscess of hard palate. Taste sour after milk; bitter; sweetish when coughing. Mouth drawn to the left. Speech difficult, stutters. Salivation saltish or sweetish. Nursing sore mouth with sore breast.

THROAT: Dry; glistening. Sensation of a cotton or something like it hanging in throat. Burning in esophagus. Stricture of esophagus. Tonsils and uvula swollen, uvula elongated.

STOMACH: CRAVES COLD DRINK WHICH > but ARE VOMITED IN A LITTLE WHILE when it becomes warm in the stomach. Post-operative vomiting after chloroform. *Regurgitates ingesta,* by mouthfuls. Pain in stomach, > cold drinks. *Hunger—ravenous;* nightly; before the attack of sickness. Waterbrash. Food scarcely swallowed comes up again; spasm of esophagus at the cardiac end. Vomiting of bile, blood, coffee-ground. Ulcer of stomach. Burning in stomach, < eating. Craves salt, acid and spicy things; what is refused when offered. EMPTY *hollow feeling in stomach;* and as if hanging down, < emotions. Tremor, fluttering or something rolling over in stomach. Waterbrash. Unable to drink water, during pregnancy, the sight of water makes her vomit, has to close her eyes when taking bath. Nausea on putting hands in warm water. Stomach cold as if frozen.

ABDOMEN: Pressure above epigastrium. Sore spot in pit of stomach. Feels cold. Rubs abdomen for relief. Stools like cooked sago, granular, *slender,* tough. Very fetid stools and flatus. Painless, copious, gray, bluish, *watery* stools *pouring out;* nervous, involuntary diarrhea after fright; *exhausting* diarrhea. Alternate diarrhea and constipation in old people. Dysentery. Anus open, prolapsed. Stricture of rectum; stools flattened. Burning in rectum. Jaundice with pneumonia or brain disease; during pregnancy; from nervous excitement; malignant; Hematogenous. Acute yellow atrophy of liver. Acute hepatitis. Large yellow spots on abdomen. Tearing in anus, > warm cloth. Discharge of blood from rectum during stool. Flatulent colic, < hot drink. Urging for stool on lying on left side.

URINARY: Profuse pale, watery urination, then weakness. Pellicle on urine. Hematuria in acute nephritis, with jaundice. Albuminuria, periodical. Bladder is full without urging.

MALE: *Irresistible desire* but impotent. Lascivious; strips himself; sexual mania. Erections feeble or none at all. Constant discharge of thin, slimy, colorless fluid from urethra.

FEMALE: Menses too early, scanty, prolonged. Leukorrhea profuse, smarting, corrosive; instead of menses. Nymphomania. Sterility from excessive voluptuousness, or with profuse or too late menses. Frequent and profuse, or short uterine bleeding in between the periods; in nursing women. Cancer of the uterus. Amenorrhea with blood spitting, bleeding from the anus or hematuria, or with milk in breast. Suppuration in mammae, with fistulous ulcer. Cancer of the breast. Uterine polypi. Left infra-mammary pains. Vagina numb during coition in spite of sexual excitement. Violent sexual desire during pregnancy and lactation. Nipple hot and sore.

RESPIRATORY: Oppressive breathing, < least motion. Tight suffocative breathing, < cough. Larynx raw, sore, furry; painful on speaking. *Voice* low, *hoarse,* < morning and evening; croupy, then bronchitis. Cough hard, wheezing, dry, violent, painful, *tickling,* hacking, exhausting; with retching; causes pain in abdomen, burning in air passages and trembling, < reading aloud, change of weather, before strangers, laughing, exertion, singing. Sputum easy, frothy, rusty, bluish, salty, sour, sweetish, or cold. Pneumonia *of left lower lung,* secondary, with sopor. *Chest* full, heavy; pains go into throat or right arm, or alternate sides; stitches in left upper chest; rattling, < cold drink. Dry hot feeling in chest with cough which is at first dry then loose. Asthma after cough. Repeated hemoptysis. Tuberculosis in tall, slender, rapidly growing persons. Congestion in lungs. Feeling as of skin in larynx.

HEART: Violent palpitation with anxiety from least thing; during goitre. Dilatation of heart from fatty degeneration or endo-carditis. Heart weak. Pulse rapid, small, soft. Feeling of warmth in heart. Yellow spots on chest.

NECK & BACK: Back pains as if broken, impeding all motion. Cramp, *burning, between* scapulae. Spinal irritation, < heat. Pain moves forward from left *scapula.* Burning spot in lumbar region, > rubbing. Pain in sacrum after confinement. Stitching pain from coccyx goes up the spine to occiput, < during stool.

EXTREMITIES: Ascending sensory and motor paralysis from ends of fingers and toes. Can scarcely hold anything with his hands. Tearing left shoulder at night. *Numb arms, hands, fingers* and toes. Palms burn. Hands and arms cold during diarrhea. Paralyzing stitches in hips, then move up to back. Pain in tibia; periosteitis. Ankles feels as if about to break, easy dislocation. *Tottery;* stumbles easily. Suppressed foot-sweat. Icy cold feet. Toes cramp. Joints suddenly give way. Periodical contraction of fingers like cramp. Weakness and trembling of limbs on every exertion. Post-diphtheritic paralysis, with formication of hands and feet. Knees cold in bed. Legs heavy, feet feel glued to the floor. Walks with legs apart (waddling), stands with legs widely separated.

SKIN: Small wounds bleed much; they heal and break out again and bleed. Brownish or blood red spots here and there. Ecchymosis. Purpura hemorrhagica. Fungus hematodes. Skin burns on shaving. Fatty cysts. Thin, foul, bloody pus. Ulcers bleed during menses.

SLEEP: Drowsiness; coma vigil. Sleepy by day, sleepless before midnight. Sleepless, cannot close the eyes, from internal heat. Short naps and frequent wakings. Somnambulism. Dreams of fire, of hemorrhage; Lewd dreams. Feels in the morning as if he had not slept enough.

FEVER: Chilly in warm room, down back. Craves ice during the chill. *Burning heat, local, up back.* Hectic. Sweat early morning, sticky; without relief. Painless fevers.

COMPLEMENTARY: Lyc; Sang; Sep.

RELATED: Bry; Caust; Con; Puls; Rhus-t; Sil.

PHYSOSTIGMA

GENERALITIES: Motor nerves in spinal cord are affected by this remedy, causing fluttering tremor in the muscles. Muscles do not respond to the will and/or draw into knots, even the intestines are seen twisted in knots. Spinal irritation; sensitive vertebrae; weakness of the lower limbs coming from a spot between hips. Loss of sensibility to pain. *Weakness*, followed by complete paralysis, though the muscular contractility is not impaired. Rigidity of muscles. *Horror of cold water;* drinks or bathing; cold water feels too cold. Averse to bathing. Shuddering, < every draft. Floating sensation. Darting pain here and there. Flushes of heat, < palms. Ataxic gait, shooting pains go down the limbs. Tetanus. Trismus. *Tremors.* Ill effects of emotions, grief, injury, blow. Progressive muscular paralysis. General paralysis of the insane.

WORSE: Change of temperature. *Eyestrain.* Bathing. Heat and cold. Descending. Motion. Stepping. Jar, misstep.

BETTER: Lying on abdomen or with head low. Exerting the will. Closing eyes. Sleep.

MIND: Active even during sleep. Nothing was right; too many things in the room, continually counting them. Paralytic state of mind and body, from grief.

HEAD: Sensation as if brain falls to side lain on; wavering in brain. Vertigo, stumbles on ascending or descending steps. Pain from forehead down nose. Sensation of a band about the head, a tight cap on head. Heartbeats felt in head on lying down. Tremors in head.

EYES: *Twitching of eye muscles.* Pain over orbits, cannot bear to raise eyelids. Accommodation affected, astigmatism. Glaucoma, esp. after injury. Pupils contracted. Post-diphtheritic paralysis of eye. Eyelids tense, cannot close or open them. Bloodshot eyes, with burning. Nightblindness. Muscae volitantes; flashes of light. Increasing myopia. Vision trembling.

EAR: Sudden pain from throat to middle ear, < eructation. Pain in the ear (R) when writing.

NOSE: *Twitching of muscles of nose.*

FACE: Lips numb; licks them. Lockjaw.

MOUTH: Teeth feel rough. Tongue feels oily, scalded,

swollen, in chorea. Loose skin feeling at roof of mouth. Thick leathery saliva.

THROAT: Feels a ball coming up throat. Strong heart-beats felt in throat. As if swallowed a large piece of food felt at epigastrium.

STOMACH: Hiccough, with short breath, > sleep.

ABDOMEN: Navel sore, bloated, red. Hypogastrium sore, bloated, < standing. Gripe in right hypochondrium. Groins pain alternately. Colicky pains, < diarrhoea, > extending legs.

FEMALE: Numbness of womb with pain in back. leuko-rrhea, < during the day-time when exercising. Sighing, < when leukorrhea is worse. Menses irregular; with palpitation.

HEART: Seems to flutter in throat or over whole body, or in head.

NECK & BACK: Creeping numbness from occiput down spine. *Sensitive spine.*

EXTREMITIES: Jerking limbs. Offensive odor from hands. Pain in deltoid (right), > violent motion. Pain in right popliteal space. Flushes of heat in palms.

SLEEP: *Attacks of overpowering sleepiness*, with feeling as if to lose consciousness.

FEVER: Every movement and draft causes shuddering. Easy sweat, with excitement.

RELATED: Agar; Gels; Nux-v.

PHYTOLACCA

GENERALITIES: This long and deep-acting remedy prominently affects the *glands*, esp. MAMMARY, tonsils; in addition it has a powerful action upon the muscles of

NECK *and back, fibrous tissue,* tendons and joints, osseous tissues, periosteum, THROAT, *digestive tract* and *right side.* SORENESS, HARD ACHING, restlessness and prostration are the guiding symptoms. Aching all over the body—in eyeballs, *kidneys, neck,* shoulders, *back,* forearms, *below knees. Bluish-red parts*—throat, glands, etc. Spreading pains. Pains come and go suddenly, change places; *rheumatism; after tonsillitis.* Discharges are *shreddy,* stringy—stools, menses, etc. Hard and painful nodes. Syphilitic bone-pains. Tetanus; general muscular rigidity; alternate spasms and relaxation of muscles. Hastens suppuration. Pus watery, fetid, ichorous. Obesity. Retarded dentition. Everything affects the mammae.

WORSE: Exposure to damp cold weather or changes of weather. *Raising up. Motion. Swallowing hot drinks;* heat. Cold night. At menses. Rain. Stepping down from height.

BETTER: Lying on abdomen or left side. Rest. Dry weather.

MIND: Loss of personal delicacy; complete shamelessness and indifference to exposure of her person. Indifferent to life. Feels faint on rising. Refuses food inspite of continuous insistence. Great fear, she is sure she will die. Digust for business.

HEAD: Vertigo on rising. Pain from frontal region backwards. Brain feels sore, head beaten. Pains come on every time it rains. Nausea and headache > eating, but returns soon with vomiting which < headache, but > nausea.

EYES: Profuse hot lacrimation. Smarting. Green vision. Fistula lacrimalis. Eyeballs ache on reading and writing. Motion of one eye only, independent of the other. Orbital cellulitis. Lids feel hot as if on fire.

EARS: *Pain in both the ears, < swallowing.*

NOSE: Feels heavy. Flow from one nostril while the other is stopped, alternately. Acrid coryza. Obstruction when riding.

FACE: Yellowish, sickly. Aching malar bones. Glands swollen at the angle of jaw. Jaws ache, as in mumps. Lips everted and firm. Chin drawn closely to sternum. Mumps.

MOUTH: *Disposition to bite the teeth together.* Difficult dentition, > on biting something hard. *Tongue* fiery red at tip, feels burnt or *pain at root;* protruded. Much stringy saliva. Very painful small ulcers on side of cheek, cannot chew on that side. Sensation of dryness, with cough.

THROAT: Dark red or bluish red. White gray spots on fauces. Sore, *very painful on swallowing, dark,* puffy, burning. Feels a stick, h*ot ball* or lump in throat. Tonsils swollen, like dark washleather on tonsils. Hard throbbing in right tonsil. Quinsy. Diphtheria. Cannot swallow anything hot. Follicular pharyngitis. Hoarseness and sore throat after diphtheria.

STOMACH: Violent vomiting with retching, desires death to relieve vomiting; every few minutes. Hunger soon after eating. Easy vomiting without nausea. Pain, < deep breathing.

ABDOMEN: Heavy aching pain in hypochondrium, < lying on affected side, > leukorrhea. Chronic hepatitis. Continuous urging to stools even in sleep. Dysentery—passage only of mucus and blood or like scraping from the intestines. Bloody discharges, with heat in rectum. Cancer of rectum. Constipation of the aged and those with weak heart. Diarrhea after lemonade.

URINARY: Hard ache in kidney with scanty, suppressed urine. Dark red urine; chalky sediment. Albuminuria after diphtheria, scarlatina. Urine stains the clothes yellow.

MALE: Spermatic cord sore. Shooting from perineum to penis. Painful induration of testicles.

FEMALE: Menses with flow of saliva and tears. HEAVY, STONY, HARD, SWOLLEN OR TENDER MAMMAE, *paining during suckling;* spreading all over the body. *Hard nodes in breast;* with enlarged axillary glands. Nipples; cracked, very sensitive; inverted. Irritable breast before and during menses. Dysmenorrhea in barren women with erosion of cervix; membranous. Galactorrhea. Bloody, watery discharge from mammae. Affection of old cicatrices in mammae.

RESPIRATORY: Panting breathing. Hoarseness. Cough with burning in trachea.

HEART: Shocks of pain in cardiac region. Pain leaves heart and goes into right arm. Sensation as if heart leaped into the throat. Fatty heart.

NECK & BACK: *Neck stiff.* Aching pain in lumbar and sacral region. Pain streaking up and down the spine.

EXTREMITIES: *Right arm numb* and fuzzy. Pain and stiffness in (right) shoulder with inability to raise the arm. Pain flies like electric shock. Hips and thighs pain on change of weather. Aching and weakness in humerus (R), < motion and extension. Aching tibiae. Aching heels, > elevating feet. Neuralgia of toes. Sharp, cutting, drawing pains in the hips; legs drawn up, cannot touch floor. Painful, hard, shiny swelling of fingerjoints.

SKIN: Dry, harsh, shrivelled. Disposition to boils. Venereal buboes. Warts. Lipoma. Corns. Barber's itch. Ringworm.

COMPLEMENTARY: Sil.

RELATED: Bry; Kali-bi; *Kali-i; Merc;* Rhus-t.

PICRIC ACID

GENERALITIES: This acid acts upon *brain, spinal cord, lumbar region,* occiput, *kidneys* and sexual organs. *Weakness; heavy tired feeling;* in body and mind. Degeneration of the spinal cord with paralysis. Spasms from myelitis. Easy prostration. Progressive pernicious anemia. Prickling as of needles. *Burning* in many parts, *along spine,* in legs. Cachexia. Worn out persons—mentally and physically. Numbness. Formication. Neurasthenia. Acute ascending paralysis. Uremia with complete anuria. Type-writer's palsy.

WORSE: *Exertion—mental,* physical. Seminal losses. Heat; of summer. Fatigue. Study. Mental shock.

BETTER: Rest. Cold. *Bandaging.* In sun.

MIND: Lack of willpower to undertake anything. Dread of failure in examination. All this after prolonged mental strain and anxiety. Feels stairs or ground coming up to meet him. Lascivious thoughts in presence of any woman. Although enjoy the society of men, idea of marriage unendurable. Sits still and listless, does not take interest in surroundings.

HEAD: *Heaviness in occiput,* felt down spine and *lower limbs.* Headache, < mental exertion, > nosebleed, bandaging; with sexual excitement and violent erection. Brain-fag. Headache during daytime, > in sleep. Headache of businessmen, teachers and students; from grief and other depressing emotions.

EYES: Yellow. Chronic conjunctivitis, with thick yellow discharge.

EARS: Painful boils in meatus.

STOMACH: Bitter taste with thirst. Aversion to food. Vomits suddenly without warning; vomitus bright yellow, bitter.

ABDOMEN: Oily burning stools. diarrhea from mental exertion. Burning in rectum while passing stools. Stool thin, yellow. Jaundice with itching.

URINARY: Urine ammoniacal. Dribbling urine. Uremia with complete anuria. Diabetes, albuminuria. Enlargement of prostate gland.

MALE: Lascivious thoughts in presence of any woman. Priapism, penis distended. Hard erection with pain in testicles moves up spermatic cord. Extreme prostration from frequent seminal emissions. Impotency, with tendency to boil and carbuncle.

FEMALE: Extreme exhaustion at her menstrual periods.

NECK & BACK: Painful boils on nape of neck. Backache with languor, patient is unable to sit straight, and burning along spine, < study. Keeps legs wide apart when standing. Aching, tired legs. Writer's cramps or palsy. Back seems as if bandaged, also limbs. Anesthesia of legs as if one has on elastic stockings. Legs weak, heavy like lead, lifts with difficulty.

SKIN: Jaundice. Small painful, sore boils, esp. on neck.

SLEEP: Sleepiness. Sleep sound but unrefreshing. Sleepy during day and sleepless during night.

RELATED: Gels; Ox-ac; Phos; Phos-ac.

PILOCARPUS (See JABORANDI)

PIPER METHYSTICUM

GENERALITIES: Kava-kava is an intoxicant which produces liveliness and inclination to do more work without fatigue. *All symptoms, esp. pains are > for a time by diverting attention,* changing position or topic of conversation.

PLANTAGO MAJOR

GENERALITIES: Affects the *nerves,* causing neuralgia of *ears, teeth, face of shingles. Pains are sharp, shifting, play between ear and teeth.* Soreness. Produces digust for tobacco in chewers and smokers. Pyorrhea. Ill effects of bruise, burn, cut, punctured wound, snake bite. Can be applied locally for neuralgia. Sensation of a foreign body between ears, in the groins, etc.

WORSE: Night. Warm room.

BETTER: Sleep. Eating.

HEAD: Feels as if brain turned over. Headache with toothache. Sense of something lying in the head through one ear to the other.

EYES: Sharp pain in the eyes reflex from decayed teeth. Sensation of hair before eye (left).

EARS: Neuralgic earache, pain goes from one ear to the other through the head. Earache with toothache. Hearing more acute; loud noises go through one. Sensation of a body between ears.

NOSE: Sudden discharge of yellow-colored water from the nose.

FACE: Periodical prosopalgia, < 7 a.m. to 2 p.m., with lacrimation, photophobia. Pain radiating to temples and lower jaw.

MOUTH: *Saliva flows with pain.* Teeth feel too long. Toothache, > eating. *Dirty taste.*

ABDOMEN: Bowels seem cold. Colic > eating. Diarrhea with brown, frothy, watery stools. Painful piles, can hardly stand.

URINARY: *Frequent passage of large quantity of pale urine,* < night, with thirst (diabetes). Enuresis.

FEMALE: Neuralgia of nipples.

BACK: Throbbing between scapulae. Cold sweat on sacrum.

EXTREMITIES: Numb tremulous legs.

SKIN: Itching and burning. Sensitive.

SLEEP: Gloomy dreams exciting tears.

RELATED: Arn; Ferr-p; Puls.

PLATINUM

GENERALITIES: This proud metal is a WOMAN'S remedy, esp. *prim old maids.* Many and various symptoms reflex from ovaries and uterus or sexual organs. It affects the nerves, vagus, sensory and trifacial, causing *violent, cramping*, squeezing, thrusting or *numbing pains;* then spasms. Spasm alternates with dyspnea. Oversensitive *mind* and nerves. Localized coldness of single parts—eyes, ears, etc., or *numbness* of scalp, face, coccyx, calves, etc. Hemorrhage; with black clots and fluid blood. Tremors, painful. *Irregular* spasms, congestion of blood. *Alternate mental* and physical or *sexual symptoms.* Pains increase and decrease gradually. *Bandaged feeling. Sticky discharges*—tears, stools, menses, etc. Hysterical spasms. Catalepsy during menses. Tonic and clonic spasms, with laughter. Ill effects of fright, vexation, bereavement, fit of passion, sexual excess, prolonged hemorrhage, masturbation, (before puberty). Sensation of pricking. Violent shocks as from pain. Contortion of limbs. Epilepsy; catalepsy. Perverted sexual desire.

WORSE: Sexual EMOTIONS, *coition,* chagrin. TOUCH. *Nerve exhaustion.* Fasting. During menses. Sitting. Standing. Bending backward.

BETTER: *Walking in open air.* Sunshine. Stretching.

MIND: Laughs at wrong time. Unkind; abrupt and quarrelsome. *Disordered sense of proportion—objects* seem smaller strange, frightful. Sensation of dread and horror; fears death which seems to be very near. Screams for help. Changing mood, weeps and laughs alternately. CONTEMPT. *Hauteur;* looks with disdain upon everyone and everything. Feels tall and stately. *Proud and erotic.* Impulse to kill her own child her husband (on seeing a knife) whom she secretly dislikes, or passionately loves. Whistles, sings, dances. Wounded pride or sexual excitement brings on mental symptoms. Weeps with pain. She feels she does not belong to her own family; everything seems changed. Lone, deserted feeling. Bad humor, yet weeps. Thinks her husband will never return, something will happen to him. Fault-finding. Unchaste talk. Mental troubles > at twilight and suppressed menses. Serious over matters that are not serious; irritable about trifling things. Sits in a corner, broods and says nothing.

HEAD: Tense, pressing pain. Numbness with headache. Clavus. Tense scalp. Headache with leukorrhea. Sensation of water in forehead.

EYES: Feel cold. Twitching of the eyelids. Objects look smaller than they are.

EARS: Sensation of coldness; feel numb; symptoms extend to cheek and lips.

NOSE: Crampy pain at the root of nose with redness of face. Nose numb.

FACE: Coldness, creeping and numbness in whole right side of face. Grimaces. Boring in the jaws. Cramps in jaws. Lock-jaw. Malar bones numb.

MOUTH: Pulsating pain in teeth. Scalded sensation of tongue. Mouth feels cold. Sweet taste on tip of the tongue.

STOMACH: Repugnance to food from sadness. Ravenous hunger. Hasty eating, eats everything around her or detests it. Loss of appetite after first mouthful.

ABDOMEN: Painter's colic. Pain in umbilical region extending to the back, turns and twists in all possible positions. Stools hard, black; passed in small portions; with great straining, adhere to rectum like soft clay. Constipation of tourists; of pregnancy. Crawling, itching anus in evening. Voluptuous crawling.

MALE: Voluptuous crawling, tickling, of genitals, itching, with excessive sexual desire. Ill effects of masturbation before puberty. Perverted sexual desire.

FEMALE: *Painfully sensitive genitals* with itching, tickling or crawling. Excessive sexual desire, esp. in virgins, that leads to masturbation. Nymphomania, < in puerperal state. Menses dark, thick, profuse, clotted, too early, too short, with dragging, after abortion. Ovaritis with burning pains, with sterility. Dysmenorrhea with shrieks and jerks. Vaginismus from excessive sensitiveness of sexual organs, coition is impossible. Pruritus vulvae with voluptuous tingling. Prolapsus uteri. Induration; cancer of uterus. Fibroid. leukorrhea like white of egg, only by day, < after urination; rising from seat. Sterility from excessive sexual excitement. Erotomania. Frequent sensation as if menses would appear. Amenorrhea in emigrants.

BACK: Bruised backache, < pressure, on bending backwards. Numbness in sacrum and coccyx as from a blow.

EXTREMITIES: Cramp in calves. Thighs tight, as if bandaged. Distorted fingers. Numbness of little finger, or fingers. Limbs feel weary, numb. Paralytic weakness.

SKIN: Tingling, prickling, itching.

SLEEP: Spasmodic yawning. Sleeps on back with knees drawn up and spread apart; wants to uncover entirely.

RELATED: Cupr; Ign; Plb; Stann.

PLUMBUM METALLICUM

GENERALITIES: Lead produces a general sclerotic condition. It affects the MUSCLES, NERVES, SPINAL CORD, *abdomen,* navel, *kidneys,* blood vessels and blood. Symptoms appear *slowly, insidiously, progressively,* often with violent side effects of very changeable and incoherent character, coming in single parts, etc. Paralysis—hysterical, infantile, of single parts (wrist— drop), flaccid, with hyperesthesia; < touch. Convulsive trembling and jerking of the limbs. Emaciation; of limbs, with plump body; of paralyzed parts, of single parts; after neuralgia. Impulse to stretch with abdominal distress. *Retraction; of abdomen; anus; testes;* navel, etc. Anaesthesia is as marked as excessive hyperaesthesia. VIOLENT CONTRACTION. *Retraction*; sense of a string pulling back or in. Exaggerates her condition. Lightning pains that extort cries. *Convulsion;* chronic epilepsy with marked aura; with hemorrhage. Boring; cramps. Progressive muscular atrophy. Multiple sclerosis; spinal sclerosis. Constriction in internal organs. Anemia; jaundice; arteriosclerosis; hypertension. Small aneurisms all over the body. Dropsical swelling. Gout. Ill effects of repelled eruptions. Sexual excess. Marasmus of infants in apparently hopeless cases, abdomen large and hard, and constipation extreme. Perception slow, comprehension is difficult. Tremors, followed by paralysis. Arthralgia.

WORSE: Clear weather. Open air. *Exertion*. Motion. In a room full of company. Grasping smooth objects. Touch.

BETTER: Hard pressure. Rubbing. Stretching limbs.

MIND: *Taciturn.* Timid, restless and anxious. Frantic—bites, strikes. Quiet and melancholic. Fears of assassination, poisoning; thinks every one about her is a murderer. Stupid, imbecile. Delirium, nocturnal, alternating with colic or pain in the limbs. Amnesic aphasia.

Physical labor exhausts the mind. Slow perception. Weakness, or loss of memory. Increasing slowness and apathy. Inclined to cheat and deceive. Feigns sickness or exaggerates her condition. Hysteric only while being watched. Screams from time to time. Fright without cause. Delirium from hearing music.

HEAD: Ache, as if a ball was rising from the throat into the head. Hair dry, falls from beard. Fainting in room full of people, or on going from one room to another.

EYES: Yellow or deep bluish red sclerotics. Optic neuritis; central scotoma. Paralysis of upper lid. Sudden loss of sight after fainting. Pupils contracted. Glaucoma from spinal affection. Profuse hot lacrimation.

EARS: Tinnitus. Occasional sudden deafness. Hears music with frightful delirium.

NOSE: Loss of smell, with epilepsy. Nose-cold.

FACE: Pale and cachectic. Twitching of side of face (right). Cheeks sunken. Skin greasy, shiny. Swelling of face, one side.

MOUTH: Yellow inside the mouth. Distinct blue line along the margins of the gums. Gums pale, swollen. Tongue trembling; seems paralyzed. Hard tubercles on gums. Sticky saliva. Sweet taste. Aphthae; fetid ulcers. Loud motion of lower jaw and frightful grinding of teeth. Saliva blue.

THROAT: Dysphagia, fluids can be swallowed, solids come back into the mouth. Stricture of esophagus from spasm. Paralysis of gullet, with inability to swallow. Globus hystericus.

STOMACH: Foul or fecal eructations. Vomiting of fecal matter, with colic and constipation. Gastralgia, > hard pressure, bending backward. Periodical or persistent vomiting of food. Vomiting of brown black liquid or green mucus.

ABDOMEN: NAVEL FEELS RETRACTED. *Colic* accompanies many symptoms. Abdominal pains radiate to all parts of the body. Boring or sensation as if forced through a narrow place. Hernia at navel. Abdomen tense or retracted. *Anus feels drawn up or painfully contracted.* Stools granular *hard black balls like sheep-dung,* passed with an urging cramp in anus. *Stubborn constipation or colic of infants.* Abdomen is drawn into uneven lumps. Intussusception. Neuralgia of rectum. Prolapsus ani, with paralysis.

URINARY: Urine profuse but flows slowly, drop by drop. Chronic interstitial nephritis. Contracted kidney. Paralysis of bladder, difficult urination or retention; suppression. Uremia. Albuminuria. Diabetes mellitus.

MALE: Testicles drawn up, feel constricted. Loss of sexual power. Frequent pollution.

FEMALE: Vaginismus. Induration of mammary glands. Tendency to abortion from undeveloped uterus. Feeling of lack of room for fetus in uterus. Breasts become momentarily harder or smaller, with colic. Menorrhagia, with a sensation of a string pulling from abdomen to back. Ovarian pain > stretching legs. Vulva and vagina hypersensitive. Cannot pass urine in pregnancy, from lack of sensation or paralysis.

HEART: Weak. Pulse, wiry; slow, sinks even to 40. Painful constriction of peripheral arteries.

EXTREMITIES: Wrist-drop. Weakness and painful lameness of arms and hands. Pain in atrophied limbs, alternating with colic. Pain in right big toe. Paralysis of lower limbs, after parturition. Lightning-like pain, > by pressure. Sciatica with muscular atrophy. Wooden feet sensation. Arms shaky when attempting to use them.

SKIN: Bluish; red spots. Yellow. Dry. Oversensitive to open air. Bed-sore. Dry, burning ulcers. Gangrene. Small wounds easily get inflamed and suppurate. Skin wrinkled, shrivelled and drawn over the bones. Blisters, corns, bunions.

SLEEP: Takes odd positions during sleep. Falls asleep while speaking.

FEVER: Coldness from exertion. General cold sweat during stools. Feet cold only when walking.

COMPLEMENTARY: Rhus-t; Thall.

RELATED: Op.

PODOPHYLLUM

GENERALITIES: Considered as a vegetable mercury, it is a remedy for *bilious* constitution. It chiefly affects the *duodenum,* liver, intestines, RECTUM; right side, ovary, scapula, throat. Alternating condition—diarrhea alternating with constipation, headache alternating with diarrhea. Many troubles during pregnancy. Sudden shocks from jerking pains. Much drowsiness and desire to stretch. Sphincters relaxed.

WORSE: Early Morning. *Eating. Hot weather.* Dentition. Drinking. Acid fruits. Milk. Before, during and after stool. Motion. Mercury.

BETTER: *Rubbing or stroking liver.* Lying on abdomen.

MIND: Whining. Loquacity during chill and fever, afterwards forgets of what has passed. Imagines he is going to die or be very ill. Fidgety and restless, cannot sit still.

HEAD: Rolling of head from side to side with moaning during dentition, from business worry. Headache alternating with or > by diarrhea. Darting pain in forehead, must close the eyes.

EYES: Lids half-closed. Jaundiced.

FACE: Hot, cheeks flushed, during diarrhoea. Jaundiced.

MOUTH: Offensive odor. Burning, rough or flabby, indented tongue. Intense desire to press the gums together; grinding of the teeth at night. Bitter taste. Tongue broad, large, moist; coated as if mustard spread on it. Loss of taste, could not tell sweet from sour. Everything tastes sour or putrid.

THROAT: Feeling of lump in esophagus.

STOMACH: Craves acids which disagree. Vomits hot froth, milk (infants). Hot sour eructations; smelling like rotten eggs. *Constant gagging.* Thirst for large quantities of cold water. Gagging in infantile diarrhea.

ABDOMEN: *Liver* and whole abdominal viscera are sore, < during vomiting. Diarrhoea before and during menses. *Painful liver, > rubbing. Weak, empty, sinking or sick feeling after stools.* Rubs for relief. GURGLING THROUGH BOWELS, THEN PRPFISE, PUTRID stools, dirty, GUSH OUT PAINLESSLY. *Stools; white, like water, foaming, with meal-like sediment;* run right through the diaper; then weakness. Summer diarrhea. Stools; involuntary, during sleep, when passing flatus. Diarrhea alternating with other symptoms. Constipation—pale, hard, chalky stools. Jaundice with gall-stone. *Rectum* raw, sore, weak; *prolapsed* before stools, after parturition, during pregnancy, on vomiting, on sneezing, from mental excitement. Moist foul piles. Morning diarrhea. Diarrhea, > lying on abdomen, < while being bathed or washed (children), eating canned, acid fruits, milk.

URINARY: Frequent urination at night during pregnancy. Enuresis. Diabetes mellitus and insipidus.

MALE: Diseases of prostate gland associated with rectal troubles.

FEMALE: Pain in the region of the ovaries (right), moves down the crural nerve, < stretching the legs. Ovarian tumor with pain extending to shoulder. Prolapse of uterus on straining or over-lifting; after parturition. Sensation as if the genitals would come out during stool. Can lie comfortably only on the abdomen during early months of pregnancy. Menorrhagia from straining. Swelling of labia during pregnancy.

HEART: Palpitation with a clucking sensation rising up to the throat, from emotions.

EXTREMITIES: Pain in right inguinal region, shoots down inner thigh to knee. Paralytic weakness of left side. Cramps in calves with stool. Pain along ulnar nerve of both arms.

SKIN: Moist, warm; jaundiced.

SLEEP: Moaning and whining during sleep. Sleepy after paroxysms of malaria.

FEVER: Chill at 7 a.m. Loquacity during fever. Sweat; profuse with sleep, offensive.

COMPLEMENTARY: Nat-m.

RELATED: Aloe; Chin; Merc.

POLYGONUM

GENERALITIES: Acts upon the genito-urinary organs and the *intestines* causing CUTTING PAINS along ureters, ovarian ducts, up spine, with bearing down. *Pulsating,* flashing, wandering pains in prostate. Coldness alternating or coinciding with heat in the same or another part, burning in chest with cold feeling in pit of stomach, etc. Smarting discharges.

WORSE: Cold; damp. Pressure of clothes.

HEAD: Acute pulsative pain in temples.

EYES: Puffiness under eyes (right). Lids twitch when closed and when lying down.

EAR: Acute pain on bending head down, > bending backward.

FACE: Coldness in right side of face when pain is most severe in left.

MOUTH: Itching, burning palate, wants to scratch it. Tongue feels swollen.

ABDOMEN: Cold feeling in stomach, with burning in chest. Nausea felt in abdomen. Cutting pain with great rumbling as if whole intestinal contents were in a fluid state. Interior of anus studded with itching eminences. Hemorrhoids with itching.

URINARY: Nephritic colic; with *grinding, griping, cutting* BELLYACHE. Cutting pain along ureters. Urine scanty, dribbling, dark, or calcareous adherent sediment. Nephritis, suppurative. Cystitis.

MALE: Scrotum excoriated. Pulsating, burning pain in prostate on urinating. Pain in testes and spermatic cord when urinating.

FEMALE: Cutting pain along the fallopian tubes, with bearing down, as if hips were drawn together. Metrorrhagia; amenorrhea in young girls. Shooting pain through the breasts.

EXTREMITIES: Aching lower limbs. Sore pain in heels. Feet alternately hot and cold.

SKIN: Urticaria. Superficial ulcers and sores on lower limbs at climacteric.

RELATED: Calc.

POTHOS FOETIDUS

GENERALITIES: A remedy for asthmatic complaints, < by inhalation of dust and relieved by stool. Absence of mind. Headache in small spots, with throbbing in temporal arteries. Red swelling across the nose. Pain in throat while sneezing. Tongue numb. Abdomen distended. Erratic spasmodic pains.

BETTER: Open air.

PRUNUS SPINOSA

GENERALITIES: This remedy specially acts on the *nerves — respiratory,* orbital; and on urinary organs. *Pains* are shooting, pressing outwards, lightning — like,wandering, CAUSING SHORT BREATH. Neuralgia. Cramps. Edema. Pains, after shingles. Nerve paralysis. Compensatory effects. Ill effects of sun, sprain, over-lifting. Dropsy caused by defective heart.

WORSE: Touch; pressure. Motion. Jarring. Stooping. Ascending.

BETTER: Bending double.

MIND: Restlessness, walks about constantly, cannot remain in one place.

HEAD: Shooting from frontal bone (right) through brain to occiput. Headache from heat of sun.

EYES: Ciliary neuralgia; pain in *eyeballs as if bursting,* or pressed apart, > lacrimation.

MOUTH: Teeth feel pulled out. Toothache, > by biting teeth together.

URINARY: Cramp in bladder from pressure of flatus; must double up to urinate. Urgent desire to urinate; urine reaches glans penis and then returns with violent pain and spasm and tenesmus in rectum. Neuralgic dysuria. Glans pains on urinating. Must press a long time before urine appears. Pulsating pudendum. Stream of urine thin like a thread, or forked.

MALE: Pulsation in glans from jar of walking.

FEMALE: Leukorrhea acrid, watery, purulent, staining yellow. Menses thin, watery, too early, too copious, with sacral pain.

RESPIRATORY: *Short breath* with pains. Feeling as if air inhaled did not reach the pit of stomach, has to yawn and try to take a deep inspiration to force the air down to that point. Air hunger.

HEART: Hypertrophied. Knocking at heart with labored breathing, < least motion. Cardiac *dropsy*. Throbbing of carotid arteries. Angina pectoris.

BACK: Feeling of a lump below the left scapula.

EXTREMITIES: Edema of feet. Itching at the tips of fingers as if frozen. Thumb feels sprained hindering writing.

SKIN: Herpes zoster. Dropsy.

FEVER: Night sweat.

RELATED: Laur.

PSORINUM

GENERALITIES: Dr. Hahnemann prepared this nosode from sero-purulent matter of scabies vesicles. The therapeutic field of action is found in the so-called psoric manifestations—when there is a *lack of reaction in chronic diseases*, when well-related remedies fail to relieve or to permanently improve; also when Sulphur seems indicated but fails to relieve. Clears up confused cases. It chiefly affects the SKIN FOLDS, *sebaceous glands*, EARS, BOWELS, *respiration,* right side. It is adapted to dirty persons with filthy smelling body even after a bath; pale, sickly, delicate, unhealthy looking children, who have a disagreeable smell around them; nervous; restless persons who are easily startled. Prostration. Feels sick all over. RECURRENCE. FOUL *discharges, odor of the body,* stools, eruptions, sweat. Stubborn foot-sweat. Secretions thick. *Weak, tender* and thin. *Easily takes cold, chilled.* Clothing seems large or he feels pushed down when walking in the sun. HUNGRY or UNUSUALLY WELL BEFORE AN ATTACK. *Wants to wash parts. Weakness remaining* after acute diseases or independent of any organic disease, after loss of fluids. Feels good and bad by turns. Ill effects of infectious disease lasting for years, emotion, over-lifting, injury, blow, sprain, dislocation. Looseness; of joints, of teeth, etc. Eruptions disappear in summer, appear in winter. Wears warm clothes even in summer. Washes his hands and feet constantly. Sick babies will not sleep day and night but worry, fret and cry; or are good and play all day, troublesome, screaming all night. Difficulty in breathing when standing in open air, wants to go home and lie down.

WORSE: COLD. *Open air; washing. Weather changing, stormy. Heat* of bed, *woollens*, of exertion. SUPPRESSION. Contact of his own limbs. Periodically, yearly. Full moon.

BETTER: *Lying with head low,* or quietly. Eating. Washing. Nosebleed. Hard pressure. Profuse sweating.

MIND: ANXIETY. Foreboding. *Despair of recovery, great despondency; hopelessness.* Joyous. Melancholy, religious; *gloomy*. Horrid thoughts; suicidal tendency. Feels himself poor; his business is going to be a failure though it is prosperous. Fear of fire, of being alone, of becoming insane, etc. Aversion to work. Children very fretful day and night. Peevish, irritable, noisy; easily startled. Severe ailments from even slight emotion. Dull, beclouded mind. Difficult thinking. Feels restless for days before a thunderstorm.

HEAD: *Aches* as from a heavy blow, with suppressed menses. *Headache follows visual* disturbances; alternates with other complaints, > nosebleed. Head feels separated from the body. *Sensitive to drafts about head, wants it covered,* in hot weather. Twitching in temples. Dull, dry, tangled hair. Humid eruptions on scalp. Migraine. Spots of white skin, with white lock of hair.

EYES: Gummy. Everted eyelids. Sensation as if something were moving or fingers playing before eyes. Recurring ophthalmia. Objects tremble, then get dark. Darkness before eyes.

EARS: Raw, red, oozing; scabs around the ears. Humid sore behind the ears. *Putrid otorrhea.* Red wax. Intolerable itching. Otorrhea, with headache, with offensive watery diarrhea. Illusory noises; as if he heard with ears not his own.

NOSE: Hay fever. Red small pimples on nose. Recurring cold.

FACE: Pale, sickly, dirty, fuzzy or puffy. Red small pimples on. Acne rosacea. Swelling of the upper lip. Down on face.

MOUTH: Teeth feel loose, then pain < touch. Tip of tongue feels scalded. *Filthy taste.* Gums, bleed, spongy, settled away from the teeth. Pyorrhea. Obstinate cracks in the corners of lips. Taste bitter, > eating or drinking.

STOMACH: Loss of appetite after illness with great thirst. Very hungry always, during headaches; must have something to eat in the middle of the night. Eructations sour, rancid, tasting and smelling like rotten egg. Ravenous appetite, yet grows thin. Desires beer, acids. Aversion to pork. Vomiting of pregnancy when not relieved by other drugs. Waterbrash when lying down.

ABDOMEN: Flatulence, with disorder of liver. Colic, > eating and passing fetid flatus. Flatus like bad egg. Pain in liver, < sneezing. STOOLS DARK, BROWN, HORRIBLY PUTRID, GUSHING, *of penetrating odor* going through the whole house. Cholera infantum. Constipation of infants. Stools soft, but difficult. Involuntary stools, during sleep. Hemorrhage from rectum in old women. He has to go several times to pass normal stools. Chronic diarrhea, early morning, urgent. Burning in rectum.

URINARY: Bed-wetting, < full moon; obstinate cases. Has to pass urine several times, from weakness of bladder.

MALE: Offensive genitals. Griping in testis. Chronic gonorrhea, painless discharge from urethra staining yellow. Aversion to coition. Want of enjoyment, no emission during coition.

FEMALE: Leukorrhea gushing, lumpy, fetid, with violent pain in sacrum and debility. Dysmenorrhea, near climaxis. Menses early and profuse. Obstinate vomiting during pregnancy. Fetus moves too violently. When after an abortion the woman gets on her feet, the flow starts anew. Breasts swollen, nipples red. Burning and itching pimples around nipples. Eruptions on mammae causing excoriation.

RESPIRATORY: Dyspnea, < sitting up, > lying down and keeping arms spread apart. Feeling of ulceration under sternum. Cough returns every winter. Hay fever regularly returning every year. Bloody expectoration, with hot sensation in chest. Cough, < lying down, drinking. Chest pain extends to shoulder, < cold drink.

HEART: Gurgling at the heart, < lying down, Cardiac murmur, mitral regurgitation. Pericarditis. Pulse weak, irregular.

BACK: Lumbarache, < standing or walking.

EXTREMITIES: Joints feel loose, as if they would not hold together. Eruptions around finger nails. Hot itching soles. Fetid foot sweat. Eruptions around joints make walking difficult.

SKIN: *Dirty,* rough, scabby, greasy; *breaks out* in folds. Intolerable itching, < heat of bed; he scratches raw or until it bleeds. Urticaria, < exertion. Excrescences disappear in summer only to occur again in winter. Constantly recurring body lice. Condylomata on edges of skin. Enlarged glands. Oily skin.

SLEEP: Dreams vivid, continue after waking.

FEVER: Heat, with steaming sweat. *Sweat easy,* profuse, < night; cold sweat on palms.

COMPLEMENTARY: Sep; *Sulph;* Tub.

RELATED: Graph; Mang; *Phos;* Sulph.

PTELEA

GENERALITIES: Suitable in liver and stomach affections, associated with pain in limbs. Taste bitter, and eructations either bitter or like rotten eggs. Aching and heaviness in the region of liver, < lying on left side. Better eating sour things. Breath hot, burns the nostrils. Edema of feet and legs with liver affections.

WORSE: Cheese, meat, pudding.

PULEX

GENERALITIES: Common flea produces, marked urinary and female symptoms. Cannot retain urine, must attend the call immediately. Stain of menses and leukorrhea very hard to wash out. Feeling as if cotton ball inside the vagina.

WORSE: Left side. Moving about.

BETTER: Sitting or lying down.

MIND: Very impatient, irritable.

EYES: Eyes feel enlarged.

FACE: Wrinkled like that of an old man.

THROAT: Sensation as if a were thread hanging in throat.

STOMACH: Thirst, esp. during headache.

URINARY: Flow of urine stops suddenly followed by pain. Urine scanty with frequent urging, pressure in bladder and tenesmus in urethra.

FEMALE: Salivation during menses. Menses delayed. Intense burning in vagina.

FEVER: Feels a glow all over, like being over steam. Chilly while sitting beside the fire.

PULSATILLA

GENERALITIES: On account of its CHANGING, SHIFTING SYMPTOMS this remedy is known as a weather cock remedy. It affects the MIND, VEINS, MUCOUS MEMBRANES, *respiration* and one side. *Symptoms rise to a certain pitch, then suddenly cease.* It is pre-eminently a remedy for females—mild, gentle, plethoric yielding disposition, who cry readily and weep when talking. Symptoms appear on one side *or go to side lain on*. THIRSTLESSNESS, CHILLINESS AND SHORTNESS OF BREATH, with digestive or menstrual disorders. Chilliness with pains. Burning, stitching pains, numbness. MUCOUS DISCHARGES ARE PROFUSE, BLAND, THICK, YELLOWISH-GREEN. Changing and contradictory symptoms having no head or tail to them. Alternations. *Metastasis.* Hemorrhage passive, vicarious; blood dark, easily coagulating. Venocity, varicose veins. *Heaviness.* Scraping. Jerking, tearing, ulcerative pains; wandering pains. *Numbness* partial— hands, feet, etc.; of the part lain on; of suffering part. Ill effects—of SUPPRESSION OF otorrhea, menses, lochia, milk, etc.; eating ice-cream, pork, fat, pastry mixed diet. Chilly but craves for open air. Pale chilly blondes. Anemia. Never well since puberty. Chorea from amenorrhea or dysmenorrhea. The longer he lies in the morning the longer he wishes to lie. *Cannot lie with head low.* Child wants to be carried slowly. Symptoms in distant parts of the body cause dyspnea. Sensation of distension in size, as if one part or every part were growing too large during pain. Bandaged sensation. Wearing of flannels or woollens cause itching and eruptions. Prophylactic for measles. Epilepsy with absent or irregular menses. Emaciation of suffering parts. Pulsation through whole body.

WORSE: WARMTH OF AIR, ROOM, *clothes,* BED. *Getting feet wet.* EVENING. REST. BEGINNING MOTION. LYING *on one side (left).* EATING—*long after,* RICH FOODS, fat, ice, eggs. PUBERTY. PREGNANCY. *Before menses.* Iron. Quinine. Hanging down limbs. Tea. Thunderstorm. Sun. Twilight.

BETTER: COLD FRESH OPEN AIR; cold food, drink. Uncovering. *Gentle motion.* ERECT POSTURE. Continued motion. *After a good cry.* Changing sides. Pressure. Rubbing. Lying with head high.

MIND: MILD, TIMID, EMOTIONAL, AND TERAFUL. Disgusted at everything. Discouraged. Easily offended. Whining. Craves sympathy. Children like fuss and caress. Morbid dread of the opposite sex, marriage; thinks that sexual intercourse is a sinful act. Given to extremes of pleasure and pain. Easily moved to tears and laughter after eating. Religious melancholy. Fear to be alone, of dark, of ghosts in the evening, therefore wants to hide or run. Capricious. Miserly. Suspicious. Very irritable, touchy; feels slighted or fears slight. Answers yes or no by nodding her head. Imagines that certain articles of food are not good for the human race. Sad from disagreeable news. Mania from suppressed menses.

HEAD: Aches; from overwork, suppressed sexual excitement, indigestion; starts in vertex. Occipital ache, < coughing. Semilateral headaches, pulsating, bursting; with scalding lacrimation of the affected side. Vertigo, < sitting, looking up, with nausea and gastric or menstrual disturbances. Vertigo before, during, after or due to suppressed menses. Profuse sweat on scalp. Headache of schoolgirls at puberty. Headache, > walking in open air. Head seems heavy. Cannot hold head upright, cannot raise it.

EYES: Dimness of vision, with a sensation as though there were something covering the eyes which the patient wishes to rub or wipe, < wind. Thick, yellow, profuse bland discharge. Ophthalmia—neonatorum, gonorrheal, from amenorrhea. Fistula lacrimalis discharging pus on pressure. Acrid lacrimation. Styes, recurrent. Blepharitis. Conjunctivitis from cold. Blind attacks before menses. Amaurosis, paralysis of the optic nerve. Itching, burning in eyes, causing rubbing. Weeping eyes.

EARS: Ache, < night. Deafness as if ears were stopped up; can hear better in a car and in a warm room. Otorrhea; discharge–of pus, blood, thick yellow humor, offensive; after exanthemata. External ear red and swollen and feels as if something pushed out from the ear. Mumps, esp. metastatic to the breast or testes. Lobes of ear swollen.

NOSE: Loss of smell with catarrh. Foul discharge or odor before the nose. Coryza; obstruction of nose, < lying down or in a room, > going out in the open air. Green, orange—colored, fetid, urinous nasal discharge; chronic bland yellow discharge. Nose-bleed before and during menses and from suppressed menses.

FACE: Pale. Neuralgia with profuse lacrimation, < chewing, talking, or with hot or cold things in the mouth. Lips cracked, peeling, swollen. *Licks lips. Crack in center of lower lip.* Acne in young girls.

MOUTH: Breath offensive. *Dry or slimy, without thirst.* Drawing toothache, > cold. *Taste bad in a.m.,* lost, of; from coryza. Taste greasy, bloody, sweet, alternating. Tongue yellow, white; feels scalded. Much sweet saliva. Food leaves an after-taste. Taste bitter, esp. of bread. Diminished taste of all food. Saliva tenacious, frothy, cotton-like.

THROAT: *Food lodges in throat.* Dry; sore with sense of dysphagia. Sensation of worm wriggling up, or of sulphur vapor when coughing.

STOMACH: *Aversion to water, fat,* pork, bread, milk, smoking, warm food and drink. Craves acids or what disagrees, refreshing things, pungent things, herring, cheese. Food tastes, too salty. Onions disagree. Sudden loathing, < eating. Eructations taste of food which remains a long time. Nausea. Heart burn. *Thirstlessness* with nearly all complaints. Vomiting. of food eaten long before. Visible pulsations in the pit of stomach. Stitching pain, < walking or mis-step. *Weight as of a stone.* Stomach DERANGED; FEELS HEAVY. Hiccough when smoking tobacco. Hunger but does not know for what.

ABDOMEN: Cutting, pulsation, in epigastrium. Painful, distended; loud, rumbling. Pressure as that from a stone. Feeling of numbness. Pains extend into groins.

Stools changeable, no two stools alike; green, bilious. Diarrhea < after midnight. Two or three normal stools daily. Hard painful lumps in both groins. Blind piles, < menses, lying down. Diarrhea in jaundice, with sensation of heat. Discharge of blood from rectum even when not at stool. Diarrhea after fright.

URINARY: *Urination;* involuntary on lying down, laughing, coughing, sneezing, hearing sudden noise, after pleasurable surprise, shock, passing flatus, during sleep esp. in little girls. Hematuria after urination. Heavy pressure or cramp in bladder after urination. Sensation of a stone rolling in the bladder. Urine dribbles when angry. Urging to urinate when lying on back. Stricture of urethra, urine comes in drops or stops and starts.

MALE: Burning down left spermatic cord. Acute prostatitis; enlarged prostate. Orchitis - gonorrheal or from sitting on cold stone. Epididymitis. Testicles hang low down. Bloody emissions. Thick yellow discharge, late stage of gonorrhea.

FEMALE: *Amenorrhea* from wet feet, nervous debility or anemia. *Feels as if menstruating.* Menses *dark,* thick, TOO LATE, SCANTY after bathing; clotted, changeable, intermittent, irregular, vicarious. DELAYED at puberty. Dysmenorrhea. Leucorrhea milky, thick like cream, acrid with pain in the back and exhaustion. Weak labor pains. Bearing down < lying. Afterpains too long and too violent. Mammae sore, aching; lumps in girls before puberty. Thin milky fluid escapes from mammae in virgins before puberty. *Milk suppressed, scanty.* Postpartum secondary hemorrhage from retained placenta. Weeps every time the child is put to breast. Swelling of breasts after weaning. Galactorrhoea. Secretion of milk during menses. Malposition of fetus.

RESPIRATORY: SHORT BREATH, < lying on left side; smothering sensation on lying down < *if heated, open air*

Cough; loose in the morning, dry in the evening and at night; *must sit up in bed* to get relief. *Expectoration* thick, purulent, slimy; sweet, saltish, better as it loosens up. Cough dry, hacking from tickling in epigastrium. *Chest oppressed* as by a load. Soreness, or stitch beneath clavicles. Hoarseness comes and goes. Asthma from suppression. Cough after measles.

HEART: Palpitation, < lying on left side. Anxious palpitation with amenorrhea, from emotion, after dinner. Catching pain, with short breath, > by pressure of hand and walking.

BACK: Semsation as if cold water was poured down the back. Pain in back and small of black as if from prolonged stooping. Curvature of the upper part of the spine. Shooting pain in the nape and back. Backache, < lying on back, > lying on sides or change of position, esp. so during pregnancy. Back feels bandaged. Pain in sacrum on sitting.

EXTREMITIES: Rapidly shifting pain in limbs. Arms feel broken and dislocated. Elbows numb. *Joints swollen,* red. Dorsum of foot swollen, edematous. Pain down lower limbs, alternating sides. Legs heavy. Sticking in tibia, < lying, > cool air and walking. Cold sweat on legs. Foul foot-sweat. *Veins full, varicose*, painful. Milk-leg. Periosteitis. White swelling of knee. Inclination to stretch the feet. Numbness in legs when remains standing for long.

SKIN: Glands swollen. Ulcer with hard, red, glistening areola. Varicose. Itches on being heated. Urticaria after rich food, with diarrhea, from delayed menses, after undressing. Measles.

SLEEP: Great sleepiness during day, *wakes confused,* languid, unrefreshed. Lies, with hands over head or crossed on abdomen, and feet drawn up. Dreams, frightful, disgusting, voluptuous, confused, of cats, etc. Chattering in sleep. Talks, whines or screams during sleep.

FEVER: *Chilly, yet averse to heat;* IN WARM ROOM, *with pain,* on lying down at night. One-sided coldness with numbness. Pains during sweat. One hand cold. Partial sweat. Feverish, hot; body temperature normal. Erratic temperature in fever.

COMPLEMENTARY: *Ars;* Kali-bi; Sep; Sil; Zinc.

RELATED: Ap; Cimic; Graph; Ham; Kali-bi; Kali-s; Nat-s.

PYROGEN

GENERALITIES: This nosode is prepared from decomposed lean beef allowed to stand in the sun for two weeks, or from septic pus. It is, therefore, a remedy for all types of *septic states* when BLOOD is disorganised, heart becomes weak and muscles prostrated. Aching. BRUISED, SORE and *prostrative,* yet restless. Discharges are horribly foul; taste, odor of body, menses, sweat, vomiting, etc. *Rosy, red streaks;* lymphangitis. *Bone-pains.* Abscess recurrent, with pain and violent burning. Chronic complaints that date back to septic conditions; dissecting wounds, sewer-gas poisoning, ptomaine poisoning, puerperal fever. After-effects of miscarriage; remote effects of typhoid fever, diphtheria, chronic malaria, where the best selected remedy fails to relieve or permanently improve, esp. in latent pyogenic processes.

WORSE: Cold, damp. Motion. Sitting. Moving eyes.

BETTER: Heat. *Hot bath,* drink. Pressure. Stretching. Changing position. Hard rocking. Walking.

MIND: Active brain, making speeches and writing articles at night. *Loquacious*; thinks and talks faster than ever before. Sensation as if she covered the whole bed. Feels one person when lying on one side and another person when turning, on the other side. *Sensitive,* anxious, confused. Sense of duality; feels crowded with arms and legs. Hallucination, that he is very wealthy. Full of anxiety and insane notions. Bed feels hard. Talks or whispers to herself; pains in sleep.

HEAD: Painless throbbing. Violent throbbing headache, > bandaging. Rolls head from side to side. Sensation of a cap on the head. Cold sweat on forehead.

EYES: Balls sore (left), < looking up and moving eyes. Photophobia.

EARS: Red; cold. Ringing like a bell.

NOSE: Cold. Fan-like motion of the alae nasi. Disgust at his own body odor. Sneezing every time when hand is out from under the covers.

FACE: Hectic flush from 3 to 4 p.m.; lasting till midnight; then covered with large drops of cold perspiration.

MOUTH: Tongue fiery red, brown streak down the centre, smooth, large, flabby. Taste sweetish; terribly fetid. Horribly offensive breath.

THROAT: Dry. Diphtheria with extreme fetor.

STOMACH: Vomiting persistent, brownish, coffee grounds, offensive, fecal, with impacted or obstructed bowels. Vomits water when it becomes warm in stomach. Nausea, > by very hot drinks, and vomiting. Great thirst for small quantities of cold drinks but the least liquid is instantly rejected.

ABDOMEN: Horribly offensive, brown-black painless involuntary stools. Constipation with complete inertia. Stools large, black, small black balls, very offensive.

URINARY: Adhesive, red, slimy sediment. Urination twice a day, scanty. Urging to urinate before fever. Urine clear like water. Tenesmus of bladder and rectum.

MALE: Testes hang down, relaxed; scrotum looks and feels thin.

FEMALE: Septic puerperal infection. Fever at each menstrual period. Menses horribly offensive. Pelvic cellulitis. Prolapsus uteri, > holding the head and straining. Lochia suppressed, followed by fever, chill and profuse fetid sweat. Pains in the region of left nipple.

RESPIRATORY: Pain in lung (right), < coughing, talking. Neglected pneumonia. Cough, > sitting, < lying down.

HEART: Purring, feels as if tired, big, or *full*. Consciousness of heart. Throbbing felt in head and ears, preventing sleep. PULSE QUICK, OUT OF ALL PROPORTION TO TEMPERATURE, OR THE REVERSE. *Heart* failure threatens in septic and zymotic states.

NECK & BACK: Throbbing in vessels of neck. Weak feeling in the back.

EXTREMITIES: Aching in all limbs and bones. Nails threaten to fly off or feel loose. Automatic movement of arm and leg (right). Pain in shoulder (right), < coughing, talking.

SKIN: Pale. Cold. Obstinate varicosis. Offensive ulcers of old persons. Rapid decubitus of septic origin. Small cut or injury becomes much swollen and inflamed.

SLEEP: Whispers in sleep. Sleepless from brain activity.

FEVER: Chilly, wants to breathe heat of fire. Chills start between scapulae, *felt in bones,* with sweat, at night. Slowly advancing, hectic sweat without relief. Cold or hot. *Quickly oscillating temperature.*

RELATED: Anthr; Ars; Bapt; Echin.

RADIUM

GENERALITIES: Radium bromide is found effective in skin affections, rheumatism and gout; nerves are affected causing *suddenly* shifting or electric pains; must lie down. *Dull, hard, aching pains all over, deep in joints;* very restless, had to keep moving about. *Dry burning heat,* as if on fire, through the entire body; craves cold air. Electric-like shock through the body, during sleep. Weakness, lassitude, tiredness. Late appearance of symptoms. *Constriction* of chest, heart, etc., with air hunger. Numbness, < stretching the part. Necrotic changes. Effects of x-ray burn. Removes small nevi, moles, ulcers. Cancer. *Lymphoid tissue.*

WORSE: *Motion. Shaving.* Washing. Smoking. Getting up.

BETTER: Open air. *Hot bath.* Cold drink. Continued motion. After sleep. Pressure. Eating.

MIND: Fear of being alone, of the dark, wants to have someone near. Cross. Easily vexed.

HEAD: Pain over right eye spreading to occiput and vertex, > heat. Vertigo, with pain in occiput. Pain in vertex and occiput, with severe aching in lumbar region.

EYES: Red, smarting, < reading. Sensation of pieces of cotton in eyes, > rubbing.

EARS: Sound of rushing water, > lying on face.

NOSE: Itching and dryness of nasal cavity. Burning.

FACE: Flushed. Aching pain in angle of right lower jaw. Violent trifacial neuralgia. Acne rosacea.

MOUTH: Dry. Breath seems hot. Metallic taste. Pricking at the tip of tongue.

THROAT: Sore, raw, with earache. Feeling in throat as after eating pepper.

STOMACH: Craves pork. Aversion to sweets, ice-cream which she is usually very fond of. Usual food not relished; sour things taste good.

ABDOMEN: Abdominal symptoms alternating with chest or ear symptoms. Nausea, > eating. Colic, > bending double and passing stools. Rectum sore, prolapsed. Stools at noon; soft, dark, or offensive, slate- colored.

URINARY: Dysuria, then erection. Nephritis with rheumatism.

MALE: Eczema of penis and inner surface of thighs. Itching.

FEMALE: Aching over pubes during menses. Right breast sore, > hard rubbing. *Itching genitals.* Menses last one day, then bloody leukorrhea. Uterine hemorrhage, when *Ipecac* fails. Lochia putrid, scanty or suppressed. Leukorrhea; white and scanty, curdy and cheesy.

RESPIRATORY: Persistent cough from tickling in throat pit, < lying, smoking, > eating and open air, sitting up, exercise. Tightness of chest, feels as if she could not get enough air. Chest pain alternating with indigestion and stuffed up feeling.

HEART: Constriction. Awakes with palpitation. Pulse rapid, irregular, fluttering. Blood pressure low.

NECK & BACK: Pain and lameness in cervical vertebrae, < dropping head forward, > standing and sitting erect. Weak between scapulae. Ascending lumbar pain, > exercise, walking. Lumbo-sacral bone pains, > hot bath, < going upstairs.

EXTREMITIES: Deep pain in joints—knees and ankles. Limbs feel hard and brittle as if they would break. Rheumatism of the hands. Cold. Numb.

SKIN: *Irritable, thick, burning, itching;* moist if scratched, < face and genitals. Branny scabs. Scabby on ears.

Eczema. Psoriasis. Scleroderma. Callosities. Cancer. Dermatitis.

SLEEP: Awakes panting, with palpitation. Dreams vivid, of fire, seem true.

FEVER: Cold sensation internally with chattering of teeth.

RELATED: *Phos;* Puls; *Rhus-r.*

RANUNCULUS BULBOSUS

GENERALITIES: It is a *painful* remedy, affecting NERVES, *muscles,* eyes, *serous membranes,* CHEST, *skin,* fingers, toes, and left side. THE PAINS are *stitching,* stabbing, shooting, extorting tears. Pain with shuddering; can not rest in any position. Burning, biting, *bruised soreness,* or *soreness* as of *deep ulceration. Sore spots.* Neuralgia. Sudden weakness and fainting. Trembling from anger. Distended feeling. Sensitive to air and touch. Burning in small spots from sedentary living. Shocks through the whole body. Chronic sciatica. Bad effects of alcoholic stimulants. Epilepsy of drunkards. Feels a cold wet cloth esp. on chest, < on going into cold air.

WORSE: AIR - *damp; cold,* open; drafts. *Change* of temperature, position. Alcohol. *Motion* of *arms.* Breathing. Touch. Eating. Fright, vexation, anger. Rainy and stormy weather. Standing.

BETTER: Standing. Sitting bent forward.

MIND: Great fear of ghosts in the evening, dares not to be alone. Quarrelsome. Depression of spirit, and desire to die. Delirium tremens, with hiccough.

HEAD: Feels too large and distended. Aching in forehead and vertex as if pressed asunder, with nausea and sleepiness. Creeping sensation in scalp. Tic (right) to ear.

EYES: Smarting as from smoke. Balls sore on moving them. Day and night blindness. Herpes on cornea with intense pain, photophobia and lacrimation. Hemiopia during pregnancy. Lids burn.

NOSE: Crawling and tingling in nostrils, in posterior nares; Tries to relieve it by hawking and blowing the nose.

MOUTH: Crawling on palate; wants to scratch it. Cramp, spasm of lips. Increased saliva. Butter tastes too sweet.

THROAT: Scraping, burning down the throat.

STOMACH: Spasmodic hiccough of drunkards.

ABDOMEN: Hypochondria bruised. Tenderness to pressure. Pinching colic, alternating with chest pain. Jaundice. Itching of body, esp. palms.

RESPIRATORY: Anxious, oppressed breathing, with desire to draw deep breath. Dyspnea, from anger. Small sore spot as from subcutaneous ulceration in chest. SHARP, CUTTING, STITCHING in chest, bilateral. Chilliness in chest when walking in open air; on breathing cold air. Pleurodynia. Pleurisy; adhesion after intercostal neuralgia.

BACK: Muscular pain along inner edge of left scapula from sitting bent, from needlework, typewriting, piano playing, extending through lower half of left chest. Scapula adherent. Muscles of neck rigidly contracted, can speak only by moving shoulders up and down.

EXTREMITIES: Crawling and tingling in fingers. Itching palms. Sudden jerking, stitching pain in forearm (R) while writing. Pain in heels as if pinched by boots.

SKIN: BLUISH VESICLES. Burning and intense itching, < touch. Shingles. Pemphigus. Horny scabs. Corrosive ichor. Flat, burning, stinging ulcers. Corns smart or burn, < touch.

FEVER: *Chilliness*, < open air.

RELATED: Canth; Rhus-t.

RANUNCULUS SCLERATUS

GENERALITIES: More acrid and irritating than *Ran-b.*, causing rawness, *burning-smarting, eating, gnawing or boring pains.* CHEST, *skin*, vertex and right side are specially affected. Pains cause fainting or shortness of breath. Feels sore all over. Periodical affections. Convulsive twitches. Sensation as of a plug.

WORSE: Motion. *Evening.* Deep breathing. Touch. Letting limb hang down.

BETTER: After midnight, *pains.*

MIND: Indolence and aversion to mental occupation.

HEAD: Gnawing pain in small spot on vertex, or either temples. Biting, itching on scalp.

NOSE: Fluent coryza with sneezing, with burning urination.

FACE: Sensation as if covered with cobwebs.

MOUTH: Blunt teeth, with toothache. Mapped tongue. Burning and rawness of tongue; denuded patches. Tongue cracks and peels off.

THROAT: Burning, scraping in throat.

STOMACH: Nausea, < after midnight. Pain with fainting.

ABDOMEN: Plug sensation behind umbilicus. Pain over region of liver as if diarrhea would set in.

RESPIRATORY: *Stitches in chest muscles;* chest with sternum is sensitive to touch. Sensation of a *plug forced between ribs,* < deep breathing. Sore, burning behind sternum.

HEART: Feels a plug in heart.

EXTREMITIES: Gout of fingers and toes. Gnawing in knee, left palm. Corns with burning soreness, < hanging down feet. Sudden stitches in big toes, passing into burning.

SKIN: *Yellow vesicles. Bullae* with acrid content. Pemphigus.

SLEEP: Dreadful dreams of dead bodies, snakes, fights.

RELATED: Ars; Arum-t.

RAPHANUS

GENERALITIES: Wild radish produces hysterical, mental and uterine symptoms. Numbness, changing places. Globus—as if hot ball from uterus goes up to the throat. Drinks more than urinates. Retained flatus, cannot be passed up and down; post-operative gas pain. Nymphomania, with aversion to her own sex and children, esp. girls. Sexual insomnia. Vomiting of fecal matter. Coldness of one foot. Epilepsy, reflex from removal of an adherent prepuce, the healing being delayed by furious priapism. Urine thick like milk.

RATANHIA

GENERALITIES: *Anal and rectal symptoms* are very marked; affects *teeth and nipples.* Pains here and there. *Sense of constriction. Hemorrhage,* passive. Pinworms. Dark, thin, scrawny persons. Cracks, *fissures.* Acts as a tonic for delicate and nervous women to prevent miscarriage, and in those who have never been able to go full term.

WORSE: Night. Anxiety, uneasiness of mind. Exertion. Touch. Straining at stool.

BETTER: Cool bathing. Hot bath. Walking in open air. Exercise.

MIND: Irritable, peevish and quarrelsome.

HEAD: Pain in middle of forehead as if brain would fall out. Bursting headache when straining at stool or after stools.

EYES: Lids feel stiff. Very rapid twitching of eyelids. Pterygium.

MOUTH: Feels as if cool air came from teeth. Toothache, < at night, must walk about. Cobweb sensation about the right side of the mouth.

STOMACH: *Cutting* or griping pain, > eructations. Violent painful hiccough.

ABDOMEN: *Constriction,* or *sharp splinter-like pain* in *rectum*; stool is forced with great straining and followed by prolonged *aching burning,* > hot water. Fissure of anus, with great constriction and burning like fire. Dry, itching anus. Pinworms. Ascarides. Discharge of blood from rectum with or without stool.

FEMALE: Metrorrhagia. Cracks in nipples, in nursing women. Compelled to get up at night and walk about during pregnancy, with toothache.

CHEST: Pain in the ribs on stepping.

RELATED: Nit-ac; Paeon.

RHEUM

GENERALITIES: Rhubarb is a remedy for sucklings and children, esp. during dentition, and suits pregnant and nursing women. It affects liver, duodenum, *bile ducts* and intestines. *Sourness* is very marked; the child smells sour, washing does not remove it. Colicky children who are always *screaming* and crying. Sour, taste, vomit, stool, sweat, etc. Difficult dentition. Requires very little sleep and not much food. Sensation of crepitation.

WORSE: *Dentition*. Eating plums. Summer. Nursing women. Motion. Before, after and during stool.

BETTER: Warmth. Wrapping up. Lying bent. Odd position.

MIND: *Impatient*; child asks for different things vehemently with crying, dislikes even its favourite things. Impetuous desire for particular objects. Restless, with weeping.

HEAD: Sweat on hairy scalp; hair *wet, sopping*.

EYES: Weak when looking steadily at any object. Convulsive twitching of eyelids.

FACE: Cold sweat on face, esp. about mouth and nose, on upper lip. Forehead wrinkled. Twitching.

MOUTH: Offensive mucus in the mouth after sleep. Breath sour. Salivation with colic or diarrhea. Food tastes bitter, even sweet things. Teeth feel cold.

STOMACH: Desire for various things, but cannot eat them. Loathing after first bite. Plums and prunes disagree. Requires little food.

ABDOMEN: Colic, with screaming, > doubling up, < uncovering any part, then pappy, *sour, brown, green, fermented, slimy* or acrid stools, < eating unripe fruit, in the evening. Shivering with stools. Diarrhea only when walking. Jaundice from eating unripe fruits, with white diarrhea.

URINARY: Burning in bladder and kidney, before and during urination. Unsuccessful urging to urinate before stool.

FEMALE: Urinary complaints after abortion. Milk in nursing women yellow and bitter, infant refuses breast. Diarrhea after parturition.

BACK: Stiffness in sacrum and hips, cannot walk straight. Cutting in lumbar region, < after stools.

EXTREMITIES: Limb on which he lies falls asleep. Twitching in arms, hands and fingers. Bubbling sensation in elbow joint, from bend of knee to heel. Lameness of wrist and knee, after sprain and dislocation.

SLEEP: Restless, with whining and crying. Twitching of face and fingers. Requires very little sleep and not much food.

FEVER: Sweat on scalp, about mouth, nose, upper lip.

COMPLEMENTARY: Mag-c.

RELATED: Cham.

RHODODENDRON

GENERALITIES: Commonly known as yellow snow-rose it is a *gouty rheumatic* remedy, affecting the FIBROUS TISSUES, forearm, lower legs, small joints, *bones, genitals, nerves,* single parts. SENSITIVE TO WINDY OR STORMY WET WEATHER even if he is in the house; nervous persons who are afraid of thunder. *Tearing, zigzag,* boring, rapidly changing, descending, *paralytic pains.* Great weakness after slight exertion. Formication with sweat. Chorea before storm. Symptoms alternate. Undulating sensation.

WORSE: BEFORE STORM. *Weather—rough, windy,* cold, damp, changing, cloudy. Night. Midsummer. Wine. Rest. Eating fruit. Getting wet. Catching cold.

BETTER: After storm breaks. Heat, in sun. Motion (at once). Wrapping head.

MIND: Confused and stupid. Forgets what he is talking about; leaves out words while writing. Fear of thunder in nervous persons. Aversion to his business. Easily affected by wine.

HEAD: Ache, < early in the morning, > eating. Throbbing in right head. Drawing, tearing under scalp. Vertigo when lying in bed, > when moving about. Hair stand up as if electrified.

EYES: Ciliary neuralgia, involving orbit, eyeball and head, < before storm. Heat in eyes when using them. Red hot needles darting from within out.

EARS: Sensation of a worm. Deafness long after rising (hearing better in the morning). Noises come on after the patient has been up a few hours. Tinnitus with vertigo.

NOSE: Nostrils obstructed alternately with fluent coryza, > in open air.

FACE: Prosopalgia; violent tearing jerking pains, > eating and warmth.

MOUTH: Toothache, > eating and warmth. Toothache ceases suddenly, < again in two or three hours.

STOMACH: Heavy pressure from cold drinks. Feels full after a little food. Green, bitter vomiting after drinking cold water.

ABDOMEN: Colic at navel. Pain from rectum to genitals.

Flatus felt in back. Diarrhea < fruits; does not weaken. Sticking pain in spleen on walking fast. Undulating sensation arising from abdomen.

URINARY: Frequent urging to urinate with drawing in the region of the bladder. Pain in urethra as from subcutaneous ulceration. Urine, profuse, foul, greenish.

MALE: *Drawing from spermatic cord into abdomen and thighs.* Testes swollen, painful, drawn up, feel crushed. Glans feels crushed. Testes indurated; pain alternately. Orchitis. Itching, wrinkled, sweaty, scrotum. Hydrocele; of boys from birth.

FEMALE: Suppressed menses. Fever with headache with each menstrual period. Serous cysts in vagina. Burning in uterine region after parturition, alternating with pain in limbs; fingers spasmodically flexed.

RESPIRATORY: Bruised, sprained feeling in chest. Breathless and speechless from violent pleuritic pains, running down anterior chest.

HEART: Warm undulation at heart. Heartbeat strong.

BACK & NECK: Neck and nape stiff. Sacrum pains, < sitting.

EXTREMITIES: Bruised, sprained feeling in wrist. Hands feel warm in cold weather. Lower legs cold, skin wrinkled, feel as if asleep. Sensation of a weight hanging to feet. Rheumatic tearing in all limbs. Drawing, tearing in periosteum of long bones. Rheumatism of hot weather. Feet cold even in warm room, in bed. Pain in tendo achilles on stepping.

SLEEP: Cannot sleep unless legs are crossed. Awakes as if called.

FEVER: Formication and itching of skin with sweat.

RELATED: Rhus-t.

RHUS TOXICODENDRON

GENERALITIES: This remedy is irritating to the SKIN, esp. of face, scalp, genitals; affects the *fibrous tissue, ligaments* and joints causing RHEUMATIC SYMPTOMS; it is an infective agent producing TYPHOID-LIKE FEVER. Affections of NERVES and SPINAL CORD give rise to PARETIC EFFECTS. GLANDS are swollen, hot and painful; indurated; suppurating. Symptoms appear on the left side or go from left to right. PAINS ARE TEARING, SHOOTING, STITCHING, < AT NIGHT, CANNOT REST in any position. Parts feel sore, *bruised* and STIFF. *Pain as if the flesh was torn loose from the bone.* Dislocative sensation. Muscles twitch. *Crawling.* Numbness; of parts paralyzed. Trembling. *Burning, swelling, and lividity.* Mucous discharges are *acrid, rusty red, like meat water; musty;* causing eruptions. Infection, septicemia, carbuncles in early stage. Cellulitis; inflammation and swelling of the long bones; scraping, gnawing, tearing in periosteum. Rheumatism in cold season. Post-operative complications. Hemiplegia, right side; sensation as if gone to sleep. Infantile paralysis from exposure to cold damp. Influenza. Small pox. Stricture after inflammation. Soreness of prominent projections of bones. Paralysis after unwanted exertion, after parturition. Boils, abscesses.

WORSE: EXPOSURE TO — WET, COLD *air, draft. Chilled* when hot or sweaty. *Uncovering* parts— head, etc. BEGINNING OF MOTION. REST. BEFORE STORM. SPRAIN. *Overexertion. After Midnight.* Blows; jar. Riding. Ice. Cold drink. Side lain on.

BETTER: *Continued motion.* HEAT. Hot bath; if heated. Warm wrapping. *Rubbing.* Nosebleed. Holding affected part, abdomen, head, etc. Stretching limbs. Change of position. Warm dry weather.

MIND: *Anxious, sad*; helplessness and *profound despondency*. Low, mild delirium; incoherent talk, answers correctly but slowly, or hastily, or reluctantly. Inclination to weep, < in evening, without knowing why, with desire for solitude, fear of being poisoned. Satiety of life, thoughts of suicide, wants to drown himself. Forgetful, cannot remember the most recent events. Fear, < at night, cannot lie in bed. *Confusion*. Anxiety regarding one's children.

HEAD: Vertigo; in the aged, whirling then headache. Shattering or loose feeling in the brain < jar. Feeling as of a board strapped across the forehead. Stupefying headache. Must lie down, < least chagrin. Painfully stiff scalp > lying on it. Head heavy.

EYES: *Pain behind eyes*, < motion. *Eyelids stiff*, agglutinated, dry, firmly closed. Profuse gush of hot tears on opening lids. Pustular inflammation. Saccular conjunctiva. Photophobia. Iritis. Ptosis. Paralysis of any of the muscles of the eyeball. Vertical diplopia. Orbital cellulitis. Affection of inner surface of the eyelids.

EARS: Parotitis (left) with fever. Lobules swollen. Pain in ear with a feeling as if something were inside. Discharge of bloody pus.

NOSE: Red, sensitive tip; it drips water. Sneezing, fluent coryza. Nosebleed, < at night, stooping, at stool, in fever; which gives relief. Violent aching in bones of the nose. Breath hot, it burns nostrils.

FACE: Jaws crack on chewing. Joints painful. Facial neuralgia with chilliness. Easy dislocation of jaws. Cheek bones painful. Red spots on left cheek. *Stiff swollen face*. Lips dry, brownish, cracked at corners, crusty. Herpes on lips. Crusta lactea. Acne rosacea.

MOUTH: *Sordes on teeth*. Teeth feel loose and long. Bloody saliva runs during sleep. Tongue dry, red at center, cracked, stiff, sore, has a *triangular red tip; coated diagonally* or one side only. Feeling as if tongue covered with skin. Coppery, herby or bitter taste. Bread tastes bitter.

THROAT: Red, puffy, itching fauces. Tonsils covered with yellow membrane. Sore throat, with *swollen glands.* Difficult swallowing; of solids as from contraction, of saliva. Oesophagitis from swallowing corrosive matter.

STOMACH: Craves cold drinks though they < cough, chill, etc. Desire for cold milk, sweets, oysters. Vomits from coughing, lying on back; *fecal vomiting.* Nausea, < ice cream, after eating. Great thirst, < at night. Drowsy after eating. Great thirst, but no appetite for any kind of food. Pain in stomach after ice water.

ABDOMEN: Sore. Feeling as if water swashing in, or a lump. Colic, compelling to walk bent, > lying on abdomen. *Ileo-cecal symptoms*; appendicitis. Stools watery; frothy, or bloody, foul, *meat water-like,* slimy, gelatinous, involuntary; in sleep at night; or with tenesmus; < drinking. Dysenteric diarrhea. Piles, < lifting. Painful tenesmus without stool. Hour-glass contraction. Mucous colitis.

URINARY: Incontinence of urine, < lying, at night or sitting; in boys. Nephritis. Urine dark, turbid, high colored, scanty. Frequent, profuse urination day and night.

MALE: Scrotum thick, swollen, *edematous.* Prepuce edematous. *Intense itching of genitals.* Hydrocele from overlifting. Metastasis of mumps to testes.

FEMALE: Swelling *with intense itching of vulva.* Menses too early, profuse and protracted. Amenorrhea from getting wet; with milk in breast. Metritis; septic. Lochia thin, protracted, offensive, diminished, with shooting upwards in vagina. Prolapsus uteri from lifting or overstraining. Frequent after-pains. Violent pain in vulva during menses. Vagina sore.

RESPIRATORY: Chest pain, < using arms. Tickling behind upper sternum, causing dry, hoarse, tearing, tormenting cough, with bloody taste, < during chill, when putting hands out of bed, after midnight till morning. Hoarseness from overstraining of voice. Sudden hypostasis or edema of lungs. Pleurodynia, chest pains shoot into shoulder. Hemoptysis from overexertion, blowing wind instruments; blood bright. Rust- colored sputum. Larynx cold when breathing. Hot air from trachea.

HEART: Uncomplicated hypertrophy from violent exertion. Heart feels tired; pains go down left arm. Palpitation, < when sitting still, > walking. Trembling in heart, > walking. Pulse quick, weak, irregular, intermittent, with numbness of left arm. Left arm aches with heart disease.

NECK & BACK: Stiff neck, with painful tension when moving. *Interscapular* pain, < swallowing. Contractive or breaking backache, > hard pressure; lying on something hard; walking about or bending backwards. Lumbago. Coccyx aches into thighs.

EXTREMITIES: *Numbness*, and prickling in limbs. Arms nervous and shaky (left). Paralytic pains in elbows. Rhagades on back of hands. Palms; dry, hot, cracked or sore; washing causes burning. *Pains down back of thighs* < stools; sciatica. Legs feel dead, wooden. Cramps in calves. Involuntary limping. Soreness of condyles of bones. Limbs stiff, paralyzed. Hot painful swelling of joints. Pricking like pins in tips of fingers and palms when grasping. Pain along ulnar nerve. Ulcers; on legs; gangrenous; runs bloody water; on dropsical legs. Itching of legs and feet. Ankles swollen after too long sitting; feet swell in the evening. Paraplegia; after parturition, sexual excess; fevers. As if walking on needles. Axillary abscess, after delivery.

SKIN: *Stiff, thick,* dry, hot, burning; itching, < hairy parts. Skin *sensitive to cold air.* ERUPTIONS; *fine,* VESICULAR; *crusty, eczematous; moist* or ERYSIPELATOUS < genitals; alternating with dysentery. Pus erodes the hair. Vesicles over abscess. Milk crusts. Baker's itch. Urticaria; from getting wet; with rheumatism or during chills and fever. Shingles.

SLEEP: Awakes tired or nervous. *Dreams; of great* exertion; of blood; or fire. Yawning; frequent, violent, spasmodic; without inclination to sleep; with stretching. Restless, tossing about.

FEVER: *Easily chilled < least uncovering; with pain in limbs.* Chill as if dashed with cold water or cold water in the veins; preceded by cough; alternating with heat. Chill in single parts. Heat, with busy delirium. Typhoid. Sweat; < during pain; with sleepiness. Urticaria during fever. Wants to yawn and stretch during chill.

COMPLEMENTARY: Bry; Calc; *Mag-c;* Med; Phyt.

RELATED: Arn; Bry; Dulc.

ROBINIA

GENERALITIES: *Acridity and acidity* are marked features of this remedy. It is therefore useful for hyperchlorhydria, when the eructations and taste are sour and *vomiting is so sour that it sets the teeth on edge* or dulls them. Infants with sour smell of the body, sour stools and vomiting, of sour milk. Acid dyspepsia. Constant full frontal headache, < motion and reading. Sick headache with acid vomiting. Waterbrash. Burning in stomach and between scapulae. Flatulence. Squeezing in stomach. Heartburn and acidity, < lying down, esp. at night.

WORSE: *Eating. Night.* Fat. Cabbage. Turnip. Raw fruit. Icecream.

RELATED: Iris; Mag-c.

RUMEX CRISPUS

GENERALITIES: It affects the *nerves,* causing numerous and varied pains; neither fixed nor constant anywhere; *sharp pains;* neuralgia. *Mucous membranes of larynx,* trachea, bowels and THROAT PIT are affected, producing *dryness and sensitiveness.* Acts on joints, esp. *ankles,* skin, chest. Left-side. MUCOUS secretions decrease causing *stickiness, with burning.* Obesity. Lymphatics enlarged and secretions perverted. Every cold affects the joints.

WORSE: INHALING; COOL AIR, open air; change from warm to cold, cold to warm. Uncovering. Night. Pressure on trachea. Talking. Deep breathing or irregular breathing. Motion. Eating; after meal.

BETTER: *Covering mouth.* Wrapping up.

MIND: Low-spirited, with serious expression of the face. Indifferent about his surroundings.

HEAD: Darting sharp pain in the left side.

EYES: Burn indoors; puffed up in A.M.

NOSE: Feeling of dryness in posterior nares. Sneezing attacks; fluent coryza. Itching that extends from the end of the nose to the pharynx.

FACE: Sodden. Pale, while standing.

MOUTH: Toothache, entirely > after dinner, rinsing mouth with cold water.

THROAT: Hawks much tenacious mucus. Throat feels

hollow. Lump not > by hawking, descends and rises again after swallowing.

STOMACH: Ravenous appetite. Sensation of a hard substance in the pit of stomach. Pain in the left breast after meal. Talking < stomach symptoms. Gastralgia, aching through the back, obliged to breath deeply. Tight, suffocative heavy ache in epigastrium, going to back; clothes feel tight. Eating meat causes eructation and pruritus. Nausea, > by eructations.

ABDOMEN: Creeping near navel, > by discharge of offensive flatus. *Stools sudden, profuse, foul;* painless, brown, black or thin watery; driving him out of bed in the *morning* (5 to 9 A.M.). Diarrhea in phthisis, after catarrh. Itching in anus with sensation of a stick in rectum. Annoying rumbling flatulence, in women.

URINARY: Sudden urging; involuntary with cough.

FEMALE: Pain right ovary to back.

RESPIRATORY: EVERY BREATH OF COLD AIR CAUSES TICKLING, *as from a feather or dust* in THROAT PIT, AND CONTINUOUS COUGH, > *closing or covering the mouth or head*, < touching throat pit, lying on left side. Dry teasing cough preventing sleep. Profuse, frothy, thin expectoration. Sputum comes by mouthfuls. Dyspnea on retiring. suffocative choking. Respiration < in wind. Cough provoked by changing room, change from cold to warm and warm to cold. Pain, rawness or burning under clavicle as if the air penetrated there, < hawking. *Pain, under sternum,* under right nipple. Burning sticking pain in left chest near the heart, < deep breathing. Barking cough. Cough comes regularly at 11 P.M., 2 and 5 A.M., in children. Cough daytime only. Cough < during early pregnancy may cause miscarriage. Clavicular pain < hawking.

HEART: Feels as if suddenly stopped, followed by heavy throbbing through the chest.

BACK: Pain under *right* scapula.

EXTREMITIES: Pain in left shoulder on coughing, on raising arms. Hands cold when coughing. Spasmodic cramps in ankles and feet.

SKIN: Intense itching, < lower limbs, exposure to cold air or undressing. Acne vulgaris on back.

SLEEP: Sudden sleepiness.

FEVER: Sweat on waking from a sound sleep.

RELATED: Caust; Seneg.

RUTA GRAVEOLENS

GENERALITIES: This remedy has a special affinity for *fibrous tissue, flexor tendons, joints— ankles, wrists; cartilages, periosteum; uterus and skin.* It is the chief remedy for injured or bruised bones Therefore, the pains are BRUISED, SORE, ACHING, WITH RESTLESSNESS. *Feeling of intense painful weariness. Heaviness*; as of a weight in forehead or hanging to feet or lower limbs, *Sensation of a rough blunt plug in part—* head, nose, etc. *Paralytic rigidity.* Distortions. *Gnawing-burning pains,* neuralgia. Rheumatism. Formation of deposits or nodes in the periosteum, tendons and about the joints, esp. wrists. Ill effects of bruises, fractures, carrying heavy weights. Lameness after sprain. Bones brittle. Lain—on parts become sore, even in bed. Feeling of intense lassitude, weakness and despair.

WORSE: *Overexertion*, injury, *sprain*. EYE STRAIN. COLD air, *damp*, wind, wet. LYING. SITTING. *Pressure on an edge*. Stooping. During menses. Uncooked or indigestible food. Exertion, ascending, descending steps.

BETTER: *Lying on back. Warmth.* Motion. Rubbing. Scratching.

MIND: *Dissatisfied with himself* and others, and disposed to weep. Suspicious, imagines that he is always being deceived. Fretful; quarrels and contradicts.

HEAD: Aches as if a nail is driven into it. Stitches, < reading.

EYES: Red, hot and painful, from reading fine print, sewing. *Vision dim.* Lacrymation. Itching inner canthi. Asthenopia. Spasm in lower eyelids, when it ceases. lacrimation starts.

EAR: Pain as from a blunt piece of wood.

NOSE: Sweat on nose. Pressive aching at the root of nose with epistaxis.

MOUTH: Cramps in tongue, causing embarrassment of speech. Woody taste.

STOMACH: Sudden nausea while eating, with vomiting of food. Burning-gnawing pain. Dyspepsia from carrying heavy weight. Violent thirst for ice cold water. Nausea felt in rectum. Tension in stomach, > drinking milk.

ABDOMEN: Urging to stool, but only *rectum prolapses.* Prolapse of rectum; on stooping, after delivery, during stools hard or soft. Feces often escape when stooping. Painful swelling of the spleen. Cancer of lower bowel. Stricture of rectum.

URINARY: Constant pressure on bladder as if it is full or moving up and down. Constant urging, can hardly retain urine if forcibly retained, she could not pass it afterwards, with severe pain.

FEMALE: Corrosive leukorrhea after irregular or suppressed menses.

RESPIRATORY: Short breath, with tightness of chest.

Weak feeling in chest after thick, yellow sputum. Painful spot on sternum. Ill effects of mechanical injury to chest.

NECK & BACK: Weak, bruised feeling in small of back, hips and lower limbs in A.M. Coldness of spine downwards. Backache, > lying on back and pressure.

EXTREMITIES: *Thighs feel broken,* < when stretching the legs. Sore tendons. Totters; stumbles easily. Pains as if deep in long bones, must walk about. Nodes in palms. Ganglion of the wrist. Bursae. Pain in bones of the feet, cannot step heavily on them. Contraction, of fingers, feet, toes. Hamstrings feel shortened. Cracking in joints, < walking in open air. Sciatica, < lying down, at night, > during daytime. Legs give out on attempt to rise from a chair, has to make several attempts. Paralytic weakness of legs, after spraining the back. Legs feel weak, knees give way while ascending and descending stairs. Ankles swollen.

SKIN: *Easily chaffed* from walking, riding; also in children. Erosive itching. Fat, smooth, painful warts on palms. Itching after eating meat.

SLEEP: Wakes frequently. Vivid, confused dreams. Yawns, stretches and extends hands.

FEVER: Frequent attacks of quick flush of heat. Glowing heat on face, skin, etc.

COMPLEMENTARY: *Calc-p.*

RELATED: Arn; Phyt; Ran-s; Symph.

SABADILLA

GENERALITIES: MUCOUS MEMBRANES OF NOSE, *lacrimal glands,* ANUS and digestive tract are affected by this remedy. NERVES are affected producing weakness, nervousness; startled easily. Nervous symptoms reflex from worms; twitching, convulsive trembling or catalepsy. *Formication*. Alternate nervous and bodily symptoms. Hysteria after fright. Ill effects of fright, mental exertion, thinking. Worms; causing convulsion, nymphomania, etc. Imaginary diseases. Cutting pain in bones.

WORSE: COLD air, drink. *Periodically*— every week, two weeks, four weeks, *same hour,* forenoon, new and full moon. Odors. Undeveloped exanthemata. Mental exertion.

BETTER: *Open air. Heat.* Eating. Swallowing. Quick motion of affected part.

MIND: Miserable. Timid. Easily startled. Erroneous (fixed) ideas about himself— imagines he is very sick, that parts are sunken, limbs are crooked, chin is elongated, one side larger than the other, she has a cancer or is pregnant. No response to questions, loss of consciousness, then he jumps up and runs recklessly through the room. Rage. Mania, > washing head in cold water.

HEAD: Vertigo, with sensation as though all things were turning around each other— sudden on waking at night, or rising from stooping, with black vision and faintness, > resting head on table. Unilateral head pains, or alternating sides, < thinking, > eating. Burning, itching, crawling on hairy scalp, > scratching. Headache in schoolgirls.

EYES: Lids red, burning. *Lacrimation*; < during pain, sneezing, coughing, yawning, when walking in open air, during chill.

EARS: Difficulty of hearing, as if there were bands over ear.

NOSE: *Persistent* VIOLENT, or ABORTIVE SNEEZING. ITCHING, tickling, rubs or picks at it. Nose dry. Tickling in nose spreads over the whole body then dyspnea. Hay fever. Influenza. *Sensitive smell.* One or the other nostril stuffed up. Fluent coryza. Discharge is worse from the odor of flowers, even thinking of flowers increases the discharge. Cannot tolerate the smell of garlic. Stubborn, lingering coryza. Hawks bright red blood from nasopharynx.

FACE: Feels hot, fiery red. Lips hot, burn as if scalded. Cracking of jaw joint on opening the mouth wide.

MOUTH: Sensation as if mouth and tongue burnt. Itching of the soft palate. Sweetish taste. Cannot bear anything hot or cold in mouth.

THROAT: Cannot protrude tongue in sore throat. Feels a *lump,* morsel, thread or skin hanging in throat, with constant inclination to swallow. Sore throat, left to right, < empty swallowing, > hot drink. Tonsillitis after coryza.

STOMACH: Craves hot things, sweets, milk. No relish for food until she takes first morsel, then she takes a good meal; especially during pregnancy. Canine hunger, for sweets and farinaceous food. Thirstless. Coldness or empty feeling. Aversion to all food, meat, sour things, coffee, garlic.

ABDOMEN: Bowels feel knotted; as if a lump or thread moved rapidly in abdomen. Burning, frothy, loose, brown, floating stools. *Crawling, itching at anus,* alternating with itching in nose or ears. Pinworms.

FEMALE: Nymphomania from worms. Menses too late, come by fits and starts, intermit, sometimes stronger sometimes weaker.

RESPIRATORY: Violent coughing attacks; muffled, < anger, with lacrimation. Asthmatic breathing with itching skin, nose and anus. Red spots on chest. Pleurisy with great paralytic debility.

HEART: Palpitation, with pulsations through whole body.

EXTREMITIES: Upward jerking of arms. Cracks between and under toes. Cutting pain in bones. Thick, deformed horny nails. Red spots on arms and hands. Yellow spots on fingers. Swelling of feet, with painful soles.

SKIN: Itching with asthmatic breathing. Dry like parchment.

SLEEP: Comes on when thinking, meditating, reading.

FEVER: Shivering as a concomitant. Thirst after chill only. Chill from below upwards. Lacrimation with chill.

COMPLEMENTARY: Sep.

RELATED: Ars; Puls; Urt-u.

SABAL SERRULATA

GENERALITIES: Genito-urinary organs, esp. *prostate, ovaries, mammae,* bladder and urethra are specially influenced by this medicine. It is soothing to the mucous membranes and is tonic, nutritive and stimulating to the overworked brain (use 1x). Sharp, stinging wandering, pains. Homeopathic catheter for retention of urine due to enlarged prostate. Nervous women and *old men. Debility.* Nervous irritability, with loss of sexual appetite in both sexes. Sexual neurotics.

WORSE: Cold, damp, cloudy weather. Sympathy. Before menses.

BETTER: After sleep.

MIND: Irritability and depression; sympathy made her angry. Broods over her own suffering or symptoms. Apathy. Indifference. Fears to fall asleep lest something should happen. Starts up with fear when dozing.

HEAD: Sharp, darting pains here and there going and coming suddenly. Pain runs up the nose and centers in forehead. Headache of weak persons.

EYES: Iritis when prostate gland is involved.

EARS: Hearing diminished; voices seem far off.

STOMACH: Constant desire for milk which is usually disliked. Acidity. Eructations.

ABDOMEN: Pain goes into thighs, radiating to different directions, settling in ovaries.

URINARY: Constant desire to pass water at night. Enuresis from any exertion—lifting, laughing, etc. Difficult urination; smarting, burning in urethra. Slimy urinary sediment. Heavy aching pain and sense of coldness in bladder extending to external genitals. Cystitis from prostate hypertrophy.

MALE: Testes drawn up, painful. *Genitals cold. Enlarged or congested prostate; senile prostate.* Wasting of testes and loss of sexual power. Painful erection or emission of semen during coition. Sexual neurotics. Epididymitis. Impotency. Semen thick, causes hot feeling along the cord.

FEMALE: Ovaries tender and enlarged; ovarian pains runs down the thighs. Vulva feels open. Female sexual neurotics, suppressed or perverted sexual inclination. Mammae sore, tender and full, < cold bath; or small and *undeveloped. Genitals cold.* One breast smaller than other. Sexual passion furious.

RESPIRATORY: Profuse expectoration with discharge from the nose. Chronic bronchitis. Wheezing cough, worse lying down, till 6 A.M.

BACK: Aches after coition. Pain in sacral region before commencement of menses.

SLEEP: Fears to fall asleep, lest something should happen; starts up with this fear when he is dozing.

RELATED: Sep; Sil.

SABINA

GENERALITIES: FEMALE PELVIC ORGANS, *esp. uterus,* are mostly affected by this remedy. In addition it affects the *fibrous tissue of small joints,* serous membranes and heels. It is suitable for hot-blooded women with gouty—rheumatic diathesis and *hemorrhagic tendency*—epistaxis, hematuria, etc. Tendency to abortion, esp. at the third month. Violent pulsations, wants windows open. Heaviness and indolence of body, wants to lie down. Red shiny swelling of affected parts. Acutely inflamed arthritic nodes. Sense of fullness. Wart—like growths. Pain increases suddenly and decreases slowly.

WORSE: *Night.* HEAT of bed, room; exertion. Pregnancy. Climacteric. Foggy weather. Stooping. Letting limbs hang down. Taking a deep breath. Music.

BETTER: Cold. Cool open air. Exhalation.

MIND: Music is intolerable, produces nervousness. Melancholic. Sad.

HEAD: *Bursting headaches,* appear suddenly, diminish slowly and return frequently. Vertigo with suppressed menses.

MOUTH: Toothache, < only when chewing. Drawing pain in the muscles of jaws. Bitter taste to food, esp. milk or coffee.

STOMACH: Desire for lemonade. Heartburn. Pain from epigastrium to back.

ABDOMEN: Plethoric. Quivering as if something were alive, resembling fetal movement. Hemorrhoids with discharge of bright red blood causing pain from sacrum to pubes. Piles alternate with pain in limbs.

URINARY: Vesical irritability, with gouty diathesis. Bloody urine, with much urging. Throbbing, burning at the region of kidneys.

MALE: Sexual desire increased, with violent continuous erections. Sycotic excrescences with burning soreness. Hard swelling on dorsum of penis.

FEMALE: *Itching genitals;* almost insatiable desire for coition. Menses too profuse, too early; *gushing of hot, bright, watery blood* mixed with dark clots, < least motion but often > by walking. Menses, with pain in joints, WITH PAIN FROM SACRUM TO PUBES or *reverse,* or *shooting up from vagina*. Bleeding between periods with sexual excitement. Leukorrhea foul, acrid, thick, yellow, from suppressed menses or copious menses, with itching of pudenda. Leukorrhea during pregnancy. Pruritus of pregnancy. Retained placenta. Severe afterpains. Promotes expulsion of moles. Crawling in nipples. Hemorrhage after abortion. Ovaritis and metritis after abortion; Premature labor. Dysmenorrhea, > lying flat on the back, with limbs extended. Voluptuous itching in nipples.

HEART: Violent pulsation in blood vessels in whole body.

BACK: Pain from lumbar region to pubis or reverse.

EXTREMITIES: Swelling, redness and stitches in right big toe. Shooting in heels. Diminishes knots, and enlargements and varices in veins. Intermittent aching in the solar part of the heels.

SKIN: Foul, itching-burning, moist figwarts. Black pores in skin, esp. face.

FEVER: Intolerable burning heat of whole body, with great restlessness.

COMPLEMENTARY: Thuj.

RELATED: Ars; Caul; Puls.

SALICYLICUM ACIDUM

GENERALITIES: In ordinary practice it is used as an acute rheumatic remedy. In homeopathy it is useful in Meniere's disease. Roaring and ringing in ears. Deafness with vertigo. Effects of suppressed footsweat.

WORSE: Motion. Night. Cold air.

SALIX NIGRA

GENERALITIES: It reduces the irritability of sexual organs of both the sexes. Satyriasis and erotomania. Seminal emission in presence of women or when talking with her. Libidinous thoughts and dreams. Use material dose of tincture—30 drops.

SAMBUCUS NIGRA

GENERALITIES: It acts upon *respiratory* organs, kidneys and the skin. *Profuse sweat or shortness of breath* accompanies many symptoms. Edematous swelling in various parts of the body, esp. legs, instep and feet. Snuffles in infants preventing breathing and nursing. General trembling with anxiety. Ill effects of fright, grief, anxeity, excessive sexual indulgence. Suits persons previously robust and fleshy suddenly becoming emaciated.

WORSE: Dry cold air. Cold drink while heated. Head low. Eating fruits. Lying down. Rest.

BETTER: Pressure over a sharp edge. Motion. Wrapping up. Sitting up in bed.

MIND: Constant fretfulness. Easily frightened. Fright followed by suffocative attacks. Sees images when shutting eyes.

EYES: Half open in sleep. Photophobia.

NOSE: Dry coryza with snuffles in infants.

MOUTH: Half open in sleep.

FACE: Pale, bluish, puffy, < coughing. Hot with icy cold feet.

URINARY: Acute nephritis. Dropsical symptoms with vomiting of bile, and distress in stomach after eating. Profuse urination with a sensation of heat in the body. Urine frequent and scanty.

MALE: Hydrocele from injury.

FEMALE: Debilitating sweats after childbirth.

RESPIRATORY: SUDDEN SUFFOCATION or *strangling cough* on falling to sleep, or *waking him at midnight with violent sweat,* < fright. Whistling breathing in spasms of glottis. Screeching voice. Croup. Spell of coughing before fever.

EXTREMITIES: Icy cold feet. Hands become blue. Dropsy of legs and feet.

FEVER: *Dry burning heat during sleep,* but *copious sweating on awakening. Sweat with cough.* Debilitating sweat, < night.

RELATED: Bell; Brom.

SANGUINARIA CANADENSIS

GENERALITIES: Commonly known as blood root, it is a RIGHT SIDED remedy, affecting the head, LIVER, chest and deltoid. It produces 'VASO-MOTOR DISTURBANCES, as is seen in circumscribed *redness* of the cheeks, abdomen, tongue, etc.; *congestion of blood* to head, chest, abdomen, etc.; flushes of heat and general pulsations. BURNING HEAT AND EBULLITIONS. Mucous membranes become dry. *Burning* in throat, under sternum, spots or stitches in chest, palms and soles. Burnt feeling, in tongue. *Symptoms ascend or end in bilious vomiting.* Internal rawness. Acrid blood-streaked or foul discharge. Lies on back with head elevated. Climacteric disorders. Bilious. Pains increase and decrease with the sun. Sudden stopping of catarrh of respiratory tract followed by diarrhea. Polypi—nasal, uterine. Fungus excrescences. Sick and faint from odor of flowers. Pains in places where bones are least covered.

WORSE: *Periodically—with sun,* weekly, night. *Climaxis. Odors. Jar.* Light. Sweets. Motion. Looking up. Touch. Raising arms.

BETTER: *Sleep.* Lying on back. Vomiting. Cool air. Passing flatus. Sour things. Lying on left side.

MIND: Irritable, morose. Grumbling. Borrows trouble. Lassitude, indisposed to move or make any mental effort.

HEAD: Pain over right eye, or ASCENDING FROM OCCIPUT TO OVER RIGHT EYE. Hemicrania, increases and decreases with the sun. Distension of veins in the temples. Pain in the occiput like a flash of lightning. Vertigo, $<$ looking up and moving head rapidly. Headache if he goes without food. Headache $>$ by sleep, vomiting and passing of copious urine.

EYES: Burning. Eyeballs painful on moving them. Hard swelling over eyebrows. Lacrimation with coryza, tears hot.

EARS: Burning. Earache with headache. Humming and roaring in the ear; painfully sensitive to sounds at climaxis.

NOSE: *Pain at the root of nose.* Coryza; stopped, then diarrhea. Nasal polypi. Rose-cold, with subsequent asthma. Sensitive to odors. Loss or perverted sense of smell, smell in nose like roasted onion.

FACE: *Redness and burning of cheeks.* Hectic flush, red cheeks. Neuralgia in upper jaw, radiating, > by kneeling down and pressing the head firmly on the floor. Fulness and tenderness behind angle of jaw.

MOUTH: Burnt feeling in tongue. Anterior tongue looks red like raw beef. Sweet things taste bitter. Palate feels scalded. Toothache from picking teeth.

THROAT: Sore, swollen (right); pains go to ear and chest. Burning, < eating sweet things. Dryness of singers.

STOMACH: Craves spices; knows not for what. Aversion to butter. Nausea with salivation, < sneezing or blowing nose, > eating; nausea followed by urticaria. Spitting of bile; gastroduodenal catarrh. Stomach pains radiate to right shoulder.

ABDOMEN : Tension of epigastrium. Feeling of hot water pouring from breast to abdomen, followed by diarrhea. Bilious, liquid, gushing stools. Flatulent distension with escape of flatus from vagina. Jaundice. Cancer of rectum.

URINARY: Urine dark yellow with jaundice. Copious and frequent, clear, < at night.

FEMALE: Climacteric disorders; esp. flushes of heat and fetid, acrid leukorrhea. Soreness under nipple (right). Menses; offensive, profuse. Uterine polypi. Mammae; sore and enlarged; at climaxis.

RESPIRATORY: Larynx, full and dry; in singers. Cough raises foul air; is dry; from tickling behind the sternum; must sit up in bed; with passing flatus up and down which >. Expectoration tough, rusty, purulent, which <. Burning in chest, sensation as of hot steam extending to abdomen, with cough. Cough after influenza or whooping cough, returns after every fresh cold. Pain in right chest (from breast) to shoulder. Pneumonia. Phthisis. Asthma; from disturbed digestion, with acrid eructations.

HEART: Weak feelling; irregular action.

EXTREMITIES: Itching in axilla, < before menses. Cutting pain or stiffness in right deltoid, < raising or turning arm. Rheumatism of right shoulder and left hip joint. Pain in shoulder, < night. Pain in bone near surface. Neuritis, > by touching the part. Burning of palms and soles, < covers; at climaxis. Palms wrinkled. Aching and swelling of ball of thumb (r). Pain in arm, > swinging arm to and fro.

SKIN: Dry, of jaundice. Acne, with scanty menses. Prickling heat spreading over body.

FEVER: *Flushes of heat rising into face and head;* with headache. Sweat, burning, scanty.

COMPLEMENTARY: Ant-t; Phos.

RELATED: Bell; Phos.

SANICULA (Aqua)

GENERALITIES: This mineral spring water affects the *nutrition, female organs, rectum, neck and skin.* Patients are thin and look old, esp. children. *Marasmus.* Body smells like old cheese. Child kicks off covers at night; wants to lie on something hard though thin. Clothes feell cold, damp. Enlarged feeling; in throat, vagina, etc. Thick acrid yellow pus. Cannot bear to have one part touch another; or cannot lie near another person. Bursting; in perineum, bowels, bladder, vertex, chest. Car or sea sickness. Shifting pains.

WORSE: Strain. *Motion;* raising arm; putting hands behind. Descending. Cold wind on occiput or neck. Jarring.

BETTER: Open air. Warmth. Vomiting.

MIND: Headstrong, obstinate, touchy children. Constant desire to look behind. Irritable - least word or action would upset her. Misconstrues everything. Crossness quickly alternating with playfulness in children. Dread of downward motion. Fear of the dark. Does not want to be touched. Restless; desire to go from place to place. Instability of purpose.

HEAD: Cannot bear cold air on occiput and neck. Profuse sweat on occiput and neck, < during sleep. Electric crackling in hair when combed. Profuse scaly dandruff; falling of hair. Bursting in vertex. Sensation as if cold cloth around brain. Small boils on head that do not mature.

EYES: Lids stick to the balls. Lacrimation in cold open air or after cold application. Dandruff of the eyebrows.

NOSE: Fluent coryza, < eating. Water smells like old musty rain water.

MOUTH: Tongue; large, flabby, burning, must protrude to keep it cool; ringworm on tongue. Mouth and palate covered with ulcers; white aphthae. Sides of tongue turn up. Tongue adheres to the roof.

THROAT: Cold, icy sensation, peppermint–like; feels too large. Can swallow solids better than fluids.

STOMACH: Child wants to nurse all the time yet loses flesh. Craves salt, bacon or ice-cold milk. Thirst little and often; water is vomited as soon as it reaches the stomach. Vomiting of curdy milk. Falls asleep after vomiting. Eating causes urging for stool, must leave the table.

ABDOMEN: Loud gurgling in pot-bellied children. *Stool of one large heavy mass;* foul like rotten cheese; dry, small balls, must be removed, or stool crumbles at the verge of anus. Bursting pain in perineum during stool. Stools misshapen, changeable, involuntary.

URINARY: Child cries before urinating, strains to urinate while at stool. Briny urine. Bursting in bladder with urgent call to pass urine. Frequent, profuse, sudden urination; urging ceases if desire is resisted. Urine stains diaper red.

MALE: Briny odor of the genitals few hours after coition.

FEMALE: Leukorrhea with strong odor of fish-brine, < stools. Bearing down as if contents of pelvis would escape, < jar, walking. Supports the relaxed parts by placing the hand against vulva, > rest. Vagina feels large. Os cervix feels open and dilated.

NECK & BACK: Neck weak and emaciated, child cannot hold its head. *Stiff backache,* < least turning, raising arms or *putting hands behind him;* must turn whole body to look around, sits head forward to ease the pain. Cold lumbar spine. Lumbago, > lying on right side. Lumbar vertebrae feel dislocated or as if were gliding past each other. Back feels broken in two pieces. Sensation of damp cloth on sacrum.

EXTREMITIES: Pain in shoulder, < raising arms or putting them behind back. Cold clammy hands and feet. Burning of palms and soles. Cramps in feet. Foul foot-sweat chafes toes, destroys shoes or stiffens the hose. Feet feel as if in cold water. Hands become sweaty when putting them together.

SKIN: Dry, brownish, flabby, < neck. Fissured hands and fingers. Skin about neck wrinkled and hangs in folds. Tendency to small boils which do not mature.

SLEEP: On awakening child rubs eyes and nose with its fist. Dreams of robbers.

FEVER: Sweat sticky.

RELATED: Lyc; Psor; Sulph.

SANTONINUM

GENERALITIES: This favorite anthelmintic produces color–blindness and yellow vision.

SARSAPARILLA

GENERALITIES: This remedy was used as restorative and blood-purifier after exhausting course of mercury. It meets syphilitic, sycotic and psoric constitutions. Its chief center of action is on the *genito-urinary organs;* skin, bones, right lower extremity. It suits *thin, frail, shrivelled,* old-looking persons, esp. children with large abdomen. Marasmus, emaciation. Parts feel screwed together. Nightly bone pains. Pains-shoot in different directions and are accompanied by depression and anxiety. Pain as if salt were put upon the wound. Lithic diathesis. Itching eruptions following hot weather and vaccination. *Very sore gouty nodes.* Rheumatism. Clears the complexion.

WORSE: *At the close of urination.* Spring. Cold, wet. Mercury. Night. Suppressed gonorrhea. Yawning. Motion. Going up and down the stairs.

BETTER: Uncovering neck and chest. Standing.

MIND: Depression and anxiety from pain. Easily offended. Taciturn. Despondent, gloomy, without any cause.

HEAD: Pains from occiput to eyes, or to root of nose. Sensation of a ball striking in head when talking; of a painful tight band around the head; removes the hat involuntarily without >.

EYES: Foggy vision, < seminal emission. Itch–like eruptions on eyelids.

EARS: Words reverberate.

NOSE: Stoppage for years. Swelling at the root of nose.

FACE: Eruptions on face and upper lips, < during menses. Yellow, wrinkled, old-looking.

MOUTH: Aphthae; salivation. Offensive breath. Pain in jaw, < bending head back.

STOMACH: After a meal sensation of emptiness as while fasting or else nausea or disgust when thinking of what has been eaten. Drinking water causes vomiting.

ABDOMEN: Colic and backache at the same time, with diarrhea. Rumbling with sensation of emptiness. Sand in stool. Moist eruptions and soreness in groins before menses. Cholera infantum. Obstinate constipation with frequent want to urinate.

URINARY: *Painful urination, extorts screams,* < at the close of urination. Can pass urine only when standing during the day, but at night urine flows freely in bed. It dribbles while sitting. Urging to urinate before menses. Passes drops of blood or white acrid material at the close of urination. Sand on diaper. Air passes from bladder during urination. *Crusty urinary sediment.* Pain in urethra going back to abdomen. Jerking along the urethra. Renal colic (R). Pus in urine.

MALE: Genitals moist and offensive. Semen bloody. Spermatic cord painful after emission, swollen after unrequited sexual excitement. Herpes preputialis. Jerking along urethra. Itching on scrotum and perineum.

FEMALE: Nipples retracted or cracked, small and shrivelled. Menses late and scanty. Dysmenorrhea, characterized by retracted nipples, or sore breast.

NECK & BACK: Emaciation of neck. Pain from small of back down the spermatic cord after emission. Backache with colic.

EXTREMITIES: Cutting under nails. *Deep cracks* on fingers and toes, < sides. Ulcerated fingertips. Affection of any kind in right lower extremity.

SKIN: Emaciated, shrivelled, lies in folds; *blotchy*, hard. Itching scaly spots. Irritating pus. Copper-colored eruptions. Ecchymoses in old age. Edema. New skin cracks and burns.

SLEEP: Yawning; complaints concomitant to yawning.

FEVER: Chill starts from region of bladder, moves to back.

COMPLEMENTARY: Merc; Sep.

RELATED: Calc; Petr.

SCILLA MARITIMA (Squilla)

GENERALITIES: Red sea-onion affects the *serous* and *mucous membranes* of respiratory and digestive tracts and acts also on *kidneys, heart*, and spleen. It is slow-acting medicine and is useful for those conditions which require several days to reach their maximum. Exudations and profuse secretions. Dropsy with *profuse urine.* Gurgling. Cardio-urinary effects. Action is just like Digitalis; follows Digitalis when it fails to relieve dropsical conditions.

WORSE: *Early morning*. Motion. Uncovering. Inspiration. Old people. Coughing.

BETTER: Rest. Sitting up. Expectoration of even a small quantity.

MIND: Angry about trifles. Aversion to mental and bodily labor.

EYES: Left eye looks much smaller than right. Child rubs eyes and face much, as if to relieve itching, in brain affections, measles. Feels as if swimming in cold water. Tears with cough. Staring look, eyes wide open.

NOSE: Violent sneezing, with fluent acrid coryza. Sneezing during cough. Copious running, < in morning.

FACE: Child rubs the face with fist during cough. Lips; twitch, covered with yellow crusts, black, cracked.

MOUTH: Black spots on teeth. *Taste sweet;* of food, esp. soup and meat; bitter to bread. Thirst for cold drink. Drinks in sips during dyspnea.

STOMACH: Pressure as from a stone. Pains > lying on left side.

ABDOMEN: Rumbling and gurgling in paroxysms above pubic region, > eating. Aching in hypochondria. Painful diseases of the spleen. Stools; dark, brown, frothy, very offensive. Ascites with scanty urine.

URINARY: Frequent or sudden urging to urinate, passes much urine. Involuntary urination when coughing. Bloody urine. Feces escape when urinating.

MALE: Erotic pollutions.

RESPIRATORY: COUGH stubborn, dry, *rattling;* disturbs sleep; *cough with sneezing, coryza, lacrimation, spurting of urine* or stools, or heat; ends in gagging, < cold drinks; inspiration. Child rubs face and eyes during cough. Cough < morning and evening. Cough dry, always followed by the need to clear the nose. Expectoration; easy, heavy, difficult, in small round balls, of sweetish taste, white or reddish, offensive. Dyspnea with stictching pain in chest and cramps in abdominal muscles. In asthma drinks in sips; *stitches* in chest (left). Cough with enlarged spleen or with pain in the region. Loose morning cough is more severe than dry evening cough. Pleurisy. Broncho-pneumonia.

HEART: Cardiac stimulant. Pulse small and slow, slightly hard.

NECK & BACK: Bubbling beneath scapula.

EXTREMITIES: Nails become brittle and split. Feet get sore from standing. Tender feet of shop girls. Hands and feet cold, body hot.

SKIN: Small red spots all over the body with pricking pain.

FEVER: Heat with aversion to uncover. Sweat absent.

COMPLIMENTARY: Ant-c.

RELATED: Ars; Bar-c; Nux-v; Rhus-t; Sil.

SCOPARIUS

GENERALITIES: It is a *heart tonic*. Affects the *kidneys*; cord, muscles and left side. It increases the strength of the heart, reduces blood pressure. Irregular heart action from influenza or other infectious diseases. Relieves the *congestion of kidneys* enabling them to eliminate and relieve the distress upon the heart. Heavy aching.

WORSE: Turning on left side.

BETTER: Cold air. Rapid motion. Passing flatus.

ABDOMEN: Stomach and bowels seem to be filled with stones or a firm mass. *Flatulency* with much mental depression. Colic, then bright acrid foaming stools followed by burning in anus.

URINARY: *Very profuse,* bright foaming urine, then burning in pudendum.

HEART: Anxious oppression, radiating to left shoulder and neck. Palpitation with congestion to head. Angina pectoris. Tobacco heart.

EXTREMITIES: Deadness of right arm and fingers.

SKIN: Barber's itch.

RELATED: Phos.

SECALE CORNUTUM

GENERALITIES: This vegetable nosode called ergot, contracts the *muscles* of BLOOD VESSELS and UTERUS, decomposes the BLOOD producing *hemorrhage* which is thin, fetid, watery, black, oozing continuously. *Twitchings;* spasms with fingers spread apart. Gnawing and *cramps* with stiffness in single parts or after pains. *Numbness.* Insufferable *tingling, crawling*, starting in face, on back, in the limbs, in fingertips, > rubbing. *Sensation of burning* in the whole body or as if sparks falling on them here and there. *Discharges are dark, thin, foul and exhausting.* Tetanic spasms with full consciousness. Rapid emaciation; of paralyzed part, with much appetite and excessive thirst. Loss of power of voluntary motion. Feels as if walking on velvet. Coldness, but does not want to be covered up. Convulsive jerks and starts in the paralyzed limbs. Neuralgia caused by pressure of distended veins. Varicoses. Thrombosis. Lymphoid tumors. Sensation of deadness in any part. Gangrene–traumatic, from application of leeches or mustard, > cold. It is suited to irritable plethoric subjects or to thin, scrawny, feeble women of cachectic appearance; to very old decrepit persons. Petechiae. Small wounds bleed much. Everything feels loose and open. Contracted arterioles. Chronic, sharp, stinging neuralgic pains, which burn like fire, > application of heat. Paralysis–with distorted limbs, of lower extremities, of one side, of one arm or one leg, with tingling, numbness and prickling. Paralysis after spasms. Restlessness, extreme debility, and prostration. Collapse.

WORSE: WARMTH. Just before or during menses. Pregnancy. Loss of fluids. COVERS. Touch. Eating. Sexual excess. After abortion. Smokers.

BETTER: *Cold bathing,* uncovering, fanning. Rocking.

Forcible stretching. Lying doubled up in bed. After vomiting.

MIND: Weakness of mind after spasm, after exhausting coition. Madness, inclination to bite or drown himself. *Maniacal fear;* tears at the genitals, inserts her finger into the vagina and scratches until it bleeds, all idea of modesty lost. Laughs, claps her hand over head, seems besides herself.

HEAD: Feels light or heavy with tingling in legs. Twisting of head to and fro. Falling of hair.

EYES: Sparks before the eyes. Senile, incipient cataract, esp. in women. Sunken; surrounded by blue rings. Paralysis of upper lid; from coal gas. Tears suppressed. Double or triple vision. Blindness. Diabetic retinitis.

EARS: Hardness of hearing, after cholera.

NOSE: Bleeds persistently; blood dark; with great prostration–in old people, drunkards or young women.

FACE: Distorted or sunken, pale, pinched. Wild look. Tingling or twitching in face which spreads all over the body. Lock-jaw.

MOUTH: Tongue dry, cracked, exudes blood inky black. Tongue stiff with tingling at tip; feels paralyzed; stuttering indistinct speech.

THROAT: Painful tingling, burning. Post–diphtheritic paralysis.

STOMACH: *Thirst unquenchable.* Unnatural ravenous appetite, craves sour things and lemonade. Vomiting; of dark brown, coffee-ground fluid. Empty retchings. Burning. Nausea, easy vomiting. Hematemesis.

ABDOMEN: Excessively inflated and tight; *wants uncovered.* Empty feeling in hypogastrium, or bearing down, must 'lie doubled up in bed. Gushing, offensive, painless, watery, olive green or bloody stools, with collapse; icy coldness and intolerance of being covered. Anus feels loose, and wide open, feces pass involuntarily. Twitching of abdominal muscles. Formation of large lumps and swelling in abdomen.

URINARY: Enuresis in old people. Bloody urine, white cheesy deposit. Urine; suppressed, pale, watery. Retention, with unsuccessful urging.

FEMALE: Menses; irregular, copious, dark. Continuous oozing of watery, fetid, blood until next period. Inert uterus, or *bearing down* with coldness. Contracted uterus, hour-glass contraction. Brownish, offensive, continuous leukorrhoea. Threatened abortion at the third month. Dark, offensive, green lochia. Septic placenta. Metritis. Gangrene of female organs. Severe after-pains. Suppression of milk, with stinging in mammae. Never well since abortion. Vagina hot or cool. Puerperal fever. Prolapse of uterus after forceps delivery.

RESPIRATORY: Pains through chest on pressing spine. Burning in lungs.

HEART: Palpitation of heart after sexual excess in males. Pulse intermittent.

NECK & BACK: Tingling in back extending to fingers and toes. Pressure on affected portion causes pain there as well as through the chest. Myelitis.

EXTREMITIES: Limbs cold. Bluish fingers and toes. *Cramps* in hands; legs and feet. *Fingers spread apart,* bent backwards or clenched, look water-soaked. Fingers of smokers feel fuzzy. Cramps in calves. Trembling, staggering or shuffling gait, as if feet were dragged along. Toes drawn up. Locomotor ataxia. Paraplegia. Hands and feet of smokers cold and dry.

SKIN: Boils with green pus, matures slowly. Bloody blisters. Skin *cold, dry*, wrinkled or bluish, < over affected part. Raynaud's disease. Edema neonatorum. Ulcers foul, indolent; varicose. Twitchings or quivering in skin. Formication under the skin.

SLEEP: Insomnia of drug and liquor habituals. Deep, lethargic.

FEVER: Internal Burning With Icy Coldness Externally, Yet Averse to Being Covered, < *abdomen*. Heat as of sparks. Erysipelas. Cold or foul sweat destroys shoes.

COMPLIMENTARY: Ars; Thuj.

RELATED: Chin; Merc; Nux-m; Puls; Ust.

SELENIUM

GENERALITIES: This element is found associated with Sulphur and Tellurium, and is a constant constituent of bones and teeth. It has marked effects on the *nerves* of Genito-Urinary Organs and supraorbital nerves (left); Larynx and liver are also affected. Patient becomes *easily debilitated* by heat or hot weather, a little mental or physical exertion makes him sleepy. Debility after exhausting diseases, after fever. Senility, early. *Emaciation* of single parts–face, hands, thighs, etc. Pulsation in the whole body, esp. in abdomen, < eating. Cramps, then stiffness. Biting, here and there. Ill effects of debauchery, tea, sugar, salt, lemonade, loss of vital fluids, masturbation, sexual excess, over-study. Troubles in general accompanying escape of semen, esp. when straining at stool.

WORSE: *Hot days.* Loss of sleep; night watching. Touch. *After sleep. Singing. Draft of air*, even if warm. After stools. Coition. Wine.

BETTER: After sunset. Inhaling cool air. Drinking cold water.

MIND: Total unfitness for any kind of work. Forgetful in business; remembers all that he has forgotten during sleep. Talkativeness. When excited, stammers, pronounces some words incorrectly. Sadness. Difficult comprehension. Forgetful when awakes, and dreams of it as he falls half asleep. Lascivious thoughts, with impotency. Imagines drafts of air. Fails to understand what he hears or reads. Aversion to draft of air, warm cold or damp. Dread of society.

HEAD: Pain over left eye, < walking in the sun, strong odor like musk, rose, and tea, with increased secretion of urine. Nervous headache. Scalp feels gathered together. Falling of hair from eyebrows, whiskers and genitals. Does not want hair touched. Pain in the scalp as if hair were pulled out.

EARS: Deafness from hardened wax.

NOSE: Coryza ending in diarrhea. Inclination to bore fingers in the nose. Obstruction of nose, chronic. Full of thick glairy mucus.

FACE: Emaciated. Comedones. Greasy, shining.

MOUTH: Toothache, from drinking tea, with feeling of coldness, > taking cold water or air in mouth.

STOMACH: Thirstless. Craves stimulants, brandy, tea, etc. Aversion to saltish food. Pulsation all over the body, esp. in abdomen after eating which hinders sleep. Sweetish taste. Irresistible desire to get drunk.

ABDOMEN: Chronic liver affections. Liver enlarged, with stitching pain, < inspiration. Fine rash over liver region. Stools; very large, impacted, so hard that require mechanical aid. Filament–like hair in feces.

URINARY: Urine; involuntary. Dribbling when walking, after urination, and after stool. Coarse sand in urine. Feels biting drop forcing its way out.

MALE: *Lascivious* but impotent. Increases desire, decreases ability. Semen dribbles during sleep. *Easy loss of semen*–during coition with feeble erection but long–continued voluptuous thrill; during stool. Semen watery, odorless. Chronic gleet. Oozing of prostatic fluid during sleep, while sitting, walking and at stool. Hydrocele.

FEMALE: Copious menses of dark color. Throbbing in abdomen during pregnancy, < eating.

RESPIRATORY: *Voice hoarse* as soon as he begins to sing, talk or read; affected by every cold. Voice rattles. Nodes on vocal cord. Hawks up clear mucus in the morning. Frequent necessity to clear the throat in singers. Takes deep breath. Tubercular laryngitis. Dry hacking cough, < in the morning. Expectoration of lumps of bloody mucus. Weak feeling in the chest.

NECK & BACK: The back becomes almost paralytic after a temporary illness. Glands of neck large and hard. Paralytic pain in small of back, > lying on abdomen.

EXTREMITIES: Emaciation of hands, legs. Sudden sciatic pain (left) leaves soreness behind.

SKIN: Itching about ankles and fold of skin. Oily. Moist after scratching. Burning spots. Crusty eruptions on palms. Psoriasis of palms. Acne.

SLEEP: Awakes early and at the same hour.

FEVER: *Sweat* profuse, yellow, *leaves a salty deposit which* stiffens the linen or makes the hair stiff and wiry, < in genitals.

RELATED: Calc-c; Merc; Nat-m; Nux-v; Sep; Sulph.

SENECIO

GENERALITIES: In eclectic practice it is considered as a regulator of menstrual function. Therefore, it has a marked action on FEMALE and URINARY ORGANS, esp. bladder. Affection of *mucous glands* causes catarrhal condition of mucous membranes, esp. of vagina, bladder and respiratory tract. Lack of reaction in genito-urinary tract. *Debilitating* or vicarious discharges. Tightness in nose, throat, etc. Muscles draw into a knot. Globus. Ill effects of suppresed or delayed menses, wounds. *Nervous, pale, weak and sleepless hysterical women. Hemorrhagic* tendency, esp. with suppressed or delayed menses. Dropsy after hemorrhage.

WORSE: Puberty. Sexual excitement. Dampness. Cold open air. Sitting, must move about (mind).

BETTER: Menstruation.

MIND: Very irritable, whining. Inability to fix mind upon any one subject. Self–centered. Elated and sad alternately.

HEAD: Wave-like sensation of dizziness from occiput to sinciput. Sharp pain over left eye and through left temple. Headache precedes leukorrhea and irritation in bladder.

EYES: Tears cause itching.

EARS: Itching in eustachian tube.

NOSE: Burning in nostrils. Sneezing, with burning in nose. Tightness in nasal passage. Epistaxis or nasal catarrh takes the place of menses when suppressed from any cause. Coryza with nosebleed.

FACE: Twitching about mouth.

THROAT: Feels dry and tight, wants to swallow; though painful.

STOMACH: Aversion to all food, esp. sweets and coffee which she was very fond of. Nausea and vomiting of renal origin. Sensation of a ball rising from stomach to throat.

ABDOMEN: Pain about umbilical region, spreading in all directions > stools, bending double. Ascites from suppressed menses. Stools thin, watery, mingled with hard lumps of feces or thin, dark, bloody with tenesmus.

URINARY: Heat in neck of bladder and constant urging with renal pain. Urine bloody, very hot, or with much mucous sediment. Renal colic (right). Nephritis. *Dysuria* in women with dysmenorrhoea or uterine displacement, and in children with headache.

MALE: Lascivious dreams, with involuntary emissions. Prostate gland enlarged, feels hard and swollen to touch.

FEMALE: *Functional amenorrhea* of young girls with backache. Menses retarded, suppressed, with concomitant symptoms; dropsy, cough, backache, etc. Profuse flow of mucus from vagina from sexual excitation. Sexual irritation causing itching, burning and swelling of labia. Pain from ovaries to breasts. Leukorrhea thick, yellow, profuse, *flows down thighs.* Feels as if menses would come. Burning in left nipple. Menorrhagia, copious flow continues until she becomes anemic. Dysmenorrhea after abortion.

RESPIRATORY: Tickling cough with blood-streaked sputum, with suppressed menses. Hemoptysis with suppressed menses. Loose cough with copious mucous expectoration and labored breathing.

BACK: *Lumbar backache, as if about to break, with amenorrhoea.* Renal disease.

EXTREMITIES: Wandering rheumatic pains, periodical. Feet cold in bed. Brittle nails.

SKIN: Dry.

SLEEP: Many dreams; erotic. Sleepless women with uterine troubles and amenorrhea. Drowsy during day.

FEVER: Hectic fever, with anorexia.

RELATED: Puls; Sep.

SENEGA

GENERALITIES: Known as snake-root, it affects the MUCOUS MEMBRANES causing catarrhal symptoms esp. of the respiratory tract and bladder. *Eyes,* serous membranes of CHEST, muscles, and the left side are also affected. It is suited to plethoric persons or persons tending to obesity; tall, slender, sprightly women; old persons; *fat, chubby children.* Paretic states esp., of occular muscles and distinct eye symptoms. Circumscribed spots left in chest after inflammation. Weakness seems to originate in the chest. Faintness when walking in open air. Burning in *air passages.* Laxity of tissues. Profuse albuminous secretions. Ill effects of poisonous bites. Sprains. Sensation of trembling, without visible trembling.

WORSE: *Open air,* wind, inhaling cold air. *Touch.* Pressure. *Rest.* Looking fixedly. Walking in open air (dyspnea, cough). Rubbing.

BETTER: Bending head backwards (vision). Sweat. Walking in open air (pains).

MIND: Anxiety with hasty respiration. Readily takes offense.

HEAD: Bursting pain in forehead going into eyes, > cool open air.

EYES: Balls feel distended or like balls of ice. Eyes tremble and water when looking fixedly or reading. Objects look shaded. Lacrimation, ptosis and diplopia, > bending head backwards. Blepharitis, lids dry and crusty. Oculomotor paralysis. Absorbs fragments of lens after operations. Flickering, must wipe eyes frequently. Opacity of vitreous humor. Iritis. Specks upon cornea. Stitches in eye (right), < coughing.

EARS: Aching in the ear when chewing.

NOSE: Sneezes so often and so violently that the head grows dizzy and heavy. Nostrils feel peppery.

FACE: Paralysis of the left side. Pimples in the corners of lips with burning.

MOUTH: Dry *scraping in mouth*, < talking. Taste metallic, like urine.

THROAT: Dry scraping, < talking. Hawks viscid mucus in detached small clots.

STOMACH: Loathing and nausea with inclination to vomit.

URINARY: Urine foamy, acrid; increased or decreased in amount; with mucous shreds. Scalding before and after urination.

RESPIRATORY: *Dry scraping in chest,* < talking. Hoarse, unsteady voice, < talking and sexual losses, suddenly when reading aloud. Cough incessant, strangling, violent, shaking, choking, ends in sneezing, < lying on right side or evening. *Loose rattle in chest* but the clear, *profuse sputum is tough and slips back.* Albuminous or blood-streaked sputum. *Chest sore* from coughing, pressure, sneezing or moving arms, in spots; as if bruised; shifting pain on stooping. Crushing weight, or weakness starts in chest; chest feels too narrow. Exudation in pleura. Hydrothorax. Burning in chest before or after coughing. Asthmatic bronchitis of old people, with chronic nephritis or emphysema. Vocal cords partially paralyzed. Pleuro-pneumonia.

RELATED: Calc-c; Caust; Hep; Lyc; Phos; Sulph.

SEPIA

GENERALITIES: Inky juice of cuttle fish, known as Indian ink, is supposed to be pre-eminently a woman's remedy, though the first symptoms were found by Dr. Hahnemann accidentally in a male artist. It affects the *venous circulation* esp. of the FEMALE PELVIC ORGANS, of *portal system* and of digestive tract. Venous stasis and thereby ptosis of viscera is a marked feature. It is suited to young persons of both sexes, of nervous and delicate constitution, who are disposed to sexual excitement or worn out by sexual excess. Children who take cold easily when the weather changes. Relaxed, plethoric females. Weak, pot-bellied mothers with yellow complexion. Affections in pregnant women. Females dragged down by overwork, loss of vital fluids, excess of sexual indulgence, who are subject to *prolapse, uterine troubles. Symptoms settle* in back, in ileo-cecal region, ovaries, etc. and upward to head. Bearing down in pelvic region. Shuddering from pain. *Sudden prostration. Weak, empty,* hollow feeling in epigaastrium, chest muscles, lumbar back, hips, knees, etc. or sensation of fulness. *Sensation of a lump* or *something rolling over internally*. Violent ebullition of blood with pulsation throughout the body. Fits of uneasiness and hysterical spasm. Spasms–clonic, tonic, cataleptic. Short walk fatigues much. Jerking in muscles. Burning pains in different parts of the body. Bleeding. Milky secretions. Fainting fits. Fidgety. Tendency to abortion from 5-7th month. Tubercular patients with chronic hepatic troubles and uterine reflexes. Feels cold even in a warm room. Ill effects of anger and vexation, blows, injury, overlifting, falls, jar, getting wet, laundry work, boiled milk, fat, pork, tobacco. Faints while kneeling in the church. Diseased conditions which drag on, linger. Warty growths. Atrophy of children, face like old man, big belly, dry flabby skin. Rheumatism–chronic cases or obstinate remains of acute.

WORSE: Cold Air, north wind, snowy air, snowfall, wet. *Sexual excess*. Before menses. *Pregnancy*. Abortion. Morning and evening. After first sleep. Falling to sleep. Sitting, standing. Kneeling. Jarring. Stooping. Coitus. Before thunderstorm. Touch. Ascending. Rubbing. Lifting. Scratching. Washing clothes.

BETTER: Violent Motion. *Warmth* of bed. Pressure. Hot application. Crossing or drawing limbs up. After sleep. Cold drinks, cold bath; open air.

MIND: Angry, sensitive, irritable, easily offended, and miserable. Wants to commit suicide. Nervous, so she wants to hold on to something or to scream. She says and does strange things. Nobody knows what she will do next. Anxious fear *over trifles*. Aversion to family, to those loved best, to sympathy, to *company*, yet dreads to be alone. Repugnance to customary business; digust of life. Stiffled affections. *Poor memory*. Makes mistakes while writing or reading. *Sad*. Irritability, *alternating with indifference* or sulkiness. Sad over her health and domestic affairs. Constantly worries, frets and cries about her real or imaginary illness. Sexually–minded. Weeps when telling her symptoms. Miserly. *Stupid*, wants to go away. *Indifference*. Takes pleasure in teasing others. Feels unfortunate without cause. Sits quietly and answers only in yes or no. Women hate men and men hate women. Breaks down in spells of weeping.

HEAD: Fits of vertigo, < walking in open air, least movement of arms; or a sensation as if something rolling round the head. *Headache*–shooting, stinging pain; within out or upwards; over left eye; heavy on vertex, alternating side of occiput, < lying on painful side, indoors; with nausea and vomiting. Headache in terrible shocks at menstrual time with scanty flow, with desire for coition. Jerking of head backward and forward, involuntary, with open fontanelles in children; hysterical or from pain. Hair fall out after chronic headache; at climaxis. Root of hair sensitive to combing. Pimples on forehead along the margins of hair. Vertex cold, and heavy. Hemicrania. Jaundice, with headache. Screams with pain. Headache, < shopping, mental labor, > meals.

EYES: *Drooping eyelids.* Sees black spots, veil, points, sparks, flashes, zigzags and streaks of light before eyes, then collapse. Tarsi red, itching; cancer. Vanishing of sight during menses, > lying. Tarsal tumor. Vision dimmed from sexual excess, masturbation and uterine disease. Cannot tolerate reflected light. Arrests cataract in women. Falling out feeling in eyes. Epithelioma of eyelids. Eyes red with styes.

EARS: Herpes behind ears, on lobe of ears, nape of neck. Oversensitive to noise, esp. music. Sudden deafness, as if caused by plug in ears. Discharge thick yellow pus, offensive. Swelling of and eruptions on external ear.

NOSE: Great sensitiveness to *odors,* which are repulsive; to the smell of cooking food. Pressing pain at root. BROWN, YELLOWISH, STRIPE ACROSS. Thick greenish discharge; thick foul plugs and crusts. Post-nasal dropping of heavy, lumpy discharge; must be hawked from mouth. Epistaxis; when the nose has been struck by anything even lightly; during menses, during pregnancy, with piles. Ozena. Ascending throat cold. Pain in occiput with drawing in arms and legs during cold.

FACE: Changing color. Dark circles under eyes. Chloasma. Acne < before menses. Malar bones numb. Swollen, cracked lower lip. Cancer of the lip, epithelioma. Old, wrinkled, with spots. Jerking of facial muscles while talking. Warts.

MOUTH: Mouth and tongue feel burnt. Taste cheesy, fishy, bitter, sour, putrid, offensive. Hawks foul or cheesy grains in the morning. Everything tastes too salty.

Painful teeth during pregnancy, menses and cold, < lying. Tongue dirty, becomes clear during menses.

THROAT: Sensation of a plug. Pain as if raw. Ascending throat colds. Pressure in the throat, feels neck cloth tight. Hawks foul mucus or balls in the morning.

STOMACH: *Nausea* at thought or *smell of food;* in A.M.; at the thought of coition. *Vomiting* of solid food only or of milky fluids during pregnancy, in the morning, when rinsing mouth. Longing for vinegar, acids and pickles, sweets. FAINT SINKING FEELING AT EPIGASTRIUM: *not* > eating; or a lump in. Burning in pit of stomach. Boiled milk disagrees. Acidity. Dyspepsia from over-lifting; from tobacco. Voracious appetite, or no appetite; sudden craving, sudden satiety. Sense of something twisting about the stomach and rising into the throat. Distress or pain in stomach, < vomiting. Eructations milky, sour, bitter, rancid; eructates tough, foamy mucus.

ABDOMEN: Pain in the region of liver or gall–bladder, < stooping. Liver sore and painful, > lying on right side. Falling out or heavy *bearing down feeling in hypogastrium* > by holding it or crossing legs. Pot-belly of mothers. Constipation obstinate, no urging for days. Large hard stools; *feeling of a ball in* rectum. Rectum constricted and powerless, almost constant oozing from anus. *Diarrhea*–greenish, infantile, from boiled milk, with rapid exhaustion. Piles prolapsing, < walking, bleed while walking, with sticking pain; piles of pregnancy. Stools followed by gelatinous mucus. Pains shoot up in rectum. Brown spots on abdomen. Stools are passed after prolonged straining, followed by cupful of jelly-like yellow-white, very offensive mucus. Prolapse of rectum after smoking. Sense of weight or ball in anus, not > by stool.

URINATION: Involuntary urination during first sleep, < coughing, sneezing, laughing, hearing sudden noise, fright, or inattention esp. in women, etc. Slow urination with bearing down sensation above pubis. URINE THICK, FOUL; white gritty or ADHERENT RED SANDY SEDIMENT. Urine feeble, slow. Cutting pain in bladder before urination. Urine bloody, milky. Shuddering when urging for urine is not attended to.

MALE: Sexual desire increased. Complaints after coition. Offensive perspiration on scrotum. Genitals cold. Condylomata surrounding head of penis. Impotency.

FEMALE: WEAK, DRAGGING or BEARING DOWN SENSATION, as if everything would escape from vulva, must cross limbs or hold parts to prevent protrusion. Griping, burning or sticking in uterus. Coition painful from dryness of vagina, bleeding after. Dryness of vagina and vulva after menses causing disagreeable sensation when walking. Aversion to coition, or complaints after. Menses absent; at puberty; after weaning. Labia swollen, abscessed. Leukorrhea; yellow, greenish, milky, in large lumps; in little girls; instead of menses; foul; gonorrheal; with stitches from uterus to navel; during day. Nipples cracked across the crown. Retained placenta after abortion. Sub-involution. Exhaustion after coition. Nausea and irritability on thought of coition. Amenorrhea. Metritis with pain in lumbar region and frequent urination. Motion of fetus is intolerable. Metrorhagia at the time of climaxis. Sudden flushes of heat, with weakness and sweat during climaxis. Tendency to abortion from 5th to 7th month. Severe itching in vulva causing abortion. Sterility. Mania from profuse menses.

RESPIRATORY: Dry, fatiguing cough, as if coming from stomach, < rapid change of temperature; cough with foul sputum. Whooping cough that drags on. Dyspnea, < after sleep, > rapid motion. Sensation of emptiness in chest. Hypostatic pleuritis. Brown spots on chest. Rotten–egg taste with coughing. Asthma. Chest symptoms > by pressure of hand. Neglected pneumonia.

HEART: *Circulation irregular*; seems to stagnate. Palpitation visible, ascends to occiput. An occasional hard thump of the heart. General pulsation. Ebullition at night. Overfull blood vessels. Wakes up with violent beating of heart. Tremulous feeling with flushes. Nervous palpitation, > walking fast, lying on left side.

NECK & BACK: Collar feels tight. *Aching* in inter-scapular or LUMBAR REGION, paralytic, wants to be pressed. Sudden pain in back, as if struck by a hammer, < stooping, kneeling. Pain in back, > eructations, by pressing back against something hard. Weakness in small of back when walking, from uterine disease. Everything affects the back. Icy coldness between the scapulae. Cramp in buttocks when stretching out legs.

EXTREMITIES: Hands purple. Cold hands in warm room. Tension in limbs as if they were too short. Limbs restless, twitching and jerking day and night. Knees and heels cold. Sciatica > during pregnancy; chronic, localizing in heels. Sensation of running, as from a mouse in lower limbs. Hot hands with cold feet or vice versa. A short walk fatigues much. Crippled nails. Hands sweaty. Skin in palms peels off.

SKIN: *Blotched*, raw, rough, hard or cracked, < flexures. Boil in axilla. Thick crusts on elbows. Ulcers on small joints. Epithelioma; on eyelids, lips. Wine-colored skin. Spots on skin. Ringworm, < every spring. Itching vesicles. Urticaria, < open air, > warm room. Thick crusts form upon the joints. Induration from constant pressure with purple color.

SLEEP: Talks loudly during sleep. Dreams, < if he lies on left side. Wakes frequently, or as if he has been called.

FEVER: Easily chilled. Chilly with air hunger. *Cold in spots, on vertex, between scapulae, feet. Cold in bed.* Anxious hot flushes preceded by sudden weakness. *Sweat easy,* offensive with orgasms; sweat on genitals, in *axillae,* or back between menses. Irregular fevers. Heat ascending or sensation as if hot water were poured over him.

COMPLEMENTARY: Nat-m; Nux-v; Phos; Psor; Puls; Sabad; Sulph.

RELATED: Calc-c; Caust; Con; Gels; Lil-t; Lyc; Murx; Nat-c; Nat-m; Puls.

SILICEA

GENERALITIES: Triturations are prepared from pure flint. It produces defective NUTRITION, esp. *in children,* due to imperfect assimilation. Affects the NERVES *increasing their susceptibility* causing neurasthenic states and exaggerated reflexes. Diseases of *bones* and cartilages–caries and necrosis, softening of bones. Exostosis. GLANDS are enlarged. Scrofulous rachitic children with large head, open fontanelles, *distended hot and hard abdomen,* who are slow in learing to walk *and wasted* in body, esp. *legs.* Children crawl nervously or are dragged in on their mother's arms; on running they become pale. *Stubborn suppurative processes;* fistulous openings; abscesses. *Slow, incomplete inflammation* of glands, cellular tissue and *skin, then induration. Keenly sensitive to noise, pain, cold*–hugs the fire, wants plenty of warm clothing, hates drafts. Cachectic and senile patients; persons of fair, clear complexion. *Pains are violent and sticking,* localized in ears, throat, in ulcers, etc. Tendency to easy exhaustion, and abnormal sweat. Want of vital warmth even when taking exercise. Spasms, epilepsy, feeling of coldness before the attack. Hysteria, paralysis and obstinate neuralgia caused by dissipation, hard work, with close confinement. Mal-nutrition. Arrested development. Emaciation. Want of grit, moral and physical. Proud–flesh. Cicatrices indurated, hard, nodular, shiny, glassy, tender, with shooting pain. Keloid. Dropsy in A.M. Cancer. Contracted sphincters. *Ascending effects*. Prostration of mind and body. Cerebral softening. Restless, fidgety, starts at least noise. Parts lain on go to sleep. Removes foreign bodies. Progressive locomotor ataxia. Sensation as if she were divided into halves and left side does not belong to her. Sensation of a hair on tongue; in trachea. Ill effects of vaccination, stone–cutting, loss of vital fluids, injury sprain, splinters. Intolerance of alcoholic stimulants. Nervous affections after spinal injury, esp. when pressure on spine causes pain in remote parts. Convulsion begins in the solar plexus; convulsions after vaccination. Epilepsy, aura in the solar plexus creeping into the chest and stomach. Skin is unhealthy; *every injury festers*. Discharges offensive–pus, sweat, stools, etc.

WORSE: COLD AIR, DRAFT, *damp*. Uncovering, bathing. Checked sweat, esp. *of feet*. Nervous excitement. Light. Noise. Jarring of spine. Moon changes. Night. Mental exertion. Alcohol. Touch. *Pressure*. Change of weather. Combing hair,

BETTER: WARM WRAPS to head. Summer. Wet humid weather. Profuse urination. Magnetism and electricity.

MIND: Yielding, faint–hearted. Sensitive, weeping mood. Obstinate. Stubborn, head-strong children. Cries when kindly spoken to. Fixed ideas; thinks only of pins, fears them, searches and counts them. Mental acuteness, with physical weakness and torpidity. Sullen. Compunctions of conscience about trifles. Loss of self–confidence; dreads failure, but unfounded. Starts from slight noise. Screaming violently, groaning, in epilepsy. Indifference to religion. Hopeless. Sad. Disgust for life, wishes to drown herself. Brain–fag. Cannot express himself correctly. Fidgety. Complaints from anticipation.

HEAD: Vertigo, ascends from dorsal region, < looking upward, closing eyes, lying on left side. Ascending occipital pain, > pressure. Periodical headache. Headache, then blindness. Vertex throbs. Fontanelles open, with distended abdomen. Lumps on scalp. Profuse urination > headache. Right side feels paralyzed, < coition. Headache < by exertion, study, noise, motion, jar, light, cold air, talking and straining at stool, and > by wrapping warmly and pressure. Moist crusty eruptions on the scalp. Swelling filled with grumous fluid between scalp and bone. Headache while fasting or when not eating at proper time. Migraine. Chronic headache since some severe disease. Falling of hair, premature baldness.

EYES: Affection of canthi in the region of tearducts; swelling of lacrimal fistula; stricture of lacrimal duct. Spotted vision. Objects appear pale. Aversion to daylight, it dazzles. Keratitis–pustular, perforating. Inflammation of eyes. Hypopion. Opacity of the cornea after small pox (use 30 for months). Cataract in office workers after suppressed foot sweat. Styes; to prevent their recurrence. Encysted tumors of lids. Letters run together while reading.

EARS: Roaring in ears. Hissing. Perforated drum. Itching. Caries of mastoid process. Deafness, hears again with a loud report or on blowing the nose, and coughing, < full moon. Fetid discharge. Sensitive to noise. Feeling of stoppage in the ear, > when yawning or swallowing. Crusty formations in ears. Child bores into its ears when asleep.

NOSE: Frothy nasal discharge. Coryza, with epistaxis. Perforation of septum. Dry hard crusts, bleeding when loosened. Sneezing in morning. Itching of the tip. Bone sore. Nose dry, obstructed, with loss of smell. Epistaxis in infants. Cracks in nostrils. Obstinate colds with ear affections. Nose cold.

FACE: Pale, cachectic, waxy. Enlarged parotids. Cracks in lips, on skin of face. Eruptions on chin. Swelling of maxillary glands. Indurated fissures at the corners of lips. Cancer of lower lip.

MOUTH: Feels a hair on tongue. Abscess at the root of the teeth. Boils on gums. Pyorrhea. Water tastes bad, vomits after drinking. Teeth break down, lose their enamel, become rough, carious. Tongue brown. Teeth feel too large and too long for the mouth. One–sided swelling of tongue.

THROAT: Bitter. Tonsils swollen, suppurating. Food is ejected through nose when swallowing. Pricking pain in tonsil. Hawks foul lumps. Swallowing painful, difficult, hysterical.

STOMACH: Aversion to cooked or warm food and meat, to mother's milk–vomits it. Likes icecream, ice water, feels comfortable when it is in the stomach. Water tastes bad, vomits after drinking. Induration of pylorus. Water-brash with chilliness. Voracious appetite, disappears on attempting to eat, or loathing of food. Sour eructations after eating. Sour vomiting. Gnawing, twisting pain in epigastrium, < by pressure. Feels a if a cold stone were in stomach.

ABDOMEN: Throbbing, ulcerative pain in the region of liver; abscess of liver. Colic, cutting pain with yellow hands and blue nails. *Distended, hard and hot, with thin legs,* esp. in children. Cutting, cramping pain in rectum extending to testes, < coition. Constipation, < before and during menses. Straining with soft stools, with exhaustion. Moist anus; foul flatus. *Stools come out with difficulty, when partly expeled, recedes again;* retained for fear of pain. Cracks on abdominal wall. Fissures, fistula in ano, with chest symptoms. Painful spasm of sphincter. Intensely painful hemorrhoids protrude during stool. Foul diarrhea. Fruitless urging to stool. Chronic diarrhea. Stools offensive, painless, lienteric. Tapeworm. Diarrhea after milk. Hernial tumor, tender. Ascites with great effusion, with frequent attacks of diarrhea.

URINARY: Profuse urination, > headache. Frequent urination with tenesmus. Nocturnal enuresis in children from worms. Chronic urethritis, foul discharge from urethra which is thick, curdy, purulent, bloody. Pus in urine. Nightly incontinence after a blow upon the head. Renal and vesical calculi.

MALE: Foul gonorrheal urethral discharge. After coition sensation on right side of head as if paralyzed. Itching moist spots on scrotum. Hydrocele. Nocturnal emissions. Sexual appetite increases or decreases. Prostatorrhea, < straining at stool. Chronic urethritis with twisting pain. Elephantiasis of scrotum. Extreme exhaustion after coition, takes 8 to 10 days to come to normal condition. Painful eruptions on mons veneris.

FEMALE: Increased menses with paroxysms of icy coldness over whole body. Cutting upward in vagina < urinating. Leukorrhea milky, acrid, gushing, < during urination. Itching of vulva and vagina, which are very sensitive. Bloody discharge, < nursing; between periods. Nipple retracted like a funnel, sore. Hard lumps, fistula, in mammae. Serous cyst in vagina; fistulous opening and abscess about vulva. Threatened abscess of mammae. Scirrhus, with itching. Sharp pains in mammae and uterus. Menses early, scanty. Amenorrhea for months. Too violent motion of fetus. Fistulous abscess or openings in or around vagina with thick, curdy discharge. Salpingitis, with accumulation of pus or serum which escapes from uterus from time to time. Cutting pain around the navel with leukorrhea. Watery discharge instead of menses. Abortion from weakness or they do not conceive because of weakness. Nausea during coition. Bloody discharge between periods. Sterility. Nymphomania. Itching of pudenda.

RESPIRATORY: Cough gagging, shaking, retching, < cold drink talking, lying and after waking. Dyspnea from draft on neck; chronic colds which settle in chest and bring on asthmatic attacks; being overheated or exertion. Sycotic asthma. Profuse foul, yellow, lumpy sputum; granular; offensive when broken. Cold fails to yield. Slow recovery from pneumonia. Rattling in chest. Stitches in chest through the back. Shortness of breath from manual labor, walking fast. Stone-cutter's affections. Emphysema after pleurisy. Neglected pneumonia. Painless throbbing in sternum.

HEART: Throbbing all over the body when sitting or while in motion. Palpitation; while sitting, with trembling of hand. Heart trouble from nervous exhaustion.

NECK & BACK: Spine; weak, very sensitive to drafts on back. Spina bifida. Caries of vertebra. Psoas abscess. Painful coccyx. Backache as from riding in carriages for a long time. Burning in back, when body is heated after walking in open air. Stiff neck, with headache. Painful kyphosis. Lameness in region of sacrum.

EXTREMITIES: Axillary glands swollen, enlarged. Finger–tips painful, dry as if made of paper, at night. Icy cold and sweaty feet. FOOT–SWEAT FOUL, itching, *acrid*, destroying shoes; *suppressed*. Sore ache in arch of foot. Distorted, ingrown, yellow nails. Weak ankles and feet. Calves tense and contracted. Felon, deep–seated pain. Atrophy and numbness of fingers. Parts lain on go to sleep. Bunion. Inflammation of bones. Trembling of hands when attempting to do something. Forearm lame. Legs feel paralyzed, trembling while walking. Voluptuous tingling in soles. Bruised feeling in whole body after coition or emission. Cramps in knees. Soft corns in between toes. Nails rough, yellow, crippled, brittle, white spots, blue in fever. Ulcers around the joints with thin, foul, bloody, purulent discharge or curdy particles. Slovenly gait. Rheumatism, esp. of the soles, cannot walk. Cramps in calves and soles. Enlarged bursa over patella. Distorted during convulsion. Arms (left) shake before epilepsy.

SKIN: Soggy, wilted. Acuminate eruptions. Scars suddenly become painful. Keloid. Every little injury suppurates. Leprous nodes. Coppery spots. Carbuncles. Ulcers; painfully sensitive, foul, spongy, on feet, toes, nails, > heat. Abscess of joints. Eruptions itch during daytime or evening only. Boils and pustules everywhere. Sensation of coldness in ulcer. Warty growths. Rose–colored blotches. Elephantiasis.

SLEEP: Somnambulism. Frightful dreams wake him on falling to sleep. Restless sleep. Dreams lascivious, of past events. Awakes frightened from sleep with trembling of the whole body. Talks in sleep loudly, whines or laughs. Violent yawning. Sleepy but cannot sleep. Sleep unrefreshed.

FEVER: CHILLY, < lying in bed, exertion. *Coldness of painful part. Icy chill.* SWEAT *profuse,* on *upper part of the body, head or affected part, at night,* foul, easy, acrid, as soon as she falls asleep. Hectic fever.

COMPLEMENTARY: Fl-ac; Phos; Thuj.

RELATED: Calc; Hep; Kali-p.

SOLIDAGO VIRGA

GENERALITIES: Diseases arising from or complicated with DEFFECTIVE FUNCTION OF KIDNEYS are very likely to be benefited by this remedy. It affects the digestive tract, lower limbs and blood. Feeling of weakness; chilliness alternating with heat. Hemorrhage. Takes cold easily. Chronic nephritis. Uremic asthma.

WORSE: Pressure.

BETTER: Profuse urination.

EYES: Red with enlarged prostate gland.

NOSE: Paroxysms of sneezing, with abundant mucous discharge.

MOUTH: Continuous bitter taste. Tongue heavily coated, clears when urine becomes normal.

ABDOMEN: Profuse, involuntary mucous stools.

URINARY: *Urine; dark and scanty* or clear, *stinking,* voided with difficulty; albuminous, mucous, phosphatic. Affections of any other part or organ complicated with these symptoms will probably find their remedy in *Solidago. Kidneys sore and tender, ache,* feel distended. Pain in kidneys extends forward to abdomen, bladder, down the thighs. Chronic nephritis. Cystitis. Inflamed or enlarged prostate gland obstructing flow of urine.

FEMALE: Uterine enlargement, organ pressed down upon the bladder. Fibroid tumor.

RESPIRATORY: Bronchitis, cough with much purulent expectoration, which may be blood-streaked; oppressed breathing. Continuous, dyspnea. Asthma with nightly dysuria.

BACK: Lumbarache, makes her sick all over.

SKIN: *Petechiae on lower limbs* with edema and itching. Gangrene, diabetic. Eczema, < suppressed urine.

SPIGELIA

GENERALITIES: Known as pink root, it markedly affects the NERVES–TRIFACIAL, HEART, EYES, *teeth,* fibrous tissue and LEFT SIDE. It produces *combined heart and eye symptoms* or the latter as an accompaniment. PAINS are *violent,* burning like hot needle or wire, jerking, tearing, stitching, *radiating* to other parts. Neuralgia. Sun pain. It is adapted to anemic, debilitated, rheumatic and scrofulous subjects. Very sensitive to touch, parts touched or bruised feel chilly or touch causes tingling or *shuddering* through the body. Children afflicted with worms refer to navel as the most painful part. Body feels light while *walking, heavy* and sore when rising from a seat.

WORSE: TOUCH, MOTION. *Jar.* Periodically; with the sun. Tobacco. Coition. Raising arms. After eating. Thinking of it. Stooping. Blowing nose. Expiration.

BETTER: Lying on right side with head high. Inspiring. Steady pressure. While eating.

MIND: Afraid of pointed things–pins, needles. Restless and anxious. Sits as if lost in thought, stares at a single object. Gloomy, suicidal mood. Easily offended.

HEAD: Pain from left side of occiput to over left eye, < stooping, making a false step, opening mouth. *Vertigo, the feet feel higher than head,* < looking down, must look straight ahead, standing, walking. Supra-orbital neuralgia. Feels too large.

EYES: *Feel too large.* Severe pain in around and eyes, extending deep into socket, < thinking of them. Squint with worms. Eyes red, *sore,* drawing ache; yellow rings about. Pain as if needles were thrust in. Lacrimation profuse from affected side, acrid. Difficulty in raising the eyelids with painful sensation of stiffness. Inclination to wink. Difficult to fit glasses, no settled focus, no fixed vision; latent errors of vision. Eso-and exophoria. Pricking in lids. Everted eyelids.

EARS: Periodical deafness; ears feel as if stuffed.

NOSE: Chronic catarrh with post-nasal droppings. Tickling and itching of nose. Dry anteriorly. Flow of water during prosopalgia.

FACE: Prosopalgia involving eye, zygoma, cheek, teeth; temples, < touch, stooping, from morning until sunset, drinking tea; suddenly going and coming.

MOUTH: *Breath offensive.* Toothache, < after eating and cold, when thinking of it, > tobacco smoke. Tongue coated yellow or white; burning or stitches; cracked.

STOMACH: Aversion to tobacco-smoke and snuff. Ravenous hunger. Nausea with sensation of a worm rising in throat.

ABDOMEN: Colic, with pinching pain in the umbilical region. Stools of only large lumps of mucus. Itching, tickling in anus and rectum. Worms. Very offensive flatus. Faints at stool.

URINARY: Urine copious with frequent urging, mostly at night.

RESPIRATORY: Dyspnea, < moving in bed, raising arms, must lie on right side, with head high. Hydro-thorax. Heart disease. Stitches in chest, < least motion or when breathing. Trembling in chest.

HEART: PALPITATION *violent, audible*; attending other symptoms. *Violent sticking* or compressive pain radiating to throat, arms, scapula, < least motion or bending double. Palpitation with foul odor from mouth. Soreness, purring, cracking in the region of heart. Pericarditis. Angina pectoris with craving for hot water which >. Rheumatic carditis. Pulse; intermittent, with nervous palpitation; weak tremulous irregular. Throbbing of carotids and subclavian arteries.

NECK & BACK: Neck stiff; pain moves into right temple or pain from left shoulder to neck. Cutting about the left scapula.

EXTREMITIES: Left arm numb. Pulsation in patellae.

FEVER: Heat, flushes at night, in back. Sweat offensive, cold on upper part of the body, hands.

COMPLEMENTARY: Calc.

RELATED: Cact.

SPONGIA

GENERALITIES: Toasted sponge contains small percentage of iodine. It affects the HEART, esp. valves and larynx, trachea and glands, esp. ductless. It is suited to fair women and children, of LAX FIBRE, flabby and scrofulous constitution. *Exhaustion and heaviness of body* with slight exertion, he must lie down. Orgasm of blood to chest, face, etc. Feels stuffed up. Hard swelling of glands (ductless). Numbness of lower half of the body. Dryness of mucous membranes of tongue, larynx, trachea, throat. Clothes feel uncomfortable. Anxiety with pain in the region of heart or dyspnea. Stiff, in ability to move. Faint when losing her breath, on raising hands above head.

WORSE: DRY COLD *wind. Roused from sleep.* After sleep. *Exertion.* Raising the arms. Before 12 p.m. Full moon. Sweets.

BETTER: Lying with head low. Eating or drinking a little. Warm things. Descending.

MIND: Irresistible desire to sing with excessive mirth followed by sadness. Fear of future; tired of life. Anxiety, fear of death, with suffocation. Timidity, fear and terror. Weeps with the dreams in whooping cough, heat and sweat. Despondent about loss of sexual power. Obstinate and improper behavior.

HEAD: Sensation as if hair were standing on end, on vertex.

EYES: Protruding; staring. Diplopia, > lying down. Red with lacrimation and burning.

NOSE: Dry coryza; nose feels stuffed up. Nose pinched, cold. Nostrils wide open–fan like motion.

FACE: *Terrified; anxious expression.* Blue lips. Pale from exercise instead of ruddy glow. Cold sweat on chin. Chin numb.

MOUTH: Tongue dry, brown. Taste sweetish.

THROAT: Taste bitter. Thyroid gland swollen even with the chin. Soreness of the throat, < eating sweet things. Clears throat constantly. Throat symptoms > lying on back. Goitre with suffocative spells, < touching neck, or pressure; or with heart–pain. Swallows water in small quantity and with difficulty. Numb externally.

STOMACH: Thirst with hunger. Cannot bear tight clothing around. Stomach feels flaccid as if standing open. Desire for dainties.

ABDOMEN: Violent action of abdominal muscles during inspiration. Viscera drawn up against diaphragm. Pain in abdomen instead of menses.

MALE: Painful swelling of spermatic cord and testicles. Screwing, squeezing or stitches. Testes hard and swollen. Genitals hot. Fistulous opening in scrotum with little thick white discharge.

FEMALE: Awakes with suffocative spells during menses. Asthma with absent menses. Hunger and palpitation of heart before menses. Pain in sacrum before menses or instead of menses.

RESPIRATORY: Hoarseness with many complaints– cough, coryza, etc. Larynx painful, dry, constricted, < touch, singing, talking or swallowing. He grasps it. Suffocation as from a plug, valve or leaf in larynx, *wakes him with violent painful palpitation,* blue lips and heavy sweat. Noisy, whistling inspiration on falling to sleep. Anxious, *gasping breathing.* Cough Hollow, Barking, Crowing, Sawing or Tight. Croupy cough wakes him with burning in chest and throat, < cold drink, excitement, sweets, drinking cold milk, > drinking or eating warm things. Voice gives way when singing or talking. Feels as if he had to breathe through a dry sponge. Chest weak, can scarcely talk; choking on falling to sleep. Asthma. Diphtheria. Croup. Profuse mucous expectoration, difficult to raise, swallows it again; smelling like milk. Tuberculosis beginning in apex. *Fullness in chest.* Oppression of breathing, > eating a little. Asthma, must throw head back, worse full moon. Sensation as if air were passing into glands of neck on breathing.

HEART: *Violent palpitation* with dyspnea; awakes suddenly at night with pain and suffocation, with fear and terror. *Blood surging to neck, head and face* with closure of eyelids and tears. Valvular insufficiency. Aneurism of aorta. Rheumatic endocarditis. Hypertrophy of heart with asthmatic symptoms. Pulse frequent, hard, full or feeble. Angina pectoris.

NECK & BACK: Feels a cord about neck. Pain in sacrum instead of menses.

EXTREMITIES: Fingertips numb. Numbness of lower half of the body. Thighs numb and cold. Pain in the knees when rising from kneeling. Thickening of joints after rheumatic fever.

SKIN: Swelling and induration of glands. Biting itching of the whole body.

SLEEP: Awakes in fright and feels as if suffocating, with terror and fear.

FEVER: *Heat* in flushes with anxiety, cardiac pain, would rather die, with cold moist thighs, < thinking of it. Heat and sudden weakness after walking in open air, he must lie down.

COMPLEMENTARY: Hep.

RELATED: Iod; Led.

STANNUM

GENERALITIES: The chief action of tin is centered upon NERVOUS SYSTEM, causing EXTREME WEAKNESS which is esp. felt in CHEST, *throat*, stomach, upper arms and thighs. The patient is unable even to talk, drops into a chair instead of sitting down, trembles on moving. Weakness is felt much more on going downstairs than going up. *Paralytic heaviness or weakness.* Spasm–hysterical, with pain in abdomen and diaphragm. Epileptic, spasm with tossing of limbs, clenching of thumbs, opisthotonos, unconsciousness and sexual complications. Affections of MUCOUS MEMBRANES produce yellow, *muco-purulent secretions.* PAINS INCREASE GRADUALLY AND GRADUALLY SUBSIDE. *Pressive, drawing pains.* Neuralgia, diaphragmatic; suppressed. Cramps. Hysteria. Emaciation. Repeated short attacks. Ill effects of emotion, fright, masturbation, dentition, overusing voice. Girdle sensation with yawning. Child wants to be carried across shoulders. Trembling more from slow motion or exercise. Paralysis, from worms, after spasm, emotions, onanism. Hemiplegia; part constantly moist.

WORSE: *Using voice.* Cold. 10 A.M. *Lying on right side. After gentle motion.* Warm drinks. During stool. Going downstairs. Ascending. Touch.

BETTER: Hard pressure over an edge. Coughing, expectoration. Rapid motion. Lying across something hard. Bending double.

MIND: Very sensitive to what others say about her. ANXIOUS, *nervous, sad,* < before menses. *Miserable and discouraged.* Cannot get rid of an idea once fixed in her mind. Taciturn and dislike of society. Sudden fits of passion. Forgetful and absent–minded. Uneasy, knows not what to do with himself. Hopeless, despondent; feels like crying all the time but crying <.

HEAD: Severe, painful constriction in forehead and temples. Pressive stupefying headache. Jarring of walking resounds painfully in head. Migraine of cerebral origin, > by vomiting. Violent, beating pains, as if the head would burst, with inward blows. Vertigo, all objects seem too far off.

EYES: Sunken, dull. Ptosis, returns every week.

EARS: Cracking, shrieking noise in ear when blowing the nose. Ulceration of ear-ring hole.

NOSE: Oversensitive to smell.

FACE: Pale. Prosopalgia. Malar neuralgia; at menses.

MOUTH: Tickling at the root of the tongue. Taste sour, sweet, bitter, to all food except water.

THROAT: Efforts to detach adhesive mucus cause nausea. Cutting pain when swallowing. Nausea felt in throat. Dry. Smarting.

STOMACH: Smell of cooking causes nausea and vomiting Vomiting, violent, of blood, bile; early in the morning, with odor of ingesta. Sensation of emptiness in stomach. Uneasy feeling.

ABDOMEN: Burning in liver. Diaphragmatic neuralgia, hysterical. Cutting, pinching colic; with hunger and diarrhea, which exhausts, > hard pressure. Passes worms. Spasmodic pain in abdomen, hysterical. Colic in children, > by carrying them on shoulder. Constipation–stools dry, hard, knotty, insufficient, and green. Monday constipation, i.e., occurring after working days.

URINARY: Insensibility of the bladder; only the sense of fullness indicates the necessity to urinate. Atony of bladder.

MALE: Sexual excitement. Voluptuous feeling in genitals ending in emission which exhausts.

FEMALE: Increased sexual desire; easy orgasm. Scratching of distant parts (of arms) produce an intolerable sensation of pleasure in genital organs producing orgasm. Bearing down in uterine region. Prolapsus uteri and vagina, < stools. Strong odor of body during menses. Menses, early and profuse. Mania erotica before menses. Leukorrhea gushing with much debility; of yellow-white or transparent mucus. Child refuses mother's milk. Uterine symptoms with a weak, drawn sensation in the chest. Pain in vagina goes to spine.

RESPIRATORY: Voice deep, hollow, hoarse, > hawking mucus. Much mucus in trachea. *Cough,* < laughing, singing, talking, lying on right side. *Expectoration easy; quantities of sweet,* saltish, sour, putrid or bright yellow pus or ball of mucus. *Short breath from* every *effort;* must loosen clothes. Takes deep breath. *Chest* feels raw or *hollow.* Hemoptysis with copious expectoration. Stitches in left side of chest when breathing or lying on that side; knife–like pain below left axilla. Catarrhal phthisis. Bronchiectasis. Retching with coughing. Cannot walk, or do anything without coughing.

EXTREMITIES: Swelling of the hands and ankles. Paralytic weakness; drops things. Limbs suddenly give out when attempting to sit down. Tremulous knees. Fingers jerk when holding pen. Neuritis. Typewriters' paralysis.

Contraction of fingers, retraction of thumbs. Cramps in hands, cannot let go the broom. Using voice or singing causes weakness in upper arm, which extends all over the body. Aching in deltoid from reading.

SLEEP: Moaning, weeping and plaintive lamentations during sleep. Sleeps with one leg drawn up, the other stretched out.

FEVER: Chill 10 A.M., with numb fingertips. *Burning palms and soles*. Hectic. Debilitating, musty sweat at 4 A.M.

COMPLEMENTARY: Puls.

RELATED: Calc; Kali-c; Lach; Nat-m; Phos; Sulph.

STANNUM IODIDE

GENERALITIES: It is valuable in chronic chest diseases, characterized by plastic tissue changes, and persistent inclination to cough excited by tickling, dry spot in throat, (apparently at the root of the tongue), beginning with a weak–sounding cough with short breath, soon gathers strength and sound and causes raising of free, copious, pale yellowish expectoration which at first relieves but is soon followed by a feeling of dryness, weakness in chest and throat, and increased oppression. It is indicated in cases that "hang fire' and need an alternative. Use low potency–2x or 3x.

STAPHYSAGRIA

GENERALITIES: Nervous affections *with trembling* is marked feature of this remedy. It produces physical, moral, *sexual disturbances,* provokes excess and irregular sexual appetite and a tendency to masturbation and the physical state corresponding to the effect of that habit. Acts on TEETH, URINARY ORGANS, *fibrous tissue* of eyelids and tarsi, skin, glands and right deltoid. *Morbidly sensitive*–the least word that seems wrong hurts her very much; special senses become irritable, cannot tolerate touch, odor, noise, taste. Squeezing, or *stinging-smarting pains,* as if cut. Pains that move into teeth. *Sphincters* lacerated and stretched. LACERATED TISSUE–perineum etc. Stitch pains remaining after operation. Ill effects of anger and insult, reserved, anger, injury, fall, clean cut wound, operation wound, sexual abuse and excess, dentition, tobacco, mercury. Painful swelling of glands. Arthritic nodosities on joints. Swelling and suppuration of bones and periosteum. Exostosis. Warts. Condylomata. Hemiplegia after anger. Stiffness and sensation of fatigue in all joints. Whole body painful with feeling of weakness.

WORSE: *Emotions, chagrin, vexation, indignation, quarrel. Sexual excess. Onanism. Touch. Cold drink. Laceration.* Stretching part. Coition. After urinating, when not urinating. Night. New moon, before full moon.

BETTER: Warmth. Rest. *Break-fast.* Coition.

MIND: Violent outburst of passion. *Always angry.* Gloomy and petulant, throws things. Child cries for many things and refuses them when offered. Poor memory. Dwells on sexual matters. Unsatisfied sexual urge in widows. Snappish; sensitive mentally and physically. Hypochondriasis. Imagines insult. Irritable, nervous, excitable and violent. Great indignation about the things done by others or by himself, grieves about the consequences. Believes he will lose his fortune, his wife will leave him. Ailments from reserved displeasure. Very sensitive to what others say about her. Sadness without any cause, with irritability. Illness after scolding or punishment in children. Want of self–control. Fear; afraid of his own shadow.

HEAD: Compressive, stupefying headache, > much yawning, leaning head against something. Brain feels squeezed or torn. Sensation of a heavy load or round ball in forehead. Moist, foul, eroding milk–crust, < occiput. Dandruff. Head lice. Falling of hair. Vertigo, > by walking about in a circle, or turning rapidly on heels. Cerebrum feels numb and occiput feels hollow. Hair fall off from occiput and around ears.

EYES: Feel dry, with lacrimation. Nodes on lids. Styes, recurrent. Blepharitis. Bursting, burning pain in eyeballs of syphilitic iritis. *Sunken* with blue rings around. Hot tears run off the eyes (left) on looking at the sun.

EARS: Hardness of hearing from enlarged tonsils, in children from adenoids.

NOSE: Coryza now thick now thin, with ulceration. Frequent sneezing without coryza.

FACE: *Sickly, peaked* nose Neuralgia from caries, pains go into the eyes. Sub-maxillary glands painful with or without swelling; abscess. Prosopalgia, pain starts from lips over to face, < mastication.

MOUTH: *Teeth loose, black, crumbling,* show dark streaks, < eating and during menses, > hard pressure and heat. Pale bleeding gums. Pyorrhea. Musty taste. Exceedingly tender decayed teeth on being filled. Teeth decay as soon as they erupt. Fistula dentalis. Stomatitis. Thrush.

THROAT: Swallows continuously while talking. Tonsils swollen, stitch runs into ear on swallowing. Induration and hypertrophy of tonsils, with nasal voice.

STOMACH: *Hungry* even when stomach is full. Desire for bread, stimulants, tobacco, milk. Feels as if stomach were hanging down relaxed. Nausea, specially after operations.

ABDOMEN: Feeling of weakness in abdomen, as if it would drop, wants to hold it up. Severe pain after abdominal operation. Swollen (in children) with much flatus. Biliary colic after anger. Flatus hot, smells like rotten eggs. Dysenteric stools, < after least food or drink. Diarrhea from drinking cold water. Piles very sensitive to touch. Dysentery in weak, ailing, pot–bellied children.

URINARY: Frequent urging to urinate with scanty or profuse discharge of watery urine; urinates in thin stream or drop by drop. Sensation as if a drop of urine rolling continuously along the urethra, < after walking or riding, > urinating. Burning in urethra when not urinating. Ineffectual urging in *newly married women;* in pregnancy. After urination, urging as if the bladder was not empty. Cystocele.

MALE: Persistently dwells on sexual subjects. Sexual neurasthenia. Priapism. Seminal emission followed by great prostration. Dyspnea, < during or after coition. Voluptuous itching of scrotum. Prostatitis, pain extends from anus to urethra. Soft humid excrescences behind corona glandis. Enlarged prostate with piles. Orchitis from mumps. Atrophy of testicles.

FEMALE: Sexual desire increased. Painful sensitiveness of genital organs. < sitting down. Ovarian pain going into thighs, < pressure, coition. Salpingitis. Amenorrhea from indignation. Granular vegetations of vagina. Itching or sensitive vulva. Menses with aching around hips and loss of power in limbs. First coition is very painful causing acute mental and bodily suffering.

RESPIRATORY: Dyspnea with constriction at close of coition or after seminal emission. Cough, < cleaning teeth, tobacco smoke, eating meat. Cough alternating with sciatica.

HEART: Tremulous palpitation when listening to music.

NECK & BACK: Pain in small of the back as after overlifting, < coition, in morning and rising from a seat.

EXTREMITIES: Fine tearing or numb fingertips. Bones of fingers imperfectly developed; osteitis of fingers. Arthritic nodes on finger–joints. Crural neuralgia. Feel beaten and painful. Knees weak. Shuffling gait. Buttocks ache while sitting.

SKIN: Pain precedes shingles. Skin symptoms alternating with joint–pains. Biting, itching as from vermin, changing place on scratching. Eczema with thick scabs, itching violently. Dry pedunculated figwarts. Ulcers, new growth, extremely sensitive, touch may bring on convulsion.

SLEEP: Violent yawning and stretching bring tears to the eyes. Child wakes, pushes everything away and wants everybody to go out, calls for mother often. Amorous dreams with emission. Sleepy all day, awake all night. Body aches all over.

FEVER: Wants to uncover. Sweat profuse, cold, smelling like rotten egg, with a desire to uncover. Inability to sweat.

COMPLEMENTARY: Caust; Coloc.

RELATED: Cham; Merc.

STICTA

GENERALITIES: Commonly known as lung-wort, it is a remedy for coryza, bronchial catarrh, *nervous* and rheumatic disturbances. General feeling of dulness and lassitude as when a cold is coming. *Rheumatic stiffness, nervous,* sense of levitation of different parts. Painful dry mucous membranes. Diagonal pains. Hysteria, chorea, after loss of blood. Ill effects of fall, hemorrhages.

WORSE: *Night.* Lying down. Motion. Change of temperature.

BETTER: Free discharges. Open air.

MIND: Feels as if she must talk about everything and anything; whether listened to or not. Lively, kicks her heels up. Feels as if floating in air.

HEAD: Aches before catarrhal discharge appears. Heaviness of forehead.

EYES: Burning of eyelids with soreness of eyeballs on closing lids or turning eyes.

NOSE: *Pressure or stuffy fullness at the root of nose.* Constant need to blow the nose but no discharge. Painful dryness of mucous membranes. Coryza which dries up soon, forming scabs difficult to dislodge. Hay fever, incessant sneezing.

THROAT: Dry; dropping of mucus posteriorly.

STOMACH & ABDOMEN: Diarrhea, frothy, in morning.

URINARY: Profuse urination, with sore painful bladder.

FEMALE: Absence of milk after delivery.

RESPIRATORY: Tickling high up in pharynx. *Incessant dry hacking cough prevents sleep, < coughing,* inspiration, towards evening, when tired; after measles, colds, influenza, whooping cough. Air passages numb. Pulsation from right side of sternum down to abdomen. Bronchitis. Pain from sternum to spine, < motion.

NECK & BACK: Sore stiff neck, pain in shoulder. Restless hands and feet. Legs feel floating in the air. *Rheumatism.* Red spots on affected joints. Bursitis, esp. about the knee. Cold moist limbs. Profuse sweat on hands. Chorea–like spasms.

SLEEP: Sleepless from nervousness, cough, after surgical operation.

RELATED: Elap; Guai; Sang; Thuj.

STRAMONIUM

GENERALITIES : Thorn-apple or datura expends its force of action on the BRAIN, producing marked and persistent disorder of the mental faculty; hallucination, fixed notion, terrifying delirium, etc. Therefore it is a remedy of TERRORS; it *however, does not in its ordinary effect cause actual pain. Secretions are suppressed,* passes neither urine nor stool. Throat, skin and spinal nerves are affected as well. Increases the mobility of the muscles of expression and of locomotion; the motions may be *graceful,* rhythmic, or *disorderly* of head and arms. Trembling of limbs. Parkinsonism. Nervous tremors. Convulsions, spasms < at night, after masturbation. Paralysis of one side, convulsions of the other side, or unilateral paralysis; with twitching. Chorea, epilepsy; from fright. Hysteria, weeping, laughing, with sexual excitement. Catalepsy, limbs can be moved by others. Tonic and clonic spasm alternately. Traumatic neuritis. General paralysis of the insane. Ill effects of shock, fright, sun, childbirth, suppression. Hydrophobia. Delusions as to size and distance. Sensation as if limbs were separated from body.

WORSE: *Glistening objects* (mirror, surface of water). Fright. *After sleep.* Dark. Cloudy days. Swallowing. *Suppression.* Intemperance. Touch.

BETTER: LIGHT. *Company. Warmth.*

MIND: Awakes terrified, knows no one, screams with fright, clings to those near him (child). DREAD OF DARKNESS, and has a horror of glistening objects. Praying, singing, devoutly; beseeching, entreating, ceaseless *talking. Fearful* hallucination which terrify the patient; sees ghosts, vividly brilliant or hideous phantoms, animals jumping sideways out of ground or running to him. *Wildly excited* as in night terror. Does all sorts of crazy things. *Active variable delirium;* delirium tremens. Raving MANIA *with cold sweat.* Religious insanity. The talk by others is intolerable. Self–accusation. *Loss of reason* or of speech. Strange absurd ideas–thinks himself tall, double, lying crosswise, one half of the body cut off, etc. Desires company; shy, hides himself or tries to escape. Talks in foreign tongue. Laughs at night, weeps during day. Proud, haughty; merry exaltation. Lascivious talk. Limbs feel separated from the body. Fear and anxiety on hearing water run. Aversion to all fluids. Maniac, curses, tears ones clothes with teeth. Violent speech. Exposes the part. Stupid; imbecile. Sits silent, eyes on ground, picking at her clothes. Wants to kill people or himself. Anxiety when going through a tunnel. Exalted states alternating with settled melancholy. Everything, everybody seem new. Wife thinks husband neglecting her, man thinks his wife faithless.

HEAD: Vertigo, < walking in dark or with eyes closed. Jerks head up from pillow and drops it again during unconsciousness, delirium, puerperal fever, etc. Headache with tendency to speak incoherently. Head bent backward in vertigo, supports head with hands while bending or rising; after sunstroke. Meningitis from suppressed ear discharge. Headache from sun.

EYES: Fixed, sparkling, *staring,* wide open. Squint. Half open in sleep. Diplopia. *Lacrimation* with headache, fever, otalgia. Night–blindness. Green vision. Hallucination in which everything looks jumbled. *All objects look black,* crooked, small or large. Squint in brain affections, during convulsions, < terror, fear. Sight darkened. Pupils dilated.

EAR: Sensation as if air rushing out of ear. Deafness. Hallucinations of hearing.

NOSE: Alae nasi white.

FACE: *Red, bloated,* hot. Expression rapidly changing–now flushed, now pale; a sardonic grin, then expression of terror. Forehead wrinkled, frowning, in brain diseases. Thinks face elongated. Lips dry, glued together. Chewing motion. Lock-jaw.

MOUTH: *Fine red dots on tongue. Tongue* dry, parched, swollen; hangs out of the mouth. Taste bitter to food. Stammering. Aphasia. Constantly spits saliva. Dribbling of viscid saliva. Grinding of the teeth.

THROAT: Dry with great thirst, *yet dreads water,* it chokes him. Up and down movement of larynx as in swallowing. Sensation as if boiling water rising. Swallowing, difficult; hasty.

STOMACH: Food tastes like straw. Vomiting of greenish substance. Great desire for acids, lemon juice >. Hiccough obstinate.

ABDOMEN: *Putrid, dark, painless,* involuntary *diarrhea,* with squint and pale face. Cholera infantum. Stools suppressed.

URINARY: Suppression of urine, esp. during typhoid, bladder empty. Loss of power of bladder in the aged, stream flows slowly, cannot make haste. Rigor during urination.

MALE: Sexual passion exalted with indecent speech and action. Hands constantly kept on genitals.

FEMALE: Nymphomania; lewd talking; sings obscene songs. Excessive menses, preceded by sexual excitement. Loquacity and singing during menses. Menses have a strong smell as of semen. Puerperal convulsions, mania, with mental symptoms and profuse sweating. Hands constantly kept on genitals. Sobs and moans after menses. Excessive menstrual flow.

RESPIRATORY: Inspiration slow, expiration quick. Spasmodic cough of drunkards; whooping. Voice hoarse and croaking; suddenly fails in higher tone. Spasms, twitching of larynx. Nervous asthma. Cough, < looking at light, fire, or bright objects. Cough with jerking of lower limbs, when sitting.

HEART: Feeble; pulse irregular. Cardiac affections with constriction of chest and mental symptoms.

NECK & BACK: Neck stiff, cannot bend it backwards. Drawing pain in the back. Spine sensitive, slightest pressure causes outcries and ravings. Opisthotonos.

EXTREMITIES: Graceful and rhythmic motions. Clasps hands over head. Hands open and shut. Wringing of hands. Staggering gait. Misses step of stairs while descending. Violent pain in hip. Trembling of limbs. Inside of right thigh red and swollen. Abscess of left hip-joint, with violent pain. Hemiplegia, with convulsions in unparalysed parts. Heels numb, sometimes painful.

SKIN: Crawling as if from movement of many bugs. Non-appearance of exanthemata. Shining red flush. Chronic abscess, fistulae. Fiery red patches on skin. Abscesses and tumor with severe pain. Burn and scalds.

SLEEP: Comatose. Weeping in dream. *Awakes in fear* or screaming. Lies on back with thighs and knees flexed. Sleepless in darkness. Frightful dreams. Laughs, screams, starts during sleep.

FEVER: Profuse sweat which does not relieve. Violent fever. Cold sweat during spasm.

RELATED: Bell; Hyos; Op.

STRONTIUM CARBONICUM

GENERALITIES: Affects the *circulation* causing congestive tension. Heart, kidneys, marrow, *ankles* and right side are also affected. *Pains are fleeting,* can hardly tell where they are, seemingly felt in marrow of bones, increase and decrease gradually or make the patient faint and sick all over. Burning, *gnawing*. Violent involuntary starts of the body. *Immobility* of one side. Sense of *paralytic weakness*. Emaciation. Prostration or shock after surgical operation. Numbness. Soreness. Formication in limbs. Edema, esp. about the ankles as a concomitant. High blood pressure; arteriosclerosis. Affections of bones, esp. of femur. Chronic sequelae of hemorrhages. Rheumatic pains. Chronic sprain. Stenosis; of oesophagus. Neuritis, < cold. Coldness in spots, on calves. Pain and itching alternate.

WORSE: COLD; *uncovering. Walking.* Sprain. *Bleeding.* Evening. Change of weather. Stooping. Touch. Rubbing.

BETTER: *Heat and light.* Sun. Wraps. Hot bath.

MIND: Excessive forgetfulness. Apprehension as from bad conscience. Depression of spirits. Irritable; suddenly becomes angry, beats anything that comes in his way.

HEAD: Ache moves into upper jaw, with vertigo and nausea. Violent pain in nape extending upwards, > wraps. Distensive pressure on entire head. Aching eyebrows.

EYES: Burning and red. Photophobia remaining after operation, objects appear covered with blood. Green. spots before the eyes in the dark. Pain and lacrimation on using eyes, with dancing and alternation of colors of objects looked at.

NOSE: Itching, redness and burning of nose. Bloody crusts.

FACE: Red with burning heat or very pale every time the patient walks.

MOUTH: *Feels numb* and dry in A.M; on waking. Teeth feel as if screwed together.

STOMACH: Pressure in stomach during digestion. Hiccough causes chest pain. Food tastes insipid. Craving for bread and beer. Aversion to meat.

ABDOMEN: Colic in umbilical region. Hard, knotty stools evacuated slowly with much effort, then burning in anus lasting for a long time. Diarrhea, < at night, with constant urging, exhausting, of yellow water; with griping, > towards morning. Periodical diarrhea.

URINARY: Pale urine with strong smell of ammonia.

RESPIRATORY: Pressure as of a load on chest. Pain in the left breast with oppression, < after meals.

HEART: *Feels smothered.* Heart–block.

EXTREMITIES: Hands numb. Cramp in calves and soles. *Ankles sprained or puffed* as a concomitant. Chronic spasms, esp. of ankle joints. Sciatica with edema of ankle. Immobility of the limbs of one side only, like paralysis. Gnawing as if in marrow of the bones. Diarrhea during rheumatism.

SKIN: Moist itching–burning eruptions, > in open air, esp. in warm sunshine.

FEVER: *Flushes of heat* in face, yet aversion *to uncovering.* Profuse perspiration at night; climacteric.

RELATED: Calc; Rhus-t.

STROPHANTHUS HISPIDUS

GENERALITIES: Used as an arrow poison, it increases the contractile power of all striped muscles, esp. of HEART, increasing the systole and diminishing the rapidity. It can be used with advantage to tone the heart and run off dropsical effusions. Has no cumulative action–safe for corpulent aged persons, with rigid arteries. Functional disturbances of heart from alcohol, tobacco, tea. Mitral regurgitation. Arterio-sclerosis. Twitching of the muscles. *Stitching pains. Undulating* sensation in whole body. Throbbings. *Rapid alternation* of symptoms with slow pulse. Faintness. Anemia with palpitation and breathlessness Goitre, exophthalmic. Increased secretions. Abolishes the taste for alcohol.

WORSE: Exertion. Tobacco. Tea. Alcohol.

MIND: *Fear of ordeal.* Feels lifted up during sleep. Precociously loquacious children.

HEAD: Vertigo with swimming vision. Senile undulations in head.

EYES: Glimmering vision. Pupils rapidly dilate and contract every few minutes. Brilliant.

FACE: Flushed; red spots. Lips scarlet.

THROAT: Seems constricted. Burning compelling empty swallowing.

STOMACH: Craving for coffee. Loss of appetite. Nausea with disgust for alcohol. Loathing of food, followed by choking and vomiting after eating.

ABDOMEN: Rumbling and pinching at navel. Diarrhea with burning and tenesmus in anus.

URINARY: Urine, increased secretion or scanty, albuminous.

HEART: Weak, *aching* or anguish at heart. *Sense of lively action.* Chronic nervous palpitation and arrest of breathing. Stitches and twitches at apex beat. Pulse; rapid, alternating with slow, weak, small, irregular beats. Cardiac dyspnoea.

EXTREMITIES: Heaviness and pain in forearms and fingers. Itching and stitching in both feet.

SKIN: *Hives*, chronic, receding.

RELATED: Apoc; *Glon; Ign;* Spig.

STRYCHNINUM

GENERALITIES: Spasmodic rigidity is the key-note of this alkaloid obtained from the seeds of nux vomica. Tetanic convulsions with opisthotonos; tetanus; violent jerking, twitching and trembling are the characteristic symptoms which it produces. Inability to take deep breath, fixation of chest walls. Athetosis. Spine is cold. Gushing sweat from head and chest.

WORSE: Touch. Noise. Motion.

BETTER: Lying on back.

SUCCINUM

GENERALITIES: A fossil resin known as amber, it produces nervous and hysterical symptoms. Fear of train and closed places.

SULPHONAL

GENERALITIES: This coal–tar product produces ataxic symptoms; staggering gait, anesthesia of legs with absence of knee–jerks.

SULPHUR

GENERALITIES: Sulph. is a product of volcanic eruptions, found free in nature and was used from remote times to remove skin affections. Therefore, it is a great anti-psoric remedy. It causes *irregular distribution of* CIRCULATION causing LOCAL BURNING, THROBBING, or CONGESTION; flushes of head, rush of blood to head, chest, heart. REDNESS OF ORIFICES or of single parts is another prominent feature due to irregular circulation–LIPS, ears, nose, eyelids, anus, vulva. NUTRITION is affected on account of defective assimilation. In spite of voracious appetite, the patient *emaciates* (esp. children). Child looks dried, a little old man, big head, big belly, with emaciated limbs. It is often of great use in beginning the treatment of CHRONIC DISEASE and in finishing acute ones, or when the REACTION IS DEFICIENT, when the carefully selected remedy fails to act. Mucous discharges and exhalations are *acrid, blood–streaked, offensive* and cause itching. Serous effusions or deposits are absorbed slowly. It has an elective affinity for SKIN where it produces heat and burning with ITCHING. Patient is unable to walk erect. STOOP–SHOULDERED UNWASHED looking, TALL AND LEAN; BODY OFFENSIVE in spite of washing. Aversion to being washed; always < after the bath. Dirty, filthy people prone to skin affections. *Complaints that relapse*. Glandular swellings, indurated and suppurating. *Weak faint spells* frequently during the day after nursing or night–watching, with great sleepiness. *Empty,* sinking feeling. Sensation of overfulness, roughness, or numbness. Epilepsy with feeling that a mouse is running up the arms to back before the fit. Child jumps, starts and screams fearfully. ASCENDING EFFECTS, rushes of blood, flushes of heat, vertigo, etc. Ragged philosopher, dirty–looking persons who are always speculating on religious or philosophical subjects. Everything affects the epigastrium. Burning in VERTEX AND SOLES. Rheumatism. Scrofula. Psora. Chronic alcoholism; dropsy and other ailments of drunkards. Ill effects of fall, blow, sprain, sun. Always desires to keep his bowels clean. Slight pressure causes pain, swelling and suppuration. Induration of tissues from constant pressure, corns, bedsore, etc. Bunion. Never well since chest trouble. Thinks bed is too small to hold him. Feels as if swinging or standing on wavering ground. Coal–miner's affections. Chorea; chronic, after suppressed eruptions.

WORSE: SUPPRESSION. BATHING. Milk. HEATED BY OVEREXERTION, IN BED, by woollens, etc. *Atmospheric changes. Talking. Periodically;* 11 A.M. *Climacteric.* Full moon. *Standing,* stooping. Reaching high. Sweets. Looking down. Crossing running water. Vaccination. Suppressed piles.

BETTER: Open air. Motion. Drawing up affected limb. Sweating. Dry warm weather. Lying on right side. Walking. Dry heat.

MIND: *Dull; difficult thinking;* misplaces or cannot find proper words when talking or writing. *Lazy, hungry,* and *always tired.* Childish peevishness in grown up–people. *Hopeful dreamers.* Mean. Prying. Easily excited. Foolish happiness and pride, thinks himself in possession of beautiful things, everything looks pretty which the patient takes a fancy to, even rags seem beautiful, or thinks himself immensely wealthy. Very selfish; no regard for others. Too lazy to rouse himself and too unhappy to live. Strong tendency to religious and philosophical reveries, with fixed ideas. Disgust up to nausea about any effluvia arising in his own body. Obstinate. Dislikes to have anyone near him. Tired of life. Strong impulsive tendency to suicide by drowning or leaping from a window (in epileptic fits, < during menses). Aversion to do mental or physical work. Loafs. Thinks that he is giving wrong things to people causing their death. Fault–finding. Aversion to business. Melancholy. Sad. Absentminded. Wishing to touch something with inability to do so. Philosophical mania, wants to know who made this or that and how, tries to reason without any hope of discovery or possible answer. Imagines himself a great man, though ignorant, despises literary men and education. Weeps without cause, or after slightest provocation, < consolation.

HEAD: Vertigo in forehead < when crossing a river, stooping, with headache. *Vertex* hot, *throbs*, heavy, sore. Pain, chill, pressure, etc. ascends *from nape* to *vertex*. Sick headache recurring periodically, on every Sunday, preceded by photopsia. Sensation as of a band about head or pain deep in brain. Hot head with cold feet. Hair dry, cold, hard; falling off, < washing. Sweaty scalp. Fontanelles remain open too long. Hydrocephalus with convulsion, red face and pupils dilated. Head bent forward when walking.

EYES: Burning. Cutting as from sand. Bursting pain in eyeballs. Trembling of eyes, quivering of eyelids. Objects seem more distant than they are. *Halo about light.* Obscuration of vision like black gauze before eyes. Retinitis caused by overuse of eyes. Painful inflammation of eye from presence of foreign body. Photophobia. Keratitis; cornea like ground glass. Agglutination of lids. Oily tears. Styes and tarsal tumors. Eczema of lids. Trachoma. Opacity of vitreous.

EARS: Deafness preceded by oversensitiveness of hearing, < after eating and blowing nose. Swashing as of water. Purulent offensive otorrhea; catarrhal discharge every eighth day. Ears very red in children. Feels as if sounds do not come through the ear but through forehead.

NOSE: Obstructed on alternate sides. Fluent burning coryza, < out of doors, stopped indoors. Tip of nose or wings red, swollen, < cold. Smell before nose as from an old catarrh. Epistaxis, < at night, on lying on right side. Sensitive to smell. Imaginary odors. Freckles and black pores on nose. Frequent sneezing.

FACE: Pale, sickly, OLD LOOKING. Circumscribed redness of cheeks. Freckled, spotted. *Lips bright red*, swollen (upper), dry, rough, cracked, burning, twitching or trembling. Swollen veins on forehead. Acne. Mumps.

MOUTH: Teeth sensitive, tender. Jerking, shooting, throbbing pains in teeth. Grinding of the teeth. Gums swollen, bleeding. Tongue dry, tremulous with red tip and borders. Taste sour, sweetish, foul, bitter, in morning. Saliva profuse, with nauseous taste. Nursing sore mouth. Food tastes like straw or too salty. Aphthae, thrush.

THROAT: Sensation of a lump, hair or splinter, or vapour rising. Ball seems to rise and close the pharynx. External redness. Swollen sensation. Dry, exciting cough.

STOMACH: *Drinks much eats little.* Eructations tasting like bad egg, < eating or at night. Complete loss of appetite or ravenous appetite. Feels hungry but when comes to the table he loathes the food, turns away from it. Eats anything and everything. Aversion to meat. Desire for sweets, for raw food. Food tastes too salty. Milk causes sour taste and sour eructation. SUDDENLY HUNGRY AND WEAK at 11 A.M.; empty *weak feeling at epigastrium.* Eructations on pressing over stomach. Headache or feels tired if he does not eat often. Vomiting of undigested food or sour vomiting. Nausea during pregnancy. Sweets disagree. Heaviness in stomach.

ABDOMEN: SORE, very sensitive to pressure. Stitches in region of spleen, < coughing or deep inspiration. Stitches in region of liver. Biliary colic, and chronic or relapsing jaundice. Intestines feel as if strung in knots, < bending forward. Abdomen heavy, as from a lump. Feels as if something moving alive–the fist of a child. Colic after eating or drinking, obliging one to bend double, < sweet things. Bearing–down against rectum. Pain, urging and itching in rectum. *Hemorrhoidal habitus,* during pregnancy. Piles external and internal, great bunches that are sore, tender, raw, burn, bleed and smart. Holds stools back from pain. DIARRHEA–HURRIED, EARLY MORNING, changing, mushy, *foul, painless,* watery, grayish, frothy, < milk. Diarrhea alternating with constipation. Habitual constipation. Odor of stool follows him as if he had soiled himself. *Redness around the anus,* with itching. Diarrhea of infants with pale face, profuse sweating, drowsiness, half–open eyes, suppression of urine, spasms of limbs. The child wakes up screaming. Colicky babies. Involuntary stool on sneezing or laughing, with emission of flatus. Big belly, emaciated limbs (children). Eczema about navel. Stools flat and thin.

URINARY: Itching, burning in urethra during micturition lasting till long after. Sudden call to urinate, must hurry. Frequent urination, esp. at night. Bed–wetting in scrofulous, untidy children. Mucus and pus in urine. Great quantities of colorless urine, greasy particles upon it. Urination involuntary while passing flatus or on coughing. Painful ineffectual efforts to urinate; retention; every cold settles in the bladder. Stream thin, intermits.

MALE: Testes hang low. Seminal emission, with burning in urethra. Penis cold. Sexual power weak; impotence.

Induration of testes. Foetid sweat on genitals. Exhaustion in the morning after seminal emission. Backache and weakness of the limbs after coition with sadness and irritability. Discharge of prostatic fluid after urination and stool. Seminal emission on touching a woman. Semen, odorless, watery. Hydrocele. Prepuce stiff, hard like leather; copious fetid smegma causes itching.

FEMALE: Vulva and vagina burn, itch, and are sore, < sitting; is scarcely able to keep still. Sore feeling in vagina during coition. Bearing–down in pelvis towards genitals, < standing. Menses irregular, too late, short, scanty, thick, foul, black, acrid, making parts sore. Leuckorrhea of yellow mucus, burning, excoriating. Troublesome itching of vulva with pimples all around. Sharp burning in mammae. Cutting pain in uterus during menses. Weak feeling in genitals. Nipples cracked around the base, smart, burn, bleed; after nursing, pain extends to back. Puerperal sepsis with high fever, profuse sweat of whole body, tenderness of abdomen and drowsiness. Offensive genitals, with offensive sweat on thighs. Suppression of menses from slight physical or mental excitement. Amenorrhea. Prolapse of uterus from reaching high. Cancer of breast or uterus. Breasts and uterus develop imperfectly.

RESPIRATORY: DIFFICULT RESPIRATION, WANTS WINDOWS OPEN; nightly suffocative air hunger. Irregular breathing. Deep hoarse voice. *Cough* violent, in two or three incomplete bouts; tickling down in larynx. Much rattling of mucus and heat in chest, < 11 A.M. *Pain goes backward from left nipple.* Band or load sensation on chest. Red, brown spots on chest. Pleuritic exudation. Pneumonia. Greenish, sweetish, purulent expectoration. Sensation of burning or coldness in chest, extending to face. Asthma preceded by cold everytime. Feeling of weakness in chest while talking. Violent cough with headache, < lying on back. Sensation as if a rivet passes through upper third of left lung. Shooting pains in chest extending to back, < coughing, lying on back and deep breathing. Neglected pneumonia.

HEART: Seems to big. Palpitation, < lying, night, in bed, ascent. Pulse more rapid in morning than in the evening. Pericarditis with effusion. Sharp pains go through chest in between shoulders.

NECK & BACK: Muscles of neck weak, child cannot hold head. Boils on neck. Neck stiff. Sensation as if vertebrae glide over each other or crack on bending backwards. Aching between scapulae. *Lumbar pains;* to stomach; *walks bent* from pain in the back, he can straighten up only after moving. Supports weight on hands when sitting. Coccyx pains during stools. Aching in small of back, < when urinating. Curvature of spine.

EXTREMITIES: Heavy shoulders. Sweat in armpit smelling like garlic. Left arm numb, < lying. Numb fingers. Palms dry, burn, crack, peel. Eczema, warts, on palms. Tense hamstring (left). Cramp in calf (left). SOLES BURN, WANTS THEM UNCOVERED, at night; cold in bed; dry. Hot sweaty hands. Heaviness, paretic feeling in limbs. *Jerks one limb on dropping to sleep.* Poplitiae tight on stooping. Swelling of the joints with hydrarthrosis. Joints stiff. Tremulous sensation in hands when writing. Tuberculosis of the knee and hip joints. Ulcers around the nails. Whitlow with rapid swelling of the finger, redness, stiffness and excessive burning–stitching. Involuntary contraction of hands as if about to grasp something. Unsteady gait.

SKIN: Eruptions almost of every kind. Skin *dry, rough, wrinkled, scaly.* ITCHING voluptuous, violent, < at night, in bed, scratching and washing. *Unhealthy,* BREAKS OUT, *festers and would not heal.* Burning when scratched; painfully sensitive to air, wind, *washing,* etc. *Eruptions alternate with other complaints*, asthma. Crops of boil.

Itch. Rhagade. Eczema. Ulcer. Creeping erysipelas. Excoriations on folds. Suppuration with air bubbles. Varicose veins ulcerate, rupture and bleed.

SLEEP: Heavy, unrefreshing. Drowsy, then migraine. Sleeps in catnaps. Drowsy by day, wakeful at night. talks, jerks and twitches during sleep. Awakes with starts or screams. Sings during sleep or wakes up singing. Vivid dreams, remain impressed on the memory.

FEVER: Chill spreading up back. *Flushes of heat. Feels too hot.* Heat with general throbbing between scapulae. Sweat on single parts–in axillae, hands and feet. Profuse sweat at night with sulphur odor. Sweat without relief. Remittent fever. Septic, puerperal fever.

COMPLEMENTARY: Acon; Aloe; Ars; Bell; Calc; Merc; Nux-v; Puls; Pyrog; Rhus-t; Sep; Sul-i.

RELATED: Graph; Psor; Sel; Syph.

SULPHURICUM ACIDUM

GENERALITIES: Weakness or debility common to all acids is felt more by the action of this acid, esp. in DIGESTIVE TRACT, giving a very relaxed feeling in the stomach, with a craving for stimulants. Weakness is out of proportion to the disease from some deep–seated dyscrasia. It affects the *blood* and blood-vessels, causing *hemorrhage*–violent, thin black blood from all orifices. Veins (of feet) distended. Purpura hemorrhagica. Removes long–lasting black and blue spots, with soreness and stiffness of the part, after trauma; follows Arnica. TREMBLING INTERNAL, wants to be held. *Sourness* of the body, stomach. Suited to *topers,* old persons, esp. women in climacteric years, weak children with no other complaint. *Profuse acrid or stringy discharges.* Parts feel stiff and tight. *Pains increase gradually and end abruptly. Feels a blunt plug being driven in. Great painfulness.* Pains felt during sleep. Disappear on waking. Gnawing pains. Lead–poisoning. Gangrene following mechanical injury. Burning, darting pains. Shocks as from pain. Ulcers become red and blue, and painful. Writer's cramp.

WORSE: *Open air. Cold. Alcohol. Injury;* surgical operation. Concussion of brain. ODOR OF COFFEE. *Climacteric.* Towards evening. Excessive heat or cold. Touch. Pressure. Sprain. Lifting arms. Drinking cold water.

BETTER: Hot drink. *Hands near head.* Moderate temperature. Warmth.

MIND: *Must do everything in great hurry.* Sullen, impatient, angry, because things move so slowly. Fretful and *irritable* over the slightest cause, nervous fatigue and tendency to take fright. Vacillating and morose. Unwilling to answer questions, says yes or no with difficulty. Constant crying or weeping. Thinks no one does anything to please him. Seriousness alternating with buffoonery.

HEAD: Brain feels loose in forehead falling from side to side, < walking in open air, > sitting quiet in room. Compressive pain in occiput, > by holding hand near head. Thrust in temples (right) as if a plug were driven in. Electric–like shock in forehead, temples. Hair falls out, turn grey.

EYES: Intra-ocular hemorrhage following trauma. Eyelids difficult to open. Sensation of a lump in outer canthi which moves to inner canthi on closing eye and returns on opening. Eyes smart, burn. Lacrimation while reading.

EARS: Feeling as if a leaf were lying before ear.

NOSE: Oozing of dark thin blood, < odor of coffee; in old people.

FACE: *Deathly pale* or wrinkled. Feels white of an egg had dried on it.

MOUTH: Aphthae during protracted disease, esp. in children with marasmus. Gums bleed easily. Offensive breath. Pyorrhea. Destruction of teeth in diabetes mellitus. Bloody saliva from mouth. Ulcers spread rapidly.

THROAT: Sore. Stringy lemon-yellow mucus hangs from posterior nares in diphtheria. Looks white-washed. Liquids regurgitate on swallowing.

STOMACH: Heartburn. Sour eructations, sets teeth on edge. Craves brandy and fruits. Hiccough, of drunkards; *nausea*, with shivering. Vomiting sour of drunkards, < lying on left side. Weak, relaxed feeling at stomach, < after stools. Drinks chill the stomach, and are rejected unless mixed with liquor. Vomits mucus instead of food. Coughs before vomiting, during pregnancy. Sweats after eating, esp. warm food. Averse to smell of coffee.

ABDOMEN: Colic with sensation as if hernia would protrude. Spleen enlarged, hard, painful on coughing. *Diarrhea* of very foul, green, black or *hacked* stools; stools orange yellow. Diarrhea from unripe fruit and oysters; from least indigestion. Piles ooze moisture. Rectum feels as if it has a big ball; hemorrhoidal tumor prevents stools. Sinking sense in abdomen after stools.

URINARY: Pain in the bladder if urging for urinating is not attended to. Hematuria.

FEMALE: Distressing nightmares before menses, or after menses. Erosion of cervix in the aged, easily bleeding. Flushes of heat followed by sweat and a feeling of tremor all over the body during climacteric. Menses too early and too profuse. Acrid, burning leukorrhea. Gangrene of vagina, after prolapse. Prolapse of vagina and uterus from weakness.

RESPIRATORY: Cough, then eructations or vomiting. Bloody expectoration during climaxis. Larynx moves up and down violently and rapid motion of alae nasi during dyspnea, > hanging down legs.

BACK: Weakness of spine, cannot sit or stand. Large abscess on right side of neck.

EXTREMITIES: Fingers jerk while writing. Writers, cramp. Knees painfully weak. Ankles weak, cannot walk. Jerking of fingers during sleep. Jerking of the tendons.

SKIN: Cicatrices turn red and blue and become painful. Ecchymoses. Carbuncles, boils, gangrene. Itching all over the body. Nodular urticaria. Bed–sore; abscess.

FEVER: HOT *flushes*, more in upper parts, then trembling or cold sweat, < after warm ingesta, < upper parts, > motion. Drenching sweats. Disproportionate weakness during fevers like typhoid.

COMPLEMENTARY: Puls.

RELATED: Ars; Lach; Sep.

SULPHUR IODATUM

GENERALITIES: Obstinate skin affections; painless enlargement of glands; infiltration of tissues with thickening and induration after inflammation are marked features of Sul-i. *Weakness as from influenza.* Prostration, sensitive to everything. Faint and sick. *Raw burning heat internally with external coldness.* Acrid discharges. Single parts, fingers etc., turn white and insensible. *Suppuration. Favors reabsorption.*

WORSE: *Exertion* even slight. *Heat.* Lying on right side. Before storm. Night. Stooping.

BETTER: Cool air. Standing. Expectoration. Winter.

MIND: Dread of exertion. Doubtful. Hurried, impatient, sad.

HEAD: Ache, > sundown. Hair seems erect. Vertigo, < stooping, binding of the hair, fasting, before and during menses.

EYES: Zigzag before vision.

FACE: Suppurating acne. Parotid hypertrophy after mumps.

MOUTH: Teeth feel soft. Tongue *glazed;* thickened after inflammation. Raw, dry, wants to moisten it. Cold sores on lips.

THROAT: Raw, dry; painful in swallowing. Uvula and tonsils enlarged and red.

STOMACH: Anorexia. Tremor in epigastrium on exertion. Appetite increased in marasmus of children.

ABDOMEN: Mesenteric disease. Stubborn constipation. Bright yellow stools. Foul anal discharge.

URINARY: Urine scanty, purulent; brown sand in urine. Smells like raspberries. Stricture after gonorrhea, painful urination, stream twisted. Burning at the end of penis, dull pain in prostate.

MALE: Testes soft. Deficient erections. Prepuce cracked. Hydrocele of small boys.

FEMALE: Irregular menses and copious thick, burning, leukorrhea, < before and after menses.

RESPIRATORY: Breathing asthmatic, irregular, rattling and suffocative. Spasmodic Cough < a.m. Expectoration greenish, purulent, copious, viscid and yellow. Chest constricted, dropsy of pleura, and eruptions on chest.

EXTREMITIES: Aching soreness below knees. Soles of feet ache, burn and become sore when standing.

SKIN: *Itching.* Ulcers. Moist eczema. Acne, suppurating. Barbers' itch.

FOLLOWS: Sulph.

SUMBUL

GENERALITIES: Musk root as its name implies closely resembles in its odor to musk. Therefore like Moschus it is the remedy for hysterical and *nervous affections*. It affects heart causing nervous palpitation. The patient is nervous, irritable and sleepless. Tendency to faint from slightest cause. Chorea, constant jerking of the head and limbs with protrusion of the tongue. Feels hot water flowing through parts. Yellow tenacious discharges. Numbness on becoming cold of left side. Neuralgia. Early senility. Sclerosed arteries. Flushings, climacteric.

WORSE: Motion. Climacteric. Music. Cold. Thinking of symptoms. Inspiration.

BETTER: Gentle motion. Warmth.

MIND: Emotional and fidgety. Weeps and laughs by turns. Faintness from hearing music. Fear of becoming insane.

NOSE: Tenacious yellow mucus from nose.

FACE: Sensation of a hair or cobweb on face. Neuralgia. Idiotic expression.

MOUTH: Tongue feels rough as if scraped.

THROAT: *Choking constriction,* constant swallowing, hysterical.

STOMACH: Burning waterbrash.

ABDOMEN: Full, distended and painful.

FEMALE: Sexual excitability. Ovarian neuralgia. Pulling like a string in breast (right). Climacteric flushes. Screwing pain in region of uterus (left side).

URINARY: Oily pellicle on urine.

RESPIRATORY: Short breath on any exertion. Asthma–cardiac, hysterical. Oppressed tightness in left chest, as if clogged.

HEART: Nervous palpitation in hysterical subjects or at climaxis, < least exertion and thinking of it. Sensation as if heart were beating in water. Neuralgia around left breast simulating angina pectoris. Cardiac asthma. High blood pressure due to arteriosclerosis.

BACK: Trickling along spine.

EXTREMITIES: Left arm aches, heavy, numb, weary.

SKIN: Pale; cold. Internal itching.

SLEEP: Dreams of falling, of coitus, followed by sudden profuse emission.

COMPLEMENTARY: Lact-v.

RELATED: Asaf; Mosch.

SYMPHORICARPUS RACEMOSA

GENERALITIES: Highly recommended remedy for persistent vomiting of pregnancy. Aversion to all food. Nausea, < during menses, by motion, better by lying on back. Smell and thought of food repugnant.

SYMPHYTUM

GENERALITIES: Common name Knit–bone or bone-set gives the indication for this remedy. *Injuries* to CARTILAGES PERIOSTEUM with excessive pain. Painful old injuries. Comminuted FRACTURE. Pricking, stitching pains remaining after wound is healed, < touch. Irritable stump after operation. Non-union of fracture. Penetrating wound to perineum. *Deficient callus*. Affects the joints. Arthralgia of knee. External application disposes the swelling due to injury. Psoas abscess. Sarcomatous tumor.

WORSE: Injury. Blow from blunt instrument. Touch. Sexual excess.

HEAD: Ache changing place.

EYES: *Injury to the eyes* from blunt instrument, blow, knock, etc.; eyelids spasmodically close.

FACE: *Injuries to face*. Malignant growth of right antrum.

STOMACH: Ulcer of the stomach. Pain about navel, < sitting.

BACK: Backache from excessive sexual indulgence, wrestling, viplent motion. Caries of vertebrae.

SKIN: Cold.

RELATED: Arn; Calc-p.

SYPHILINUM

GENERALITIES: A nosode prepared from syphilitic virus. It affects the *mucous membranes, nerves* and *bones. In chronic cases* when *reaction is poor* and the indicated remedy gives partial relief, esp. when there is hereditary tendency to alcoholism or Syphilitic Taint. Great weakness with very few symptoms, or utter *prostration and debility* in the morning on waking. *Multiphase symptoms. Ulceration* stubborn. Dwarfed, shrivelled up, old–looking babies and children, bald head, pouting lips and big belly. Foul odor of the body. Violent, or linear pains. *Succession of abscess.* Foul or green pus. Knots in muscles. Pains or other conditions < and > gradually. Epilepsy < after menses. Foetid discharges. Persistent pains in any part of the body. Cold pain. Crying infants who begin crying immediately after birth. Slowly advancing hemiplegia. Sensation as of hot water in blood vessels. Bones sore; caries, curvature. Exostoses. Glands enlarged. Hodgkin's disease. *Sawing pain in bones.*

WORSE: NIGHT. *Sundown to sunrise.* Damp. Extreme heat or cold. Every alternate full moon. During thunder-storm. In any position. Motion. Raising arms laterally. Squatting. Winter. Summer. Sea–shore. Protruding tongue.

BETTER: Continued or slow motion. Changing position. High altitude. Applied heat. During day.

MIND: *Hopeless despair of recovery. Antisocial. Horrid depression.* Cross, irritable, peevish. Feels as if going insane or being paralyzed. Far–away feeling; says he is not himself and he cannot feel like himself, with apathy and indifference to future. *Impulse to wash hands.* Terrible dread of night. Loss of memory, does not remember faces, names, events, places, etc. but remembers everything previous to his disease. Very nervous, laughs or weeps without cause. Does not want to be soothed. Nightly delirium. Syphilitic insanity. *Aversion to company.* Sad and lamenting.

HEAD: *Deep crushing head pain* across the base or temples. Linear head pain. Beats head against wall. Feels pulled back. Cerebral softening. Hair falls profusely. Vertex bursting. Tubercles all over the scalp.

EYES: Chronic recurrent phlyctenular keratitis, > cool bathing. Intense photophobia and lacrimation. Ophthalmia neonatorum. Glimmering vision. Vertical *diplopia. Ptosis.* Feeling of cold air blowing on the eye. Squint. Amaurosis; atrophy of optic nerve. Spots on cornea.

EARS: Deafness without any obvious cause; nervous deafness with cachexia. Calcareous deposit on tympanum. Abscess of the middle ear.

NOSE: Ozena–offensive, thick yellow-green discharge. Painful to inhaled air. Sinuses painful. Green lumps from posterior nares. *Snuffles.* Caries of bones. Septum perforated. Saddle across the bridge of the nose to which

Sepia saddle is but a shadow. Attacks of fluent coryza. Itching nostrils.

FACE: Pale, wrinkled; old look. Twitching of muscles. Pain over eye (right), < protruding tongue. Paralysis of one side with difficult speech and mastication, twitching of eyes and lids.

MOUTH: *Teeth feel sticky.* Sensation of a worm in mouth. Teeth cupped in children. Feeling as if teeth, had all got out of place. Teeth decay at the edge of gums. Tongue; coated, indented; deep longitudinal cracks along center, ulcers smart and burn. Putrid taste before epileptic fit. *Excessive flow of saliva, runs out of mouth during sleep.* Aphasia. Paralysis of tongue. Toothache, > pressing them together, < hot or cold things.

THROAT: Sore right to left, < cold drink. Chronic hypertrophy of tonsils with syphilitic taint.

STOMACH: Capricious appetite. *Craves alcoholic liquor.* Aversion to meat. Total loss of appetite for months. No food agrees or satisfies him. Vomiting for weeks or months.

ABDOMEN: Obstinate constipation. Rectum seems tied up with strictures. Fissures in anus and rectum. Water from enema escapes with pain. Diarrhea bilious, painless < sea shore. Drives her out of bed about 5 A.M.

URINARY: Urine frothy, scanty, yellow. Nocturnal enuresis. Passes urine better while standing. Urinates only once during 24 hours but profuse.

MALE: Nodular formation in testes, spermatic cord and scrotum. Chancres. Aching of genitals, cannot sit still.

FEMALE: Menses having putrid meat-like odor. Yellow, offensive, *acrid leukorrhea so profuse,* it soaks through napkins and runs to the heels; with ovarian pain; in sickly nervous women; with itching of the genitals.

Habitual abortion. Mammae sensitive to touch, feel sore. Ulcers on the vulva with ovarian pain; sensitive to touch. Cutting pain in ovary during coition at the moment of orgasm.

RESPIRATORY: Cough dry at night, < lying on right side. Aphonia before menses. Chronic asthma < in summer, during thunderstorm, at night, in humid weather. Continuous pain in the larynx, < touch.

HEART: Pain from base to apex of heart. Large soft pulse. Sensation of hot water flowing in the veins.

NECK & BACK: Neck feels short. Pain in the back in the region of kidney, < after urinating. Pain at coccyx with sensation as if it is swollen, < sitting.

EXTREMITIES: Pain at the insertion of deltoid, < from raising arm laterally. Pain in front. Affections of *middle fingers*. Osteo-sarcoma in center of tibia. Itching eruptions about elbows. *Cold pain* in legs. Festination. *Bones pain as if sawed.* Bilateral exostoses sore and painful. Shin bones painful, > pouring cold water. Sciatica, < at night. Muscles knotted in rheumatism. Soles painful with feeling of contraction, < standing on them. Cannot sit on low chair or squat.

SKIN: Swollen and blotched. Biting as by bugs. Wandering erysipelas. Conical crusts. Bullae. White or pock–mark cicatrices. Distorted nails. Coppery spots.

SLEEP: *Sleeplessness.*

FEVER: Chilly. Sweats at night, with exhaustion.

RELATED: Aur; Kal-i; Merc; Nit-ac.

TABACUM

GENERALITIES: Tobacco, though widely used as snuff, for smoking and chewing, is used as medicine only in homeopathy. Vagus, sympathetic, cerebro-spinal nerves and HEART are prominently affected. It produces complete *prostration and relaxation* of the entire muscular system, with *free secretions*–vomiting, sweat; lacrimation, salivation, etc. *Constriction of the muscles of hollow organs*–throat, bladder, rectum, chest, etc. Cramps then paralysis of bowels, heart, etc. Convulsion, head firmly drawn back. Jerking throughout the body. Trembling. Faintness. Stormy, dangerous cases with rapid changes. Pains < from heat. Excessive emaciation esp. of the muscles of back and cheeks. Gait slow and shuffling, unsteady; difficulty in ascending stairs. Angina pectoris with coronary sclerosis and high tension. Feeling of seasickness. Tetanus. Paralysis of sphincters. Slides in bed. Effects of sunstroke. Palliative for bee-sting and mosquito bites.

WORSE: MOTION *of boat, riding* Lying; on left side. Opening eyes. Evening. Extremes of heat or cold.

BETTER: *Cold* application. Fresh air. Twilight. Uncovering abdomen. Weeping. Vomiting.

MIND: Very despondent. *Indifferent.* Morose; sensation of extreme wretchedness. Forgetful; slow perception. Confusion. Mental fag. Idiotic; epileptic idiocy. Silly talk. Feels as if someone were coming to arrest him or murder him.

HEAD: *Excessive vertigo* with copious sweat (cold), < on opening eyes. Sudden pain as if struck by a hammer, < while passing urine. Tight feeling as from a band. Periodical sick headache.

EYES: Loss of sight on looking steadily at any white object. Sudden loss of vision without lesion, followed by atrophy of optic nerve. Central color scotoma. Dim sight, sees through a veil. Retina retains the image too long.

EARS: Hearing music causes pain in the ears. Meniere's disease with feeling of sea-sickness.

NOSE: Secretion increased.

FACE: *Deathly pale*, blue, *pinched*, sunken. Covered with cold sweat. One cheek hot and glowing, other pale. Spasms of the lower jaw. Pain in maxillary joint, < laughing. Lips retracted. Emaciation of face.

MOUTH: Salivation. *Spits much*, with other complaints. Speech difficult.

THROAT: Violent constriction of throat in angina pectoris.

STOMACH: *Deathly nausea and violent vomiting, < least motion,* > uncovering abdomen; nausea with much spitting and during pregnancy. Sea-sickness. Terrible faint, *sinking feeling at pit of stomach.* Vomiting of fecal matter. Retching. Acidity.

ABDOMEN: Pressure in hepatic region as from a heavy body. *Wants it uncovered,* it lessens nausea, vomiting and other distresses. Horrible colic, must shriek, with weakness. Involuntary watery or thick curdled stools like sour milk. Cholera infantum. Intestinal obstruction. Strangulated hernia. *Sinking feeling in epigastrium,* with dreadful faint sensation. Retraction of navel; abdominal muscles contracted. Habitual constipation.

URINARY: Renal colic with cold sweat and deathly nausea. Paralysis of sphincters, urine dribbles. Enuresis.

MALE: Nocturnal emissions. Impotency. Hyperesthesia and neuralgia of penis.

FEMALE: Morning sickness. In climacteric period and during menses excessive sense of wretchedness. Leukorrhea of serous fluid, < after menses. Severe itching of the whole body during pregnancy.

RESPIRATORY: Violent constriction of chest. Cough dry, teasing, must take a swallow of cold water followed by hiccough or with hiccough.

HEART: Violent palpitation, < lying on left side. Twisting about the heart. Angina pectoris with nausea, cold sweat and collapse. Unsteady heartbeat. Acute dilatation caused by shock or physical exertion. Pulse thready, intermittent, hard, cord–like, imperceptible.

NECK & BACK: Head drawn back in convulsions. Neck stiff. Emaciation of the muscles of back. Pain in the small of back, < lying, > while walking. Heat down spine.

EXTREMITIES: Finger tips fuzzy. Cramp in single finger, < washing. Legs and hands icy cold. Formication.

SKIN: Itching as from flea–bites.

SLEEP: Insomnia with dilated heart. Nightmare. Stupefying sleep at night.

FEVER: *Icy cold skin.* Heat down spine, of one cheek; internal. Sudden *cold sweat* with chill, angina pectoris, renal colic, etc.

COMPLEMENTARY: Op.

RELATED: Ars; Gels; Verat.

TARAXACUM

GENERALITIES: Affecting *liver* it is a bilious remedy. Feeling of *sickness* and exhaustion, inclined to sit or lie down. Stitching pains. Jaundice, gall–stone, enlarged indurated liver.

WORSE: *Rest.* Sitting. Standing. Lying down.

BETTER: Walking. Touch.

MIND: Depression. Constant muttering to himself. Shuns labor, but after beginning works well. Inclined to talk, laugh, and be merry.

HEAD: Ache due to gastric disturbances. Vertex feels very hot.

MOUTH: Tongue coated, *with raw patches; mapped*. Taste bitter, sour. Salivation with sensation of larynx being pressed shut.

THROAT: Hawks sour mucus.

STOMACH: Gastric, bilious attacks. Loss of appetite. Bitter eructations.

ABDOMEN: Sensation of bubbles bursting in bowels. Hysterical tympanitis. Liver enlarged and indurated. Bilious diarrhea. Stools white. Jaundice. Pain in the region of liver and spleen.

URINARY: Urination painless, urging, frequent, copious discharge.

FEMALE: Menses suppressed.

NECK & BACK: Tearing pain from ear down to neck. Sternomastoid muscle very painful to touch.

EXTREMITIES: Limbs restless. Fingertips cold (a guiding symptom). Jerking pain in calf (right), > on touch. Tearing pains in limbs. Neuralgia of knee, > pressure. Toes burn.

FEVER: Chilly after eating, esp. after drinks. Profuse night–sweats.

RELATED: Nux-v.

TARENTULA CUBENSIS

GENERALITIES: The poison of this spider affects the cellular tissues. It is a toxemic medicine useful in septic conditions, when incubation is slow but further progress is *rapid, with alarming prostration, atrocious burning or sharp stinging pain. Board–like* HARDNESS OF AFFECTED PART and *copious sweat.* Diphtheria with intense fever and numb aching. Malignancy. Carbuncle. *Bluish,* painful abscess. *Felon.* Remedy for *pain of death, soothes the last agony.* Paralysis then convulsions Bubonic plague. Gangrene.

WORSE: Cold drinks. Exertion. Night.

BETTER: Tobacco smoking.

MIND: Nervous restlessness.

HEAD: Fullness in head. Meningitis.

STOMACH: Tendency to vomit.

URINARY: Cannot hold urine on coughing. Retention of urine. Urine hot, thick.

FEMALE: Pruritus vulvae.

RESPIRATORY: Spasmodic difficulty of breathing. Shattering cough; pertussis.

EXTREMITIES: Trembling hands. *Fidgety feet.* Unsteady gait.

SKIN: Feels puffed all over. *Purple discoloration.* Pungent burning. Senile ulcer.

SLEEP: Drowsiness. Prevented by harsh cough.

FEVER: *Pungent heat of surface.*

RELATED: Anthraci; Lat-m.

TARENTULA HISPANIA

GENERALITIES: 'Tarantism' is the term applied to the dancing mania set up in persons bitten by the Tarn; the cure is music and dancing. These symptoms give a key–note indication of this remedy. It affects the NERVES which are highly strung producing remarkable nervous symptoms–hysteria, chorea, many times reflex from generative sphere. HEART, *spine,* RESPIRATION and right side are also prominently affected. Symptoms appear suddenly with VIOLENCE. The patient is *restless, fidgety, hurried,* in constant motion, though walking <. *Rolls on ground from side to side,* strikes vehemently with his feet or rolls the head and rubs it to relieve her distress. Quivering, *jerking, trembling, twitching. Synalgias* or associated pains–pain headache with pain in uterus, throat with eye pain, face pain with stomach pain, pain in the ear with hiccough, etc.; or pains from sexual excitement. Violent pain, neuralgia, as if thousands of needles were pricking. Deep septic conditions; abscess, evacuates pus rapidly. Noma. Emaciation, < of face. Ill effects of unrequited love, bad news, scolding, punishment, fall, sepsis. Can: run better than walk. Irregular movements. Numbness with prickling. Emaciation, as if the flesh fairly fell off the bones. Cancer; fibrous tumor. Its action is similar to Ars. in many symptoms, therefore, when *Ars.* seems indicated but fails, it is advisable to give Tarent.

WORSE: Periodically, yearly, at the same hour. TOUCH. *Cold. Noise. Damp.* Evening. After menses. Coitus. Washing head. Seeing others in trouble. Hands in cold water. Music.

BETTER: Relaxation. *Rubbing. Sweating.* Smoking. Music. *Open air.* Riding in a carriage. In the sun. Bright color.

MIND: Aversion to colors black, red, yellow, *green.* Dances up and down. Fits of nervous laughter, then screaming. *Suddenly* changing mood, fancy or strength. *Lacks control. Erratic.* Impulsive. Moral depravity. Crafty, *cunning.* Selfish. Destructive, destroys whatever she can lay hand on, tears her clothes, etc. Hateful. Adroit. Throws things away. Malingering; when there are no observers there is no hysteria; when attention is directed to her, she begins to twitch, feigns fainting, insensibility, but looks sideways to observe the effect on those around her. Desire to strike herself or others. Laughs, mocks, runs, dances, jesticulates, jokes, cries, sings till hoarse or exhausted. Kleptomania. Angry despair. Death agony. Ungrateful. Melancholy. Discontended. Mental symptoms > P.M., after eating.

HEAD: Vertigo, < carrying burden on head. Sensation a of needles pricking the brain. Heavy pain in temples extending to face and neck, with nausea and impatience. Violent crushing *headache* as accompaniment to many ailment. Wants hair brushed, pulled, or head rubbed. Meningitis. Sensation as if cold water were poured on head and body. Vertigo at night, when descending stairs.

EYES: Itching of the eyes with thick tears. Stitching in eyes as from sand or thorn. Photophobia. One pupil dilated other contracted. Eyes wide open spasmodically, staring. Sees ghosts, faces, flashes.

EARS: Snapping, cracking in ears (right) with pain and hiccough. Noises; ringing, < on waking, in the morning.

NOSE: Epistaxis > throbbing carotids and fullness of head.

FACE: Fiery red, bloated. Expression of terror. Wrinkled.

MOUTH: Dry. Tongue drawn backward preventing speech.

STOMACH: Craving for sand or raw food. Aversion to meat, bread. Gastric disturbances are accompanied by sympathetic pain in head, face, teeth, etc. Thirst for cold water. Bitter eructations, hysterical. Vomits all food eaten.

ABDOMEN: Burning in hypogastrium with great weight, interferes with walking. Stools oily, black, offensive, excited by washing head. Severe constipation not relieved by purgatives or enema. Constipation with involuntary passing of urine on coughing or any effort.

URINARY: Urine foul, with sandy sediment. Incontinence on laughing, coughing, etc. Diabetes mellitus. Polyuria.

MALE: Extreme sexual excitement. Lasciviousness almost to insanity, < coition. Prostatic ailments after masturbation. Seminal emission hot, bloody. *Sensitive genitals.* Indolent tumor of testicles.

FEMALE: *Itching* vulva and vagina, < scratching. Pruritus vulvae. Violent nymphomania, < coitus. Dry, hot, RAW, menses. Profuse with erotic spasms. Menses early. Sensation of motion in uterus like due to fetus, or burning. Anguish, malaise in sexual organs. Expulsion of gas from uterus. Cancer of cervix. Leukorrhea of clear acrid sticky lumps. Ovaries sensitive to pressure.

RESPIRATORY: Attacks of SUFFOCATION with crying, screaming and restlessness, must have fresh air, < coughing. Cough gagging, when expectorating, fatiguing, < after coition, noise, > smoking.

HEART: Twists around, takes sudden jumps. Trembling and thumping of heart as from bad news or fright. Diseases of heart < by wetting hands in cold water. Chorea cordis, with arm symptoms. Pulse hard, infrequent, irregular.

NECK & BACK: *Painfully sensitive spine,* touch excites pain in chest, heart, etc. Coccygodynia, > standing, < slightest movement, touch. Tumors around vertebral column.

EXTREMITIES: Restless arms, *keeps hands busy,* picks fingers. Legs restless, impulse to walk. Festination. Can run better than walk. Cold moist feet and hands. Soles itching. Sawing bone pains. Extraordinary contractions, movements erratic. Weak legs, cannot plant them firmly, they do not obey will. Kneeling difficult.

SKIN: *Purplish.* Ecchymosed spots. Cold spots, or feels cold matter flowing or dropping on part. Carbuncle. Deep abscess. Helps evacuation of pus. Dry eczema (after the failure of Ars. and Sulph.), itching. Sensation of insects creeping and crawling.

SLEEP: *Sleepless* before midnight from excitement. Dreams sad, with weeping.

FEVER: *Alternate chill and heat.* General heat with cold feet. Septic fever. Sweat profuse, excoriating.

COMPLEMENTARY: Ars.

RELATED: Agar; Mygal.

TELLURIUM

GENERALITIES: This metal irritates the skin, affects *the spinal* column, ears and eyes; produces neuralgic pain, notably sciatica. *Discharges* are *acrid,* excites itching, vesicates any part of the skin it touches. The odor of the body and sweat is offensive and garlic–like; ear discharge smells of fish–brine. Salt taste, mucus from throat, pus, etc. Sharp quick pain, then soreness. *Numbness.* Sense of retention. Periosteitis. Linear pains. Ill effects of spinal injury, fall.

WORSE: *Touch. Lying on affected part. Cold.* Empty swallowing. Spinal injuries. Weekly. Cold weather. Friction. Stooping. Laughing. Coughing. Straining at stool.

MIND: Fear of being touched in sensitive place. Neglectful and forgetful.

HEAD: Vertigo, < when falling to sleep, > lying perfectly quiet. Linear head pains.

EYES: Lids thickened, inflamed, itching. Pterygium. Watery eyes. Cataract following ocular lesions. Feels lashes of lower lids turned in.

EARS: *Inflamed, bluish, puffy.* Hearing impaired from injury to membrana tympani. Otorrhea of fish-brine odor. Eczema behind the ears with thick crust. Itching, swelling, throbbing in meatus. Constant pain deep in ear.

NOSE: Fluent coryza with lacrimation and hoarseness, < when walking in open air, but > after being in open air for some time. Hawks salty mucus from posterior nares.

FACE: Twitching and distortion of facial muscles, < when talking. Pain jerks angle of mouth up. Sudden flush of redness. Barber's itch.

MOUTH: Breath has odor of garlic.

THROAT: Sore on empty swallowing, > after eating or drinking.

STOMACH: Craving for apples. Rancid belchings. Retching ends in yawning. Vomits after eating rice. Sensation of weakness or emptiness.

ABDOMEN: Pinching. Flatus stinking, offensive. Itching of anus and perineum after every stool.

RESPIRATORY: Pain in the muscles of chest, as if sprained, < raising arms. Cough causes pain in the small of back. Pain in region of clavicle. Bubbling in lungs (R).

HEART: Dull pain over heart, > lying on back.

NECK & BACK: Numbness of nape and occiput. *Painful sensitiveness of spine* (from last cervical to fifth dorsal).

Pain in sacrum passing into right thigh, < coughing, laughing; pressing at stool.

EXTREMITIES: Deep sciatic pain, < coughing, sneezing, straining at stools, lying. Sensitive spine. Contraction of tendons in the bend of knee. Fetid foot–sweat. Sweat in axilla smelling like garlic.

SKIN ; Circular, eruptions, lesions. Ringworm, cover the whole body–lower limbs, single parts, scrotum, perineum, etc. Itching pricking; as from bug-bites. Burning in old scar. Barber's itch. Itching, < in cool air.

SLEEP: Yawning after retching or with belching. Drowsy after meals.

FEVER: Chilly with pain. Chill felt down spine while lying on back. Sweat on spots with itching.

RELATED: All-c; Sel.

TEREBINTHINA

GENERALITIES: Oil of turpentine has a selective affinity for *mucous membranes* of KIDNEY and bladder, *as also for respiration,* bronchi, heart and blood. HEMORRHAGE passive, black, offensive, oozing from mucous membranes. Affection of kidneys with rheumatism. *Aching, soreness* and *stiffness* of muscles. *Purpura hemorrhagica.* Pain *excites urination.* Pain along large nerves with sensation of coldness in the nerves, or occasionally felt like hot water running through a tube. *Burning* in various parts–tip of tongue, epigastrium, small of back, kidney, *uterus,* etc. Exhausted, *sensitive* and tired. Disturbed sense of equilibrium. Ill effects of alcohol, fall, strain, tooth extraction. Every trifle bruises him.

WORSE: *Dampness.* Cold. Night. Lying. Pressure.

BETTER: Motion. Stooping.

MIND: Difficult concentration; intense irritability, children fly into temper during dentition. Coma.

HEAD: Sensation of a band around the head. Dull headache with colic.

EYES: Blindness from alcohol. Opens eyes when swallowing in coma. Eyes dark red face red on affected side.

EARS: Own voice sounds unnatural. Noise in ears as striking of a clock. Loud talking is very painful.

NOSE: Passive epistaxis in children. Discharge of serum without coryza.

FACE: Pale, earthy, sunken. Hot flushes followed by sweat.

MOUTH: Tongue smooth, glossy, sore, red; burning in tip. STOMACH: Nausea and vomiting, with intense burning. Burning in epigastric. Nausea > loose stool. Aversion to meat Aphthae from mouth to anus. Breath cold, foul.

ABDOMEN: *Bruised soreness. Flatulence. Tympanites.* Ascites. Profuse mucous stools–watery, green, fetid. Bloody stool. Worms. Bleeding from ulcer in the intestine. Bowels feel drawn towards spine. Diarrhea, with tetanic spasms.

URINARY: Burning, drawing pain, in region of kidney. *Burning* or pain along ureters. Strangury with *bloody* urine. Urine *smoky* with coffee–ground, or thick, yellow, slimy, muddy sediment; odor of violets. Nephritis after exanthemata with violent *bronchitis.* Cystitis. Bleeding bladder. Pains alternate between navel and bladder, > walking. Urine scanty, suppressed, during dentition.

FEMALE: Intense burning in uterine region, with metrorrhagia. Metritis. Uterine disease after wearing pessary.

RESPIRATORY: Burning and tightness across chest.

Bronchial asthma or catarrh with profuse expectoration. Hemoptysis. Bloody expectoration. Bronchitis of children with drowsiness and retention of urine. Dyspnea.

HEART: Pulse rapid, small, thready, intermittent.

BACK: Backache and soreness in kidney affection.

EXTREMITIES: Hands feel swollen. Cramp in knees. Intense pain along the larger nerves, < damp weather. Stands with feet apart, has no power of balancing the body. Muscles stiff, walks bent like an old man. Brachial or sub-scapular neuralgia. Feeling as if pitching forward while walking.

SKIN: Purpura hemorrhagica, advancing. General sensibility increased. Unbroken chilblains with excessive itching and pulsations.

SLEEP: *Drowsiness;* with retaining of urine etc.

FEVER: Heat under the skin. Cold sweat on legs.

RELATED: Canth; Erig; Phos.

THALLIUM

GENERALITIES: This rare metal is useful for most horrible neuralgic, spasmodic shooting pains. Pains like electric shock. Numbness or formication starting in the fingers and toes extending to lower limbs involving lower abdomen and perineum. Paralysis of lower limbs. Locomotor ataxia. Tremors. Falling of hair with great rapidity after acute or exhausting diseases. Muscular atrophy.

THERIDION

GENERALITIES: Poison of this orange spider produces *hypersensitiveness of* N*ERVES*, *esp. to* N*OISE which* PENETRATES THE BODY, *affects* the teeth, causes nausea, chill and pain all over, strikes the painful parts, etc. It causes *spinal irritation*, and affects the *bones* causing caries, necrosis. Tubercular diathesis. When the best remedy fails to act, esp. in caries and necrosis. Rachitis. Bones feel broken. Phthisis. Water feels too cold. Bounding internally. Burning pains. Seasickness. Sense of duality. Effects of sunstroke. Hysteria during puberty and at climaxis. Infantile atrophy; glands enlarged with marasmus. Nodes on various parts, esp. buttocks.

WORSE: NOISE. *Touch*. CLOSING EYES. Least motion. Exertion. *Jar. Riding.* Cold. Washing clothes. Coitus. Sun.

BETTER: Rest in horizontal position. Warmth.

MIND: Time passes too quickly. Startled by the least thing. Fruitless activity; finds pleasure in nothing. Hysteria. Talkativeness and hilarity. Want of self–confidence.

HEAD: *Vertigo with nausea,* < stooping, least movement, CLOSING *eyes, kneeling.* Headache felt during sleep, < jarring. Headache with nausea and vomiting at climaxis. Head feels thick, thinks it belongs to another, that she can lift it off, or she would like to remove it. Migraine. Headache, < after stool. Joyous during headache. Cannot lie down with headache. Faints after washing clothes.

EYES: Glittering vision on stooping. Luminous vibrations before eyes, blurred vision then affections of head and weakness.

EARS: Every sound, however least, penetrates her whole body, esp. teeth. Gushing noise in both ears like waterfall.

NOSE: Pain over root of nose. Chronic catarrh; yellow-green, thick, offensive, discharge. Ozena. Post-nasal catarrh.

FACE: Pale. Jaws immovable in the morning.

MOUTH: Remains open involuntarily, cannot close. Froth before the mouth with shaking chill. Cold water is too cold. To the teeth. Mouth feels furred, benumbed. Lock-jaw at a.m. on waking. Bites tip of tongue during sleep.

STOMACH: Constant desire to eat and drink but knows not what. Craves oranges and bananas, tobacco smoke, wine, acid fruits and drinks. Nausea, < least motion, looking steadily at one object, noise. Nausea and retching, > drinking warm water.

ABDOMEN: Violent burning in liver region. Abscess of liver. Pain in the groins after coitus, motion, and drawing up the limbs.

URINARY: Increased urination at night, does not pass much during day.

MALE: Seminal emission during afternoon sleep. Gonorrhea. Prostate enlarged, sense of a lump and heaviness in perineum, < at every step.

FEMALE: Hysteria during puberty, at climaxis. Menses suppressed.

RESPIRATORY: *Pain at end of left floating rib. Cough* jerks body together, head forward and knees upward. Too much air seems to enter the chest. Stitches high up in chest going back through apex of left lung. Phthisis. Breathing difficult going up and down stairs.

HEART: Anxiety about the heart; sharp pain radiates to arm and left shoulder. Pulse slow with vertigo.

NECK & BACK: Spine is sensitive to pressure and jar, sits sideways in a chair, to avoid pressure.

EXTREMITIES: Burning in upper arm. Restless feeling in hands, wrings them. Stinging from elbow to shoulder. Lies or sits with feet crossed, cannot uncross them.

SKIN: *Stinging thrusts in skin.* Itching.

FEVER: Foam at mouth with shaking chill. Internal coldness. Cold sweat easily excited.

RELATED: Asar; Sil.

THIOSINAMINUM

GENERALITIES: A chemical derived from oil of mustard, it acts as a resolvent externally and internally for cicatrices, adhesions, strictures, tumors, enlarged glands. Should be given in half grain doses 2 or 3 times a day of 2x attenuation.

THUJA OCCIDENTALIS

GENERALITIES: Dr. Hahnemann found Thuja an antidote to sycotic miasm. It acts chiefly on the mucous membranes of GENITO-URINARY *tract*, intestines, SKIN, *mind, nerves, glands,* occiput, left side. It is the remedy for *soft, exuberant, fungoid tissue*–polypi, condylomata, warts which are pediculated, black, suppressed. Hydrogenoid or lymphatic constitution. Great prostration and rapid emaciation. The patient is *exhausted* and *soft,* body feels thin and delicate, frail. Deadness of the affected part. Discharges are foul, acrid, *musty, rancid* or of *sweetish odor. Trickling* in urethra. Burning, sticking, numbing, drawing or *wandering pains,* < warmth. Oily stools, skin, sweat. Flesh feels as if beaten off the bones. Edema about the joints. Jerking of the upper part of the body of spinal origin; chorea. Sensation of lightness of body when walking. Vaccinosis–never well since vaccination–neuralgia, skin troubles, etc. Crying babies with a sycotic taint inherited from the father, from congenital inguinal hernia. Pains keep radiating from their original site. Neurasthenia, prostatic. Rheumatism. Paralysis. Suppressed gonorrhea. Ill effects of tobacco. Suppressed sycosis, figwarts. Aneurism by anastomosis; swelling of the blood-vessels. Stitching, tearing pains in the glands as if they were being torn to pieces.

WORSE: COLD; DAMP heat; of bed. Periodically, 3 A.M. and 3 P.M., yearly. Increasing moon. Moonlight. During menses. Urinating. Tea. Coffee. Sweets. Fat food. Onions. Sun. Chewing. Bright light. Mercury. Syphilis. Stretching. Coitus. Closing eyes.

BETTER: Warm wrapping, air, wind. *Free secretions. Sneezing*. Motion. Crossing legs. Touch. Drawing up limbs. Rubbing. Scratching.

MIND: *Fixed ideas*–as if a strange person were at his side, soul and body were separated, body fragile, made of glass, *as if a living thing were inside,* being in the hands of a stronger power. *Hurried* with ill humor; talks hastily; swallows words. Sad. Aversion to life. Overexcited, angry or anxious about trifles. Music causes weeping and trembling of feet. Nervous, begins to twitch on approach of strangers. Cannot concentrate. Insane women will not be touched or approached. Fear on seeing green stripes. Speech slow, hunts for words. Irritable, jealous, quarrelsome towards husband or mother, controls herself among strangers and doctors. Cretinism. Mental depression after child–birth. Walks in a circle in room.

HEAD: Vertigo as from motion of a swing; everything seems to jump on closing eyes, looking upwards or sideways.

Pain as if pierced by a nail. Headache, < sexual excess, tea, > bending head backwards. Tearing, jerking pain. White scaly dandruff. Hair get dry, split and fall out. Sweat smelling like honey.

EYES: Blood–red; full of tears; stand open. Lids heavy as lead. Jagged iris. Iritis. Scleritis. Styes and tarsal tumors. Feels as if cold air were streaming out of the head through eye, > when warmly covered. Photopsies, beyond visual field. Floating (green) stripes. Exophthalmos; from tumor behind eyeball.

EARS: Otorrhea watery, purulent, putrid. Cracking when empty swallowing. Noise in ear as from boiling water.

NOSE: *Bloody* scabs; briny odor in nose. Blows thick, green mucus. Epistaxis, < after being over-heated.

FACE: Pale, waxy, *shiny*, dark under eyes. Netted with spider–like veins. Boring in malar bones (left), > by touch. Skin greasy. Neuralgia from suppressed gonorrhea or eczema of ear. Tumor on cheek.

MOUTH: Teeth decay at the edge of gums, crumble, turn yellow. Gnawing pain in teeth, < cold, tea and blowing nose. Pyorrhea. Ranula. Varicose veins on tongue and mouth. Aphthae; ulcers in the mouth. White blisters on sides close to the root of tongue, painfully sore. Frequently bites the tongue from swelling of it. Sweetish taste with gonorrhea. Becomes dry while chewing food.

THROAT: Much mucus in throat hawked up with difficulty.

STOMACH: *Noisy swallowing*; loud belchings. Rancid or greasy eructations. Aversion to potatoes and fresh meat. Onions disagree. Tea–drinker's dyspepsia. Unable to eat breakfast. Desires cold drinks and salt.

ABDOMEN: Big, puffed; protrudes here and there as from arm of fetus; motions as if something alive (in old maids). Induration in abdomen. Rumbling flatulence; upper part drawn in. Soreness of navel. Cutting, squeezing in hypogastrium. Ileus. Gurgling in bowels, then painless watery grass–green stools. Stools gurgle or pop out, < breakfast. Stools hard, oily, black, lump, mixed with gushing water; hurried, explosive, gassy, spraying. Cutting, squeezing in groins. Piles swollen, painful. Anus fissured, warty, oozing. Perineum moist. Tenesmus with rigidity of penis. Perineal fistula.

URINARY: Cutting, squeezing in *bladder* and urethra. Bladder feels paralyzed, must wait for urination, which is frequent, hasty, with pain in other parts; urging with profuse flow. Urine burns, dribbles, is foul. Feels as if a drop is running down urethra after urination. Forward cutting in urethra on urinating. Urinary stream split and small. Pains from left kidney to epigastrium, < motion. Lithemia. Diabetes mellitus. Involuntary urination at night when coughing. Foamy urine.

MALE: Gonorrhea, scalding when urinating. Rheumatism from checked gonorrhea. Prostatic enlargement. Offensive genitals; sweetish smelling sweat on scrotum. Testes feel bruised; left one drawn up. Swelling of prepuce. Excrescences of prepuce and glans. Chordee, < at night. Semen offensive.

FEMALE: *Vagina very sensitive,* prevents coition; itching. Left ovary inflamed with tearing pain < menses. Leukorrhea profuse, thick, greenish, from one period to another. Erosion of cervix. Fetus moves violently, awakes her. Abortion at the 3rd month. Cauliflower-like excrescences, bleeding easily. Recto-vaginal fistula. Sweaty organs before menses. Retracted nipples. Menses too early, too short.

RESPIRATORY: Short difficult breathing, < deep breathing and talking. Cough only during the day, < as soon as he eats or drinks anything cold. Expectoration easy when lying down; green, taste like old cheese. Asthma, < night. Asthma of sycotic children. Chest pains take various directions. Skin of clavicles blue. Brown spots on chest. Polypus of vocal cord. In asthma, if *Ars.* fails to cure even though seems indicated, *Thuj.* and *Nat-s.* will cure.

HEART: Anxious palpitation on waking in the morning.

NECK & BACK: Pulsation in the back. Pressing pain over kidney region. Atrophy of long muscles. Spine curved. Stands bent forward. Blood–boils.

EXTREMITIES: Cracking in joints when stretching them. Fingers cold, numb, as if dead, on waking at night. Crawling or inflamed finger or toe tips. Hip–joints give way when walking. Limbs feel paralyzed. Knees restless. Nails *painful,* brittle, crumbling, discolored, distorted. Coxalgia with *tender soles.* Foul, acrid foot–sweat. Nails ribbed, soft. Ingrowing toe nails.

SKIN: Brown, *spotted, dirty,* hairy. Eruptions itch or burn violently, < cold bathing. Moist foul polypi. Nevi. Eruptions only on covered parts. Ulcers flat, with sunken apices. Luxurient growth of hair on parts otherwise not covered with hair. Herpes zoster.

SLEEP: Sleepless when lying on left side. Persistent insomnia. Dreams of death; of falling from a height.

FEVER: Shaking chill with yawning, < urinating, not > by heat. Heat rises into chest with *icy cold hands,* nose–bleed or cough. Sweat only on uncovered parts; with dry heat on covered one, with cold hands, > washing. Sweat *profuse on genitals,* gushing, < company. Sweat foul, oily, pungent, sweetish, sometimes garlicky, staining yellow.

COMPLEMENTARY: Med; Nat-m; Nat-s; Nit-ac; Puls; Sabin; Sil.

RELATED: Asaf; Calc-c; Ign; Kali-c; Lyc; Merc.

THYMOL

GENERALITIES: Considered to be a specific for hook–worm disease. Sexual neurasthenia.

THYROIDINUM

GENERALITIES: A sarcode prepared from dried thyroid gland of sheep or calf. Thyroid has close connection with the HEART. Moreover it exercises a general regulating influence on the mechanism of the organs of *nutrition, growth and development.* It affects the central nervous system, skin of the left side. A state of puffiness and obesity. Feels tired and sick, easy fatigue, wants to lie down. Fainting fits, nervous tremor of face and limbs. Stabbing, splitting, clutching sensation. Choking. Rapid emaciation. Goitre. Tingling. Myxedema, with loss of hair and cretinism. Arrested development of children. Infantile wasting. Undescended testicles in boys. Thyroid weakness causes decided craving for large quantities of sugar. Acromegaly; delayed union of fractures. TETANY, < cold. Hystero-epilepsy. Sensation as of a cold wind blowing on the body. Rheumatoid arthritis. Edema. Mammary tumor. Low blood pressure.

WORSE: Least exertion or cold. Stooping.

BETTER: Lying on abdomen or reclining position.

MIND: Stupor alternating with restless melancholy. Weeps, undresses. Homicidal tendency. Suspicious. Idea of persecution. Ill–tempered, goes into a rage over trifles, < opposition. Grumbling continuously. Laughing in a way peculiar to herself.

HEAD: Feeling of lightness in brain. Persistent frontal headache; heaviness over eyes. Falling of hair.

EYES: Exophthalmic goiter. Progressive loss of sight with central scotoma.

EARS: Sclerosis of ossicles.

NOSE: Dry indoors, runs outdoors.

FACE: Flushed. Lips dry, red, burn, with free desquamation.

MOUTH: Tongue thickly coated; metallic taste at tip.

THROAT: Dry, burning. Sensation as of a splinter stuck across the throat.

STOMACH: Desire for sweets and thirst for cold water. Vomiting of pregnancy.

ABDOMEN: Cutting in liver, < deep breathing. Rolling flatulence with gurgling, then loose gassy stool. Bearing and aching from pelvis to anterior thigh.

URINARY: Increased flow of urine. Diabetes mellitus. Urine smells of violets. Enuresis of weakly children.

FEMALE: Amenorrhea. Gnawing in uterus. Agalactia. Vomiting of pregnancy. Uterine fibroid. Mammary tumor. Puerperal convulsions, insanity.

RESPIRATORY: Larynx dry. Dry painful cough on entering a warm room, from cool air. Breathlessness, > lying in recumbent position.

HEART: *Palpitation,* < least exertion; hammering; beats felt in ear. Tachycardia. Heart pains radiate to axilla; clutching, constricting, < lying down; causes short breath. Hypertrophy after hard labor. Blood seems rushing downwards. Jumping sensation at heart. Large veins on arms and hands. Valvular diseases of heart.

EXTREMITIES: Quivering of limbs; tremors. Numbness; left fingers, then right leg. Left hand icy cold. Cold clammy hands. Abnormal growth of limbs due to excessive exertion.

SKIN: Very dry. Itching without eruptions. Psoriasis with adiposity. Icthyosis. Itching with jaundice. Peeling of skin of lower limbs. Brawny swelling. Symmetrical serpignous eruptions.

FEVER: Hot flushes, then chill or drenching sweat. Oily, musty sweat.

RELATED: Calc; Glon.

TILIA EUROPA

GENERALITIES: It causes weakness of the *muscles* and affects the female genital and urinary organs. Intense *soreness* of abdomen, *uterus,* etc. Bearing or dragging–down pains in genito-urinary and rectal region. Bed feels too hard. Edema. Neuralgia. Rheumatism. Hemorrhage of thin pale blood. THE MORE HE SWEATS THE GREATER THE PAIN.

WORSE: SWEATING. Drafts. Talking. After sleep. Walking. Sneezing.

BETTER: In cool room. Walking about in open air.

MIND: Love-sick. Dread of society.

HEAD: Neuralgia (right to left) with veil before eyes.

EYES: Sees as if a gauze before eyes. Feels as if a piece of cold iron pressed through right eye causing burning.

NOSE: Much sneezing with fluent coryza. Epistaxis.

ABDOMEN: Soreness with warm sweat which gives no relief. Peritonitis.

URINARY: Heavy dragging pain in urethra. Scanty urine.

FEMALE: Intense sore feeling about uterus; bearing down with hot sweat which does not relieve. Soreness and redness of external genitals. Puerperal metritis.

RESPIRATORY: Cough from tickling in throat.

SKIN: Urticaria. Intense itching and burning like fire after scratching.

SLEEP: *Sleepy,* < during pain.

FEVER: Profuse warm sweat soon after falling aslep without relief.

RELATED: Ap; Calc; Lil-t.

TRIFOLIUM PRATENSE

GENERALITIES: Sensation in lungs as if breathing hot air full of impurities. Preventive for mumps. Retards progress of cancerous tumor before ulceration has taken place. Use mother tincture.

TRILLIUM

GENERALITIES: Common name Birth-root, it gives the indication for its use. It is a *hemorrhagic* remedy–hemorrhage of all kinds–antepartum, postpartum, climacteric, fibroid tumour. Blood gushing, bright red, *with great faintness and dizziness. Relaxation* of pelvic region.

WORSE: *Motion.* Climaxis. Sitting erect.

BETTER: Exertion in open air. Tight bandage. Bending forward.

HEAD: Dull pain, < noise, walking, coughing, > bending forward.

EYES: Feel too large and about to fall out from their sockets. Everything looks blue.

NOSE: Profuse nosebleed.

MOUTH: Bleeding after extraction of teeth.

ABDOMEN: *Faintness and sinking* at stomach. Chronic diarrhea with bloody discharge. Dysentery with passing of almost pure blood.

FEMALE: Uterine hemorrhage with sensation as though *the bones of hips, back and thighs are forced* apart or falling to pieces, > tight bandaging. Bleeding with faintness and sinking at stomach. Menses every two weeks. Varices of pregnancy. Dribbling of urine after labor. Profuse long-lasting bloody lochial discharge. Leuckorrhea profuse, yellow, sticky.

COMPLEMENTARY: Calc-p.

RELATED: Sabin.

TROMBIDIUM

GENERALITIES: Specific in the treatment of dysentery, < by food and drink. Brown, thin, bloody stools, much pain before and after stool. Stools only after eating. Mucous discharge from nose while eating dinner.

TUBERCULINUM

GENERALITIES: This nosode is prepared either from tubercular abscess or from a glycerine extract of pure cultivation of tubercular bacilli. It affects the *mind,* LUNGS, occiput, glands and larynx. Very valuable in the treatment of incipient tuberculosis. The symptoms are *constantly changing,* begin suddenly, cease suddenly, *or of obscure nature* and when well–selected remedy fails to improve. Weakness, emaciation with good appetite.

Patient takes cold easily on slightest exposure which ends in diarrhea. Very susceptible to change of weather. Relapsing states. Always tired, motion causes intense fatigue. Increasing exhaustion and lowered vitality. Rapid breakdown. Adapted to light–complexioned, narrow–chested subjects. Scrofula; enlargement of the glands. Adenoids. TUBERCULAR TAINT. Quiverings. Mentally deficient children. Epilepsy. Neurasthenia. Very sensitive mentally and physically. Nervous weakness. Trembling. *Clothes felt damp.* When *Tub.* fails *Syph.* often follows favorably producing a reaction. This remedy should not be given when the heart is weak. Bruised pain throughout the body. Bones painful. Formication. Faintings.

WORSE: CLOSED ROOM. Motion. *Exertion.* Weather *changing*; DAMP; cold. Draft. *Awakening.* Noise. Thinking of it. Mental excitement. Music. *Pressure of waist–band.* Standing. Periodically.

BETTER: Cool wind. Open air. Motion.

MIND: SENSITIVE to music. *Every trifle irritates,* < awakening. Fits of violent temper, wants to fight, throws things at anyone even without a cause. *Dissatisfied;* always wants a change. Wants to travel, does not want to remain in one place long, wants to do something different, to find a new doctor. Weary of life. Aversion to mental work. Reckless. Fear of animals, dogs. Whines and complains with very little ailment. Desire to use foul language, curse and swear. Changing moods. Confusion; everything in the room seems strange. Nocturnal hallucinations, awakes frightened. Children awake screaming, with restlessness. Anxious. Hopeless. Loquacious; during fever. Contradictory–mania and melancholia, insomnia and stupor.

HEAD: *Deep* violent head pains; tears hair or beats head with fist or dashes against the wall or floor, < motion.

Shooting from over eyes (right) through the head to back of ear (left) or from right frontal protuberance to right occipital region. Brain feels loose. Meningitis. Sensitive scalp. Plica polonica (matted hair). Periodical headaches.

EYES: Eczema of margins of eyelids. Sore, bruised eyeballs, < turning them. Meningitis with squint.

EARS: Persistent offensive otorrhea. Perforation of tympanum with ragged edges.

NOSE: Crops of small boils, very painful successively appear in nose, green fetid pus. Sweat on nose. Cold ending in diarrhea.

FACE: Old, edematous, pale. Aching in malar bones.

MOUTH: Feeling as if the teeth were all jammed together and too many for his mouth. Teeth sensitive to air. *Delayed dentitition.* Dryness, stickiness. Black blisters on lips.

THROAT: Hawks mucus after eating. Adenoids. Dryness of the posterior nares. Enlarged tonsils.

STOMACH: *Craves cold milk* or sweets. Aversion to meat, to all food. All–gone hungry sensation which drives one to eat.

ABDOMEN: Early morning sudden diarrhea. Stools brown, *foul*, watery, discharged with much force. Tabes mesenterica. Diarrhea of children running for weeks with wasting, exhaustion and bluish pallor. Tearing in rectum on coughing. Inguinal glands indurated and visible. Drum–belly. Chronic diarrhea, with excessive sweat. Constipation, stools large and hard, then diarrhea. Spleen region bulging out; stitching pain in sides after running.

URINARY: Must strain at stool to pass water. Bed–wetting. Sticky urine sediment.

FEMALE: Menses soon after childbirth; menses too early, too profuse, long–lasting. Dysmenorrhea, pain increases with the flow. Mammary tumor, benign. Retraction of nipples. Amenorrhea. Severe pain in breast at the beginning of menses.

RESPIRATORY: SENSATION OF SUFFOCATION even with plenty of fresh air; longs for cold air. Hoarseness, > talking. Cough dry, hard, more during sleep and dyspnea. Cough with chill and red face, < evening, raising arms. Mucus rattle in chest without expectoration. Sore spot in chest. Asthma. Pneumonia after influenza. Profuse expectoration. Thick yellow or yellow–green sputum.

HEART: Heaviness and pressure over the heart. Palpitation on taking deep breath, after evening meal.

NECK & BACK: Tension in nape. Pain in back, with palpitation. Chill between shoulders or up back.

EXTREMITIES: Hands and arms feel lame, unable to write or raise a cup or a glass. Fingertips brown. Sensation of fatigue in limbs. Cold feet in bed. Limbs feel weak or paralyzed, < dinner. Acute articular rheumatism. Pains in ulnar nerve.

SKIN: Dry, *harsh,* sensitive, easily tanned; itching in cool air. Branny scale. Psoriasis. Chronic eczema. Itching changes places on rubbing.

SLEEP: Dream vivid, of shame, frightful. Awakes in horror. Shuddering sensation on falling to sleep. Restless at night and screams in sleep.

FEVER: Chilly when beginning to sleep yet wants fresh air. Heat on cheek of affected side, in spots. Flushes of heat, < eating. Burning in genitals. Sweat easy, cold, clammy; on upper parts, on hands; stains yellow < coughing. Wants covers in all stages.

COMPLEMENTARY: Bell; Calc; Kali-s; Psor; Sep; Sulph.

RELATED: Bar-c; Calc-p; Phos; Puls; Sil.

URANIUM NITRICUM

GENERALITIES: A remedy for glycosuria and increased urine. Excessive thirst, nausea, vomiting, excessive appetite. Diabetes mellitus and insipidus. Great emaciation. Debility. Tendency to ascites and general dropsy. Nephritis. High blood pressure. Burning in stomach; gastric ulcer. Incontinence of urine. Burning in urethra while passing urine. Impotency with nightly emissions. Menses suppressed during diabetes.

WORSE: At night.

BETTER: Deep breathing.

URTICA URENS

GENERALITIES: As its common name Stinging Nettle implies, it produces stinging or *stinging-burning* pains. Affects the MAMMARY GLANDS, *genito-urinary* organs, liver and spleen. Urinous odor of the body. Uric acid diathesis. *Urticaria* associated or alternating with rheumatism. Hemorrhage. Ill effects of *burn,* bee-sting, eating shell-fish, suppressed milk, urticaria. Angio-neurotic edema.

WORSE: Snow air; cold moist air. Cool bath. Yearly. Touch. Lying on arm.

HEAD: Headache with stitches in spleen.

ABDOMEN: Stools small, painful. Mucus mixed with white matter like boiled white of an egg. Intense itching of anus from pinworms. Vomiting, from suppression of urticaria.

URINARY: Acrid urine causing itching. Gravel. *Uric acid toxemia.* Urine suppressed.

MALE: Itching, burning of genitals keeps him awake.

FEMALE: *Pruritus* vulvae; itching, stinging; edema of the parts. *Diminished secretion of milk* after parturition. Swelling of the breast with stinging, burning pain. Arrests the flow of milk after weaning.

RESPIRATORY: Hemoptysis after violent exertion.

EXTREMITIES: Continuous pain in deltoid (right), could not put on the coat, < rotating arm inwards. Acute gout.

SKIN: Itching, raised red blotches. Nettlerash, every year same season. Prickly heat. *Hives* elevated, with rheumatism, after shell–fish, with pinworms. Vesicles. Burn and scald of the first degree with intense burning, itching. Apply locally.

FEVER: Sweatiness at night with vertigo, with throbbing all over the body.

RELATED: Form; Nat-m; Oci.

USTILAGO MAYDIS

GENERALITIES: Corn-smut affects the *female sexual organs,* skin, hair and nails. Congestive, passive or *slow bleeding* or in clots; blood dark but watery. *Dark hemorrhage.* Sensation of a *knot* in uterus, bowels, throat, etc. *Loss of hair and nails.* Prostration from sexual abuse. Adapted to tall thin women at climaxis.

WORSE: Climacteric. Touch. Motion.

MIND: Great depression of spirits. Weeps frequently.

HEAD: Sticky secretion matting the hair. Milk–crust. Vertigo with profuse menses. Nervous headache from menstrual irregularities.

ABDOMEN: Pain as if intestines were tied in a knot, Colicky pain, > by hard stools or constipation.

MALE: Irresistible desire to masturbation. Erotic fancies. Emisson every night and even when talking to a woman.

FEMALE: Vicarious menstruation, from lungs and bowels. Menses half liquid half clotted, bright red, < slightest provocation. Menorrhagia, of climaxis, after abortion. Oozing of dark blood, clotted, forming large black strings. Cervix spongy, easily bleeding. Acute ovarian pain (left). Burning distress in ovaries (right). Soreness of uterus and ovary (left). Pain shoots down thighs. Foul yellow or brown leukorrhea. Pain constant under left breast, at margin of ribs, between periods. Hypertrophy of uterus; sub-involution. Uterus feels drawn into a knot. Bearing–down pain when child nurses. Fibroid. Tumors have been noted to have disappeared after its use. Menses suppressed without cause with accompanying symptoms.

BACK: Sensation of boiling water flowing along the back.

EXTREMITIES: Muscular contractions of lower limbs.

SKIN: Dry, hot.

RELATED: Asaf; Bov; Sec.

VACCININUM

GENERALITIES: A nosode prepared from vaccine matter. Useful for the morbid chronic states known as vaccinosis. Neuralgia. Inveterate skin eruptions; new growth; sycotic conditions.

RELATED: Maland; Thuj.

VALERIANA

GENERALITIES: Produces over-sensitiveness of NERVES–*spinal*, genito-urinary. Affects the *mind*, muscles, calf, heels, tendo-achilles. *Mental and physical dispositions change suddenly*; and go to extreme. Pains are darting, tearing, *move outwards,* felt here and there or come and go, jump from one place to another. *Illusions* of vision, hearing, smell, or taste. Sensation of floating, duality, of a ball or plug. *Want of reaction.* Alternating symptoms. Agitation of all nerves–jerks, twitches, trembling. Restlessness, *impulse to move,* cannot keep still. *Weak single parts*–eyes, arms, wrists, popliteus, etc. Globus. Sensation of a thread hanging down from esophagus. NERVOUS, *irritable and weak* hysterical women in whom the intellectual faculties predominate and who suffer from neuralgia. Red parts turn white. Slight injury causes spasm. Early bed-sore. Epileptic fits. Paralysis and contraction of limbs, hysterical. Constant heat and uneasiness.

WORSE: REST. STANDING. *Excitement.* Evening. Open air; draft of air. Fasting. Darkness. Stooping.

BETTER: *Changing position.* Walking about. Rubbing. After sleep. Meals, breakfast.

MIND: Mental disturbances pass from one extreme of emotion to another, from greatest joy to deepest sorrow, from murmur to grumbling. Impatient, quickly passes from one subject to another. Erroneous ideas, thinks she is someone else, as if all around were strange and disagreeable. Wriggles or squirms about. Anger. Inclined to faint. Hysteria; dreads being alone and in the dark. Madness, raving, swearing. Sees, imagines animals, men.

HEAD: Aches in jerks, > moving about, < sunshine.

Coldness in upper head. Vertigo on stooping. Feels light like floating.

EYES: Brightness and light before eyes in dark room. Vision sharp. Objects seem too near. Wild look

EARS: Illusions of hearing, imagined he heard the bell tinkle. otalgia, < draft and cold.

FACE: Pain appears suddenly, jerks. Muscles twitch. Cheeks red and hot in open air.

MOUTH: Rancid greasy taste. Nausea felt in throat. Tongue thickly coated.

THROAT: Sensation of a thread with salivation and vomiting.

STOMACH: Eructations like bad eggs. Hunger with nausea as if from navel. Child vomits curdled milk in large lumps after nursing, after mother's anger. Sensation of something warm rising from the stomach and causing suffocation. Cramps in stomach.

ABDOMEN: Bloated. Cramps. *Flatulency*–hysterical. Thin, watery, diarrhea with lumps of curdled milk and violent screaming in children. Cramps, after eating, in bed at night. Draws abdomen in involuntarily.

URINARY: *Urine increased and more frequent;* in nervous women.

RESPIRATORY: Choking in throat on falling asleep. Wakes as if suffocating. Spasmodic asthma.

HEART: Stitching in heart with quick, small and weak pulse.

EXTREMITIES: Crampy pain, electric–like shock in humerus (left), wakes from sleep. Heels pain when sitting or constantly. Sciatica pain, < when standing, sitting and resting, > walking and rubbing. Constant jerking. Tensive pain in the calves, < crossing legs. Cramp in biceps (right) while writing. Cramp of hands and feet prevents sleep. Pain from calf to heel. Legs feel light after walking.

SLEEP: Sleepless, with nightly itching and muscular spasms, from nervous excitement.

FEVER: Chills go down back from occiput. Fever composed of disagreeable heat only. Sudden gushes of sweat mostly on forehead. Body ice–cold with nausea and vomiting.

RELATED: Asaf, Ign.

VANADIUM

GENERALITIES: A remedy for degenerative conditions of liver and arteries. Fatty degeneration of heart and liver. Arterio-sclerosis. Deeply pigmented patches on forehead in liver affections. Profound weakness.

VARIOLINUM

GENERALITIES: This nosode prepared from lymph of small pox pustule has proved an efficient preventive against small pox contagion and vaccinal infection. Modifies and aids in the cure of small pox. *General aching in the muscles, < in back, occiput and legs.* Calcareous deposits in the blood-vessels, spinal cord.

WORSE: Motion. *Vaccination.*

MIND: Morbid fear of small pox.

HEAD: Crazy feeling in the brain. Headache with icy coldness of feet and hands.

EYES: Green vision on rising.

MOUTH: Tongue protrudes during sleep. Foul metallic taste. Offensive mouth.

STOMACH: Every odor nauseates. Wants to regurgitate food. Vomiting of milk immediately after drinking it.

ABDOMEN: Tympanites, pouting upwards; she looks pregnant.

BACK: *Breaking backache.* Pains from back shift to abdomen.

SKIN: Sensation of bugs crawling under the skin. Eczema of palms. *Pustular eruptions;* foul. Shingles, and pain that follows. Ulcers look scooped out.

FEVER: Sensation of cold water trickling down the back. Violent chill. Intense burning fever. Foul sweat.

RELATED: Ant-t; Cimic; Maland.

VERATRUM ALBUM

GENERALITIES: White Hellebore profoundly affects the *mind,* NERVES—*abdominal, heart,* blood, blood-vessels, respiration, *vertex,* and digestive system. COPIOUS EVACUATIONS—vomiting, purging, salivation, sweat, urine, with PROFOUND PROSTRATION, COLDNESS, *blueness,* and COLLAPSE are characteristic features. EFFECTS ARE VIOLENT AND SUDDEN. It is a great FAINTING remedy—faints from emotion, least exertion, slight injury, with hemorrhage, after stool and vomiting. *Cold perspiration on the forehead* with all complaints. *Cold* as ice—breath, tongue. Tonic *spasms* or *cramps* in chest, bowels, hands, fingers, toes, soles of feet, with diarrhea. Progressive weakness and emaciation in acute diseases, whooping cough, ague, etc. Sudden sinking of strength. Paralysis after debilitating losses. Convulsions caused by religious excitement. Excessive dryness of all mucous membranes. Burning. Post-operative shock. Children feel better when carried about quickly. Blood seems to run cold; blood sepsis, pyemia. Carphology. Ill effects of fright, disappointed love, injured pride or honor; suppressed exanthema, opium, tobacco, alcohol.

WORSE: Exertion. Drinking; *cold drink*. Fright. *During pain*. Wet cold weather, change of weather. Before and during menses. Before, during, after stool. Touch, pressure. Injured pride or honor. Opium eating. Tobacco chewing.

BETTER: Warmth, covering. Walking about. Hot drink. Lying. Eating meat. Milk.

MIND: Sullen indifference. Amativeness. Haughtiness. *Delirium early,* with violence, loquacity or lewdness. Delirium during pain. Melancholy, head hangs down, sits brooding in silence, wants to be alone. Prays, curses, shrieks in turn. Desire to cut and tear things. Mania alternating with taciturnity. Insanity. Remorse. Delusion of impending misfortune. Busy restlessness. Aimless wandering from home. Deceitful, never speaks the truth. Kisses everybody before menses. Despair about position in society; feels very unlucky. Sings, whistles, laughs. Runs from place to place. Malingering, thinks herself pregnant. Puerperal mania. Nymphomania; embraces everybody, even objects. Religious mania. Talks about the faults of others or scolds. Anguish, fear of death. Despairs of her salvation. Imagines the world on fire. Swallows his own excrement. Extravagant, haughty ideas and actions. Imaginary diseases.

HEAD: Cold sweat on forehead; in all complaints. Violent pain driving him to despair, > cold. Sensation of a lump of ice on vertex. Headache; with nausea, vomiting, pale face, diarrhea, diuresis. Rubs forehead. Hair bristle, painful. Feels cold wind blowing through head. Vertex itches during headache.

EYES: Surrounded by dark rings. Turned upwards. Lacrimation with redness. Lids dry, heavy.

NOSE: Smell before nose. Tip icy cold. Nose pointed. Epistaxis from right nostril only at night in sleep.

FACE: Deathly pale on rising, *bluish*, pinched or distorted, frowning, cold; terrified look. Cheek red (left) as if burnt. Jaws cramp on chewing. Lock-jaw. Lips blue; hang down.

MOUTH: Toothache. Teeth feel heavy as if filled with lead. Grinding of the teeth. Tongue cold, pale, cool sensation as from peppermint. Taste peppermint-like. Speech lisping, stammering as if tongue was too heavy. Mouth dry, salty saliva. Water tastes bitter.

THROAT: Dry, scraping or roughness. When drinking water it seems to run outside, not going down the esophagus.

STOMACH: Burning thirst. *Craves ice water* which is vomited as soon as swallowed; wants everything cold, sour drinks, juicy fruits and salt. Vomits or eructates froth. VOMITING WITH PURGING, *violent retching*. Hiccough after hot drinks. Nausea while eating, cannot get food down without retching. Vomiting < drinking and least motion. Cold waterbrash. All fruits disagree, causes painful distension. Gnawing hunger in spite of nausea and vomiting. Voracious appetite. Potatoes and green vegetables disagree. Eating meat and drinking milk >.

ABDOMEN: Painful retraction of abdomen during vomiting. Burning pain at pit of stomach. Sinking and empty feeling. Burning or cold feeling. Watery, green, odorless or colorless (rice-water) stools or in large masses, with straining until exhausted and cold sweat. Diarrhea from drinking cold water in hot days. Peritonitis. Intussusception. Reversed peristaltic action. *Cutting colic,* as if bowels are twisted in knots, with *cramp in limbs and rapid prostration.* Cholera, morbus and infantum. Epigastrium painful. Hot coal sensation. Constipation of nursing infants or from cold weather. Stools thin like ribbon, flat.

URINARY: Urine scanty, red brown. Thick, greenish, suppressed, involuntary during cough.

FEMALE: Nymphomania before menses, from disappointed love, unsatisfied passion, in lying-in women. Dysmenorrhea with prolapse, coldness of the body, diarrhea, cold sweat, and fainting with slightest movement. Eclampsia. Puerperal mania. Menses too early, too profuse, or suppressed. Menorrhagia with nausea, vomiting, diarrhea.

RESPIRATORY: Air seems too hot. Asthma, < in damp cold weather, > bending head back. Tickling down throat into lungs. Continuous violent cough with retching, < cold drink. Rattling in chest. Neglected whooping cough with complication. Barking cough with eructations, < warm room. Involuntary urination with cough. *Loss of voice.* Cough on entering a warm room from cold.

HEART: Weak. Cutting. Visible palpitation with chorea. Pulse intermittent, feeble, slow, thready. Blood runs like cold water through venis.

NECK & BACK: Neck so weak, child can scarcely keep it erect, < whooping cough. Crampy pain between scapulae, > motion. Bruised feeling in sacral region.

EXTREMITIES: Brachial neuralgia, paralytic and bruising pain in arms. Fine burning in arms, right to left. Arms feel full and swollen. Tingling in hands and fingers. *Cramps in calves* during stool. Electric jerks in legs, must sit up and let legs hang down. Difficulty in walking like due to paralysis from debility. Pain in feet or knees as if heavy stone were tied to parts, must move about. Feet icy cold.

SKIN: Wrinkles. Feels scorched. Blue, cold.

SLEEP: Awakes at night trembling. Starts as if frightened.

FEVER: GENERAL COLDNESS. Icy *cold vertex,* nose, tongue, mouth, limbs, sweat. Internal heat with cold surface when drinking. Fevers showing external coldness only. Congestive chill with thirst.

COMPLEMENTARY: Carb-v.

RELATED: Ars; Camph; Cupr; Cyanides; Tub.

VERATRUM VIRIDE

GENERALITIES: Green American Hellebore produces VIOLENT CONGESTIVE *conditions at base of brain,* MEDULLA, *lungs,* with nausea, vomiting, and weakness. *Stomach,* heart and capillaries are also affected. Marked uneasy sensation in the whole body. Twitchings and convulsions here and there, during sleep; jerking and trembling threatened with convulsions. *Muscular prostration;* pseudo-hypertrophic muscular paralysis. General pulsations. Erratic motion; staggering. Spasm with violent shrieks, opisthotonos, before and after menses. *Burning* in different places—tongue, pharynx, gullet, skin which is cold with prickling. Uremia. Eclampsia. SUDDEN effects. *Fainting,* prostration, nausea. Numbness. Feels damp clothing on arms and legs, or clothes would not fit him, seemed they were scratching him somewhere. Suited to full-blooded plethoric persons. Effects of sunstroke. Reduces blood-pressure. Children tremble as if frightened and on verge of spasm. Chorea, twitching, contortions, unaffected by sleep; froth about the lips. Continuous jerking of the head. Sexual excitement. Lies with head low.

WORSE: Raising Up. Motion. Cold. Lying on back. After confinement. Sunstroke.

BETTER: Rubbing. Lying with head low. Eating.

MIND: Loquacity, with exaltation of ideas. Quarrelsome. Furious delirium—screams, howls, strikes, incessant muttering. Puerperal mania. Carphology. Fear of seeing her physician, of being poisoned. Suspicious.

HEAD: Vertigo with nausea and sudden prostration, > closing eyes and resting head. Head retracted. Constant jerking or nodding of the head (chorea); throbs on raising up. Aching on vertex and between eyes. Pain up occiput with dim vision and dilated pupils. Basilar meningitis. Apoplexy.

EYES: Vision; of red spots, purple, on closing eyes; unsteady vision. Pupils dilated. Wild, staring, during delirium. Blood-shot.

EARS: Deafness from moving quickly with faintness. Cold and pale.

NOSE: Pinched and blue. Rapid and continued sneezing, with worm biting feeling in mouth.

FACE: Flushed. Livid, Turgid, But Becomes Faint on sitting up. Tension across malar bones. Convulsive twitching of facial muscles. Chewing motions of the jaw.

MOUTH: Drawn at one corner. Tongue white as if bleached; dry; *with red streak down centre.* Taste like odor of semen. Odor from mouth like chloroform or ether. *Foul.* Mouth feels scalded.

THROAT: Burning in gullet; esophagitis. Sensation of a ball rising.

STOMACH: Very thirsty, drinks little which quenches for a short time. Hiccough painful, violent, constant, with spasm of oesophagus. Nausea, with vomiting and purging, smallest quantity of food or drink immediately rejected. *Violent vomiting* without nausea. Stomach seems to press against the spine. Gastritis.

ABDOMEN: Pain and soreness across just above pelvis. Cutting from navel to groin. Pain in bowels runs into scrotum. Tenesmus and burning in rectum, > during and after stool. Enteritis with high fever.

URINARY: Urine scanty with cloudy sediment. Cystitis with fever.

FEMALE: Dysmenorrhea with strangury. Suppressed menses with congestion of head. Rigid os. Puerperal fever, convulsions; with mania or mania continues after convulsions have ceased.

RESPIRATORY: Congestion of lungs. *Slow heavy breathing* as if with a load on chest. Dyspnea. Violent cough from very start. Pneumonia. Burning in chest.

HEART: Dull aching; burning. *Pulse, full, large, soft or slow* with strong or violent heartbeats. Pulsation throughout the body, more in right thigh.

NECK & BACK: Aching neck and shoulders. Cannot hold head up. Opisthotonos.

EXTREMITIES: Cramps in legs, feet, soles, fingers, toes. Vesicles on hands. Violent electric-like shocks in limbs. Convulsive twitching. Pain about the condyles. Pulsation felt in thighs. Restless hands during delirium.

SKIN: Tingling and prickling in skin. Itching in different parts, > rubbing. Cold, clammy, bluish. Erysipelas with brain symptoms.

SLEEP: Coma: Sleeplessness. Dreams of drowning, of being in water.

FEVER: *Hyperpyrexia* or rapidly oscillating temperature with sweat. Cold *clammy* or hot *sweat. Cerebrospinal*, suppurative, acute rheumatic fever. Fever high in the evening, below normal in the morning.

RELATED: Acon; Gels.

VERBASCUM

GENERALITIES: Mullein oil is prepared from flowers known to be useful locally in deafness or earache. This remedy has a marked effect on the *nerves,* esp. the inferior maxillary branch of the fifth nerve, ears, respiratory tract of bladder and left side. Soothes nervous, bronchial and urinary irritation. Produces catarrh and cold, spasmodic effects and neuralgias. Tearing, stitching, *cramping, squeezing, crushing, paralyzing* pains.

WORSE: Draft. Change of temperature. With every cold. 9 A.M. to 4 P.M. Twice a day, at same hour. Talking. Sneezing. Touch.

BETTER: Deep inspiration.

EYES: Pain in eyes as from contraction of the orbits.

EARS: Deafness. Earache. Deafness from getting water in, as during swimming, or deafness as if stopped by a valve. Numb (L).

NOSE: Coryza, with hot lacrimation.

FACE: Prosopalgia, < pressing teeth together, least movement. Pain in malar bones.

MOUTH: Copious salty water in the mouth.

ABDOMEN: Sensation of a lump, Twisting around navel. Piles obstruct stools, itching, inflamed.

URINARY: Enuresis at night, < coughing.

RESPIRATORY: *Hoarseness*; voice sounds like a trumpet. Frequent attacks of deep hollow cough with sound like a trumpet, > deep breathing. Nervous cough without waking.

RELATED: Acon; Plat; Sep.

VESPA CRABRO

GENERALITIES: Wasp produces stinging, burning pain *as if pierced with red hot needles.* Convulsion, loss of consciousness, does not answer when spoken to, looks into space, has no recollection of the attack.

WORSE: Hot stove, or in a closed room.

BETTER: Cold washing of hands.

VIBURNUM OPULUS

GENERALITIES: Common name Cramp Bark shows what this remedy produces—general *cramp,* violent spasmodic nervous effects esp. in the *females* dependent upon ovarian or uterine origin. Pains make her so nervous, she cannot keep still. Hemorrhage. Suited to tall, slender, fair-haired or dark hysterical subjects. Left-sided symptoms. Feels sick all over in pelvic complaints. Paralytic condition after convulsions.

WORSE: Fright. *Before menses.* Cold Snow air. Lying on left side. Sudden jar. Close room.

BETTER: *Rest. Pressure.* Open air.

MIND: Very nervous and irritable.

HEAD: Vertigo, < descending stairs. Feels faint on sitting up. Terrible crushing pain < left parietal region with a sensation of head opening and shutting.

EYES: Sore feeling in eyeballs

FACE: Flushed and hot.

STOMACH: Constant nausea, > by eating. No appetite.

ABDOMEN: *Excruciating crampy,* colicky pain or heavy aching in hypogastrium, > menses.

URINARY: *Frequent profuse urination* during headache, menses, hemorrhage, etc. Cannot hold water on coughing or walking. Spasmodic dysuria.

FEMALE: Menses too late, scanty, lasting a few hours, offensive. Dysmenorrhea with flatulence, loud eructations and nervousness. Spasmodic, membranous dysmenorrhea. Heavy aching feeling or *excruciating cramps* in pelvis, > menses. Frequent and very early *miscarriage,* may cause sterility. False labor pains. Violent persistent after-pains. *Uterine hemorrhage.* Leukorrhea thick, white, blood-streaked, < during stools. Consciousness of internal sexual organs. Prevents abortion when it is given before the membranes are broken. Uterine pains move around the pelvis often extending to thighs. Pelvic organs turn upside down.

RESPIRATORY: *Suffocative spells* at night, < cold, damp. Infantile asthma.

NECK & BACK: Tired backache, > pressure. Lumbago, > walking with a cane pressed or arms crossing the back. Pain in the back ends in a *cramp in uterus or goes down the thighs.*

EXTREMITIES: Cramp in calves before menses.

SKIN: Tettery spots on cheeks, arms, etc.

RELATED: Caul; Puls; Sep.

VINCA MINOR

GENERALITIES: It affects skin and hair and is effective in uterine hemorrhage. Weakness and prostration accompanies many sufferings, as if he would die. Mental exertion causes tremulous feeling and tendency to start.

WORSE: After swallowing. Anger. Stooping. Walking.

HEAD: Spots on scalp oozing foul moisture, matting hair together. Corrosive itching of scalp. Plica polonica (matted hair). Bald spots covered with short wooly hair. Hair falls out and is replaced by gray hair.

NOSE: Becomes red on being least angry. Sores in nose. Frequent nose bleeding.

THROAT: Cutting in lower esophagus which provokes swallowing.

FEMALE: Menses profuse; flowing like a stream without interruption; with great weakness; at climaxis. Passive uterine hemorrhage long after climacteric. Bleeding fibroids.

SKIN: Very sensitive, becomes red and sore from slight rubbing. Weeping eczema intermingled with foul, thick crusts. Corrosive itching.

RELATED: Ust.

VIOLA ODORATA

GENERALITIES: Sweet violet produces great *nervous debility*. Affects ears, eyes, wrist (right) and skin. Combined *eye, ear and kidney symptoms*. Worm affections in children. *Tension.* Suited to tall, thin, nervous girls. Nervous activity, then sudden exhaustion.

WORSE: Cloudy weather. Cold air. Music. Puberty. Suppressed discharges.

MIND: Inclined to weep without knowing why. Aversion to music, esp. violin. Childish behavior; despondent; refuses eating; talks in low soft voice.

HEAD: Tension in scalp extending to upper part of the face. Headache across the forehead, above the eyebrows; must knit the brows. Burning in forehead.

EYES: Pain from eyes (left) to vertex, < cough. Choroiditis. Illusions of vision—fiery, serpentine circles. Cramp in eyes. Lids tend to close without physical sleepiness.

EARS: Affections with pain in eyeballs. Otorrhea recurrent from birth. Deafness.

NOSE: Tip numb as from a blow.

STOMACH: Craves meat.

ABDOMEN: Itching at anus. Worms.

URINARY: Urine milky with strong smell. Enuresis in nervous children.

FEMALE: Dyspnea during pregnancy.

RESPIRATORY: Oppression of chest as from a weight. Difficult breathing, anxiety and palpitation. Long-lasting spells of cough during daytime only with dyspnea.

EXTREMITIES: Shoulders cold. Rheumatism of deltoid muscles and wrist (right) esp. in females. Trembling of limbs. Pressing pain in bones of fingers.

SKIN: *Dry, with moist palms.*

SLEEP: Yawning and stretching without sleepiness.

RELATED: Puls; Spig.

VIOLA TRICOLOR

GENERALITIES: *Skin of the scalp* and urinary organs are the chief centres of action of this remedy. Combined urinary symptoms with skin affection. Nervous paroxysms after suppressed crusta lactea, eczema.

WORSE: Pressure on side opposite to painful side. Winter. Cold air.

HEAD: Cracked, gummy crusts on scalp exuding profuse tenacious yellow fluid matting the hair together, with swelling of cervical glands. Milk-crusts.

URINARY: Urine offensive; smelling like cat's urine. Enuresis.

MALE: Seminal emissions with vivid dreams; at stool. Swelling of prepuce with itching.

EXTREMITIES: Articular rheumatism. Itch-like eruptions round the joints.

SKIN: Eczema of childhood. Impetigo. Large boils all over the body in scrofulous children.

RELATED: Rhus-t.

VIPERA

GENERALITIES: The poison of common German viper affects the *blood* and blood-vessels, esp. VEINS causing inflammation of veins and HEMORRHAGIC TENDENCY. Paralysis ascending; paraplegia, of foot. Multiple neuritis. Poliomyelitis. *Bursting feeling.* Climacteric affections. Goitre.

WORSE: LETTING LIMBS HANG DOWN. Yearly. Cold. Touch. Change of weather.

NOSE: *Epistaxis* with vertigo while nursing the child.

MOUTH: Tongue swollen, brownish-black, protruding. Lips blue, swollen. Speech difficult. Face swollen.

THROAT: Swelling like goitre. Edema of glottis.

ABDOMEN: *Excruciating pain in epigastrium,* < pressure. Violent pain in *enlarged liver,* extends to shoulder and hip. Jaundice with fever.

URINARY: Hematuria.

FEMALE: Climacteric hemorrhage, flow red with dark clots, continuous, with prostration and faintness. Bleeding from nursing the child.

EXTREMITIES: *Fullness and unbearable pain as if limb would burst,* must keep parts elevated, sits with feet high. Cramps or blueness of lower limbs. Shuffling gait caused by paralysis of foot. Varicose veins and acute phlebitis.

SKIN: Ulcer. Gangrene. Boil. Carbuncle with bursting sensation. Peeling off in large plates. Lymphangioma.

RELATED: Elap.

VISCUM ALBUM

GENERALITIES: Mistletoe affects the nerves and female sexual organs. General tremor as if all muscles are in fibrillary contraction. Neuralgia. Chorea from fright. Spinal pain due to uterine cause. Epilepsy, he felt a glow that rose up from feet to head. Gouty and rheumatic complaints. Blood would not clot and wounds would not heal. Sciatica with otorrhea.

WORSE: Winter; cold stormy weather. Motion. Lying on left side. Becoming chilled while hot. Suppression of menses.

MIND: Fear of telephone.

HEAD: Persistent vertigo after epileptic attack. Sudden throbbing in vertex.

ABDOMEN: Feels someone dragging her down from the waist. Sore about waist.

URINARY: Urine milky; after standing.

FEMALE: Metrorrhagia, blood partly bright and partly clotted and dark.

RESPIRATORY: Feeling of suffocation when lying on left side. Bronchial asthma connected with gout or rheumatism.

HEART: Palpitation during coitus in males. Hypertrophy. Low tension.

EXTREMITIES: Tearing, shooting pains in both thighs and upper extremities. Sciatica with otorrhea. Sensation of a spider crawling over back of hand and foot. Feels red hot coal applied to the heel. Glow sensation from foot to head. Lumbago from a chill, wants someone to press the back.

RELATED: Bufo.

XANTHOXYLUM

GENERALITIES: Commonly known as Prickly Ash, it exerts influence on nerves, female sexual organs, respiration and left side. Paralysis of single members, hemiplegia. Sudden grinding, shooting, radiating, pains; neuralgia. Neurasthenic patients who are thin, emaciated, having poor assimilation, with insomnia. Pricking sensation; shocks electric-like. Numbness of left side. Mucous membranes smart as from pepper. Floor feels soft like wool on walking. Injury to nerves.

WORSE: Sleeping. Dampness. Getting feet wet. Suppressed menses.

BETTER: Vomiting. Lying down. Drinking of ice water.

MIND: Nervous frightened feeling. Did not care if she lived or died.

HEAD: Throbbing headache; pain as if top of head would fly off. Thinks head is divided into two parts. Feels a tight band around.

THROAT: Peppery taste in mouth and throat. Feels hollow.

STOMACH: Dyspepsia from excessive eating and drinking.

FEMALE: Ovarian neuralgia with pain in hips and lower abdomen. Violent, *agonizing, grinding, dysmenorrheal* pain, not > in any position; pains go to thighs or radiate over whole body. After-pains with lochia with characteristic pains. Menses too early and profuse, thick almost black blood. Leukorrhea replaces menses. Amenorrhea.

RESPIRATORY: Constant desire to take deep breath. Oppression of chest. Dry cough day and night.

EXTREMITIES: Soreness of thighs before menses. Neuralgic shooting pains in limbs. Hemiplegia (left). Sciatica, < in summer. Coccyx very sensitive, seems elongated.

SLEEP: Dreams of flying.

RELATED: Ars; Lach.

ZINCUM METALLICUM

GENERALITIES: This remedy corresponds to the poisoning of NERVES AND BRAIN AND NERVES ARE FAGGED. Tissues are worn out faster than they can be repaired causing *depression* and *enervation.* Cannot throw thing off, cannot develop exanthemata or discharges. *Period of depression in disease.* Marked anemia; increasing *weakness,* with *restlessness* < eating. Poisoning by suppressed discharges and eruptions. *Isolated effects; formication.* One part numb another sensitive, one part hot other cold. Pain in spots between skin and flesh. Internal *trembling.* Convulsive *twitching* or *jerking,* < at night during sleep. *Spasms* from spinal injury. *Fidgety feet.* Automatic motion of mouth, arms and hands. Feels numb all over on lying down. Neuralgia after shingles, > touch. Transverse pain; shooting pain. Descending paralysis. Disabling bone pains. Chilblains, blueness of the surface. Bloody discharge. Ill effects of grief, anger, fright, night-watching, surgical operations, excessive study. Chorea esp. of feet, from fright or suppressed eruptions, < during sleep. Ill effects of concussion of brain.

WORSE: EXHAUSTION, mental or physical. *Noise. Touch.* Wine. After being heated. Suppressed eruptions, menses, discharges. Sweet things. Milk. After eating.

BETTER: *Motion.* Hard pressure. Warm open air. *Free Discharges,* menses, etc. Rubbing, scratching. Eating.

MIND: Repeats all questions before answering them. Fears arrest on account of supposed crime. Fretful, peevish; *cries* if vexed or moved during sleep (children). Easily startled; excited or intoxicated. *Forgetful. Screams* with pain. Averse to conversation, work. *Sensitive* to others talking and noise. Stares as if frightened on walking. And rolls head from side to side. Muddled. Brainfag. Weeps when angry. Lethargic. Thinks of death calmly.

HEAD: Violent vertigo with stupor. *Headache* of varying intensity. *Pressive pain on vertex, at the root of nose,* extending to eyes with weak vision, < warmth, > hard pressure, open air. Heavy aching pain in temples, < biting. Dragging down to back from occiput; feels a blow on occiput, then weak legs. Crashing in head on falling to sleep. Rolls head, bores in pillow and grinds teeth. Occiput hot, forehead cold. Hair falls from vertex. Hair brittle, bristling, sensitive. Brain paralysis. Vertex bald with soreness of scalp. Headache, of overtaxed school children; from drinking small quantity of wine. Headache with dim vision, < heat. Meningitis. Hydrocephalus after infantile cholera or diarrhea.

EYES: Itching and soreness of lids and inner angles. Conjunctivitis, < inner canthi. Feel drawn together. Lacrimation on eating. Pterygium. Rolling of eyes. Squint. Sees luminous bodies or intense burning after operation.

EARS: Frequent acute stitches in boys. Otorrhea of fetid pus. Itching, > boring into it.

NOSE: Swollen. Pressure upon the root. Dry, sore.

FACE: Pale alternating with redness. Bluish; miserable. Lips sticky, dry, cracked.

MOUTH: Grinds the teeth. Bleeding gums. Echo-speech. Herpes in mouth from sea-bathing. Bitter or bloody taste.

THROAT: Pain in muscles of throat externally while swallowing. Pain in fauces when yawning. Bitter taste in.

STOMACH: Ravenous hunger about 11 a.m. Heartburn, < sugar. Great haste when eating or drinking, cannot eat fast enough. Loss of appetite with clean tongue. Feels as if a worm crawling up to the throat from the pit of stomach causing coughing. Sweetish rising into throat with sweet taste. Globus hystericus rising from pit of stomach. Aversion to meat esp. veal, sweets, cooked or warm food. Wine < liquids are vomited immediately after drinking.

ABDOMEN: Sensation of a lump in liver region or at Navel. Hypogastric flatulence. Liver enlarged, hard and sore. Reflex symptoms from floating kidneys. Piles drawn down, > heat, < walking. Stools; large, dry, difficult, followed by involuntary urination. Itching at anus during stool. Ulceration of piles. Cholera-like diarrhea of infants. Nervous diarrhoea. Affections of brain from sudden stoppage of diarrhea. Constipation of newborn. Hot, putrid flatus. Neuralgia; of spleen; intercostal. Jerking from groins to penis.

URINARY: Violent urging, but urinates only in odd positions—bending backwards, crossing limbs, etc. Hysterical retention. Bleeding after urination. Pressive cutting about kidneys. Unable to retain the urine unless the feet are in constant motion. Floating kidney. Involuntary urination when walking, coughing or sneezing. Vicarious bleeding from suppressed menses.

MALE: Easy sexual excitement; emission too rapid or difficult during embrace. Discharge of prostatic fluid without cause. Grasps the genitals with cough etc. Falling of public hair. Sadness after emission. Swelling of testicles with retraction. Neuralgia of testes, < walking.

FEMALE: Sexual desire increased. Desire for masturbation during menses. Nymphomania of lying-in women; from suppressed lochia. Profuse lumpy menses. Menses flow more at night. Itching of vulva during menses causing masturbation. Varicose veins during pregnancy. Breasts painful, nipples sore. All complaints better during menstrual flow. Pain in ovary (left). Restlessness, sadness, coldness of the body, sensitiveness of the spine and fidgety feet—all these symptoms are found in women's complaints. Mammae and genitals painful with suppressed menses.

RESPIRATORY: Dyspnea, < flatulence, > expectoration. Debilitating spasmodic cough, < eating sweet things. Constricted chest. Dry cough before and during menses. Child fumbles the genitals while coughing.

HEART: Feels presence of a cap over the heart. Hard heartbeat. Irregular spasmodic action of the heart; occasional one violent thump. Violent pulsations during heat.

NECK & BACK: Nape of neck feels weary and tired from writing or any mental exertion. Neck feels lame, then stupor. *Burning along whole spine, < sitting. Aching in spine, small of the back,* < turning in bed, sitting or in the act of sitting down, and stooping. Spine sensitive, cannot bear it touched. Cutting pain in inter-scapular region, > eructations. Dull aching pain about last dorsal or first lumbar vertebra. Weakness in lumbar region, < standing.

EXTREMITIES: Pains in the limbs on becoming heated. Weakness and trembling of the hands when writing, during menses. Eczema on hand. Transverse pain esp. in upper limbs. CANNOT KEEP FEET AND LEGS STILL. Cramps when cold. Toes feel swollen, sore; tips ache. Soles sensitive. Bones of the feet fell broken. Stumbling, spastic gait; totters while walking in the dark and with closed eyes. Chronic painful varicoses. Lightning-like pain in locomotor ataxia; sweaty feet with sore toes. Formication of feet and legs as of insects crawling over the skin, prevents sleep, > rubbing and pressure. Hysterical contractions, drawing the fingers out of shape. Burning in tibia. Paralysis of feet. Ulcerative pain in heel, < walking. Pain in deltoid, < raising arm.

SKIN: Itching of thighs and hollow of knees. Eczema; in the anemic and neurotic; eczema of hands. Varicose veins of legs and genital organs. Formication.

SLEEP: Broken, unrefreshing. Loud screaming in sleep without being aware of it. Jerks and starts on falling to sleep. Somnambulism after suppressed emotions.

FEVER: Chilliness in the back as if fever would appear. Hands and legs become cold. Profuse sweat at night. Sweaty feet.

COMPLEMENTARY: Puls; Sep; Sulph.

RELATED: Hep; Ign; Kali-p; Lach; Pic-ac.

ZINC ARSENITE

GENERALITIES: It involves the *lumbar region* and lower limbs. Chorea. Profound exhaustion on slight exertion. Occipital pain. Blue vision. Burning in *bladder.* Numb right arm then left, > writing. Lumbar pain < *exertion,* sitting, jarring or standing. Soles ache when tired, > pressure.

WORSE: 10 A.M. and 3 P.M. Slight exertion.

ZINC CHROMATE

GENERALITIES: Acts upon *ears, nose,* throat, of left side. Aching, gnawing, grinding pain. Wandering, shock-like pain. Catching stitches that impede motion.

WORSE: MOTION. Lying on back. Washing head.

MIND: Aversion to work, cannot bring herself to it.

HEAD: Inward pressure in spot on bregma. Throbbing temples.

EYES: Vision wavering.

EARS: Throbbing behind the ears.

NOSE: Bad odor within nose. Blowing of pus and blood, and scabs.

MOUTH: Taste metallic.

STOMACH: Indefinite craving, knows not for what. Averse to even thinking of food.

ABDOMEN: Cannot tolerate her hands on abdomen.

FEMALE: Dryness of vagina with sense of coming sickness; from 10 to 12 A.M.

RESPIRATORY: Cough from tickling in throat-pit. Expectoration sweet, loose, but had to be swallowed, or tough, with spitting spells. Shooting from larynx (left) up through tonsils into ear.

HEART: Cutting at apex; at night.

BACK: Gnawing and grinding below and above left scapula.

EXTREMITIES: Feet sore. Cramps with gnawing, grinding pain in toes;, at night.

RELATED: Puls.

ZINC IODIDE

GENERALITIES: Heart valves and nerves are affected. Jerking, starting, splinter-like pains. Floating sensation. Undulating pain.

WORSE: Hard to remember what he reads.

HEAD: Vertigo, < lying on left side.

NOSE: Obstructed at night. Blowing of thick yellow lumps. Hot and dry.

THROAT: Goitre pressing inwardly. Splinter-like pains.

STOMACH: Coldness in stomach and bowels with tendency to perspire.

RESPIRATORY: Tickling in throat, the more he coughs the more the tickling. Undulating pain at border of right floating ribs.

HEART: Palpitation when lying on left side. Myocardial exhaustion.

EXTREMITIES: Lower limbs feel as if floating, < lying on left side. Cramp in calves, ankles, > pressing feet on floor.

RELATED: Stict.

ZINC PHOSPHATE

GENERALITIES: A remedy for mental depression, fatigue, trainfag of businessmen. Sexual excitement and sleeplessness. Nervousness. Paralysis. Epilepsy. Abuse of bromides. Forgetful, indolent, apprehensive, < afternoon and night. Formication all over the body. Nervous vertigo, > lying.

ZINC SULPHATE

GENERALITIES: Clears up the opacity of cornea. Trembling and convulsion.

ZINC VALERIANATE

GENERALITIES: Affects the nerves, ovaries and spine. Painful nervous effects. Neuralgia. Oversensitive, nervous and sleepless. Hysteria. Obstinate hiccough. Epilepsy without aura.

BETTER: Rubbing.

MIND: Excitable. Distressed. Groundless fear.

HEAD: Violent neuralgic intermittent headache.

EARS: Tickling over left ear.

FACE: Prosopalgia.

MOUTH: Sour taste in A.M. Smothers on attempting to eat.

ABDOMEN: Crampy pain shoots from abdomen to thighs and feet during and after menses. Dysmenorrhea, pains go down the thighs.

BACK: Aching.

FEVER: Chill after mental excitement or exertion. Cold parts burn as they warm up.

ZINGIBER

GENERALITIES: Affects the digestive tract. Complaints from eating melon and drinking impure water. Asthma of gastric origin, < towards the morning. Suppressing of urine after typhoid. Dry cough with profuse expectoration in the morning. All joints feel weak. Heels ache after standing long.

ZIZIA

GENERALITIES: Spasmodic movement of the muscles of face and extremities. Choreic twitching during sleep. Hypochondriasis, desire to commit suicide.

◆◆◆